Crosstalk between Depression, Anxiety, Dementia, and Chronic Pain: Comorbidity in Behavioral Neurology and Neuropsychiatry 2.0

Crosstalk between Depression, Anxiety, Dementia, and Chronic Pain: Comorbidity in Behavioral Neurology and Neuropsychiatry 2.0

Editor

Masaru Tanaka

MDPI • Basel • Beijing • Wuhan • Barcelona • Belgrade • Manchester • Tokyo • Cluj • Tianjin

Editor
Masaru Tanaka
ELKH-SZTE Neuroscience
Research Group
Eötvös Loránd Research Network
University of Szeged
Szeged
Hungary

Editorial Office
MDPI
St. Alban-Anlage 66
4052 Basel, Switzerland

This is a reprint of articles from the Special Issue published online in the open access journal *Biomedicines* (ISSN 2227-9059) (available at: www.mdpi.com/journal/biomedicines/special_issues/neuropsychiatry_2).

For citation purposes, cite each article independently as indicated on the article page online and as indicated below:

LastName, A.A.; LastName, B.B.; LastName, C.C. Article Title. *Journal Name* **Year**, *Volume Number*, Page Range.

ISBN 978-3-0365-8253-5 (Hbk)
ISBN 978-3-0365-8252-8 (PDF)

Contents

About the Editor

Masaru Tanaka

Masaru Tanaka, M.D., Ph.D., is a Senior Research Fellow at the Danube Neuroscience Research Laboratory, Neuroscience Research Group of Eötvös Loránd Research Network, University of Szeged (ELKH-SZTE). His scientific interests include depression, anxiety, dementia, pain, their comorbid nature, and translational research on neurological diseases and psychiatric disorders. Dr. Tanaka's current research focuses on investigating the antidepressant, anxiolytic, and nootropic effects of neuropeptides, neurohormones, tryptophan metabolites, and their analogues in animal models of neuropsychiatric diseases.

Dr. Tanaka holds several notable Editorial Board Member positions, contributing his expertise to various scientific journals. He is an Editorial Board Member for the following journals: *Frontiers in Neuroscience, Frontiers in Psychiatry, Anesthesia Research, Journal of Integrative Neuroscience, Advances in Clinical Experimental Medicine, Biology and Life Sciences,* and *Biomedicines.*

He received his Ph.D. in Medicine and an M.D. in General Medicine from the University of Szeged. Prior to that, he earned a bachelor's degree in Biophysics from the University of Illinois, Urbana-Champaign.

Preface to "Crosstalk between Depression, Anxiety, Dementia, and Chronic Pain: Comorbidity in Behavioral Neurology and Neuropsychiatry 2.0"

Depression, anxiety, cognitive impairment, and pain are prevalent mental symptoms experienced across a broad spectrum of diseases. Advances in neuroscience have significantly contributed to our understanding of these distressing symptoms. State-of-the-art brain research, employing preclinical, clinical, and computational approaches, is dedicated to unraveling the complex nature of these symptoms and their underlying mechanisms. In line with this progress, this reprint presents a compilation of the most recent studies published in the Special Issue titled, "Crosstalk between Depression, Anxiety, Dementia, and Chronic Pain: Comorbidity in Behavioral Neurology and Neuropsychiatry 2.0".

Masaru Tanaka
Editor

biomedicines

Editorial

Integrating Armchair, Bench, and Bedside Research for Behavioral Neurology and Neuropsychiatry: Editorial

Masaru Tanaka [1,*,†], Ágnes Szabó [2,3] and László Vécsei [1,2,*,†]

[1] ELKH-SZTE Neuroscience Research Group, Danube Neuroscience Research Laboratory, Eötvös Loránd Research Network, University of Szeged (ELKH-SZTE), Tisza Lajos krt. 113, H-6725 Szeged, Hungary
[2] Department of Neurology, Albert Szent-Györgyi Medical School, University of Szeged, Semmelweis u. 6, H-6725 Szeged, Hungary
[3] Doctoral School of Clinical Medicine, University of Szeged, Korányi Fasor 6, H-6720 Szeged, Hungary
* Correspondence: tanaka.masaru.1@med.u-szeged.hu (M.T.); vecsei.laszlo@med.u-szeged.hu (L.V.); Tel.: +36-62-342-361 (M.T. & L.V.)
† These authors contributed equally to this work.

Citation: Tanaka, M.; Szabó, Á.; Vécsei, L. Integrating Armchair, Bench, and Bedside Research for Behavioral Neurology and Neuropsychiatry: Editorial. *Biomedicines* **2022**, *10*, 2999. https://doi.org/10.3390/biomedicines10122999

Received: 1 November 2022
Accepted: 8 November 2022
Published: 22 November 2022

> "To learning much inclined, who went to see the Elephant (though all of them were blind) that each by observation might satisfy the mind"
>
> —John Godfrey Saxe
>
> —Tittha Sutta

Medical sciences have been steadily paving an exploratory path toward understanding the mechanisms of mental suffering, such as depression, anxiety, cognitive impairment, and pain. Such progress in contemporary research is certainly appreciable, and its tempo appears to be gaining increasing impetus. Indeed, state-of-the-art biotechnology, information science, and imaging techniques may help reveal novel findings in mental illnesses. It is no coincidence that this Special Issue, just titling common symptoms typical to not only psychiatric disorders but also common illnesses, collected 15 research papers, including seven preclinical studies, three clinical studies, one computational medicine, and four review articles covering interdisciplinary topics, including psychotherapy. This editorial introduces original research and review articles published in the Special Issue "Crosstalk between Depression, Anxiety, Dementia, and Chronic Pain: Comorbidity in Behavioral Neurology and Neuropsychiatry 2.0", the second volume of the Special Issue "Crosstalk between Depression, Anxiety, and Dementia" [1]. We discuss ongoing projects to benefit from this current driving force in behavioral neurology and neuropsychiatry.

Recent advancements in neuroscience have enabled researchers to probe the brain in larger regions, at the cellular level, and with increased receptor specificity [2–6]. Research is focused on finding scientific frameworks for understanding the neuropathophysiology of mental illnesses, exploring the molecular regulation of higher-order neural circuits and neuropathological alterations, which may lead to prefrontal cortex (PFC) dysfunction, eliciting the symptoms of mental illnesses [7–13]. The deficit in control and motor inhibition [14–16], in motor imagery or in the suppression of ongoing action [17], or in emotion perception, reactivity, and regulation [18–20], which depend on aberrant neural activity in the PFC associated with serious impulsivity problems, are characterized in neuropsychiatric disorders. Furthermore, functional alterations in the PFC affect the memory and learning abilities of psychiatric and brain-damaged patients. This evidence suggests that PFC dysfunctions cause impairment of aversive learning and emotional memory circuits, which might be transversal across many psychiatric disorders in humans and neurologic patients [21–23].

Experimental medicine employs in vitro systems as well as a wide variety of organisms [24–26]. The data collected using laboratory animals have led to significant leaps in understanding the effects of endogenous neuropeptides, neurohormones, and metabolites [27–31]. The initial step in animal research is to engineer typical animal models representing a certain human disease. Animal models are an essential tool to bridge the knowledge of data- and hypothesis-driven benchwork and its application to clinical bedside management. Nevertheless, assessing the validity of an animal model remains the greatest challenge. Model validity is determined by construct, face, and predictive validities. Construct validity ensures that a disease phenotype in modeling animals is induced by the currently understood pathomechanism of a disease.

Gene manipulation is one of the most popular methods to construct animal models of Alzheimer's disease (AD). The authors in this Special Issue employed transgenic mice models: amyloid precursor protein (APP) 23 transgenic mice that overexpress human APP with the Swedish mutation (KM670/671NL), triple-transgenic mice of AD (3xTg-AD) that harbor a *Psen1* PS1M146V mutation and the co-injected APPSwe and tauP301L transgenes (Tg(APPSwe,tauP301L)1Lfa), and the pyruvate dehydrogenase lipoamide kinase isozyme 1 K465E gene knock-in mice. Those models have good face validity, which ensures that the signs exhibited in the models resemble those of human diseases. Particularly, the 3xTg-AD model displays that the accumulation of tau and amyloid plaques in the brain increases with age.

Muntsant and Giménez-Llort revealed an increasing APP level in genetic load- and aging-dependent manners, correlating with cognitive impairment and anxiety-like behaviors [32]. Giménez-Llort and colleagues investigated the chronological and behavioral aging of APP23 transgenic mice. The survival curves were better in male than in female APP23 mice and wild types. Age-related differences were observed, and variables related to stress, thigmotaxis, frailty, and cognition were more prominent in male APP23 mice in 12-, 18-, and 24-month-old time points compared to those of the wild-type counterparts. Muntsant and colleagues investigated the genetic and aging interactions of 3xTg-AD [33]. The study revealed an increased APP level in a genetic load-dependent manner, convergent synaptophysin and choline acetyltransferase levels, cognitive impairment coupled with the activation of the hypophysis–pituitary–adrenal axis, anxiety-like behaviors elicited by genetic load, and systemic organ injuries, showing the presence of the genetic- and aging-dependent vulnerability and compensation in AD [34]. Castillo-Mariqueo and colleagues conducted longitudinal and cross-sectional studies to assess physical and behavioral variables in 3xTg-AD, concluding that the transgenes modify functional trainings, especially in survival, physical resistance, and motor learning [35]. Santana-Santana and colleagues studied the impact of gender and the pyruvate dehydrogenase lipoamide kinase isozyme 1 K465E knock-in gene on behaviors by comparing homozygous, heterozygous, and wild-type mice. The difference between gender and the transgenic mice was observed in an anxiogenic environment during the middle age of the mice. The male transgenic mice showed increased anxiety. The authors concluded that various negative emotional valence, such as anxiety, were elicited by the interaction of sex and PI3K/Akt signaling [36]. Furthermore, gene manipulation is applied to construct animal models of other neuropsychiatric pathogenesis, including neurodevelopmental disorders and the decreased resilience of neuroplasticity as a pathogenesis of neuropsychiatric disorders [37,38].

Surgical intervention can simulate vascular dementia, the second most common neurocognitive disorder. Employing bilateral carotid artery stenosis in mice, Lee and colleagues reported that pro-inflammatory cytokines, rho-associated protein kinase, and mRNA levels of blood–brain barrier-related tight junction proteins were decreased; smooth muscle alpha-actin positive vessels were increased, cortex cell rearrangement was decreased, and microtubule-associated protein-2-positive neural cells was decreased in the hippocampus, simulating the clinical pathology of vascular dementia [39]. Thus, this model ensures high face validity.

Environmental risk factors also generate a disease phenotype. The chronic social defeat stress model is an ethologically valid animal model that exhibits behavioral and physiological phenotypes such as anxiety- and depression-like behaviors and the downregulation of serotonergic gene expression. Smagin and colleagues investigated the chronic effects of lithium chloride on anxiety-like behavior and the expression of serotonergic genes in the midbrain raphe nuclei of mice. The chronic lithium chloride administration elicited anxiolytic- and anxiogenic-like behaviors and the higher expression of serotonergic genes in the midbrain raphe nuclei. The authors concluded the increased expression of serotonergic genes occurs with the activation of the serotonergic system and elevated anxiety [40].

Health resilience has drawn increasing attention to one of the etiological factors of illnesses from molecular to social levels. Less mitochondrial stress resilience, the disturbance of thiol homeostasis, and contemporary lifestyles may reportedly contribute to the pathogenesis of neurological and psychiatric diseases, multiple sclerosis, and mental illnesses, respectively [41].

The prevalence of hypertension in schizophrenia (SCZ) patients and psychosis-related disorders reaches nearly 40%. Spontaneously hypertensive rat is an animal model of SCZ. Correia and colleagues reported that antipsychotics haloperidol and clozapine increased total lipids and decreased phospholipids in spontaneously hypertensive rats [42]. The findings are in line with those of SCZ patients. Thus, the spontaneously hypertensive rat model possesses high predictive validity that ensures translational ability between animal models and human disease. However, SCZ develops from heterogenic insults in the early neurodevelopmental stage, confirming the presence of various subgroups of SCZ. Vitamin D deficiency is highly prevalent in patients with SCZ; however, little is known about how vitamin D deficiency affects the disease course of SCZ, especially cognitive function. Gaebler and colleagues assess the correlation between the serum 25-OH-vitamin D levels, anticholinergic drug exposure, and neurocognitive functions in patients with SCZ, reporting a positive correlation of vitamin D levels with cognitive processing speed and a negative correlation of vitamin D levels of anticholinergic drug exposure [43]. Cognitive function, including memory and learning, is sustained by synaptic plasticity, which governs the fine-tuning of the synaptic strength and efficacy of the synaptic transmission. Carnosine is an endogenous anti-aging dipeptide, highly concentrated in brain and muscle tissues. Caruso and colleagues conducted a systematic review and a meta-analysis, concluding that a dose of 500 mg–1 g/day carnosine/anserine for 12 weeks improved cognitive function and verbal memory but not depressive symptoms [44].

Deep brain stimulation is a surgical procedure used to treat Parkinson's disease, essential tremor, epilepsy, and dystonia, which is reportedly beneficial for treatment-resistant depression. Vila-Merkle and colleagues studied the therapeutic mechanisms of deep brain stimulation of the infralimbic cortex by electrophysiological recordings in the β-carboline FG 7142-induced anxiety model. The model exhibits the predominance of certain frequency bands during the anxiogenic state and the activation of subnetworks with specific oscillatory patterns. The study reported that the deep brain stimulation of the infralimbic cortex reversed the oscillatory pattern, restoring the communication of the amygdala–hippocampal network [45].

An increasing number of studies have focused on the fact that the tryptophan (Trp)–kynurenine (KYN) metabolic system not only plays a role in the pathogenesis of diseases but also serves as a potential biomarker for environmental health [46,47]. The Trp–KYN metabolic system refers to a group of endogenous bioactive metabolites arising via the KYN metabolic pathway from an essential amino acid Trp. The metabolic system adds more implications of their versatile biological activities than the traditionally used term, the Trp–KYN pathway that produces a group of simply categorizing neurotoxic and neuroprotectant KYN molecules. Indeed, KYN metabolites exhibit a wide range of bioactive properties, frequently showing a Janus-like face depending on their concentration and environment and possibly influencing the bioenergetic resilience of mitochondria [41,48]. Tanaka and colleagues featured the Trp–KYN metabolic system with special emphasis on its interaction with the immune system, including the tolerogenic shift towards chronic low-grade inflammation, to explore the linkage between chronic low-grade inflammation, KYN metabolites, and major psychiatric disorders, including depressive disorder, bipolar disorder, substance use disorder, post-traumatic stress disorder, SCZ, and autism spectrum disorder [49–51]. In parallel, the role of diet in maintaining mental health has been explored [52]. Furthermore, the link between air pollution and the pathogenesis of depression has been proven [53]. Novel therapeutics for neuropsychiatric conditions are under extensive study [54,55].

Furthermore, the Trp–KYN metabolic system and its metabolites have been discussed as a target of potential therapeutic molecules for cognitive impairment as well as for headaches [56,57]. Tanaka and colleagues discussed the involvement of the Trp–KYN system in chronic pain, addressing the components of the pain pathway, the components-based pain mechanisms, and central and peripheral pain sensitization arising from psychosocial and behavioral factors, which have been in a discounted trend in contemporary clinical nosology [50]. Pharmacotherapy and surgical intervention have their limits due to the development of drug intolerance and contraindications. Balogh and colleagues highlighted evidence in philosophically-rich interpretations and counseling techniques of existential–phenomenological psychotherapy and meaning-centered counseling techniques, and reviewed its effectiveness in the negative-emotion-management of terminally ill patients. The authors concluded that phenomenological psychotherapy might potentially play a synergistic role with the currently prevailing medication-based approaches for treating depression and anxiety [58].

Myalgic encephalomyelitis/chronic fatigue syndrome is a fatiguing medical condition caused by heterogeneous pathogenesis; thus, it is a challenging task to subgroup for personalized treatment. Simonato and colleagues revealed that interleukin-17A, fatty acid-binding protein 2, and 3-hydroxykynurenine were higher. However, KYN and serotonin were lower in myalgic encephalomyelitis/chronic fatigue syndrome patients, concluding that the clinical traits and serum biomarkers associated with inflammation, intestinal function, and Trp metabolism deserve to be explored for the development of personalized treatment [59].

Indeed, "personalized medicine" indicates "precision medicine", which focuses on identifying an effective therapeutic approach based on the patient's phenotypes. Artificial intelligence leverages computation and inference to augment logical insights into artificial intelligence, enabling the system to reason and learn, thus potentially empowering clinical decision-making. The Research Domain Criteria Initiative attempts to reconceptualize mental disorders with multidimensional data. Komatsu and colleagues reviewed the application of economic and machine learning frameworks to neuroscience to present neural mechanisms of cognitive processes, such as decision-making, the translation of machine learning approaches to clinical sciences, and the identification of functional connectivity as disease classifiers for schizophrenia, bipolar disorder, depression, anxiety disorders, and autism spectrum disorder. The authors proposed artificial intelligence algorisms as tools for precision psychiatry, which potentially surpass the International Classification of Diseases and Diagnostic and Statistical Manual of Mental Disorders [60].

Clinical, experimental, and computational medicines have witnessed notable advances in understanding pathogenesis, making precise diagnoses, and exploring novel treatments for neuropsychiatric disorders. Research Domain Criteria is an ongoing initiative that allows a multidimensional and intersectional approach to link mental illnesses, as extreme conditions that deviate from healthy norms, to genomic, neuroscience, and behavioral sciences across reified International Classification of Diseases and Diagnostic 11 and Statistical Manual of Mental Disorders 5. Thus, the endeavor potentially provides an alternative taxonomy that complements the current system. Meanwhile, computational medicine seeks to advance healthcare by analyzing, modeling, simulating, and visualizing biological systems and medical conditions in a virtual environment in an attempt to improve preventive, diagnostic, prognostic, predictive, and therapeutic measures. Such in silico approaches employ artificial intelligence, machine learning, and deep learning to analyze patient datasets and bioinformatics databases, apply computational algorithms, and utilize big data analytics tools at molecular, cellular, and organism levels. Accordingly, science and medicine have been unintermittingly advancing, firmly reinforcing the interdisciplinary translatability and synthesizability of individual research, and thus hopefully leading to a future paradigm shift in diseases and medicine.

The blind never see the elephant, but together they might attain a closer image.

"the Elephant is very like a wall, spear, a snake, a tree, fan, rope"

"Though each was partly in the right, Additionally, all were in the wrong!"

"Additionally, prate about an Elephant Not one of them has seen!"

—in memory of Dr. Mutsuo Shimizu

Author Contributions: Conceptualization, M.T.; writing—original draft preparation, writing—review and editing, M.T. and L.V.; visualization, M.T. and Á.S.; supervision, L.V.; project administration, M.T.; funding acquisition, M.T. and L.V. All authors have read and agreed to the published version of the manuscript.

Funding: This research was funded by National Scientific Research Fund OTKA138125, MTA-JSP-050609, and ELKH-SZTE.

Acknowledgments: The graphical abstract was made by biorender.com.

Conflicts of Interest: The authors declare no conflict of interest.

Abbreviations

3xTg-AD	triple-transgenic mice of Alzheimer's disease
AD	Alzheimer's disease
APP	amyloid precursor protein
KYN	kynurenine
PFC	prefrontal cortex
SCZ	schizophrenia
Trp	tryptophan

References

1. Tanaka, M. *Crosstalk between Depression, Anxiety, and Dementia: Comorbidity in Behavioral Neurology and Neuropsychiatry*, 1st ed.; MDPI: Basel, Switzerland, 2022; pp. 1–266.
2. Nyatega, C.O.; Qiang, L.; Adamu, M.J.; Kawuwa, H.B. Gray matter, white matter and cerebrospinal fluid abnormalities in Parkinson's disease: A voxel-based morphometry study. *Front. Psychiatry* **2022**, *13*, 1027907. [CrossRef] [PubMed]
3. Nyatega, C.O.; Qiang, L.; Adamu, M.J.; Younis, A.; Kawuwa, H.B. Altered Dynamic Functional Connectivity of Cuneus in Schizophrenia Patients: A Resting-State fMRI Study. *Appl. Sci.* **2021**, *11*, 11392. [CrossRef]
4. Younis, A.; Qiang, L.; Nyatega, C.O.; Adamu, M.J.; Kawuwa, H.B. Brain Tumor Analysis Using Deep Learning and VGG-16 Ensembling Learning Approaches. *Appl. Sci.* **2022**, *12*, 7282. [CrossRef]
5. Nyatega, C.O.; Qiang, L.; Adamu, M.J.; Younis, A.; Kawuwa, H.B. Altered Striatal Functional Connectivity and Structural Dysconnectivity in Individuals with Bipolar Disorder: A resting state Magnetic Resonance Imaging Study. *Front. Psychiatry* **2022**, *13*, 1054380. [CrossRef]
6. Nyatega, C.O.; Qiang, L.; Jajere, M.A.; Kawuwa, H.B. Atypical Functional Connectivity of Limbic Network in Attention Deficit/Hyperactivity Disorder. *Clin. Schizophr. Relat. Psychoses* **2022**, *16*. [CrossRef]
7. Borgomaneri, S.; Battaglia, S.; Sciamanna, G.; Tortora, F.; Laricchiuta, D. Memories are not written in stone: Re-writing fear memories by means of non-invasive brain stimulation and optogenetic manipulations. *Neurosci. Biobehav. Rev.* **2021**, *127*, 334–352. [CrossRef]
8. Borgomaneri, S.; Battaglia, S.; Avenanti, A.; Pellegrino, G.D. Don't Hurt Me No More: State-dependent Transcranial Magnetic Stimulation for the treatment of specific phobia. *J. Affect. Disord.* **2021**, *286*, 78–79. [CrossRef]
9. Battaglia, S. Neurobiological advances of learned fear in humans. *Adv. Clin. Exp. Med.* **2022**, *31*, 217–221. [CrossRef]
10. Borgomaneri, S.; Battaglia, S.; Garofalo, S.; Tortora, F.; Avenanti, A.; di Pellegrino, G. State-Dependent TMS over Prefrontal Cortex Disrupts Fear-Memory Reconsolidation and Prevents the Return of Fear. *Curr. Biol.* **2020**, *30*, 3672–3679.e4. [CrossRef]
11. Battaglia, S.; Serio, G.; Scarpazza, C.; D'Ausilio, A.; Borgomaneri, S. Frozen in (e)motion: How reactive motor inhibition is influenced by the emotional content of stimuli in healthy and psychiatric populations. *Behav. Res. Ther.* **2021**, *146*, 103963. [CrossRef]
12. Borgomaneri, S.; Serio, G.; Battaglia, S. Please, don't do it! Fifteen years of progress of non-invasive brain stimulation in action inhibition. *Cortex* **2020**, *132*, 404–422. [CrossRef] [PubMed]

13. Battaglia, S.; Garofalo, S.; di Pellegrino, G.; Starita, F. Revaluing the Role of vmPFC in the Acquisition of Pavlovian Threat Conditioning in Humans. *J. Neurosci.* **2020**, *40*, 8491–8500. [CrossRef] [PubMed]
14. Battaglia, S.; Harrison, B.J.; Fullana, M.A. Does the human ventromedial prefrontal cortex support fear learning, fear extinction or both? A commentary on subregional contributions. *Mol. Psychiatry* **2022**, *27*, 784–786. [CrossRef] [PubMed]
15. Battaglia, S.; Cardellicchio, P.; Di Fazio, C.; Nazzi, C.; Fracasso, A.; Borgomaneri, S. Stopping in (e)motion: Reactive action inhibition when facing valence-independent emotional stimuli. *Front. Behav. Neurosci.* **2022**, *16*, 998714. [CrossRef] [PubMed]
16. Sellitto, M.; Terenzi, D.; Starita, F.; di Pellegrino, G.; Battaglia, S. The Cost of Imagined Actions in a Reward-Valuation Task. *Brain Sci.* **2022**, *12*, 582. [CrossRef]
17. Battaglia, S.; Cardellicchio, P.; Di Fazio, C.; Nazzi, C.; Fracasso, A.; Borgomaneri, S. The Influence of Vicarious Fear-Learning in "Infecting" Reactive Action Inhibition. *Front. Behav. Neurosci.* **2022**, *16*, 946263. [CrossRef]
18. Battaglia, S.; Thayer, J.F. Functional interplay between central and autonomic nervous systems in human fear conditioning. *Trends Neurosci.* **2022**, *45*, 504–506. [CrossRef]
19. Battaglia, S.; Orsolini, S.; Borgomaneri, S.; Barbieri, R.; Diciotti, S.; di Pellegrino, G. Characterizing cardiac autonomic dynamics of fear learning in humans. *Psychophysiology* **2022**, *59*, e14122. [CrossRef]
20. Ellena, G.; Battaglia, S.; Làdavas, E. The spatial effect of fearful faces in the autonomic response. *Exp. Brain Res.* **2020**, *238*, 2009–2018. [CrossRef]
21. Battaglia, S.; Fabius, J.H.; Moravkova, K.; Fracasso, A.; Borgomaneri, S. The Neurobiological Correlates of Gaze Perception in Healthy Individuals and Neurologic Patients. *Biomedicines* **2022**, *10*, 627. [CrossRef]
22. Battaglia, S.; Garofalo, S.; di Pellegrino, G. Context-dependent extinction of threat memories: Influences of healthy aging. *Sci. Rep.* **2018**, *8*, 12592. [CrossRef] [PubMed]
23. Di Gregorio, F.; La Porta, F.; Petrone, V.; Battaglia, S.; Orlandi, S.; Ippolito, G.; Romei, V.; Piperno, R.; Lullini, G. Accuracy of EEG Biomarkers in the Detection of Clinical Outcome in Disorders of Consciousness after Severe Acquired Brain Injury: Preliminary Results of a Pilot Study Using a Machine Learning Approach. *Biomedicines* **2022**, *10*, 1897. [CrossRef] [PubMed]
24. Datki, Z.; Sinka, R. Translational biomedicine-oriented exploratory research on bioactive rotifer-specific biopolymers. *Adv. Clin. Exp. Med.* **2022**, *31*, 931–935. [CrossRef] [PubMed]
25. Palotai, M.; Telegdy, G.; Tanaka, M.; Bagosi, Z.; Jászberényi, M. Neuropeptide AF induces anxiety-like and antidepressant-like behavior in mice. *Behav. Brain Res.* **2014**, *274*, 264–269. [CrossRef]
26. Lieb, A.; Thaler, G.; Fogli, B.; Trovato, O.; Posch, M.A.; Kaserer, T.; Zangrandi, L. Functional Characterization of Spinocerebellar Ataxia Associated Dynorphin A Mutant Peptides. *Biomedicines* **2021**, *9*, 1882. [CrossRef]
27. Telegdy, G.; Tanaka, M.; Schally, A.V. Effects of the growth hormone-releasing hormone (GH-RH) antagonist on brain functions in mice. *Behav. Brain Res.* **2011**, *224*, 155–158. [CrossRef]
28. Tanaka, M.; Kádár, K.; Tóth, G.; Telegdy, G. Antidepressant-like effects of urocortin 3 fragments. *Brain Res. Bull.* **2011**, *84*, 414–418. [CrossRef]
29. Tanaka, M.; Schally, A.V.; Telegdy, G. Neurotransmission of the antidepressant-like effects of the growth hormone-releasing hormone antagonist MZ-4-71. *Behav. Brain Res.* **2012**, *228*, 388–391. [CrossRef]
30. Rákosi, K.; Masaru, T.; Zarándia, M.; Telegdy, G.; Tóth, G.K. Short analogs and mimetics of human urocortin 3 display antidepressant effects in vivo. *Peptides* **2014**, *62*, 59–66. [CrossRef]
31. Telegdy, G.; Adamik, A.; Tanaka, M.; Schally, A.V. Effects of the LHRH antagonist Cetrorelix on affective and cognitive functions in rats. *Regul. Pept.* **2010**, *159*, 142–147. [CrossRef]
32. Muntsant, A.; Giménez-Llort, L. Genotype Load Modulates Amyloid Burden and Anxiety-Like Patterns in Male 3xTg-AD Survivors despite Similar Neuro-Immunoendocrine, Synaptic and Cognitive Impairments. *Biomedicines* **2021**, *9*, 715. [CrossRef] [PubMed]
33. Giménez-Llort, L.; Marin-Pardo, D.; Marazuela, P.; Hernández-Guillamón, M. Survival Bias and Crosstalk between Chronological and Behavioral Age: Age- and Genotype-Sensitivity Tests Define Behavioral Signatures in Middle-Aged, Old, and Long-Lived Mice with Normal and AD-Associated Aging. *Biomedicines* **2021**, *9*, 636. [CrossRef] [PubMed]
34. Muntsant, A.; Jiménez-Altayó, F.; Puertas-Umbert, L.; Jiménez-Xarrie, E.; Vila, E.; Giménez-Llort, L. Sex-Dependent End-of-Life Mental and Vascular Scenarios for Compensatory Mechanisms in Mice with Normal and AD-Neurodegenerative Aging. *Biomedicines* **2021**, *9*, 111. [CrossRef] [PubMed]
35. Castillo-Mariqueo, L.; Giménez-Llort, L. Impact of Behavioral Assessment and Re-Test as Functional Trainings That Modify Survival, Anxiety and Functional Profile (Physical Endurance and Motor Learning) of Old Male and Female 3xTg-AD Mice and NTg Mice with Normal Aging. *Biomedicines* **2022**, *10*, 973. [CrossRef] [PubMed]
36. Santana-Santana, M.; Bayascas, J.-R.; Giménez-Llort, L. Fine-Tuning the PI3K/Akt Signaling Pathway Intensity by Sex and Genotype-Load: Sex-Dependent Homozygotic Threshold for Somatic Growth but Feminization of Anxious Phenotype in Middle-Aged PDK1 K465E Knock-In and Heterozygous Mice. *Biomedicines* **2021**, *9*, 747. [CrossRef] [PubMed]
37. Tanaka, M.; Spekker, E.; Szabó, Á.; Polyák, H.; Vécsei, L. Modelling the neurodevelopmental pathogenesis in neuropsychiatric disorders. Bioactive kynurenines and their analogues as neuroprotective agents-in celebration of 80th birthday of Professor Peter Riederer. *J. Neural. Transm.* **2022**, *129*, 627–642. [CrossRef]
38. Tanaka, M.; Vécsei, L. Editorial of Special Issue 'Dissecting Neurological and Neuropsychiatric Diseases: Neurodegeneration and Neuroprotection'. *Int. J. Mol. Sci.* **2022**, *23*, 6991. [CrossRef]

39. Lee, E.C.; Hong, D.-Y.; Lee, D.-H.; Park, S.-W.; Lee, J.Y.; Jeong, J.H.; Kim, E.-Y.; Chung, H.-M.; Hong, K.-S.; Park, S.-P.; et al. Inflammation and Rho-Associated Protein Kinase-Induced Brain Changes in Vascular Dementia. *Biomedicines* **2022**, *10*, 446. [CrossRef]
40. Smagin, D.A.; Kovalenko, I.L.; Galyamina, A.G.; Belozertseva, I.V.; Tamkovich, N.V.; Baranov, K.O.; Kudryavtseva, N.N. Chronic Lithium Treatment Affects Anxious Behaviors and theExpression of Serotonergic Genes in Midbrain Raphe Nuclei of Defeated Male Mice. *Biomedicines* **2021**, *9*, 1293. [CrossRef]
41. Tanaka, M.; Szabó, Á.; Spekker, E.; Polyák, H.; Tóth, F.; Vécsei, L. Mitochondrial Impairment: A Common Motif in Neuropsychiatric Presentation? The Link to the Tryptophan–Kynurenine Metabolic System. *Cells* **2022**, *11*, 2607. [CrossRef]
42. Correia, B.S.B.; Nani, J.V.; Waladares Ricardo, R.; Stanisic, D.; Costa, T.B.B.C.; Hayashi, M.A.F.; Tasic, L. Effects of Psychostimulants and Antipsychotics on Serum Lipids in an Animal Model for Schizophrenia. *Biomedicines* **2021**, *9*, 235. [CrossRef] [PubMed]
43. Gaebler, A.J.; Finner-Prével, M.; Sudar, F.P.; Langer, F.H.; Keskin, F.; Gebel, A.; Zweerings, J.; Mathiak, K. The Interplay between Vitamin D, Exposure of Anticholinergic Antipsychotics and Cognition in Schizophrenia. *Biomedicines* **2022**, *10*, 1096. [CrossRef] [PubMed]
44. Caruso, G.; Godos, J.; Castellano, S.; Micek, A.; Murabito, P.; Galvano, F.; Ferri, R.; Grosso, G.; Caraci, F. The Therapeutic Potential of Carnosine/Anserine Supplementation against Cognitive Decline: A Systematic Review with Meta-Analysis. *Biomedicines* **2021**, *9*, 253. [CrossRef] [PubMed]
45. Vila-Merkle, H.; González-Martínez, A.; Campos-Jiménez, R.; Martínez-Ricós, J.; Teruel-Martí, V.; Blasco-Serra, A.; Lloret, A.; Celada, P.; Cervera-Ferri, A. The Oscillatory Profile Induced by the Anxiogenic Drug FG-7142 in the Amygdala–Hippocampal Network Is Reversed by Infralimbic Deep Brain Stimulation: Relevance for Mood Disorders. *Biomedicines* **2021**, *9*, 783. [CrossRef]
46. Török, N.; Maszlag-Török, R.; Molnár, K.; Szolnoki, Z.; Somogyvári, F.; Boda, K.; Tanaka, M.; Klivényi, P.; Vécsei, L. Single Nucleotide Polymorphisms of Indoleamine 2,3-Dioxygenase 1 Influenced the Age Onset of Parkinson's Disease. *Front. Biosci.* **2022**, *27*, 265. [CrossRef]
47. Jamshed, L.; Debnath, A.; Jamshed, S.; Wish, J.V.; Raine, J.C.; Tomy, G.T.; Thomas, P.J.; Holloway, A.C. An Emerging Cross-Species Marker for Organismal Health: Tryptophan-Kynurenine Pathway. *Int. J. Mol. Sci.* **2022**, *23*, 6300. [CrossRef]
48. Martos, D.; Tuka, B.; Tanaka, M.; Vécsei, L.; Telegdy, G. Memory Enhancement with Kynurenic Acid and Its Mechanisms in Neurotransmission. *Biomedicines* **2022**, *10*, 849. [CrossRef]
49. Tanaka, M.; Tóth, F.; Polyák, H.; Szabó, Á.; Mándi, Y.; Vécsei, L. Immune Influencers in Action: Metabolites and Enzymes of the Tryptophan-Kynurenine Metabolic Pathway. *Biomedicines* **2021**, *9*, 734. [CrossRef]
50. Tanaka, M.; Török, N.; Tóth, F.; Szabó, Á.; Vécsei, L. Co-Players in Chronic Pain: Neuroinflammation and the Tryptophan-Kynurenine Metabolic Pathway. *Biomedicines* **2021**, *9*, 897. [CrossRef]
51. Vecsei, L.; Tanaka, M. Kynurenines, anxiety, and dementia. *J. Neural. Transm.* **2021**, *128*, 1799–1800.
52. Hepsomali, P.; Coxon, C. Inflammation and diet: Focus on mental and cognitive health. *Adv. Clin. Exp. Med.* **2022**, *31*, 821–825. [CrossRef] [PubMed]
53. Gładka, A.; Zatoński, T.; Rymaszewska, J. Association between the long-term exposure to air pollution and depression. *Adv. Clin. Exp. Med.* **2022**, *31*, 1139–1152. [CrossRef] [PubMed]
54. Tanaka, M.; Török, N.; Vécsei, L. Novel Pharmaceutical Approaches in Dementia. In *NeuroPsychopharmacotherapy*; Riederer, P., Laux, G., Nagatsu, T., Le, W., Riederer, C., Eds.; Springer: Cham, Switzerland, 2022. [CrossRef]
55. Zhao, X.; Zhang, H.; Wu, Y.; Yu, C. The efficacy and safety of St. John's wort extract in depression therapy compared to SSRIs in adults: A meta-analysis of randomized clinical trials. *Adv. Clin. Exp. Med.* **2022**. *online ahead of print*. [CrossRef] [PubMed]
56. Tanaka, M.; Török, N.; Vécsei, L. Are 5-HT1 receptor agonists effective anti-migraine drugs? *Expert. Opin. Pharmacother.* **2021**, *22*, 1221–1225. [CrossRef] [PubMed]
57. Spekker, E.; Tanaka, M.; Szabó, Á.; Vécsei, L. Neurogenic Inflammation: The Participant in Migraine and Recent Advancements in Translational Research. *Biomedicines* **2022**, *10*, 76. [CrossRef] [PubMed]
58. Balogh, L.; Tanaka, M.; Török, N.; Vécsei, L.; Taguchi, S. Crosstalk between Existential Phenomenological Psychotherapy and Neurological Sciences in Mood and Anxiety Disorders. *Biomedicines* **2021**, *9*, 340. [CrossRef] [PubMed]
59. Simonato, M.; Dall'Acqua, S.; Zilli, C.; Sut, S.; Tenconi, R.; Gallo, N.; Sfriso, P.; Sartori, L.; Cavallin, F.; Fiocco, U.; et al. Tryptophan Metabolites, Cytokines, and Fatty Acid Binding Protein 2 in Myalgic Encephalomyelitis/Chronic Fatigue Syndrome. *Biomedicines* **2021**, *9*, 1724. [CrossRef] [PubMed]
60. Komatsu, H.; Watanabe, E.; Fukuchi, M. Psychiatric Neural Networks and Precision Therapeutics by Machine Learning. *Biomedicines* **2021**, *9*, 403. [CrossRef]

biomedicines

MDPI

Article

The Interplay between Vitamin D, Exposure of Anticholinergic Antipsychotics and Cognition in Schizophrenia

Arnim Johannes Gaebler [1,2,3,*], Michelle Finner-Prével [1,2], Federico Pacheco Sudar [1,2], Felizia Hannah Langer [1,2], Fatih Keskin [4], Annika Gebel [1,2], Jana Zweerings [1,2] and Klaus Mathiak [1,2]

1 Department of Psychiatry, Psychotherapy and Psychosomatics, Faculty of Medicine, RWTH Aachen University, 52062 Aachen, Germany; mfinner@ukaachen.de (M.F.-P.); fpachecosuda@ukaachen.de (F.P.S.); flanger@ukaachen.de (F.H.L.); annika.gebel@rwth-aachen.de (A.G.); jzweerings@ukaachen.de (J.Z.); kmathiak@ukaachen.de (K.M.)
2 JARA—Translational Brain Medicine, 52062 Aachen, Germany
3 Institute of Physiology, Faculty of Medicine, RWTH Aachen University, 52062 Aachen, Germany
4 Klinik Königshof, 47807 Krefeld, Germany; fkeskin@ukaachen.de
* Correspondence: agaebler@ukaachen.de; Tel.: +49-241-8089632; Fax: +49-241-8082401

Abstract: Vitamin D deficiency is a frequent finding in schizophrenia and may contribute to neurocognitive dysfunction, a core element of the disease. However, there is limited knowledge about the neuropsychological profile of vitamin D deficiency-related cognitive deficits and their underlying molecular mechanisms. As an inductor of cytochrome P450 3A4, a lack of vitamin D might aggravate cognitive deficits by increased exposure to anticholinergic antipsychotics. This cross-sectional study aims to assess the relationship between 25-OH-vitamin D-serum concentrations, anticholinergic drug exposure and neurocognitive functioning (Brief Assessment of Cognition in Schizophrenia, BACS, and Trail Making Test, TMT) in 141 patients with schizophrenia. The anticholinergic drug exposure was estimated by adjusting the concentration of each drug for its individual muscarinic receptor affinity. Using regression analysis, we observed a positive relationship between vitamin D levels and processing speed (TMT-A and BACS Symbol Coding) as well as executive functioning (TMT-B and BACS Tower of London). Moreover, a negative impact of vitamin D on anticholinergic drug exposure emerged, but the latter did not significantly affect cognition. When other cognitive items were included as regressors, the impact of vitamin D remained only significant for the TMT-A. Among the different cognitive impairments in schizophrenia, vitamin D deficiency may most directly affect processing speed, which in turn may aggravate deficits in executive functioning. This finding is not explained by a cytochrome P450-mediated increased exposure to anticholinergic antipsychotics.

Keywords: schizophrenia; vitamin D; anticholinergic drugs; antipsychotics; pharmacokinetics; cognition; processing speed; BACS

Citation: Gaebler, A.J.; Finner-Prével, M.; Sudar, F.P.; Langer, F.H.; Keskin, F.; Gebel, A.; Zweerings, J.; Mathiak, K. The Interplay between Vitamin D, Exposure of Anticholinergic Antipsychotics and Cognition in Schizophrenia. *Biomedicines* **2022**, *10*, 1096. https://doi.org/10.3390/biomedicines10051096

Academic Editors: Masaru Tanaka and Nóra Török

Received: 15 March 2022
Accepted: 4 May 2022
Published: 9 May 2022

1. Introduction

Schizophrenia is a severe mental disorder characterized by multiple disturbances of perception, emotion and cognition [1]. It represents a multifactorial disease with high heritability, typically manifests in early adulthood and is associated with functional impairment, reduced life expectancy and socioeconomic burden [2]. Symptoms can be categorized into positive symptoms such as delusions and hallucinations, negative symptoms such as affective flattening and social withdrawal as well as cognitive symptoms [1].

Cognitive dysfunction is a core element of schizophrenia and one of the major factors contributing to long-term disability in this patient cohort [3]. Cognitive deficits in schizophrenia particularly comprise deficits in processing speed, attention/vigilance, social cognition, verbal learning, visual learning, as well as working memory, reasoning/problem solving and other aspects of executive function (such as abstract thinking and cognitive flexibility) [4–6]. However, current treatment options for this symptom domain are still insufficient. Remarkably, cognitive deficits typically manifest early in the disease course—i.e., before the diagnostic criteria are fulfilled—and persist despite successful pharmacological treatment of positive symptoms [7]. Neurobiological correlates of cognitive dysfunction may be impairments of dorsolateral prefrontal cortex function and its interactions with other brain regions [5], altered hippocampal activity [8] and bottom-up consequences of early sensory processing deficits [9–13]. Given the multifactorial nature of schizophrenia and its heterogeneous clinical phenotype, several factors may be ethiopathogenetically relevant for the emergence of cognitive dysfunction in this disorder with their individual contributions varying from patient to patient [14,15]. These factors may also include iatrogenic effects such as the prescription of antipsychotics with high anticholinergic potency [16].

Schizophrenia and other severe mental disorders are associated with lower levels of vitamin D [17]. Given the abundance of vitamin D-receptors in the human body, a lack of this hormone may have consequences going far beyond its well-known role in calcium homeostasis. Indeed, vitamin D deficiency is linked to a generally higher mortality with a significant contribution of cardiovascular diseases and cancer [18]. Therefore, it may be one of the factors leading to reduced life expectancy in this vulnerable patient cohort [19]. Moreover, there is growing evidence for vitamin D deficiency as a risk factor for the development of schizophrenia [7] and its aggravating impact on psychopathology [20,21]. In particular, neonatal vitamin D deprivation is associated with increased risk of developing schizophrenia [22,23]. Accordingly, as adults, rodent models of developmental vitamin D deficiency exhibit a phenotype mimicking some aspects of schizophrenia and show altered dopaminergic neurotransmission [24]. In contrast, in rodent models of adult vitamin D deficiency, there is evidence for a predominant dysfunction of glutamatergic and GABAergic circuits [25,26] and affected animals particularly show cognitive deficits [27,28]. Similarly, a growing number of human studies suggest a contribution of vitamin D deficiency to cognitive deficits in adult patients with schizophrenia and also other mental disorders [29]. However, there is limited knowledge about the clinical profile of vitamin D-related cognitive deficits and their underlying molecular mechanisms. Converging evidence suggests that vitamin D reduces exposure to many different drugs—including antipsychotics [30]—particularly by induction of the Cytochrome P450 (CYP) isoenzyme 3A4 [31–33]. Accordingly, vitamin D deficiency might lead to a decreased elimination, i.e., an increased exposure to anticholinergic antipsychotics, which in turn may increase cognitive dysfunction in this patient cohort. In the present study, we therefore aimed to characterize the neuropsychological profile of cognitive deficits in schizophrenia related to vitamin D deficiency and address the potential contribution of a vitamin D-mediated reduction of anticholinergic drug exposure.

2. Material and Methods

2.1. Participants and Neuropsychological Assessment

Serum concentrations of 25-OH-vitamin D and neuropsychological assessments were obtained from 141 in- and out-patients with schizophrenia. Sociodemographic and clinical characteristics of the patients are given in Table 1. For the different neuropsychological tests, the number of patients who completed them varied slightly (between 130 and 139; see Table 2). In- and out-patients with schizophrenia were recruited at the Department of Psychiatry, Psychotherapy and Psychosomatics of RWTH Aachen University Hospital and four academically associated psychiatric hospitals (Alexianer Hospital, Aachen; ViaNobis Gangelt; LVR Klinik Langenfeld, LVR Klinikum Düsseldorf). The data were obtained in the framework of an interventional brain imaging study with preregistration (NCT02435095). The study was approved by the ethics committee of the North Rhine medical association (AEKNO) and the ethics committee of the RWTH Aachen University Hospital (EK 156/16). We obtained written informed consent from all participants after a complete description of the study. The intended sample size with respect to the primary outcome (gray matter change) of 574 patients could not be achieved and therefore the trial was stopped. All data presented here were obtained before any intervention.

Table 1. Sociodemographic and clinical characteristics of the sample.

Characteristic	Mean	Std
Biometrics		
Age [Years]	33.1	11.4
C (25-OH-Vitamin D3) [ng/mL]	14.5	8.9
Duration of disease	4.9	7.1
Cognitive Performance		
TMT-A [s]	35.3	15.3
TMT-B [s]	95.9	49.6
BACS—Verbal Memory	37.8	12.5
BACS—Working Memory: Correct Answers	17.6	4.4
BACS—Working Memory: Longest Sequence	6.3	1.6
BACS—Motor Speed	64.0	17.6
BACS—Fluent Speech Category	18.1	5.2
BACS—Fluent Speech Letter	20.1	7.9
BACS—Symbol Coding	44.9	13.5
BACS—Tower of London	15.0	4.2
Positive and Negative Syndrome Scale (PANSS)		
Positive Symptoms	16.1	6.9
Negative Symptoms	17.8	6.6
Global Symptoms	32.8	10.9
	N	**%**
Gender		
Female	40	28.4
Male	101	71.6

BACS = Brief Assessment of Cognition in Schizophrenia.

Table 2. Correlation analysis.

		C(25-OH-Vitamin D) [a]	C(Anticholinergic) [a]
TMT−A (in s)	Pearson's r	** −0.373	0.169
	p-value	<0.001	0.097
	N	133	61
TMT−B (in s)	Pearson's r	** −0.336	0.174
	p-value	<0.001	0.092
	N	130	60
Verbal Memory	Pearson's r	0.175	−0.124
	p-value	0.020	0.173
	N	139	60
Working Memory Correct Answers	Pearson's r	0.131	−0.048
	p-value	0.062	0.358
	N	139	60
Working Memory Longest Sequence	Pearson's r	0.204	−0.022
	p-value	0.008	0.434
	N	139	60
Motor Speed	Pearson's r	0.107	−0.122
	p-value	0.108	0.184
	N	136	57

Table 2. *Cont.*

		C(25-OH-Vitamin D) [a]	C(Anticholinergic) [a]
Fluent Speech Category	Pearson's r	0.195	0.001
	p-value	0.011	0.496
	N	137	59
Fluent Speech Letter	Pearson's r	0.136	−0.044
	p-value	0.056	0.370
	N	138	59
Symbol Coding	Pearson's r	** 0.280	−0.070
	p-value	<0.001	0.299
	N	139	59
Tower of London	Pearson's r	** 0.274	−0.103
	p-value	<0.001	0.220
	N	137	59

** Correlation remains statistically significant after Bonferroni correction for multiple testing. Given *p*-values in the table are uncorrected. Corrected *p*-values are given in the main text. [a] C (25-OH-vitamin D) and C (anticholinergic) were log-transformed, as the curve fitting revealed a logarithmic relationship.

The study employed the following inclusion criteria: diagnosis of schizophrenia according to DSM-5, age of 18–65 years, written declaration of consent, subjects being contractually and mentally capable to attend the medical staffs' orders and MRI capability. Exclusion criteria comprised: relevant somatic diseases, which could have an impact on the conduct of the study based on clinical judgement of the treating physician (e.g., epilepsy, cancer), prior to insufficiently documented drug therapy with antipsychotics, magnetic metals in and on the body, cardiac pacemakers and body piercings, pregnancy or lactation, hospitalization of the patient ordered by the court or public authorities, relationship of dependence or employment to sponsor or investigator and simultaneous participation in another clinical trial. Trained psychiatrists confirmed the diagnosis of schizophrenia according to DSM 5 criteria using the structured clinical interview for DSM disorders (SCID) and performed the clinical ratings and neuropsychological assessments. As a structured interview, the SCID was used to minimize interviewer bias. For neuropsychological assessments, the Brief Assessment of Cognition in Schizophrenia (BACS) as well as the Trail Making Test A (TMT-A) and B (TMT-B) were employed [34–36]. The BACS is a cognitive battery that was designed to assess multiple cognitive domains affected in schizophrenia in relatively a short time (about 30 to 40 min). It contains seven tests in total, assessing verbal memory, working memory (Digit sequencing), semantic (naming of animals) and lexical verbal fluency, processing speed (Symbol coding Test) and motor speed (Token motor test) as well as reasoning and problem solving (Tower of London Test). In both parts of the TMT, study participants have to connect 25 circles distributed over a sheet of paper as quickly as possible without lifting the pen or pencil from the paper. In Part A, the circles are numbered from 1 to 25, and the numbers should be connected in ascending order. In Part B, the circles include both numbers (1–13) and letters (A–L); which again should be connected in an ascending pattern (concerning the size of the number and the alphabetical order of the letters), but alternating between numbers and letters (i.e., 1-A-2-B, etc.).

2.2. *Quantification of Vitamin D Levels and Anticholinergic Drug Exposure*

Within this study, blood samples were taken throughout the year between August 2015 and March 2020. A part of the vitamin D and drug concentrations used for this analysis were already used previously [30]. According to the study protocol, all patients underwent blood sampling for the analysis of vitamin D levels. If patients were already under antipsychotic treatment, we also obtained blood samples for therapeutic drug monitoring. For clinical and organizational reasons, time-points of blood sampling slightly varied from patient to patient. Ideally, for therapeutic drug monitoring, blood samples should be collected just before intake (providing trough levels) and at steady-state conditions of the respective drug (i.e., after more than 4 elimination half-lives under the same dose). In case these conditions were not met, hospital charts were reviewed to identify accurate drug concentrations obtained during the clinical routine within a maximum temporal window of 2 months before or after the determination of vitamin D concentrations. Drug concentrations that were still outside the steady state conditions, for which the dose or time of intake could not be determined or which were obtained during the drug absorption phase (i.e., before the expected time of maximum concentration, Tmax) were excluded from the further analysis. If blood samples were not immediately collected before the next drug intake (a typical clinical situation is given for antipsychotics, which are taken as a single dose in the evening, but blood is withdrawn in the morning), expected trough levels (C_{min}) were calculated using the drug's half-life ($t_{1/2}$) and the following exponential function [37]:

$$Cmin = C(t) * e^{-ke *(tmin-t)}$$

with $C(t)$ as the drug concentration measured at time t, t_{min} as the time at C_{min}, and k_e as the elimination rate constant (k_e = ln2/$t_{1/2}$). From the final set drug through levels, dose-adjusted drug concentrations were calculated by dividing them by the given daily dose (C/D) [in (ng/mL)/(mg/day)]. If the date of TDM differed from the date of neuropsychological testing, d0, (i.e., drug levels had to be retrieved from the hospital charts), drug levels at d0 were estimated by multiplying the dose-adjusted drug concentrations with the dose given at d0.

From the total sample, 75 quality-controlled serum concentrations of different antipsychotic drugs obtained from 61 patients were available: amisulpride (N = 12), aripiprazole (N = 8), clozapine (N = 9), olanzapine (N = 16), quetiapine (N = 8) and risperidone (N = 22). The remaining patients either were not yet medicated at the time of assessment or serum concentrations did not fulfil our quality criteria. Among those 75 serum levels, 62 were corrected using the equation above.

For aripiprazole, clozapine, olanzapine, quetiapine, and risperidone, serum concentrations of their respective main metabolites were also determined, i.e., dehydroaripiprazole, norclozapine, desmethylolanzapine, norquetiapine, and 9-OH-risperidone. All drug and metabolite concentrations were analyzed in the same laboratory by Liquid Chromatography with tandem mass spectrometry (LC-MS/MS) [38]. For vitamin D levels (25-OH Vitamin D), chemiluminescent immunoassays (CLIA) were applied [39].

To control for potential pharmacokinetic confounding variables, we screened all patients for the co-prescription of drugs with known inducing or inhibiting properties on the major cytochrome P450 isoenzymes CYP1A2, CYP2B6, CYP2C8, CYP2C9, CYP2C19, CYP2D6 (only inhibitors are known) and CYP3A4 according to the suggestions by the US Food and Drug Administration [40]. We identified two patients receiving the CYP1A2-inhibitor fluvoxamine and one patient receiving the CYP2D6-inhibitor fluoxetine as a co-medication, respectively. The latter patient was not included in any pharmacokinetic analysis, as there was no TDM data available meeting our quality criteria. To assess the impact of the two remaining patients who were under co-treatment with fluvoxamine, we conducted a sub-analysis for which we removed these patients (see Section 3).

For the estimation of anticholinergic exposure, drug serum concentrations were first normalized to the upper level of the therapeutic reference range TRRmax. For risperidone, the concentration of the active moiety (parent compound + active metabolite 9-OH-risperidone) was used instead of the pure concentration of the parent compound, as the TRR is typically defined for the active moiety [37]. Normalized concentrations were adjusted for each drug's anticholinergic potency by division by the drug's M1 muscarinic receptor dissociation constant Kd and multiplication with the corresponding dissociation constant Kd of the reference substance chlorpromazine, i.e.,

$$C(\text{Anticholinergic}) = \frac{C(\text{Drug x})*\text{Kd}(\text{Chlorpromazine})}{\text{TRRmax}(\text{Drug x})*\text{Kd}(\text{Drug x})}$$

Dissociation constants (Kd) were obtained from the NIMH Psychoactive Drug Screening Program (PDSP) Database [41] Chlorpromazine, which is typically considered the first antipsychotic drug [42] and is often used to compare antipsychotic potency (chlorpromazine equivalent dose) [43], was chosen as a reference substance due to its broad receptor profile including affinity for muscarinic M1 receptors [44]. If a patient received more than one antipsychotic drug, the respective measures of anticholinergic drug exposure were added to each other.

2.3. Statistical Analysis

In order to assess the different relationships between the variables of interest, we conducted four main regression analyses:

(1) In the first regression analysis, we assessed the impact of vitamin D on cognition. Thereto, for each of the 10 cognitive items, we separately calculated a bivariate regression model with the respective item as the dependent variable and the 25-OH-vitamin D concentration as the independent variable, yielding 10 regression models in total.

(2) In the second analysis, we investigated the influence of anticholinergic drug exposure on cognition. As in the first analysis, we calculated separate bivariate regression models for each cognitive item, which served as the dependent variable, and the adjusted anticholinergic drug concentration served as the independent variable.

(3) In the third analysis, we assessed the relationship between vitamin D levels (independent variable) and anticholinergic drug exposure (dependent variable) in a single bivariate regression model. To control for potential confounders, we conducted two additional sub-analyses. In the first one, we added the number of cigarettes per day as a second independent variable to the regression model. In the second one, we removed the two patients receiving a co-treatment with the CYP1A2-inhibitor fluvoxamine.

(4) In a stepwise forward regression analysis, we used one of the three following cognitive items as the dependent variables in separate sub-analyses: TMT-A, TMT-B and the Tower of London. The remaining two cognitive items, the number of cigarettes per day as well as the log-transformed vitamin D and anticholinergic levels served as the independent variables. The independent variables with the most significant impact on the respective dependent variable were sequentially added to the model until no further significant improvement of model fit could be achieved.

(5) As a further exploratory analysis, we assessed the impact of vitamin D on an alternative measure of cognition derived from a five-factor model of the positive and negative syndrome scale (PANSS) [45,46]. This five-factor model includes a "positive", "negative", "cognitive", "emotional/depressed" and "excited" factor, with the cognitive factor being composed of item 2 of the positive symptom subscale, item 5 o the negative symptom subscale and item 11 of the general psychopathology subscale (P2N5G11).

For all regression analyses, in order to verify the linear relationship between the dependent variable and the predictors, individual scatter plots were subjected to a curve fitting analysis, which revealed that some variables had to be log-transformed to establish a linear relationship. In such cases, the respective variables were log-transformed before entering the regression analysis (see Section 3). Gaussian distribution and homoskedasticity of residuals were confirmed by inspection of histograms and Q-Q-plots. If more than one predictor was included in the analysis, absence of multicollinearity was verified by variance inflation factor (VIF), which was required to be below 4. For each of the five main analyses, we used one-tailed p-values corrected for multiple comparisons using the

Bonferroni correction. Patients with missing values were not included in the respective regression model, i.e., there was no imputation of missing values. Statistical analysis and data visualization were performed using SPSS 28 (IBM, Armonk, NY, USA), RStudio (RStudio Team (2021). RStudio: Integrated Development Environment for R. RStudio, PBC, Boston, MA, USA, Available online: http://www.rstudio.com) and GraphPad Prism 5 (GraphPad Software, San Diego, CA, USA).

3. Results

Sociodemographic characteristics of the sample are given in Table 1. Only 22% of patients exhibited sufficient vitamin D levels (>20 ng/mL), i.e., 78% of patients exhibited vitamin D insufficiency (11–20 ng/mL) or deficiency (≤10 ng/mL). For a visualization of the distribution of vitamin D levels, see Figure 1.

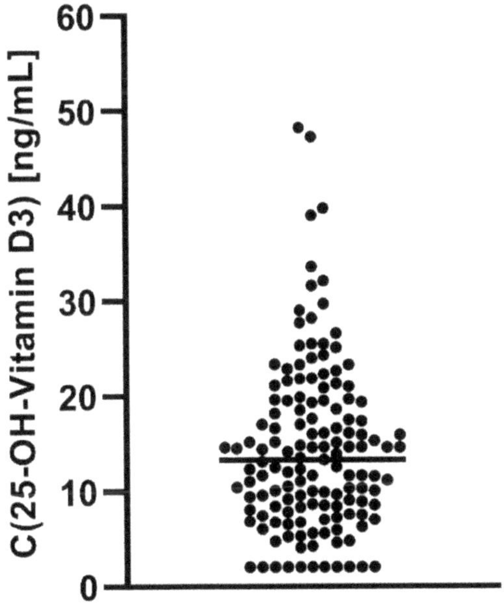

Figure 1. Distribution of 25-OH vitamin D-levels in our sample. Note the high proportions of patients following below the threshold of vitamin D insufficiency (≤20 ng/mL) and deficiency (≤10 ng/mL).

Confirming the primary hypothesis, we observed a general positive relationship between vitamin D levels and cognitive performance; i.e., patients with lower vitamin D levels exhibited more pronounced cognitive impairments (see Table 2). The curve fitting revealed that each of the different cognitive items could be best described as a function of the logarithm of the 25-OH-vitamin D-concentration (see Figure 2). After a Bonferroni correction of multiple comparisons, the impact of vitamin D on four cognitive items remained statistically significant including the TMT-A ($p < 0.001$) and the BACS Symbol Coding Test ($p = 0.004$) as measures of processing speed as well as the TMT-B ($p < 0.001$) and BACS Tower of London Test ($p = 0.006$) as measures of executive functioning with the former operationalizing cognitive flexibility and the latter planning and problem solving. Corresponding Pearson correlation coefficients addressing the correlation between the respective cognitive items and the log-transformed 25-OH-vitamin D-concentration as well as uncorrected p-values are provided in Table 2.

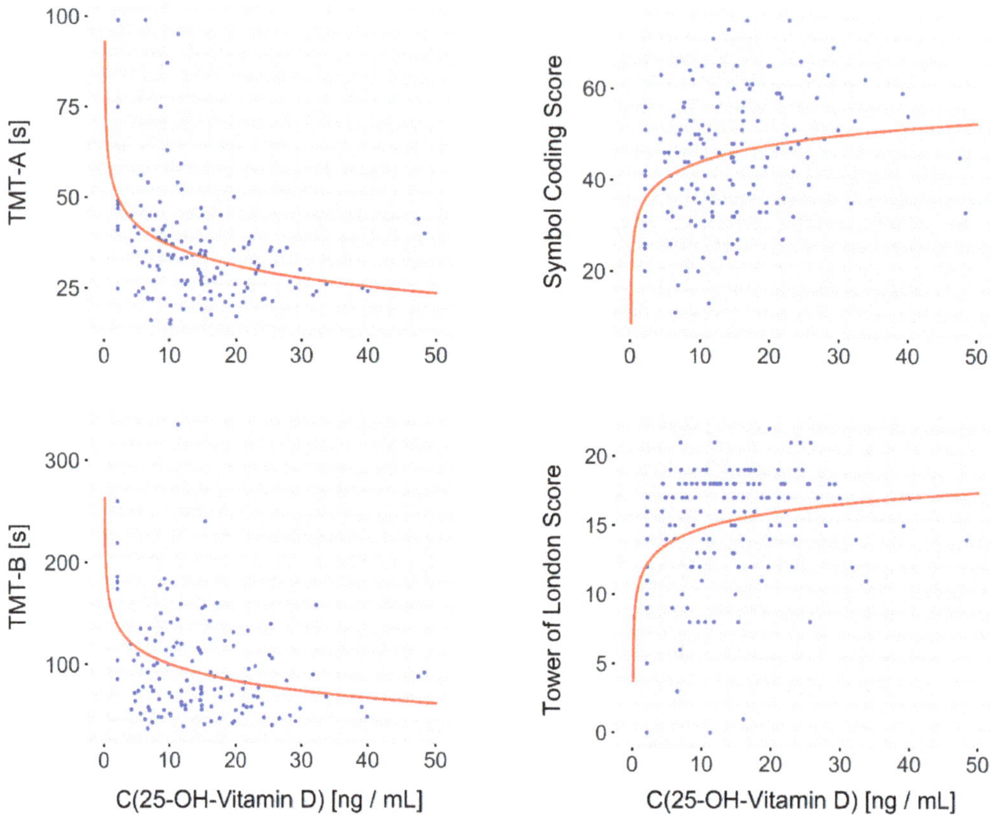

Figure 2. The relationship between 25-OH vitamin D-levels and cognition. Scatter plots and estimated regression curves are shown for the four cognitive items for which vitamin D's impact remained statistically significant after Bonferroni correction of multiple comparisons. Curve fitting indicated that each of the different cognitive items (*y*-axis) could be best described as a function of the logarithm of the 25-OH-vitamin D-concentration (*x*-axis).

Only at a trend level, a negative relationship between the estimated anticholinergic drug levels and each of the cognitive items emerged. Similar to the first regression analysis, a best curve fit could be achieved when applying a logarithmic function. However, even without correction for multiple testing, none of the regression models reached statistical significance. For detailed statistics, see Table 2. Whereas the negative effect of anti-cholinergic substances of cognition is consistent with the data, the significance of such effects seems lesser than the positive vitamin D effects.

We observed a negative association between 25-OH-vitamin D-concentration and anticholinergic drug exposure. Curve fitting revealed a best fit for logarithmic transformation of both the independent and dependent variable (see Figure 3). This association reached statistical significance (standardized beta = −0.235; p = 0.034; N = 61), confirming the pharmacokinetic relationship between vitamin D and (some) anti-cholinergic drugs. Since smoking is known to induce the cytochrome P450 isoenzyme CYP1A2, we subsequently included the number of cigarettes per day as a second predictor to assess the effect of this potential confounder on anticholinergic drug exposure. This covariate did not show any association with the dependent variable (standardized beta = −0.014; p = 0.913; N = 61), whereas the effect of vitamin D remained significant (standardized beta = −0.235; p = 0.036; N = 61). To control for further pharmacokinetic confounders, for all patients we assessed the prescription of co-medication with known inducing or inhibiting properties on the major cytochrome P450 isoenzymes. We identified two patients who received the CYP1A2-inhibitor fluvoxamine and one patient receiving the CYP2D6-inhibitor fluoxetine as a co-medication, respectively. Since for the latter patient, there was no TDM data meeting our quality criteria available, this patient was not included in the analysis. When excluding the two patients who were under co-treatment with fluvoxamine, the effect of vitamin D on anticholinergic drug levels remained significant (Pearson's $r = -0.256$; $p = 0.025$; N = 59). We therefore decided not to exclude these two patients from the further analyses.

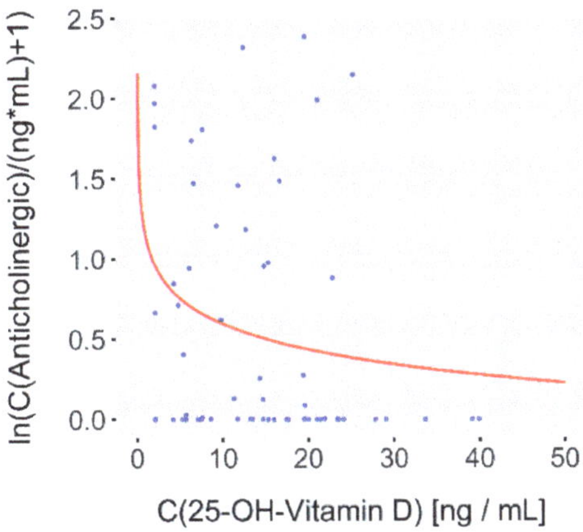

Figure 3. The relationship between 25-OH vitamin D-levels and exposure to anticholinergic antipsychotics. Scatter plot of the association between 25-OH-vitamin-concentration (x-axis) and antipsychotic drug concentrations adjusted for anticholinergic potency (y-axis). Curve fitting revealed a best fit for a log-transformation of both the dependent and independent variable.

For the stepwise regression analysis, we selected the TMT-A, TMT-B, and the Tower of London Test performance as the dependent variables, as those were the only three items—besides the Symbol Coding Test—which remained significant after correction for multiple testing. Since the Symbol Coding Test is a further measure of processing speed—just as the TMT-A—we decided to exclude it from the analysis in order to minimize the number of statistical tests. The sub-analyses revealed that for none of the three investigated cognitive scales, anticholinergic drug exposure or the daily number of cigarettes was included in the model. For the TMT-A, the best model fit could be attained ($R^2 = 0.418$) when including the Tower of London Test performance (standardized beta = −0.477; t = −4.434; $p < 0.001$) and the log-transformed 25-OH-vitamin D concentration (standardized beta = −0.319; t = −2960; $p = 0.003$). For the TMT-B, the final model ($R^2 = 0.339$) included the TMT-A (standardized beta = 0.352; t = −2.638; $p = 0.006$) and the Tower of London Test (standardized beta = −0.304; t = −2.278; $p = 0.014$). Finally, for the Tower of London Test performance ($R^2 = 0.339$), the TMT-A (standardized beta = −0.422; t = −3.389; $p < 0.001$) and the TMT-B (standardized beta = −0.283; t = −2.278; $p = 0.014$) were included in the model.

Thus, after regressing out the respective other tests, only for the TMT-A, the inclusion of log-transformed 25-OH-vitamin D concentration resulted in a significant improvement of model fit. This effect remained also significant after Bonferroni correction (p-corrected = 0.045).

Further, we investigated the relationship between vitamin D concentration and an alternative measure of cognition, namely the cognitive component of a five-factor model of the positive and negative syndrome scale (PANSS) [45,46]. Again, lower 25-OH-vitamin D levels were associated with greater cognitive impairment, and curve fitting revealed a logarithmic relationship between the dependent (i.e., the cognitive) variable and the independent variable (vitamin D concentration). (Standardized beta = −0.144; $p = 0.046$; N = 139) (see Figure 4).

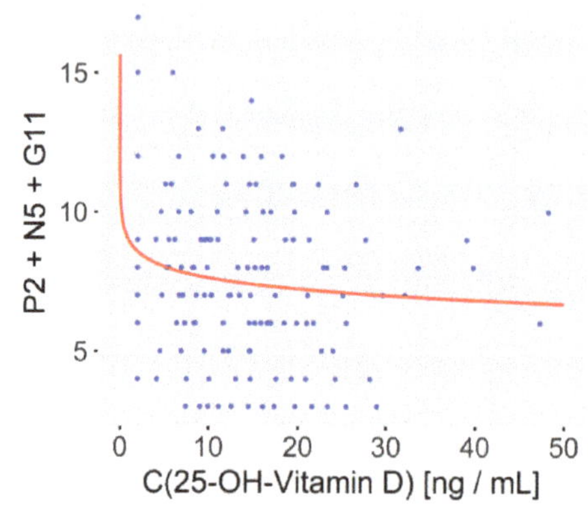

Figure 4. The relationship between 25-OH vitamin D levels and the cognitive component of the PANSS five factor model derived from items P2, N5 and G11 of the PANSS. As for the other cognitive variables, curve fitting indicated that the cognitive component (*y*-axis) could be best described as a function of the logarithm of the 25-OH-vitamin D concentration (*x*-axis).

4. Discussion

A significant proportion of patients with schizophrenia suffer from vitamin D deficiency, which may contribute to somatic comorbidity and psychopathology, particularly cognitive symptoms. The present study thus confirmed prior evidence for vitamin D deficiency as a factor contributing to neurocognitive dysfunction in schizophrenia and provided a characterization of the neuropsychological profile of vitamin D-deficiency-related cognitive deficits. We detected a strong association between vitamin D serum concentrations and processing speed as well as executive functions in patients suffering from schizophrenia. However, a stepwise regression analysis revealed that vitamin D deficiency most directly affected processing speed, while its impact on executive functioning may be better explained as a consequence of the former effect, i.e., its effect on processing speed. Cognitive dysfunction in schizophrenia comprises a well-defined set of cognitive domains, including processing speed, attention/vigilance, visual and verbal learning, and social cognition as well as working memory, reasoning/planning and other executive functions [4]. There is still controversy about the existence of a hierarchy of the different cognitive symptom domains and their causal relationship. However, several studies suggest a pivotal role of deficits in processing speed [47], which may contribute to other cognitive deficits such as working memory deficits and executive dysfunction [48]. Interestingly, our present findings suggest that vitamin D deficiency primarily affects this important cognitive domain. Previous studies addressing the neuropsychological profile of cognitive deficits related to vitamin D deficiency have yielded inconclusive results: In a cross-sectional study assessing cognitive performance in 20 patients with first episode schizophrenia and 20 healthy controls, vitamin D deficiency was associated with lower scores of a summary measure of different cognitive tests in patients with schizophrenia, only [49]. For the individual tests, only verbal fluency was significantly correlated with vitamin D levels, but not processing speed. However, insufficient power due to the small sample size (N = 20) may have biased the results. Based on the relationship between vitamin D and the TMT-A (yielding the highest effect size), a post hoc power analysis of our own data indeed suggests a minimum required sample size of 40 patients given an expected power of 80% and a one-tailed alpha-level of 0.05. For the different cognitive tests that were significantly correlated with vitamin D concentrations in our own dataset, the post hoc power analysis estimated a power of 99.8% for the TMT-A, 99.2% for the TMT-B, 96.2% for the BACS Symbol Coding Test and 95.3% for the BACS Tower of London Test, respectively, given the respective sample sizes and a one-tailed alpha-level of 0.05.

Accordingly, in a larger sample of 225 patients with psychotic disorders, Nerhus et al. observed that a low vitamin D status was significantly associated with decreased processing speed and verbal memory [50]. Similar to the present study, the strongest association was observed for processing speed. In a randomized, double-blind, placebo-controlled clinical trial, 47 patients with therapy-resistant schizophrenia and low vitamin D levels were randomly assigned to a vitamin D supplementation or placebo group [51]. After eight weeks, the vitamin D group demonstrated a significant increase in vitamin D levels and a trend towards improved cognition, particularly for attention and verbal memory. Notably, the authors applied the Montreal Cognitive Assessment (MOCA), which does not include an explicit test for processing speed [52]. Larger clinical trials are desirable to draw further conclusions on the effectiveness of vitamin D supplementation on cognitive symptoms in schizophrenia. As a neural correlate of improved cognitive performance, there is first evidence for an amelioration of hippocampal volume loss in schizophrenia mediated by vitamin D [53], but there is still limited knowledge on the molecular mechanisms of vitamin D's neurophysiological effects. A potential mechanism that we wanted to address in this study is grounded in vitamin D's impact on drug metabolism. Indeed, vitamin D has been demonstrated to increase metabolism and elimination of many different drugs including antipsychotics [30]—particularly CYP3A4 substrates. Since there is converging evidence for a negative impact of antipsychotics with high anticholinergic potency on cognition [16], we assessed whether the effect of a low vitamin D status on cognition in schizophrenia might be mediated by a reduced metabolism of anticholinergic antipsychotics. Several in vitro studies demonstrated CYP3A4 induction by vitamin D in different cell lines including primary human hepatocytes [54–56]. Human in vivo studies revealed that the supplementation of vitamin D is associated with increased elimination of the statin and CYP3A4 substrate atorvastatin [33]. Moreover, blood concentrations of the immunosuppressants tacrolimus and sirolimus—both of which are substrates of CYP3A4—show a cyclic seasonal variation, which is anti-correlated to the well-known seasonal variation of vitamin D levels [32]. Similarly, intestinal CYP3A4 expression was demonstrated to be predicted by genetic polymorphisms of the vitamin D receptor [57]. beyond CYP3A4, there is preliminary evidence suggesting that vitamin D also has inducing properties on the isoenzymes CYP2B6 and CYP2C9 —with probably minor quantitative contribution, though [54] as well as *p*-glycoprotein (*p*-gp), a renal efflux pump of xenobiotics [58]. Accordingly, vitamin D deficiency might lead to a decreased elimination, i.e., an increased exposure to anticholinergic antipsychotics, which in turn may increase cognitive dysfunction in this patient cohort. However, even though we observed a significant negative relationship between vitamin D levels and the exposure to anticholinergic antipsychotics, this finding could not explain the robust effects of vitamin D on the cognition observed in this study. Several animal studies have suggested a neurotrophic effect of vitamin D promoting neurogenesis and enhancing synaptic function in the hippocampus [59,60]. Accordingly, a human study suggested an amelioration of hippocampal volume loss in schizophrenia mediated by vitamin D (see above) [53]. Cognitive dysfunction in schizophrenia may also be related to inflammatory processes [61–63]. Indeed, increased serum concentrations of C-reactive protein (CRP), a peripheral marker of inflammation, were associated with worse cognitive performance in patients with schizophrenia [64]. Notably, vitamin D has been found to regulate the production of proinflammatory cytokines and the proliferation of proinflammatory cells, respectively [65]. Accordingly, such anti-inflammatory properties may represent a mechanism that might explain its potential benefits for cognition in schizophrenia. Statins may constitute a further candidate drug group to modulate inflammatory processes in schizophrenia [66]. Other potential molecular targets of pro-cognitive pharmacotherapy may be N-Methyl-D-Aspartate (NMDA) receptors, metabotropic glutamate receptors and the kynurenine pathway [67–69]. Cognitive deficits in schizophrenia are likely multifactorial and may require different treatment approaches for the individual patients. The identification of pathophysiologically specific molecular markers (e.g., [70,71]) obtained from easily accessible biomaterial or brain imaging endophenotypes and combined with machine learning algorithms may serve as a basis for the establishment of precision medicine in psychiatry [72].

Several test batteries have been employed to study cognitive deficits in schizophrenia (for an overview see [73]). An ideal test battery should cover most cognitive domains affected in schizophrenia within an appropriate time frame, which should be tolerable for most patients and economic for staff members administering the tests. Among the different test batteries that were used in the literature, the MATRICS Consensus Cognitive Battery (MCCB) and the Brief Assessment of Cognition in Schizophrenia (BACS) represent two well-validated and reliable instruments meeting the abovementioned criteria. The BACS, which was used in the present study, is particularly short (around 30 min for completion) while covering most of the cognitive domains that are impaired in patients with schizophrenia. It comprises seven tests in total, examining verbal memory, working memory (Digit sequencing), semantic (naming of animals) and lexical verbal fluency, processing speed (Symbol coding Test) and motor speed (Token motor test) as well as reasoning and problem solving as an aspect of executive function (Tower of London Test). It was shown to be as sensitive to cognitive impairment in schizophrenia as more extensive test batteries. Since the battery is specifically designed to measure treatment-related changes of cognitive symptoms, it provides alternate forms for some of the tests in order to minimize practice effects. Moreover, it is available in nine languages and norms are also available. In the present study, besides the BACS, we additionally administered The Trail Making Test (TMT)-A and -B, as both tests require a minimum time for completion but provide an additional measure of processing speed (TMT-A) as well as a measure of cognitive flexibility (TMT-B). The TMT, which was originally introduced as a part of the Army Individual Test Battery [74], represents one of the most popular neuropsychological tests employed by many different test batteries [75] and patients with schizophrenia have been demonstrated to exhibit significant performance deficits for both tests [76].

As stated above, a good alternative to the set of tests used in this study (BACS and TMT) may be the MCCB. It comprises 10 tests selected by experts within the framework of the NIMH Measurement and Treatment Research to Improve Cognition in Schizophrenia (MATRICS) based on more than 90 tests nominated for inclusion [77]. Notably, the TMT-A and the BACS Symbol Coding Test (both assessing processing speed) as well as an animal naming test comparable to the one which is part of the BACS are included in this battery. The remaining seven tests examine attention/vigilance (Continuous Performance Test—Identical Pairs), working memory (WMS–III Spatial Span; University of Maryland Letter-Number Span), verbal memory (Hopkins Verbal Learning Test—Revised), visual memory (Brief Visuospatial Memory Test—Revised), reasoning and problem-solving (Neuropsychological Assessment Battery—Mazes) as well as social cognition (Mayer–Salovey–Caruso Emotional Intelligence Test—Managing Emotions). Accordingly, while there is a substantial overlap between the assessed cognitive domains and administered tests of the MCCB and the set of tests employed in this study, the MCCB provides tests for attention/vigilance, visual memory, and social cognition that are not assessed explicitly by the BACS or TMT, whereas our set of tests provides additional measures of motor skills (Token motor test) and cognitive flexibility (TMT-B). Another advantage of our approach is the lower amount of time required for completion (around 30 to 40 min as compared to 60 min for the MCCB). Future studies should also investigate the relationship between vitamin D and tests of attention/vigilance, visual memory and social cognition, as provided by the MCCB.

5. Limitations

A major limitation of the present study is its cross-sectional and non-interventional nature. Accordingly, the correlations reported in the present study may in principle reflect pure epiphenomena, but not necessarily a causal relationship. Moreover, the true causal relationship may also be reverse, i.e., cognitive deficits may also lead to lower vitamin D levels. Due to the inability to perform everyday activities, patients with cognitive deficits may spend less time outdoors and therefore may be less exposed to sunlight.

This hypothesis has been also stated for elderly persons with cognitive deficits. However, according to our hypothesis, animal studies [59,60,78,79] and first randomized controlled clinical trials [51] have provided some preliminary evidence for a direct causal impact of vitamin D on cognition, Further randomized controlled clinical trials (RCTs) comparing the effects of vitamin D supplementation in comparison to a placebo group are warranted. Ideally, such studies should apply therapeutic drug monitoring during the course of the treatment in order to control for vitamin D's negative impact on antipsychotic drug exposure. From a more preventive perspective, screening for vitamin D deficiency and supplementation studies may be also relevant for persons who are at a high risk for schizophrenia [80].

Our inclusion and exclusion criteria may have caused some degree of selection bias. Such as many other studies on patients suffering from severe mental disorders, for ethical and legal reasons, we only included subjects being contractually and mentally capable to attend the medical staffs' orders and understand the study procedure. Moreover, we excluded patients whose hospitalization was ordered by the court or public authorities. As a consequence, patients with less severe psychopathology may be overrepresented in our study cohort. Moreover, due to the fact that the study was part of a larger brain imaging trial, we only considered patients who met the MRI safety criteria which are—however—not relevant for the data that were the basis of this study.

6. Conclusions

Cognitive dysfunction is a core symptom domain of schizophrenia associated with long-term disability, but limited treatment options. In the present study, we observed a significant association between serum concentrations of vitamin D—which are insufficient in many patients with schizophrenia—and cognitive performance, particularly processing speed. This relationship could not be explained by the negative impact of vitamin D on the exposure to anticholinergic antipsychotics—given its inducing effects on cytochrome P450 isoenzymes—particularly CYP3A4. Considering vitamin D's well-established effects on physical health, the growing evidence for its effects on mental health and cognition as well as the frequency of vitamin D insufficiency in schizophrenia, screening for vitamin D insufficiency and its compensation by supplementation may be beneficial for this vulnerable patient cohort.

Author Contributions: A.J.G., study design, data acquisition, analysis and interpretation; writing of manuscript; M.F.-P., data acquisition and analysis, and correction of manuscript; F.P.S., data acquisition and correction of manuscript; F.H.L., data acquisition and correction of manuscript; F.K., data acquisition and correction of manuscript; A.G., data acquisition and correction of manuscript; J.Z., data acquisition and correction of manuscript; K.M., study design, data analysis and interpretation, and correction of manuscript. All authors have read and agreed to the published version of the manuscript.

Funding: This work was supported by the Federal Ministry of Education and Research (01EE1405A-C), Germany and the international research training group (IRTG) 2150 funded by the German research foundation (DFG; project number 269953372). AJG was supported by a clinician scientist scholarship and the START grant (project number 36/20) of the Faculty of Medicine of the RWTH Aachen University.

Institutional Review Board Statement: The study was conducted according to the guidelines of the Declaration of Helsinki, and approved by the ethics committee of the North Rhine medical association (AEKNO) and by the local ethics committee of the RWTH Aachen University Hospital (EK 156/16).

Informed Consent Statement: Written informed consent was obtained from all participants, following a complete description of the study.

Data Availability Statement: Data are stored at RWTH Aachen University hospital. The data are not publicly available due to privacy and ethical restrictions.

Acknowledgments: The authors thank Manuela Das Gupta for her contribution to blood sampling, and Michelle Schlingensief, Jasmin Mühlenberg, as well as the Brain Imaging Facility of the Interdisciplinary Center for Clinical Research (IZKF) Aachen for their organizational help. Moreover, the authors thank the other members of the APIC Consortium for their contribution to the recruitment of participants and organizational help: Marc Augustin; Joachim Cordes; Emir Demirel; Thomas Dielentheis; Jan Dreher; Patrick Eisner; Frederik Hendricks; Jana Hovancakova; Peter Kaleta; Miriam Kirchner; André Kirner-Veselinovic; Sarah Lammertz; Christina Lange; Federico Maria Larcher; Laura M. Lenzen; Eva Meisenzahl-Lechner; Jutta Muysers; Andrea Neff; Michael Plum; Erik Röcher; Axel Ruttmann; Sabrina Schaffrath; Lara Schwemmer; Eva Stormanns; Antje Trauzeddel1; Lina Winkler, Michael Paulzen, Gerhard Gründer and Frank Schneider.

Conflicts of Interest: The authors declare no conflict of interest.

References

1. Kahn, R.S.; Sommer, I.E.; Murray, R.M.; Meyer-Lindenberg, A.; Weinberger, D.R.; Cannon, T.D.; O'Donovan, M.; Correll, C.U.; Kane, J.M.; van Os, J.; et al. Schizophrenia. *Nat. Rev. Dis. Primers* **2015**, *1*, 15067. [CrossRef]
2. Jauhar, S.; Johnstone, M.; McKenna, P.J. Schizophrenia. *Lancet* **2022**, *399*, 473–486. [CrossRef]
3. Fett, A.K.; Viechtbauer, W.; Dominguez, M.D.; Penn, D.L.; van Os, J.; Krabbendam, L. The relationship between neurocognition and social cognition with functional outcomes in schizophrenia: A meta-analysis. *Neurosci. Biobehav. Rev.* **2011**, *35*, 573–588. [CrossRef]
4. Heinrichs, R.W.; Zakzanis, K.K. Neurocognitive deficit in schizophrenia: A quantitative review of the evidence. *Neuropsychology* **1998**, *12*, 426–445. [CrossRef] [PubMed]
5. Barch, D.M.; Ceaser, A. Cognition in schizophrenia: Core psychological and neural mechanisms. *Trends Cogn. Sci.* **2012**, *16*, 27–34. [CrossRef]
6. Kimoto, S.; Makinodan, M.; Kishimoto, T. Neurobiology and treatment of social cognition in schizophrenia: Bridging the bed-bench gap. *Neurobiol. Dis.* **2019**, *131*, 104315. [CrossRef] [PubMed]
7. Rund, B.R. A review of longitudinal studies of cognitive functions in schizophrenia patients. *Schizophr. Bull.* **1998**, *24*, 425–435. [CrossRef]
8. Tregellas, J.R.; Smucny, J.; Harris, J.G.; Olincy, A.; Maharajh, K.; Kronberg, E.; Eichman, L.C.; Lyons, E.; Freedman, R. Intrinsic hippocampal activity as a biomarker for cognition and symptoms in schizophrenia. *Am. J. Psychiatry* **2014**, *171*, 549–556. [CrossRef]
9. Gaebler, A.J.; Mathiak, K.; Koten, J.W., Jr.; Konig, A.A.; Koush, Y.; Weyer, D.; Depner, C.; Matentzoglu, S.; Edgar, J.C.; Willmes, K.; et al. Auditory mismatch impairments are characterized by core neural dysfunctions in schizophrenia. *Brain* **2015**, *138*, 1410–1423. [CrossRef]
10. Gaebler, A.J.; Zweerings, J.; Koten, J.W.; Konig, A.A.; Turetsky, B.I.; Zvyagintsev, M.; Mathiak, K. Impaired Subcortical Detection of Auditory Changes in Schizophrenia but Not in Major Depression. *Schizophr. Bull.* **2020**, *46*, 193–201. [CrossRef]
11. Javitt, D.C. When doors of perception close: Bottom-up models of disrupted cognition in schizophrenia. *Annu. Rev. Clin. Psychol.* **2009**, *5*, 249–275. [CrossRef] [PubMed]
12. Javitt, D.C.; Sweet, R.A. Auditory dysfunction in schizophrenia: Integrating clinical and basic features. *Nat. Rev. Neurosci.* **2015**, *16*, 535–550. [CrossRef] [PubMed]
13. Nyatega, C.O.; Qiang, L.; Adamu, M.J.; Younis, A.; Kawuwa, H.B. Altered Dynamic Functional Connectivity of Cuneus in Schizophrenia Patients: A Resting-State fMRI Study. *Appl. Sci.* **2021**, *11*, 11392. [CrossRef]
14. Shafee, R.; Nanda, P.; Padmanabhan, J.L.; Tandon, N.; Alliey-Rodriguez, N.; Kalapurakkel, S.; Weiner, D.J.; Gur, R.E.; Keefe, R.S.E.; Hill, S.K.; et al. Polygenic risk for schizophrenia and measured domains of cognition in individuals with psychosis and controls. *Transl. Psychiatry* **2018**, *8*, 78. [CrossRef] [PubMed]
15. Tripathi, A.; Kar, S.K.; Shukla, R. Cognitive Deficits in Schizophrenia: Understanding the Biological Correlates and Remediation Strategies. *Clin. Psychopharmacol. Neurosci. Off. Sci. J. Korean Coll. Neuropsychopharmacol.* **2018**, *16*, 7–17. [CrossRef] [PubMed]
16. Georgiou, R.; Lamnisos, D.; Giannakou, K. Anticholinergic Burden and Cognitive Performance in Patients With Schizophrenia: A Systematic Literature Review. *Front. Psychiatry* **2021**, *12*, 779607. [CrossRef]
17. Belvederi Murri, M.; Respino, M.; Masotti, M.; Innamorati, M.; Mondelli, V.; Pariante, C.; Amore, M. Vitamin D and psychosis: Mini meta-analysis. *Schizophr. Res.* **2013**, *150*, 235–239. [CrossRef]
18. Fan, X.; Wang, J.; Song, M.; Giovannucci, E.L.; Ma, H.; Jin, G.; Hu, Z.; Shen, H.; Hang, D. Vitamin D status and risk of all-cause and cause-specific mortality in a large cohort: Results from the UK Biobank. *J. Clin. Endocrinol. Metab.* **2020**, *105*, e3606–e3619. [CrossRef]
19. Bruins, J.; Jörg, F.; van den Heuvel, E.R.; Bartels-Velthuis, A.A.; Corpeleijn, E.; Muskiet, F.A.J.; Pijnenborg, G.H.M.; Bruggeman, R. The relation of vitamin D, metabolic risk and negative symptom severity in people with psychotic disorders. *Schizophr. Res.* **2018**, *195*, 513–518. [CrossRef]
20. Yee, J.Y.; See, Y.M.; Abdul Rashid, N.A.; Neelamekam, S.; Lee, J. Association between serum levels of bioavailable vitamin D and negative symptoms in first-episode psychosis. *Psychiatry Res.* **2016**, *243*, 390–394. [CrossRef]

21. Cieslak, K.; Feingold, J.; Antonius, D.; Walsh-Messinger, J.; Dracxler, R.; Rosedale, M.; Aujero, N.; Keefe, D.; Goetz, D.; Goetz, R.; et al. Low vitamin D levels predict clinical features of schizophrenia. *Schizophr. Res.* **2014**, *159*, 543–545. [CrossRef] [PubMed]
22. McGrath, J.J.; Eyles, D.W.; Pedersen, C.B.; Anderson, C.; Ko, P.; Burne, T.H.; Norgaard-Pedersen, B.; Hougaard, D.M.; Mortensen, P.B. Neonatal vitamin D status and risk of schizophrenia: A population-based case-control study. *Arch. Gen. Psychiatry* **2010**, *67*, 889–894. [CrossRef] [PubMed]
23. Eyles, D.W.; Trzaskowski, M.; Vinkhuyzen, A.A.E.; Mattheisen, M.; Meier, S.; Gooch, H.; Anggono, V.; Cui, X.; Tan, M.C.; Burne, T.H.J.; et al. The association between neonatal vitamin D status and risk of schizophrenia. *Sci. Rep.* **2018**, *8*, 17692. [CrossRef] [PubMed]
24. Cui, X.; McGrath, J.J.; Burne, T.H.J.; Eyles, D.W. Vitamin D and schizophrenia: 20 years on. *Mol. Psychiatry* **2021**, *26*, 2708–2720. [CrossRef]
25. Groves, N.J.; Kesby, J.P.; Eyles, D.W.; McGrath, J.J.; Mackay-Sim, A.; Burne, T.H. Adult vitamin D deficiency leads to behavioural and brain neurochemical alterations in C57BL/6J and BALB/c mice. *Behav. Brain Res.* **2013**, *241*, 120–131. [CrossRef]
26. Kasatkina, L.A.; Tarasenko, A.S.; Krupko, O.O.; Kuchmerovska, T.M.; Lisakovska, O.O.; Trikash, I.O. Vitamin D deficiency induces the excitation/inhibition brain imbalance and the proinflammatory shift. *Int. J. Biochem. Cell Biol.* **2020**, *119*, 105665. [CrossRef]
27. Byrne, J.H.; Voogt, M.; Turner, K.M.; Eyles, D.W.; McGrath, J.J.; Burne, T.H. The impact of adult vitamin D deficiency on behaviour and brain function in male Sprague-Dawley rats. *PLoS ONE* **2013**, *8*, e71593. [CrossRef]
28. Taghizadeh, M.; Talaei, S.A.; Salami, M. Vitamin D deficiency impairs spatial learning in adult rats. *Iran. Biomed. J.* **2013**, *17*, 42–48. [CrossRef]
29. Roy, N.M.; Al-Harthi, L.; Sampat, N.; Al-Mujaini, R.; Mahadevan, S.; Al Adawi, S.; Essa, M.M.; Al Subhi, L.; Al-Balushi, B.; Qoronfleh, M.W. Impact of vitamin D on neurocognitive function in dementia, depression, schizophrenia and ADHD. *Front. Biosci.* **2021**, *26*, 566–611. [CrossRef]
30. Gaebler, A.J.; Finner-Prével, M.; Lammertz, S.; Schaffrath, S.; Eisner, P.; Stöhr, F.; Röcher, E.; Winkler, L.; Kaleta, P.; Lenzen, L.; et al. The negative impact of vitamin D on antipsychotic drug exposure may counteract its potential benefits in schizophrenia. *Br. J. Clin. Pharmacol.* **2022**. [CrossRef]
31. Wang, Z.; Schuetz, E.G.; Xu, Y.; Thummel, K.E. Interplay between vitamin D and the drug metabolizing enzyme CYP3A4. *J. Steroid Biochem. Mol. Biol.* **2013**, *136*, 54–58. [CrossRef] [PubMed]
32. Lindh, J.D.; Andersson, M.L.; Eliasson, E.; Björkhem-Bergman, L. Seasonal variation in blood drug concentrations and a potential relationship to vitamin D. *Drug Metab. Dispos. Biol. Fate Chem.* **2011**, *39*, 933–937. [CrossRef] [PubMed]
33. Schwartz, J.B. Effects of vitamin D supplementation in atorvastatin-treated patients: A new drug interaction with an unexpected consequence. *Clin. Pharmacol. Ther.* **2009**, *85*, 198–203. [CrossRef] [PubMed]
34. Keefe, R.S.; Goldberg, T.E.; Harvey, P.D.; Gold, J.M.; Poe, M.P.; Coughenour, L. The Brief Assessment of Cognition in Schizophrenia: Reliability, sensitivity, and comparison with a standard neurocognitive battery. *Schizophr. Res.* **2004**, *68*, 283–297. [CrossRef]
35. Arbuthnott, K.; Frank, J. Trail making test, part B as a measure of executive control: Validation using a set-switching paradigm. *J. Clin. Exp. Neuropsychol.* **2000**, *22*, 518–528. [CrossRef]
36. Corrigan, J.D.; Hinkeldey, N.S. Relationships between parts A and B of the Trail Making Test. *J. Clin. Psychol.* **1987**, *43*, 402–409. [CrossRef]
37. Hiemke, C.; Bergemann, N.; Clement, H.W.; Conca, A.; Deckert, J.; Domschke, K.; Eckermann, G.; Egberts, K.; Gerlach, M.; Greiner, C.; et al. Consensus Guidelines for Therapeutic Drug Monitoring in Neuropsychopharmacology: Update 2017. *Pharmacopsychiatry* **2018**, *51*, e1. [CrossRef]
38. Saar, E.; Beyer, J.; Gerostamoulos, D.; Drummer, O.H. The analysis of antipsychotic drugs in human matrices using LC-MS(/MS). *Drug Test. Anal.* **2012**, *4*, 376–394. [CrossRef]
39. Arneson, W.L.; Arneson, D.L. Current Methods for Routine Clinical Laboratory Testing of Vitamin D Levels. *Lab. Med.* **2013**, *44*, e38–e42. [CrossRef]
40. Administration UFaD. Drug Development and Drug Interactions: Table of Substrates, Inhibitors and Inducers. 2020. Available online: https://www.fda.gov/drugs/drug-interactions-labeling/drug-development-and-drug-interactions-table-substrates-inhibitors-and-inducers (accessed on 10 January 2022).
41. Besnard, J.; Ruda, G.F.; Setola, V.; Abecassis, K.; Rodriguiz, R.M.; Huang, X.-P.; Norval, S.; Sassano, M.F.; Shin, A.I.; Webster, L.A.; et al. Automated design of ligands to polypharmacological profiles. *Nature* **2012**, *492*, 215–220. [CrossRef]
42. Ban, T.A. Fifty years chlorpromazine: A historical perspective. *Neuropsychiatr. Dis. Treat.* **2007**, *3*, 495–500. [PubMed]
43. Davis, J.M. Dose equivalence of the antipsychotic drugs. In *Catecholamines and Schizophrenia*; Elsevier: Amsterdam, The Netherlands, 1975; pp. 65–73.
44. Wishart, D.S.; Knox, C.; Guo, A.C.; Shrivastava, S.; Hassanali, M.; Stothard, P.; Chang, Z.; Woolsey, J. DrugBank: A comprehensive resource for in silico drug discovery and exploration. *Nucleic Acids Res.* **2006**, *34*, D668–D672. [CrossRef] [PubMed]
45. Wallwork, R.S.; Fortgang, R.; Hashimoto, R.; Weinberger, D.R.; Dickinson, D. Searching for a consensus five-factor model of the Positive and Negative Syndrome Scale for schizophrenia. *Schizophr. Res.* **2012**, *137*, 246–250. [CrossRef] [PubMed]
46. Guan, H.Y.; Zhao, J.M.; Wang, K.Q.; Su, X.R.; Pan, Y.F.; Guo, J.M.; Jiang, L.; Wang, Y.H.; Liu, H.Y.; Sun, S.G.; et al. High-frequency neuronavigated rTMS effect on clinical symptoms and cognitive dysfunction: A pilot double-blind, randomized controlled study in Veterans with schizophrenia. *Transl. Psychiatry* **2020**, *10*, 79. [CrossRef] [PubMed]

47. Dickinson, D.; Ramsey, M.E.; Gold, J.M. Overlooking the obvious: A meta-analytic comparison of digit symbol coding tasks and other cognitive measures in schizophrenia. *Arch. Gen. Psychiatry* **2007**, *64*, 532–542. [CrossRef] [PubMed]
48. Leeson, V.C.; Barnes, T.R.; Harrison, M.; Matheson, E.; Harrison, I.; Mutsatsa, S.H.; Ron, M.A.; Joyce, E.M. The relationship between IQ, memory, executive function, and processing speed in recent-onset psychosis: 1-year stability and clinical outcome. *Schizophr. Bull.* **2010**, *36*, 400–409. [CrossRef] [PubMed]
49. Graham, K.A.; Keefe, R.S.; Lieberman, J.A.; Calikoglu, A.S.; Lansing, K.M.; Perkins, D.O. Relationship of low vitamin D status with positive, negative and cognitive symptom domains in people with first-episode schizophrenia. *Early Interv. Psychiatry* **2015**, *9*, 397–405. [CrossRef]
50. Nerhus, M.; Berg, A.O.; Simonsen, C.; Haram, M.; Haatveit, B.; Dahl, S.R.; Gurholt, T.P.; Bjella, T.D.; Ueland, T.; Andreassen, O.A.; et al. Vitamin D Deficiency Associated With Cognitive Functioning in Psychotic Disorders. *J. Clin. Psychiatry* **2017**, *78*, e750–e757. [CrossRef]
51. Krivoy, A.; Onn, R.; Vilner, Y.; Hochman, E.; Weizman, S.; Paz, A.; Hess, S.; Sagy, R.; Kimhi-Nesher, S.; Kalter, E.; et al. Vitamin D Supplementation in Chronic Schizophrenia Patients Treated with Clozapine: A Randomized, Double-Blind, Placebo-controlled Clinical Trial. *EBioMedicine* **2017**, *26*, 138–145. [CrossRef]
52. Julayanont, P.; Tangwongchai, S.; Hemrungrojn, S.; Tunvirachaisakul, C.; Phanthumchinda, K.; Hongsawat, J.; Suwichanarakul, P.; Thanasirorat, S.; Nasreddine, Z.S. The Montreal Cognitive Assessment-Basic: A Screening Tool for Mild Cognitive Impairment in Illiterate and Low-Educated Elderly Adults. *J. Am. Geriatr. Soc.* **2015**, *63*, 2550–2554. [CrossRef]
53. Gurholt, T.P.; Nerhus, M.; Osnes, K.; Berg, A.O.; Andreassen, O.A.; Melle, I.; Agartz, I. Hippocampus volume reduction in psychosis spectrum could be ameliorated by vitamin D. *Schizophr. Res.* **2018**, *199*, 433–435. [CrossRef] [PubMed]
54. Drocourt, L.; Ourlin, J.C.; Pascussi, J.M.; Maurel, P.; Vilarem, M.J. Expression of CYP3A4, CYP2B6, and CYP2C9 is regulated by the vitamin D receptor pathway in primary human hepatocytes. *J. Biol. Chem.* **2002**, *277*, 25125–25132. [CrossRef] [PubMed]
55. Schmiedlin-Ren, P.; Thummel, K.E.; Fisher, J.M.; Paine, M.F.; Lown, K.S.; Watkins, P.B. Expression of enzymatically active CYP3A4 by Caco-2 cells grown on extracellular matrix-coated permeable supports in the presence of 1alpha,25-dihydroxyvitamin D3. *Mol. Pharmacol.* **1997**, *51*, 741–754. [CrossRef] [PubMed]
56. Thummel, K.E.; Brimer, C.; Yasuda, K.; Thottassery, J.; Senn, T.; Lin, Y.; Ishizuka, H.; Kharasch, E.; Schuetz, J.; Schuetz, E. Transcriptional control of intestinal cytochrome P-4503A by 1alpha,25-dihydroxy vitamin D3. *Mol. Pharmacol.* **2001**, *60*, 1399–1406. [CrossRef]
57. Thirumaran, R.K.; Lamba, J.K.; Kim, R.B.; Urquhart, B.L.; Gregor, J.C.; Chande, N.; Fan, Y.; Qi, A.; Cheng, C.; Thummel, K.E.; et al. Intestinal CYP3A4 and midazolam disposition in vivo associate with VDR polymorphisms and show seasonal variation. *Biochem. Pharmacol.* **2012**, *84*, 104–112. [CrossRef]
58. Chow, E.C.; Durk, M.R.; Cummins, C.L.; Pang, K.S. 1Alpha,25-dihydroxyvitamin D3 up-regulates P-glycoprotein via the vitamin D receptor and not farnesoid X receptor in both fxr(-/-) and fxr(+/+) mice and increased renal and brain efflux of digoxin in mice in vivo. *J. Pharmacol. Exp. Ther.* **2011**, *337*, 846–859. [CrossRef]
59. Latimer, C.S.; Brewer, L.D.; Searcy, J.L.; Chen, K.-C.; Popović, J.; Kraner, S.D.; Thibault, O.; Blalock, E.M.; Landfield, P.W.; Porter, N.M. Vitamin D prevents cognitive decline and enhances hippocampal synaptic function in aging rats. *Proc. Natl. Acad. Sci. USA* **2014**, *111*, E4359–E4366. [CrossRef]
60. Becker, A.; Eyles, D.W.; McGrath, J.J.; Grecksch, G. Transient prenatal vitamin D deficiency is associated with subtle alterations in learning and memory functions in adult rats. *Behav. Brain Res.* **2005**, *161*, 306–312. [CrossRef]
61. Ribeiro-Santos, A.; Lucio Teixeira, A.; Salgado, J.V. Evidence for an immune role on cognition in schizophrenia: A systematic review. *Curr. Neuropharmacol.* **2014**, *12*, 273–280. [CrossRef]
62. Tanaka, M.; Tóth, F.; Polyák, H.; Szabó, Á.; Mándi, Y.; Vécsei, L. Immune Influencers in Action: Metabolites and Enzymes of the Tryptophan-Kynurenine Metabolic Pathway. *Biomedicines* **2021**, *9*, 734. [CrossRef]
63. Tanaka, M.; Vécsei, L. Editorial of Special Issue "Crosstalk between Depression, Anxiety, and Dementia: Comorbidity in Behavioral Neurology and Neuropsychiatry". *Biomedicines* **2021**, *9*, 517. [CrossRef] [PubMed]
64. North, H.F.; Bruggemann, J.; Cropley, V.; Swaminathan, V.; Sundram, S.; Lenroot, R.; Pereira, A.M.; Zalesky, A.; Bousman, C.; Pantelis, C.; et al. Increased peripheral inflammation in schizophrenia is associated with worse cognitive performance and related cortical thickness reductions. *Eur. Arch Psychiatry Clin. Neurosci.* **2021**, *271*, 595–607. [CrossRef] [PubMed]
65. Yin, K.; Agrawal, D.K. Vitamin D and inflammatory diseases. *J. Inflamm. Res.* **2014**, *7*, 69–87. [CrossRef]
66. Avan, R.; Sahebnasagh, A.; Hashemi, J.; Monajati, M.; Faramarzi, F.; Henney, N.C.; Montecucco, F.; Jamialahmadi, T.; Sahebkar, A. Update on Statin Treatment in Patients with Neuropsychiatric Disorders. *Life* **2021**, *11*, 1365. [CrossRef] [PubMed]
67. Wonodi, I.; Schwarcz, R. Cortical kynurenine pathway metabolism: A novel target for cognitive enhancement in Schizophrenia. *Schizophr. Bull.* **2010**, *36*, 211–218. [CrossRef] [PubMed]
68. Koola, M.M. Kynurenine pathway and cognitive impairments in schizophrenia: Pharmacogenetics of galantamine and memantine. *Schizophr. Res. Cogn.* **2016**, *4*, 4–9. [CrossRef] [PubMed]
69. Ulivieri, M.; Wierońska, J.M.; Lionetto, L.; Martinello, K.; Cieslik, P.; Chocyk, A.; Curto, M.; Di Menna, L.; Iacovelli, L.; Traficante, A.; et al. The Trace Kynurenine, Cinnabarinic Acid, Displays Potent Antipsychotic-Like Activity in Mice and Its Levels Are Reduced in the Prefrontal Cortex of Individuals Affected by Schizophrenia. *Schizophr. Bull.* **2020**, *46*, 1471–1481. [CrossRef]
70. Correia, B.S.B.; Nani, J.V.; Waladares Ricardo, R.; Stanisic, D.; Costa, T.B.B.C.; Hayashi, M.A.F.; Tasic, L. Effects of Psychostimulants and Antipsychotics on Serum Lipids in an Animal Model for Schizophrenia. *Biomedicines* **2021**, *9*, 235. [CrossRef]

71. Rog, J.; Błażewicz, A.; Juchnowicz, D.; Ludwiczuk, A.; Stelmach, E.; Kozioł, M.; Karakula, M.; Niziński, P.; Karakula-Juchnowicz, H. The Role of GPR120 Receptor in Essential Fatty Acids Metabolism in Schizophrenia. *Biomedicines* **2020**, *8*, 243. [CrossRef]
72. Komatsu, H.; Watanabe, E.; Fukuchi, M. Psychiatric Neural Networks and Precision Therapeutics by Machine Learning. *Biomedicines* **2021**, *9*, 403. [CrossRef]
73. Kraus, M.S.; Keefe, R.S.E. Cognition as an outcome measure in schizophrenia. *Br. J. Psychiatry* **2007**, *191*, s46–s51. [CrossRef] [PubMed]
74. US. Army. Army Individual Test Battery. In *Manual of Directions and Scoring*; War Department, Adjunct General's Office: Washington, DC, USA, 1944.
75. Tombaugh, T.N. Trail Making Test A and B: Normative data stratified by age and education. *Arch. Clin. Neuropsychol.* **2004**, *19*, 203–214. [CrossRef]
76. Laere, E.; Tee, S.F.; Tang, P.Y. Assessment of Cognition in Schizophrenia Using Trail Making Test: A Meta-Analysis. *Psychiatry Investig.* **2018**, *15*, 945–955. [CrossRef] [PubMed]
77. Nuechterlein, K.H.; Green, M.F. *MATRICS Consensus Cognitive Battery Manual*; MATRICS Assessment Inc.: Los Angeles, CA, USA, 2006.
78. Morello, M.; Landel, V.; Lacassagne, E.; Baranger, K.; Annweiler, C.; Féron, F.; Millet, P. Vitamin D Improves Neurogenesis and Cognition in a Mouse Model of Alzheimer's Disease. *Mol. Neurobiol.* **2018**, *55*, 6463–6479. [CrossRef] [PubMed]
79. Turner, K.M.; Young, J.W.; McGrath, J.J.; Eyles, D.W.; Burne, T.H.J. Cognitive performance and response inhibition in developmentally vitamin D (DVD)-deficient rats. *Behav. Brain Res.* **2013**, *242*, 47–53. [CrossRef] [PubMed]
80. Salazar de Pablo, G.; Woods, S.W.; Drymonitou, G.; de Diego, H.; Fusar-Poli, P. Prevalence of Individuals at Clinical High-Risk of Psychosis in the General Population and Clinical Samples: Systematic Review and Meta-Analysis. *Brain Sci.* **2021**, *11*, 1544. [CrossRef]

biomedicines

MDPI

Article

Impact of Behavioral Assessment and Re-Test as Functional Trainings That Modify Survival, Anxiety and Functional Profile (Physical Endurance and Motor Learning) of Old Male and Female 3xTg-AD Mice and NTg Mice with Normal Aging

Lidia Castillo-Mariqueo [1,2] and Lydia Giménez-Llort [1,2,*]

1 Institut de Neurociències, Universitat Autònoma de Barcelona, 08193 Barcelona, Spain; lidia.castillom@autonoma.cat
2 Department of Psychiatry and Forensic Medicine, School of Medicine, Universitat Autònoma de Barcelona, 08193 Barcelona, Spain
* Correspondence: lidia.gimenez@uab.cat

Abstract: Longitudinal approaches for disease-monitoring in old animals face survival and frailty limitations, but also assessment and re-test bias on genotype and sex effects. The present work investigated these effects on 56 variables for behavior, functional profile, and biological status of male and female 3xTg-AD mice and NTg counterparts using two designs: (1) a longitudinal design: naïve 12-month-old mice re-tested four months later; and (2) a cross-sectional design: naïve 16-month-old mice compared to those re-tested. The results confirmed the impact as (1) improvement of survival (NTg rested females), variability of gait (3xTg-AD 16-month-old re-tested and naïve females), physical endurance (3xTg-AD re-tested females), motor learning (3xTg-AD and NTg 16-month-old re-tested females), and geotaxis (3xTg-AD naïve 16-month-old males); but (2) worse anxiety (3xTg-AD 16-month-old re-tested males), HPA axis (3xTg-AD 16-month-old re-tested and naïve females) and sarcopenia (3xTg-AD 16-month-old naïve females). Males showed more functional correlations than females. The functional profile, biological status, and their correlation are discussed as relevant elements for AD-pathology. Therefore, repetition of behavioral batteries could be considered training by itse1´, with some variables sensitive to genotype, sex, and re-test. In the AD-genotype, females achieved the best performance in physical endurance and motor learning, while males showed a deterioration in most studied variables.

Keywords: Alzheimer's disease; aging; survival; anxious profile; functional profile; motor performance; frailty; training; gait; kyphosis

Citation: Castillo-Mariqueo, L.; Giménez-Llort, L. Impact of Behavioral Assessment and Re-Test as Functional Trainings That Modify Survival, Anxiety and Functional Profile (Physical Endurance and Motor Learning) of Old Male and Female 3xTg-AD Mice and NTg Mice with Normal Aging. *Biomedicines* **2022**, *10*, 973. https://doi.org/10.3390/biomedicines10050973

Academic Editors: Masaru Tanaka and Nóra Török

Received: 14 February 2022
Accepted: 11 April 2022
Published: 22 April 2022

1. Introduction

Specific motor skills impaired in old age include a broad and varied spectrum that involves a reduction in gait speed, loss of strength and muscle mass, and decline of balance [1–3]. However, aging has become increasingly recognized as a potentially modifiable risk factor for chronic disease and frailty [4,5]. The deterioration of motor performance related to cognitive dysfunction in Alzheimer's disease (AD) has recently gained importance in clinical research [6–9]. Particularly, gait impairment and its association with cognitive impairment [10] could shed light on potentialities to distinguish AD [1]. Inclusive, higher levels of Aβ and tau are associated with more significant memory decline, but not with changes in executive function [11]. The study by Sperling points out that these results could explain why some clinically active patients presented elevated tau and Aβ levels [11]. Thus, Aβ and tau proteins can serve as markers of cognitive impairment; however, they are insufficient and cannot detect all cases of dementia, especially in the early stages [11,12]. For this part, gait speed, for example, is longitudinally associated with cognitive decline, dementia, and falls in older adults [13,14], with slower gait associated with increased fall risk and poor baseline cognition [6]. However, motor dysfunctions and deterioration remain poorly explored. Consequently, functional and cognitive decline comorbidity is a warning sign for increased disability [8], a growing public health problem [15], and it is already present at preclinical stages of Alzheimer's disease [5].

On the other hand, aging is a frequent risk factor for different diseases, including dementia [16]. Recently, in a review of the literature that examined the pathophysiological basis and biomarkers of AD and other neurodegenerative diseases, it was pointed out that the predisposing factors for neuroinflammation are aging, metabolic diseases, hypertension, cerebrovascular accidents, depression and depression, dementia, among others [17]. In addition, healthy aging would be associated with chronic inflammation, contributing to a greater vulnerability to anxiety and depression [17]. Thus, cause–effect relationships can become bidirectional in the pathogenesis of multifactorial diseases, leading to a disease-prone state [18]. Age-related deficits in the ability to process contextual information and regulate responses to threat, addressing that structural and physiological alterations in the prefrontal cortex and medial temporal lobe determine cognitive changes in advanced aging, which may eventually cause patterns of cognitive dysfunction seen in patients with AD and mild cognitive impairment (MCI) [19].

Furthermore, it is known that AD is characterized by high heterogeneity in the disease's manifestation, progression, and risk factors [20]. Such a high phenotypic variability is considered one of the most significant obstacles in early diagnosis and clinical trial design [20]. Therefore, there is great interest in identifying factors driving variability used for patient stratification [20,21]. Additionally, the impact of sex on the disease varies throughout its progression [22,23]. It is important to identify the role of sex differences in the cognitive dimension if potentially more precise diagnoses and treatments should emerge [24,25], but few studies have reported differences in the psychomotor functional dimension of the disease.

In the last decade, at the translational level, the impact of interventions on age-related disability, frailty, and the onset of AD has been investigated in animal models to develop clinically relevant measures that provide indications for the approach and management of disability, frailty, and illness [26,27]. In addition, genotype and sex differences in cognitive, emotional, and locomotor performance have been studied at the preclinical level to assess the effects of promising interventions before their application in clinical settings [28–30].

Recently, our laboratory has developed a study method to identify psychomotor impairments and deficits at different stages of Alzheimer's disease [31]. Previously, we reported a functional impairment phenotype in male mice's gait and physical performance of the 3xTg-AD transgenic model in the initial, intermediate, and advanced stages of the disease. The results showed that 3xTg-AD mice show a significant functional impairment in the quantitative variables of gait and exploratory activity, movement limitations, and muscle weakness related to functional decline in the different stages of severity of the disease intensify with increasing age. In addition, signs of frailty accompany functional deterioration, and sarcopenia is evident in an advanced stage of AD, with differences in the morphological characteristics of muscle fibers and the number of fat cells [31].

Furthermore, we differentiate the disorders and postural patterns into two types of kyphosis (postural and structural) that differ in severity and limit the exploratory activity. In addition, the results indicated that the presence of bizarre gait patterns accounts for behavior similar to anxiety when 3xTg-AD mice face novelty situations and recognition of places, with circling and backward movements being the most frequent, in an already frailty setting [32,33].

The present study was designed to investigate the impact of two factors, sex, and repeated test, assessing the behavioral outputs of 3xTg-AD mice and mice with normal aging in longitudinal and transversal experimental designs. According to our previous work, a battery of psychomotor tests: gait, exploration, muscle strength, motor learning, physical endurance, and frailty status, was used [31]. In addition, phenotype of frailty and biological status (HPA axis and sarcopenia index) was also included [32,33]. Thus, in the first place, we studied the sex factor by characterizing the psychomotor phenotype of middle—(12 months) and old—(16 months) age females, that in the 3xTg-AD mice corresponds to two neuropathological stages of the disease [31], as compared to that of aged-matched males. On the other hand, long-term studies provide better insights for assessing interventions with preclinical validity, but the administration of behavioral batteries is not exempt from carryover effects. In addition, behavioral batteries and repeated tests can be considered behavioral stimulation [34]. Therefore, we aimed to investigate the effects of repeated tests on the behavioral performance of animals assessed in two scenarios: 1) in a longitudinal design, with within-subjects analysis of a set of 12-month-old animals re-tested four months later, at 16 months of age; and 2) in a transversal design, when comparing 16-month-old animals that had (re-tested) or not (naïve) that experienced the battery of tests.

2. Materials and Methods

2.1. Animals

A total of 191 male and female mice were included for the survival analysis, and ninety-six of them, homozygous 3xTg-AD (n = 54) and non-transgenic (NTg, n = 42) male and female mice of 12 to 16 months of age in a C57BL/6J background (after embryo transfer and backcrossing of at least ten generations), established at the Universitat Autònoma de Barcelona, were included in the experimental study. As previously described, the 3xTg-AD mice harboring transgenes were genetically created at the University of California at Irvine [35]. Animals were kept in groups of 3–4 mice per cage (Macrolon, 35 cm×35 cm×25 cm) filled with 5 cm of clean wood cuttings (Ecopure, Chips, Date Sand, UK; uniform cross-sectional wood granules with 2.8–1.0 mm chip size) and nesting materials (Kleenex, Art: 08834060, 21 cm×20 cm, White). In all cases, standard home cages covered with a metal grid to allow the perception of olfactory and auditory stimuli from the rest of the colony. All animals were kept under standard laboratory conditions of food and water ad libitum, 20 ± 2 °C, 12 h light cycle:dark with lights turned on at 8:00 a.m. and 50–60% relative humidity. The study complied with the ARRIVE guidelines developed by the NC3Rs and aimed to reduce the number of animals used [36].

2.2. Experimental Design

A longitudinal and a transversal study were carried out to evaluate the anxious-like and functional profiles of male and female 3xTg-AD and NTg mice. Biological variables (corticosterone and sarcopenia) of animals at the end point (16 months of age) were also included. For this purpose, animals were randomly assigned into two experimental batches (see Figure 1, Experimental design)

2.3. Behavioral Assessment and Biological Status

The assessment consisted of four consecutive evaluation steps conducted during 5 days, as follows: Day 1, bodyweight, phenotype scoring system, and frailty; Day 2, gait and exploration; Day 3, geotaxis, muscle strength, and rotarod; Days 4–5, rotarod. The procedures and protocol were based on the protocol used by Castillo-Mariqueo and Giménez-Llort [31]. Assessments were performed under dim white light (20 lx) in the light cycle (10:00 a.m. to 1:00 p.m.). Behavioral evaluations were carried out in a counterbalanced way by two independent observers, blind to the genotype. Animals were habituated to the test room 30 min before the start of the tests.

2.3.1. Survival, Bodyweight, Phenotype Scoring System, Frailty Score, and Kyphosis

Survival curves were analyzed considering the cohort of siblings from the same litter of mice included in the study, from birth to 16 months of age. A total of 191 male and female mice, NTg and 3xTg-AD were included in this analysis (NTg males = 49; NTg females = 58; 3xTg-AD males = 50; 3xTg-AD females = 34). All animals were weighed and evaluated with the phenotype scoring system that includes four subtests and scores: ledge, grip, gait, and kyphosis [37,38]. Individual measures were scored from 0 (the absence of the relevant phenotype) to 3 (the most severe manifestation) [37]. The measures can be analyzed individually or combined into a composite phenotype score [39,40]. On the other hand, frailty was assessed using an adaptation of the MCFI by Whitehead [41], which includes 30 assessment items from the clinical setting. The 12 elements with the highest incidence previously reported by our laboratory were selected [42]. Their incidence was reported through an absence (0), presence (1) score. The clinical evaluation included physical aspects, injuries and wounds, alopecia, piloerection, body and tail position, tremor, and urogenital alterations.

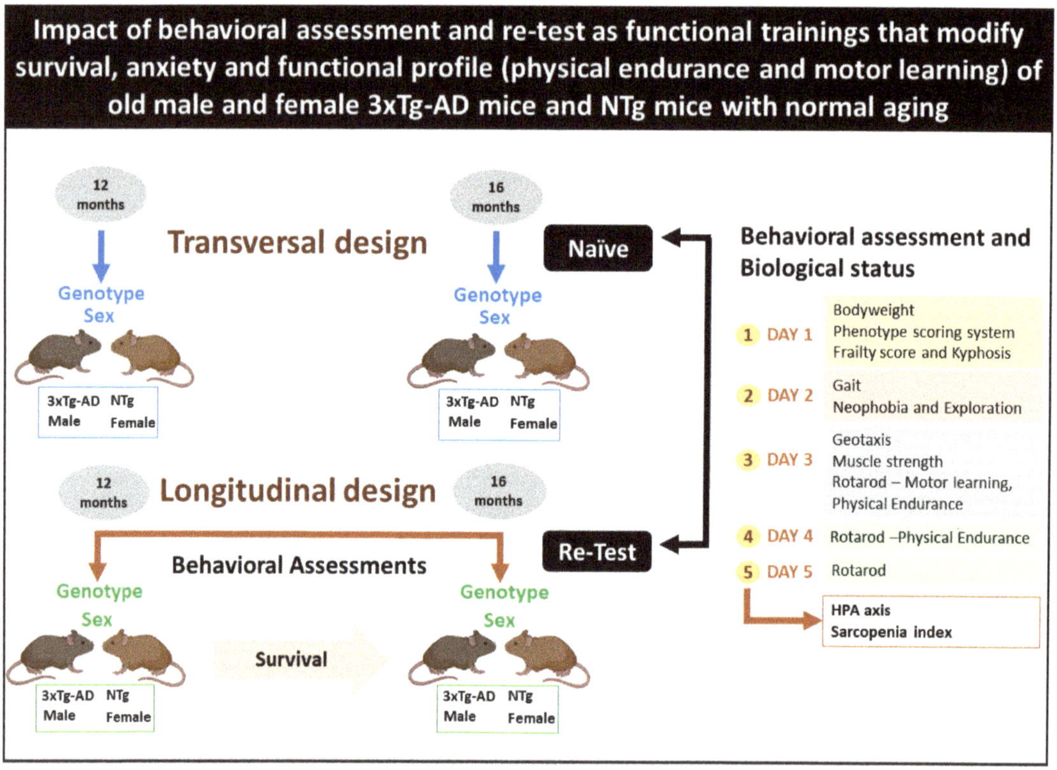

Figure 1. Experimental design. Longitudinal design: the first group was assessed in the behavioral battery at the age of 12 months and again when the animals reached 16 months of age. Transversal design: the second group was housed in standard conditions without manipulation until they were tested at 16 months of age, so they could be compared to re-tested 16 months old animals.

2.3.2. Quantitative Parameters of Gait, Neophobia, and Exploration

The quantitative parameters of the gait and exploration were recorded by filming the spontaneous gait of the mice for 1 min. Later the videos were analyzed using KINOVEA 0.8.15 free software according to the Castillo-Mariqueo and Gimenez-Llort protocol [31]. Stride length, stride length variability, speed, and cadence were included according to the methodology used by Wang et al. [43]. The examination included observation of body position, limb support, and movement. In addition, neophobia (immediate fear of a new place) was assessed by means of the corner test [44] and the recording of freezing (latency of movement), the number of explorations on the horizontal axis (visited corners), the latency and number of explorations on the vertical axis (rearings).

2.3.3. Muscular Strength—Hanger Test and Geotaxis

The muscle strength was measured in the forelimbs using the hanger test. Three trials were performed to observe the tendency of a mouse to instinctively grasp a rack or bar when suspended by the tail. In the first and second trials, grip strength was assessed by holding the animal with its front legs for 5 s at the height of 40 cm. In the third trial, the animal is suspended for 60 s in a single attempt to assess muscular endurance. This test allows discriminating grip strength and muscular endurance according to the suspension times used by mice [45]. A box with sawdust is placed under the animal to prevent a possible fall in each trial. The bar used is graduated in 5-cm blocks to obtain the distance covered when the animal moves through the bar. The latency and movement distance are recorded. Geotaxis was measured using a 10 cm × 12cm grid. A single trial registered the time it took for the animal to reach the vertical position from an inverted position at a 90° angle on the grid.

2.3.4. Motor Performance: Learning and Physical Endurance—Rotarod

Six micro training cycles were carried out during three consecutive days with a previous learning session and psychomotor coordination. The animals were trained in the Rotarod apparatus (Ugo basile®, Mouse RotaRod NG) according to a training volume established in our previous research laboratory investigations [31]. An incremental intensity of 5 to 48 rpm was applied according to individual tolerance with a maximum duration of 360 s in each microcycle with a 1-min recovery between trial.

2.3.5. Biological Status: HPA Axis and Sarcopenia Index

The animals were euthanized and the muscle tissues were necropsied. Plasma from a blood sample was obtained by centrifugation and stored and −80 °C until corticosterone analysis. Corticosterone content (ng/mL) was analyzed using a commercial kit (Corticosterone EIA Immunodiagnostic Systems Ltd., Boldon, UK). Absorbance was read at 450 nm with Varioskan LUX ESW 1.00.38 (Thermo Fisher Scientific, Massachusetts, MA, USA) [42]. The weights of the quadriceps and triceps surae muscles of the right lower extremity of each animal were recorded and kept for future analysis. The sarcopenia index [46] was applied to obtain an indirect measure of sarcopenia as a biological marker of frailty.

2.4. Statistics

Statistical analyses were performed using SPSS 15.0 software. Results were expressed as the mean ± standard error of the mean (SEM) for each task and trial. The variables recorded were analyzed with Student t-test, Chi-squared or Fisher's exact test, one-way ANOVA, and multiple regression analysis (MRA). The split-plot ANOVA design with factors genotype (G), sex (S), previous experience either as a re-test (R) in the longitudinal approach or as naïve (N) in the transversal approach, were included. Their G×S, G×R, and S×N factor interactions were also studied. *Post hoc* comparisons were run with Bonferroni corrections. Pearson's correlations were made to analyze the functional correlations with (1) corticosterone, (2) sarcopenia index, and (3) phenotype score system. The survival curve was analyzed with the Kaplan–Meier test (Log rank). In all cases, $p < 0.05$ was considered statistically significant.

3. Results

3.1. Survival, Bodyweight, Phenotype Scoring System, Frailty Score, and Kyphosis

Figure 1 shows the data obtained for survival, frailty score and postural and structural kyphosis. Thus, the animal cohort was analyzed from birth to 16 months (16 months NTg and 16 months 3xTg-AD). Only siblings from the same litter belonging to mice meeting the end-points were considered. Log rank analysis showed statistically significant differences dependent on genotype and sex (G, χ^2 (1) = 20.044, $p < 0.001$; S, χ^2 (1) = 33.531, $p < 0.001$), see Figure 2A. In this way, it was possible to observe that females of both genotypes have higher mortality than males, and that of them the NTg is even higher (days of average survival: Males, NTg = 445.05 ± 15.75, CI: 414.16–475.94; 3xTg-AD = 505.57 ± 13.04, CI: 480.01–531.13. Females, NTg = 343.60 ± 15.39, CI: 313.42–373.78; 3xTg-AD = 442.76 ± 18.40, CI: 406.69–478.83). In addition, the female NTg cohort reached 79% (46/58) of mortality and 3xTg-AD the 50% (17/34) with ages 11 to 13 months having the greatest death. For their part, NTg males reached 37% (18/49) and 3xTg-AD 24% (12/50), with 15 to 16 months being the age of greatest death. During the follow-up of the animals that started the battery at 12 months, 20 deaths were detected, the NTg males had 29% (4/14), the 3xTg-AD males a 20% (4/20), the NTg females a 35% (7/20), and 3xTg-AD females 31% (4/13), see Figure 2A.

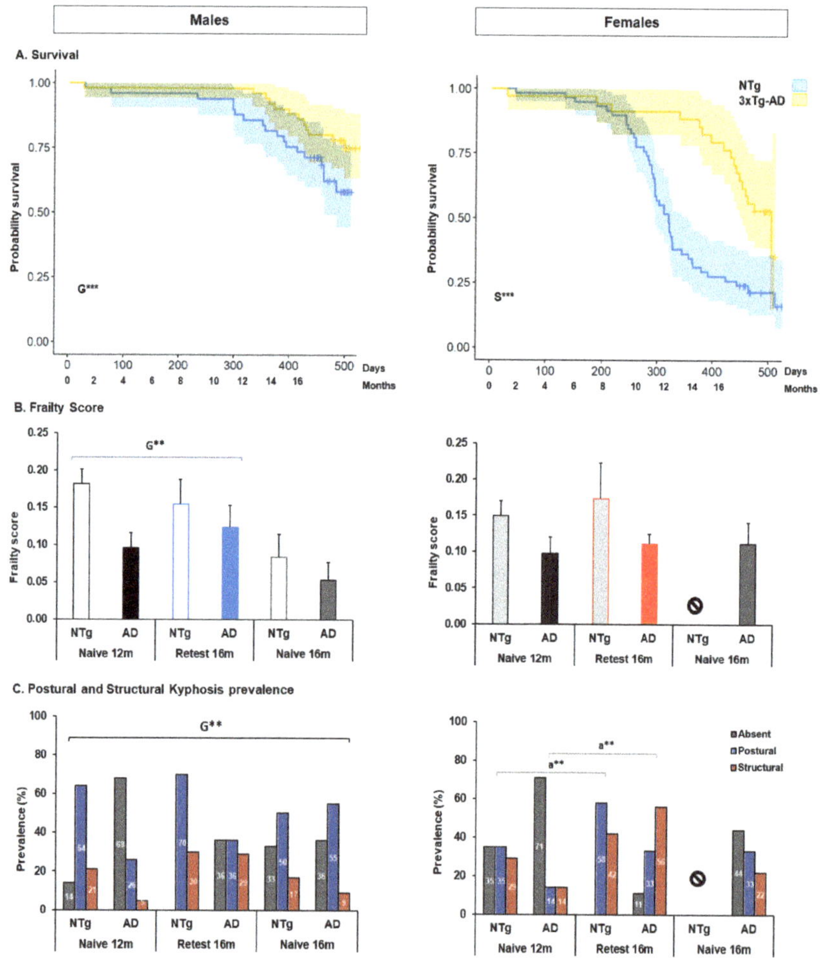

Figure 2. Survival, frailty score, and postural and structural kyphosis. (**A**) Survival. Statistics: Kaplan–Meier test—Log rank, G, genotype effect: χ^2, G*** $p < 0.001$***; S, sex effect: χ^2, S*** $p < 0.001$***. (**B**) Frailty score. Statistics: ANOVA, G, genotype effect: G** $p < 0.01$**. (**C**) Postural and structural kyphosis. Statistics: Fisher's exact test, G, genotype effect in males, G** $p < 0.01$**; a, aging effect in females: a** $p < 0.01$**. The symbol ⃠ indicates the absence of the group, and m, months.

In terms of frailty score, G effect were identified, the score is higher in NTg animals in naïve 12 months (frailty score, G, F (1, 62) = 11.159, $p = 0.001$), see Figure 2B. In addition, the severity of kyphosis has been identified, thus, in males, a higher prevalence of postural kyphosis has been observed, being higher in the case of NTg mice (severity, Fisher's exact test df (15) = 24.403, p = 0.023. G effect, Fisher's exact test df (3) = 11.842, p = 0.004). In the case of females, the highest prevalence of cases was also postural kyphosis, and this increased in 3xTg-AD mice at 16 months, being the structural type disorder in this group the one with the highest prevalence attributable to age (severity, Fisher's exact test df (12) = 22.900, p = 0.008. 3xTg-AD naïve 16 months *vs.* re-test 16 months, Fisher's exact test df (3) = 16.137, p = 0.001), see Figure 2C.

Table 1 shows the phenotype scoring system obtained in males and females. Specifically, at naïve 12 months, differences were detected in the gait, kyphosis, and total score, with G effect in kyphosis and total score showing the high deterioration in the NTg group (kyphosis, G, F (1, 62) = 13.329, p = 0.001. Total score, G, F (1, 62) = 4.078, p = 0.048). In addition, there is an interaction of the G×S in gait, with 3xTg-AD females and NTg males presenting a lower (gait score, G×S, F (1, 62) = 7.776, p = 0.007). At the 16 months re-tests, the difference in gait score is maintained without significant differences in the other parameters (gait score, G×S, F (1, 44) = 10.709, p = 0.002). In contrast to naïve 16 months, differences were observed in genotype and sex in the clasping score and gait, being measured the genotype differences only in males and sex between the 3xTg-AD group (clasping score, F (2, 30) = 4.646, p = 0.017; male 3xTg-AD naïve 16 months vs. male NTg naïve 16 months, p = 0.019. G, in male group, T student t = −2.836, p = 0.012. S, in 3xTg-AD group T student t = −2.138, p = 0.046). If we consider the change between the groups after the re-test, we have detected differences in the different scores of the phenotype scoring system. The main differences were detected in the total score, kyphosis and ledge score (re-test, total score, F (1, 141) = 15,972, p < 0.0001. Kyphosis score, F (1, 141) = 14.596, p < 0.000 and G, F (1, 141) = 5.159, p = 0.025. Ledge score, F (1, 141) = 10.435, p = 0.002). In addition, differences in total score, gait, kyphosis, and ledge score were detected between males, with effect of previous experience and genotype (total score, F (5, 80) = 3.449, K= 0.007, 3xTg-AD naïve 12 months vs. 3xTg-AD re-test 16 months, k = 0.031; R, F (1, 80) = 13.002, p = 0.001. Ledge score, R, F (1, 80) = 7.447, p = 0.008. Gait, F (5, 80) = 4.303, p = 0.002, 3xTg-AD re-test 16 months vs. 3xTg-AD naïve 16 months, p = 0.003; 3xTg-AD re-test 16 m vs. NTg naïve 16 months, p = 0.003; R, F (1, 80) = 7.461, p = 0.008; and G, F (1, 80) = 5.560, p = 0.021. Kyphosis score, F (5, 80) = 3.269, p = 0.010; R, F (1, 80) = 6.310, p = 0.014; and G, F (1, 80) = 5.225, p = 0.025). In females, differences were found in total score, kyphosis and gait with effect of previous experience and genotype (total score, F (4, 60) = 2,800, p = 0.034; R, F (1, 60) = 4.517, p = 0.038; G, F (1, 60) = 4.767, p = 0.033. Kyphosis score, F (4, 60) = 3.375, p = 0.015, 3xTg-AD naïve 12 months vs. 3xTg-AD re-test 16 months, p = 0.050; R, F (1, 60) = 7.791, p = 0.007. Gait score, F (4, 60) = 2.909, p = 0.029; G, F (1, 60) = 5.632, p = 0.021).

Table 1. Phenotype scoring system.

Phenotype Scoring System		Naïve 12-Month-Old			Re-Test 16-Month-Old			Naïve 16-Month-Old			Statistics
		Males	Females	p-Value	Males	Females	p-Value	Males	Females	p-Value	
Clasping score	NTg	0.52 ± 0.16	0.43 ± 0.08	n.s.	0.67 ± 0.20	0.69 ± 0.17	n.s.	0.25 ± 0.06	NR	g^{*}	n.s.
	AD	0.56 ± 0.17	0.62 ± 0.24		0.79 ± 0.19	0.30 ± 0.15		0.67 ± 0.18 *	0.26 ± 0.12		
Ledge score	NTg	0.40 ± 0.15	0.48 ± 0.14	n.s.	0.60 ± 0.09	0.68 ± 0.11	n.s.	0.31 ± 0.12	NR	n.s.	R^{**}
	AD	0.25 ± 0.08	0.48 ± 0.13		0.58 ± 0.16	0.51 ± 0.07		0.22 ± 0.09	0.41 ± 0.14		
Gait score	NTg	0.21 ± 0.15	0.33 ± 0.12	$G{\times}S^{**}$	0.20 ± 0.13	0.38 ± 0.15	$G{\times}S^{**}$	-	NR	$s^{\#}$	G^{*}, R^{**}, $r^{\&\&}$, $r^{\$\$}$
	AD	0.26 ± 0.10	-		$0.64 \pm 0.13^{\&\&}$	-		0.03 ± 0.03	0.44 ± 0.24		
Kyphosis score	NTg	1.07 ± 0.16	1.0 ± 0.25	G^{**}	1.30 ± 0.15	1.38 ± 0.15	n.s.	0.72 ± 0.21, $s^{\$\$}$	NR	n.s.	G^{*}, R^{***}, $r^{\&}$
	AD	0.30 ± 0.13	0.43 ± 0.20		0.95 ± 0.26	$1.37 \pm 0.27^{\&}$		0.47 ± 0.17	0.67 ± 0.28		
Total score	NTg	2.21 ± 0.37	2.24 ± 0.39	G^{*}	2.77 ± 0.37	3.14 ± 0.45	n.s.	1.28 ± 0.23	NR	n.s.	R^{***}, $r^{\&}$ G^{*}
	AD	1.37 ± 0.30	1.52 ± 0.33		$2.96 \pm 0.58^{\&}$	2.18 ± 0.32		1.39 ± 0.28	1.78 ± 0.44		

Statistics: ANOVA, G, genotype effect, G^{**} $p < 0.01$, $p < 0.05$, n.s. $p > 0.05$. R, Re-test effect, R^{***} $p < 0.001^{***}$, R^{**} $p < 0.01^{**}$, $p < 0.05^{*}$, n.s. $p > 0.05$. G×S, genotype and sex interaction effect, $G{\times}S^{**}$ $p < 0.01^{**}$, $p < 0.05^{*}$, n.s. $p > 0.05$. Bonferroni post hoc test: g, genotype, g^{*} $p < 0.05^{*}$; s, sex; \$ expressed genotype differences between sex, $s^{\$\$}$ $p < 0.01^{\$\$}$; & expressed differences between re-test groups, $r^{\&\&}$ $p < 0.01^{\&\&}$, $p < 0.05^{\&}$; \$ expressed genotype differences between re-test group, $r^{\&}$ $p < 0.05^{\&}$, and $r^{\$\$}$, between sex differences. NR indicates the absence of the group.

In bodyweight at 12 months was high in 3xTg-AD, and at 16 months it decreased in females. In addition, males naïve 16 months weighed more than re-test males at the same, see Tables S1–S3.

3.2. Quantitative Parameters of Gait, and Neophobia and Exploration

Quantitative parameters of gait are shown in Figure 3. For naïve 12 months, statistically significant differences were observed in all quantitative gait variables. Stride length showed differences in G and S, with the longest stride length in NTg males and 3xTg-AD in females. This interaction was also observed in gait speed, high in NTg mice. At the same time, the variability of gait presented differences associated with S, with females showing less than males' variability and, therefore a gait with more homogeneous steps in its trajectory. Additionally, a genotype-dependent difference was observed in cadence, where NTg mice show better performance in this variable with marked differences between males. In the re-test at 16 months, this group registered a gait performance that shows the interaction between the G×S effect in stride length and speed, with the performance of 3xTg-AD females being the one with the best performance in both variables. The re-test of this group at 16 months showed differences in cadence, increasing its performance in the group of 3xTg-AD mice of both sexes and decreasing in the NTg group, see Figure 3A–D and Tables S1–S3.

On the other hand, mice at 16 months did not show significant differences in quantitative variables of gait. Differences could only be observed between the re-test and a naïve group of males at 16 months in stride length, cadence, and speed, where the re-test NTg mice presented a high performance in speed and cadence compared to the naïve NTg mice, 3xTg-AD re-test, and naïve, but lower performance in stride length than naïve mice. In addition, differences were detected between the 3xTg-AD males and females in the variable's variability and gait speed, with the 3xTg-AD naïve and re-test females showing less variability than the 3xTg-AD males. This difference was also present in gait speed, with a better performance of re-test females followed by naïve 16 months females over 3xTg-AD males in both conditions, see Figure 3A–D and Tables S1–S3.

For its part, the neophobia and exploratory activity presented sex differences in the ratio visited corners/rearings, being higher in females of both genotypes, see Figure 4. This difference was maintained at re-test 16 months, with the higher ratio in females. In addition, the ratio in MRA of the groups showed an interaction between G×S, indicating a lower performance in 3xTg-AD re-test males at 16 months and higher in re-test females, see Figure 4B and Tables S1–S3.

As in gait, no significant differences were detected in exploratory activity between the naïve 16 months group. However, in contrast to the re-test males at 16 months, the naïve males presented high vertical activity than the re-test, see Figure 4C,D. Between the group of 3xTg-AD mice, S effect was identified in vertical activity, where naïve males presented higher activity. Movement latency was also lower in naïve males, but the same was not observed in 3xTg-AD females, see Figure 4A and Tables S1–S3.

3.3. Muscular Strength: Forelimb Grip Strength and Muscular Endurance—Hanger Test and Response to Gravity: Geotaxis

Lower muscle strength can be observed in the resistance distance in the 3xTg-AD animals at the age of 12 months, which, despite not showing statistical differences, shows a trend with less strength in the 3xTg-AD males. No statistically significant differences were detected in the rest of the variables, although a worse performance of the animals was observed, see Table S1. At 16 months re-test and 16 months naïve, no significant differences were detected.

On the other hand, significant differences in geotaxis were detected. The group of 3xTg-AD male took longer to complete the test in the re-test 16 months group in contrast to the 12 months and naïve 16 months group, see Figure 5A. Notably, at 16 months in the re-test group, an interaction was observed between the G×S of the animals, showing more significant latency in 3xTg-AD males and NTg females. G×S interaction was also observed between the group of naïve 16 months 3xTg-AD mice. In addition, there was an interaction between the G×R was detected among male mice at 16 months in contrast to naïve mice of the same age, with the test time being shorter in naïve mice, see Figure 5A and Tables S1–S3.

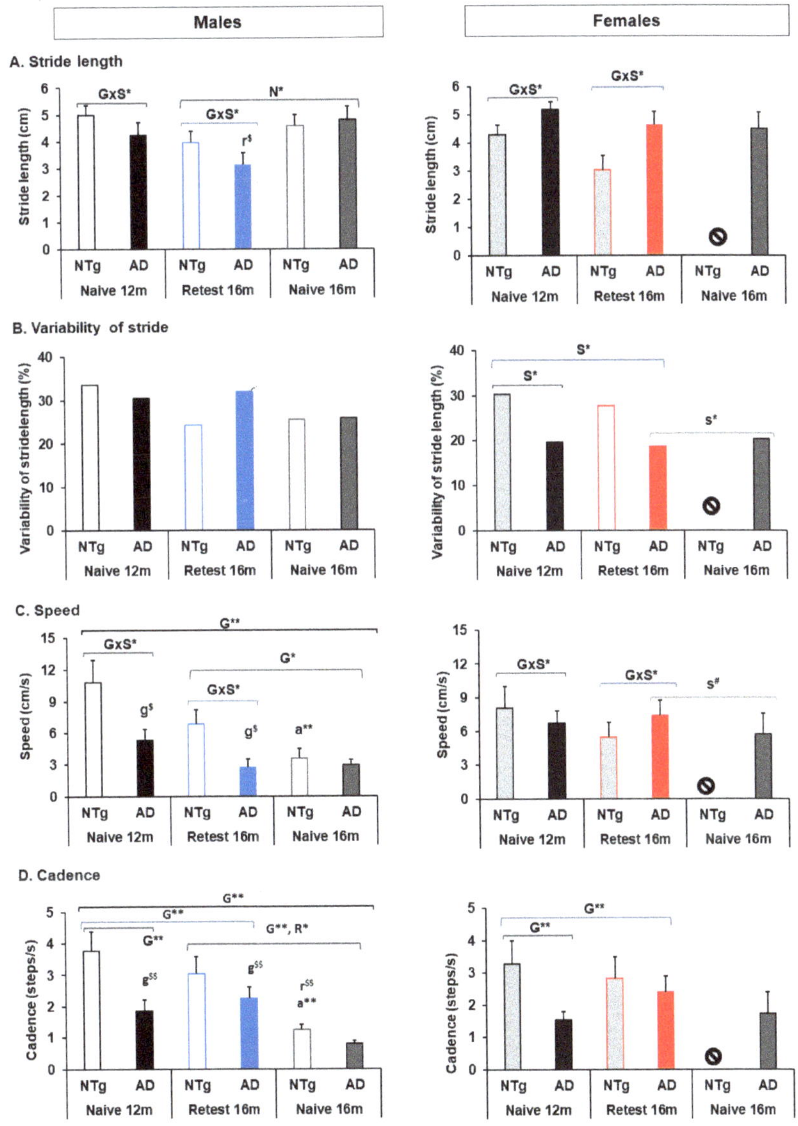

Figure 3. Quantitative parameters of gait. (**A**) Stride length, (**B**) variability of stride, (**C**) speed, (**D**) cadence. Statistics: ANOVA, G, genotype effect, G** $p < 0.01$**, G* $p < 0.05$*. S, sex effect, S* $p < 0.05$*. G×S, genotype and sex interaction effects, G×S* $p < 0.05$*. R, re-test effect, R* $p < 0.05$*. N, naïve effect, N* $p < 0.05$*. a, aging, a** $p < 0.01$**. Bonferroni *post hoc* test: g, genotype; s, sex; $ expressed genotype differences between sex, and # expressed sex differences between genotypes. The symbol ⦸ indicates the absence of the group, and m, month.

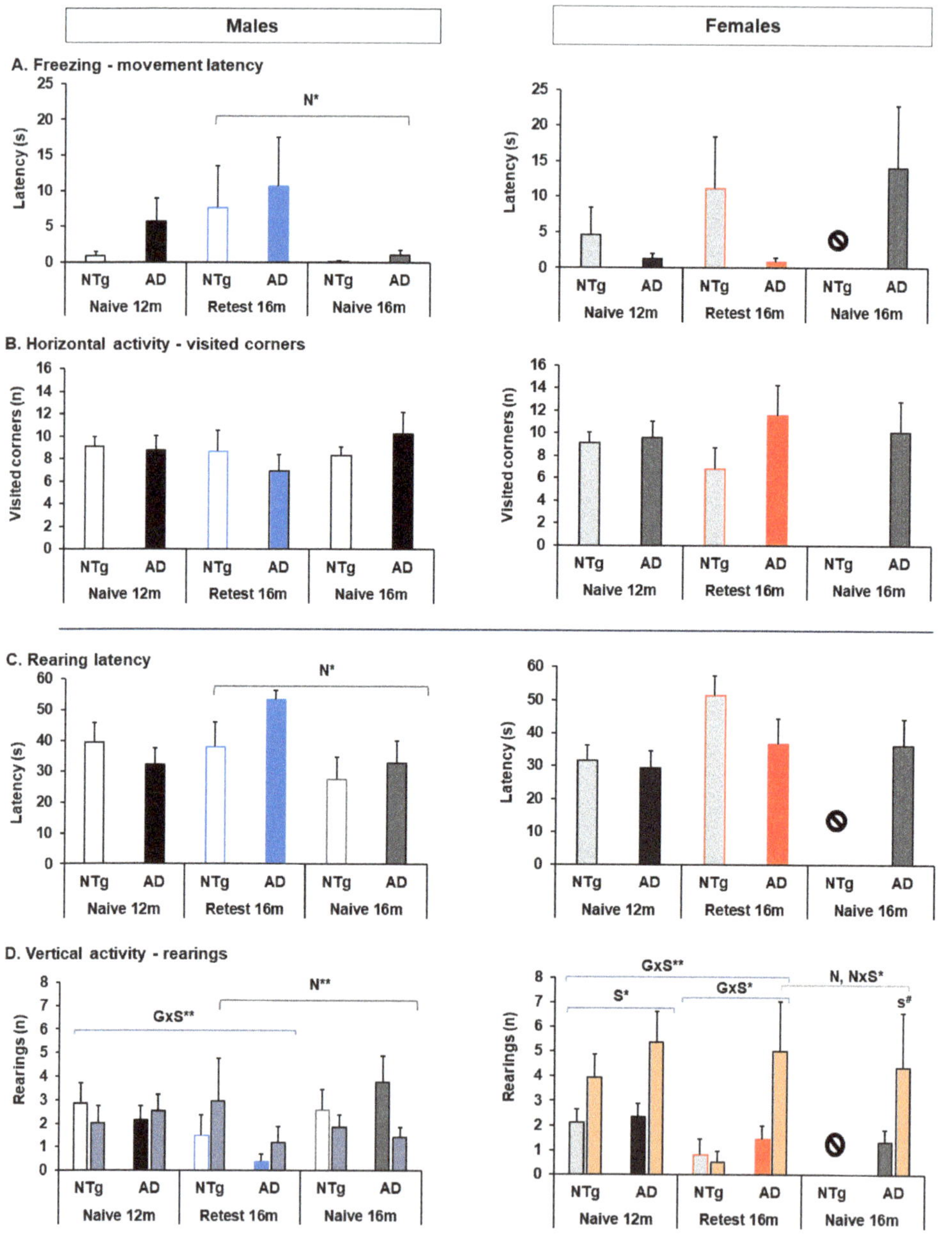

Figure 4. Ethogram of Neophobia and Exploratory activity. (**A**) Freezing, (**B**) horizontal activity, (**C**) rearing latency, (**D**) vertical activity. Statistics: ANOVA, S, sex effect, S* $p < 0.05$; G×S, genotype and sex interaction effects, G×S* $p < 0.05$*. N, naïve effects, naïve at 16 months *vs.* re-test 16 months, N** $p < 0.01$**, N* $p < 0.05$*. N×S, naïve and sex interaction effects, N×S* $p < 0.05$*. Bonferroni *post hoc* test: s, sex; and # expressed sex; differences between genotypes. The symbol ⊘ indicates the absence of the group, and m, month.

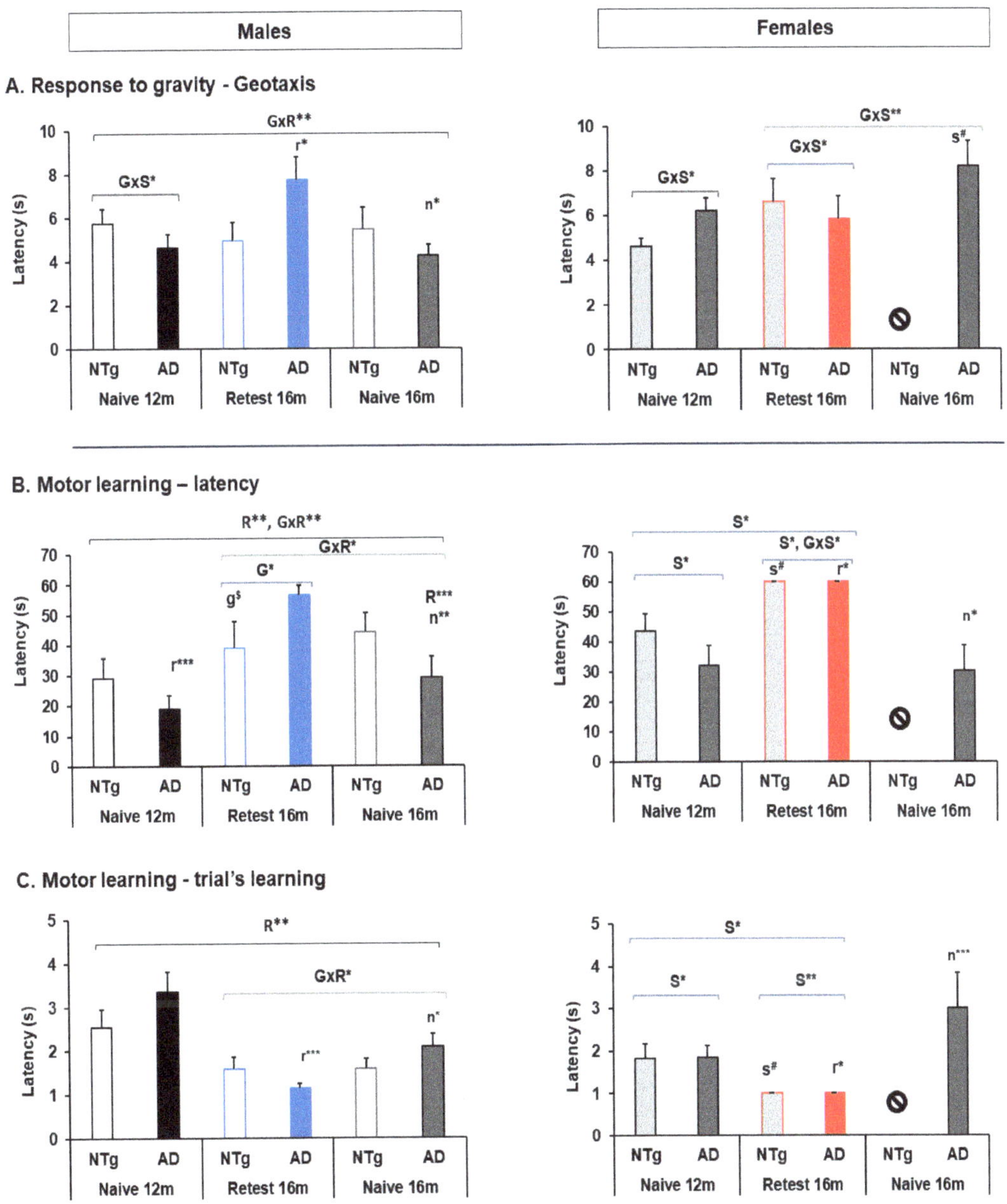

Figure 5. Geotaxis and motor learning—rotarod. (**A**) Geotaxis, (**B**) latency, (**C**) trial's learning. Statistics: ANOVA, G, genotype effect, G* $p < 0.05$. S, sex effect, S** $p < 0.01$, S* $p < 0.05$. R, Re-test effect, naïve 12 months and re-test 16 months, R** $p < 0.01$**, R* $p < 0.05$*. G×S, genotype and sex interaction effects, G×S** $p < 0.01$**, G×S* $p < 0.05$*. G×R, genotype and re-test effects, G×R** $p < 0.01$**, G×R* $p < 0.05$*. Bonferroni *post hoc* test: g, genotype, s, sex, r: re-test naïve 12 months vs.16 months, and n, naïve 16 months vs. re-test 16 months; $ expressed genotype, and # expressed sex differences between genotypes. The symbol ⊘ indicates the absence of the group, and m, month.

3.4. Motor Performance: Learning and Physical Endurance—Rotarod

The learning and motor performance tests in the Rotarod showed significant differences associated with different factors depending on the test or the group studied, see Figure 5. Among the males, significant differences were detected in learning and the number of trials between naïve and re-tests at 12 months and 16 months. In females, differences were detected in 3xTg-AD of 12 months and 16 months re-test and naïve, see Figure 5B,C and Tables S1–S3. In turn, for motor learning, the S effect plays an important role since females manage to learn earlier than males and spend more time on the wheel during the test at 12 months. At the re-test 16 months, the S effect was maintained in the number of trials, but in learning the G effect and G×S became important. In the same way, when performing MRA in the groups naïve at 12 months and re-test at 16 months, the S effect was the one that marked the statistical difference, see Figure 5B,C and Tables S1–S3. Nevertheless, there were no significant differences between the naïve 16 months group. However, between the re-test 16 months group vs. the naïve 16 months, differences were detected between males, where the R and G effects were significant. In addition, significant differences were also detected between the 3xTg-AD group, where the differences in S and R effects were the ones that obtained significance, see Figure 5B,C and Tables S1–S3.

At the same time, it is possible to differentiate physical endurance according to the interaction of G and S in the naïve 12 months, re-test 16 months, and naïve 16 months groups, see Figure 6. The NTg males have a physical endurance similar to that of 3xTg-AD females, followed by NTg females and finally 3xTg-AD males, whose performance is low and does not improve with training. This difference persisted in the re-test at 16 months. In males, differences were also detected in the physical endurance and each training days, with significance in the age of the NTg animals and the effect of Re-test in 3xTg-AD and the NTg (see Figure 6A and Tables S1–S3). In addition, on the first day of training, it was observed that 3xTg-AD males showed differences in R and aging effect among naïve mice (see Figure 6B, and Tables S1–S3). On the second day of training, the difference in G at 12 months and the effect of aging in the naïve 3xTg-AD group stand out. The changes observed on the third day of the test were recorded at 12 months, where the G has statistical significance and the R only in NTg group. For females, physical endurance was higher in the 3xTg-AD group. The re-test 16 months group had high latencies (see Figure 6A and Table S2). Differences were observed on Day 1 and Day 3, with differences was in the 16 months re-test NTg group and aging effect in the 3xTg-AD group (see Figure 6B and Table S3).

On the other hand, differences in genotype and sex were detected in the 12 months group (see Figure 6A and Table S1). In the 3 days of training, differences in effect were detected, with G distinction only on the second day (Figure 6B, and Table S1). Additionally, at 16 months in the re-test group, differences in G×S were recorded in physical endurance (see Figure 6A and Table S2). Days 2 and 3 showed differences in G×S, with no significant differences on the first day (see Figure 6B and Table S2). The re-test of this group corroborated the differences in G×S of the batch at 16 months (see Figure 6B and Table S2). However, at 16 months, groups of naïve mice did not show significant differences in this test. Yet, when comparing the re-test and naïve mice at 16 months, significant differences were detected between the group of males in physical endurance and the performance of Days 1 and 3 (see Figure 6A,B and Table S3). In addition, among the group of transgenic mice, differences in sex and re-test were detected between the groups, with the performance of the females being higher (see Figure 6A,B and Table S3).

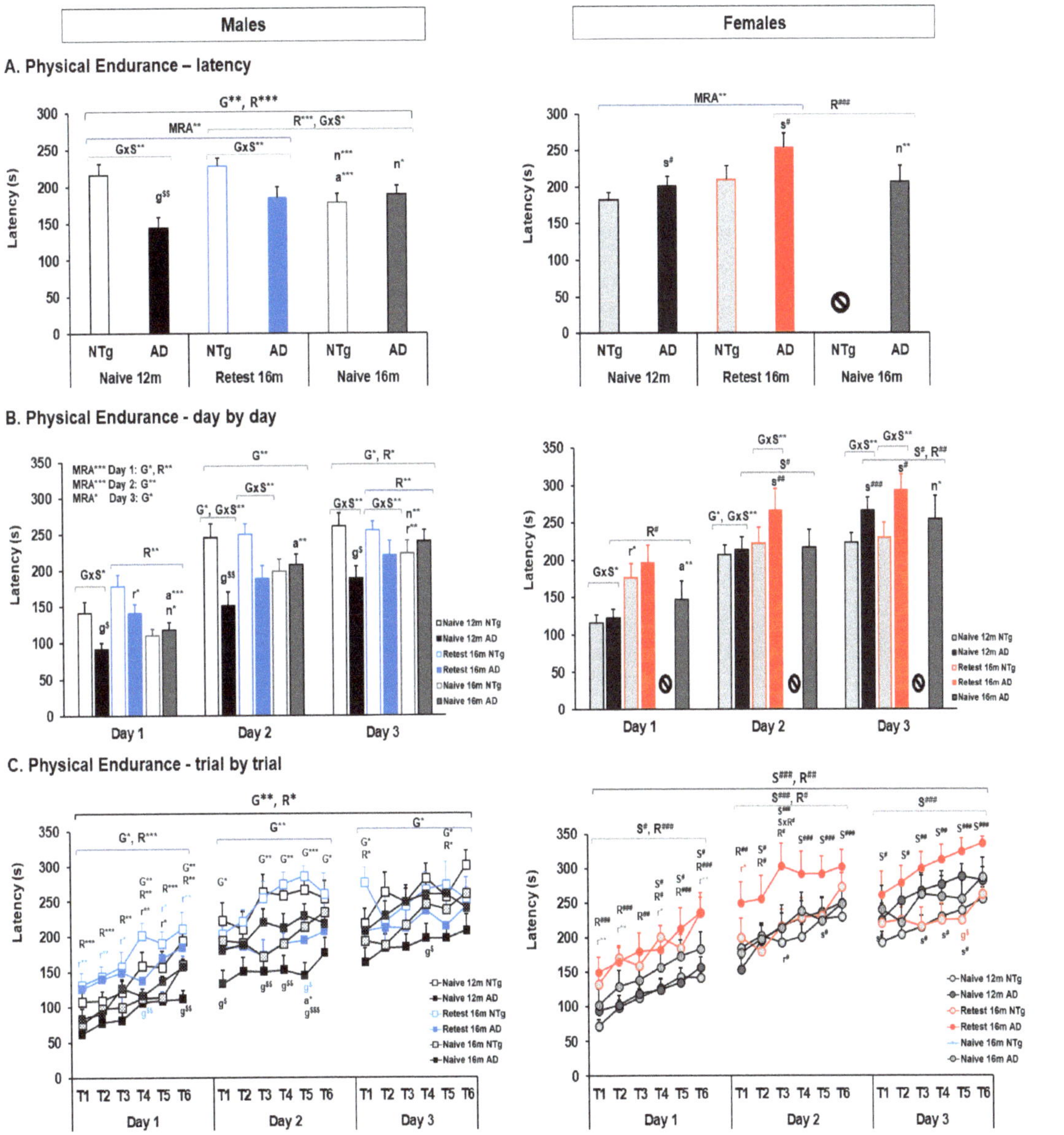

Figure 6. Physical endurance—rotarod. (**A**) Latency, (**B**) day by day, (**C**) trial by trial. Statistics: ANOVA, MRA-ANOVA, G, genotype effect, G** $p < 0.01$, G* $p < 0.05$. S, Sex effect, S*** $p < 0.001$***, S** $p < 0.01$**, S* $p < 0.05$. R, re-test effect, naïve 12 months vs. re-test 16 months, R*** $p < 0.001$***, R** $p < 0.01$**, R* $p < 0.05$*. G×S, genotype and sex effects, G×S** $p < 0.01$**, G×S* $p < 0.05$*. S×R, sex and re-test effects, S×R* $p < 0.05$*. Bonferroni *post hoc* test: g, genotype; s, sex; r: re-test, naïve 12 months vs. 16 months; n, naïve, naïve 16 months vs. re-test 16 months; $ expressed genotype, and # expressed sex differences between genotypes. The symbol ⃠ indicates the absence of the group, and m, month.

Furthermore, considering MRA between the groups, we can differentiate the effect of G, S, and R in the day-by-day and trial-by-trial tests, Table S4 shows the statistical differences from Figure 6C. The MRA analysis between males on Day 1 showed differences in G and S, see Figure 6C. It was observed that the NTg retest males improve with the repetition of the trials as well as the 3xTg-AD, but these do so to a lesser extent, and both the 12 months and 16 months naïve males have lower performance than retest. On Day 2, the genotype effect was observed here. The naïve 12 months NTg mice and the retest 16 months show a high latency in the test that increases with the execution of the trials. Naïve 16 months 3xTg-AD mice show the best performance within this group. In addition, the MRA trial-by-trial showed the differences in each trial and the animals' G and R differences. Here, it is highlighted that the first day plays an important role in the retest and then the differences of genotype. Also, among the females, significant differences were recorded in MRA trial by trial, with the 3xTg-AD retest of 16 months being the ones with the highest performance during all the test days. On the first day of training, differences in performance were obtained between the naïve 12 m NTg females and their retest 16 months, with a higher latency between the 16 months 3xTg-AD retest (Figure 6C). The second day of training did not record differences between the females, but on the third day, the highest performance of the 3xTg-AD retest 16 months was observed again.

Additionally, it is possible to differentiate females from males in the 3xTg-AD group, with females showing better performance in all tests. Thus, on Day 1 the mice differ in S and R. On the second day, the differences obtained on Day 1 are maintained, but the difference in the gender factor increases between the groups. On the third day, it is only possible to differentiate the gender factor between the groups. Specifically, the differences between the different factors have been identified in each trial. Thus, we can highlight specific differences be-tween the groups as detailed below on supplementary data for males and females. In addition, differences between 3xTg-AD males and females were detected in the following trials (see Figure 6C and Table S4).

3.5. Biological Status: HPA Axis and Sarcopenia Index

Higher differences were found in the corticosterone level in the re-test group compared to the naïve group (corticosterone, F (6, 70) = 9.817, $p < 0.001$ *post hoc:* male 3xTg-AD naïve vs. female 3xTg-AD naïve $p < 0.001$, male NTg naïve vs. male NTg re-test, $p = 0.001$). In addition, between group of males, the interaction of N had a lower level of corticosterone in the naïve group (N, F (1, 47) = 25.163, $p < 0.001$). In the 3xTg-AD group of animals, S effect and S×N interaction effects were differentiated (S, F (1, 42) = 16.456 $p < 0.001$. S×N, F (1, 42) = 4.243, $p = 0.046$), see Figure 7A.

The weight of the quadriceps and triceps sural muscles showed statistically significant differences (quadriceps, F (6, 70) = 3.203, $p = 0.008$. Triceps surae, F (6, 70) = 7.126, $p < 0.001$, *post hoc*: male naïve 3xTg-AD vs. female naïve 3xTg-AD, $p < 0.001$; female naïve 3xTg-AD vs. female re-test 3xTg-AD, $p = 0.022$). In addition, differences in the N effect were detected in male group, so, the muscle weight being greater in the naïve group in both muscles (quadriceps, N, F (1, 46) = 8.965, $p = 0.005$. Triceps surae, N, F (1, 46) = 7.267, $p = 0.008$). In the group of 3xTg-AD mice, differences in S and N were detected in the triceps surae muscle, the quadriceps muscle did not show significant differences in this analysis (triceps surae, S, F (1, 44) = 14.955, $p < 0.001$. S×N, F (1, 44) = 6.998, $p = 0.012$), see Figure 7B,C.

In the sarcopenia index, significant differences were observed in sarcopenia index-triceps surae (sarcopenia index, F (6, 70) = 3.158, $p = 0.008$, *post hoc*: male naïve 3xTg-AD vs. female naïve 3xTg-AD, $p < 0.001$; female naïve 3xTg-AD vs. female re-test 3xTg-AD, $p = 0.022$), see Figure 7E.

Furthermore, corticosterone levels were correlated with different variables, detecting a different correlation between males and females. In males, a negative correlation with the muscle weight of the quadriceps and triceps surae stands out, and a positive correlation with the variables, phenotype scoring system, frailty score, cadence and physical endurance on the first day (quadriceps, r^2 = (-) 0.141, $p = 0.008$; triceps surae, r^2 = (-) 0.098, $p = 0.03$).

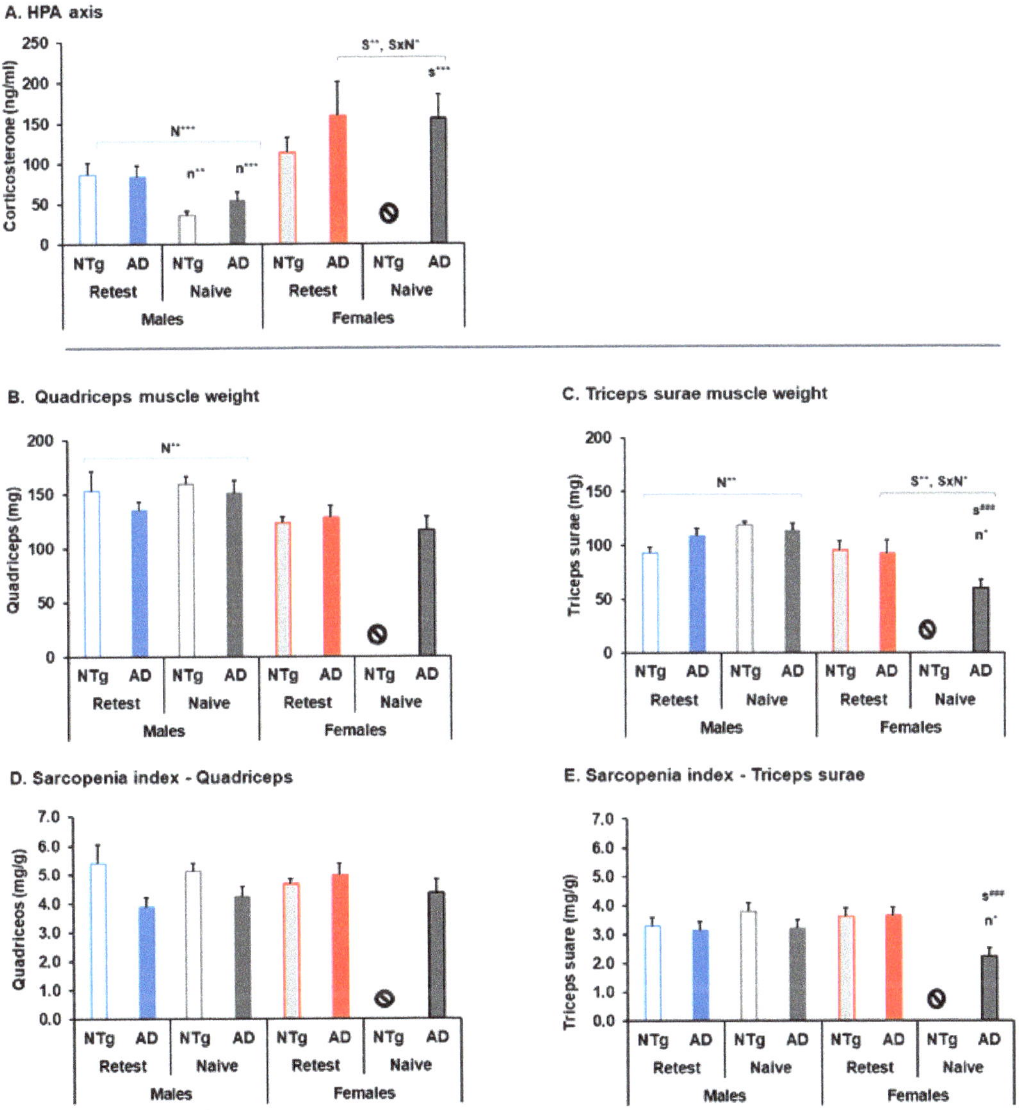

Figure 7. Biological status: HPA axis and sarcopenia index. (**A**) HPA axis, (**B**) quadriceps muscle weight, (**C**) triceps surae muscle, weight, (**D**) sarcopenia index—quadriceps, (**E**) sarcopenia index—triceps surae. Statistics: ANOVA, S, sex effect, S** $p < 0.01$**. N, naïve, naïve 16 months vs. re-test 16 months, N*** $p < 0.001$***, N** $p < 0.01$**. S×N, sex and naïve effects, S×N** $p < 0.01$**, S×N* $p < 0.05$*. Bonferroni *post hoc* test: s, sex; n: naïve, naïve 16 months vs. re-test 16 months; and # expressed sex differences between genotypes, s###, $p < 0.001$###. The symbol ⃠ indicates the absence of the group, and m, month.

Phenotype scoring system, $r^2 = 0.182$, $p = 0.002$; frailty score, $r^2 = 0.119$, $p = 0.016$; Cadence, $r^2 = 0.092$, $p = 0.036$; Physical endurance day 1, $r^2 = 0.190$, $p = 0.002$), see Figure 8A–F. In females, a positive correlation between corticosterone with performance in the rotarod on total, the second and third day were detected (physical endurance—total, $r^2 = 0.143$,

p = 0.039; physical endurance Day 2, r^2 = 0.157, p = 0.03, physical endurance Day 3, r^2 = 0.168, p = 0.024), see Figure 8G–I.

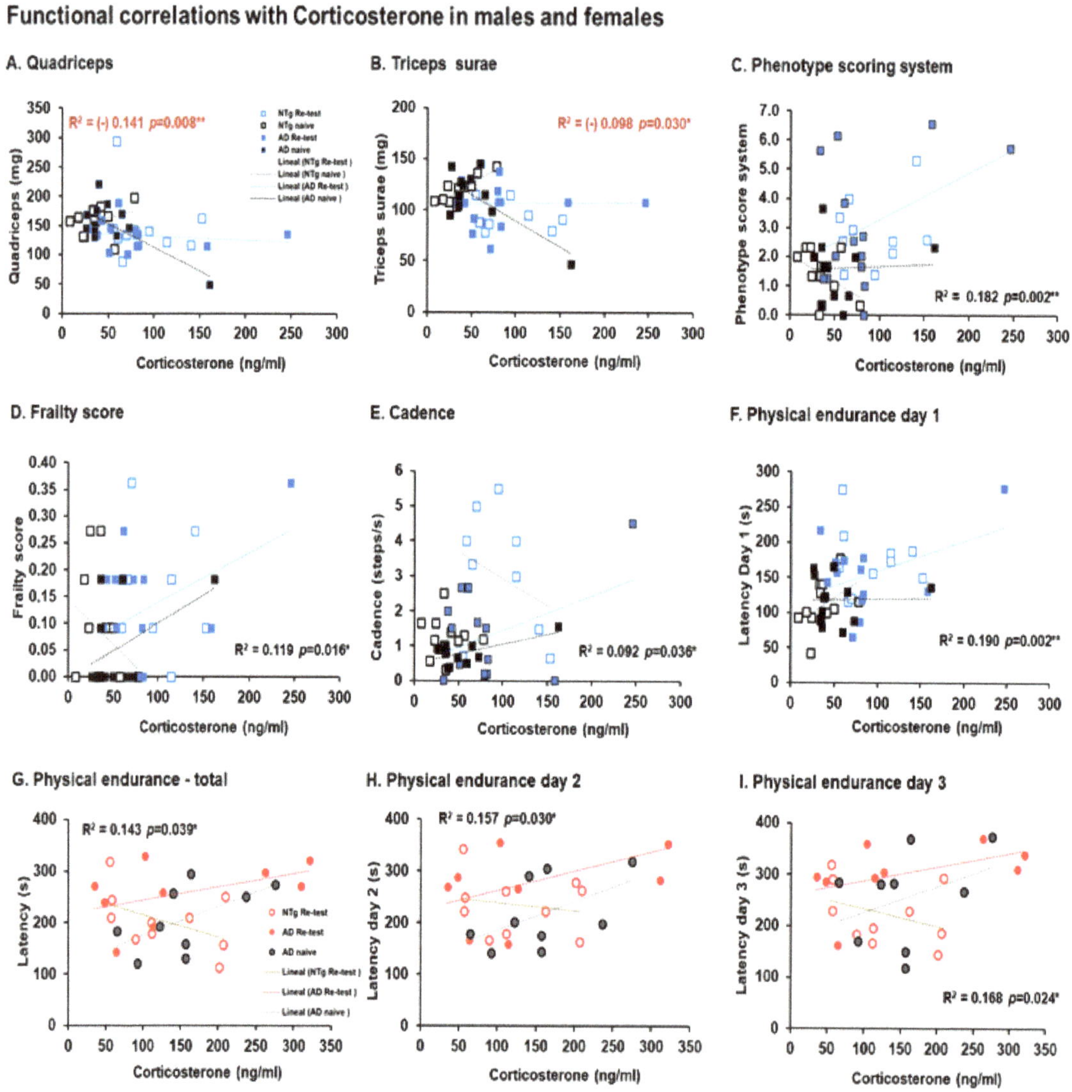

Figure 8. Functional corticosterone correlations in males and females. Pearson's Correlations analysis of corticosterone in males and females. Meaningful, Pearson's correlation in males between corticosterone and (**A**) quadriceps, (**B**) triceps surae, (**C**) phenotype scoring system, (**D**) frailty score, (**E**) cadence, and (**F**) physical endurance Day 1. Meaningful, Pearson's correlation in females between corticosterone and (**G**) physical endurance—total, (**H**) physical endurance Day 2, (**I**) physical endurance Day 3. Statistics: Pearson r^2, $^{**}p < 0.01$, $^{*}p < 0.05$.

In different way, only in male, functional correlations with sarcopenia index were detected. Thus, sarcopenia index-quadriceps correlations with physical endurance Day 1 and Day 2 (sarcopenia index-quadriceps—physical endurance Day 1, r^2 = 0.190, p = 0.002. sarcopenia index–quadriceps—physical endurance Day 2, r^2 = 0.084, p = 0.048). In addition, sarcopenia index–triceps surae correlation with the number of horizontal explorations (visited corners) (sarcopenia index–triceps surae—corners, $r^2 = (-)0.099$, $p = 0.029$), see Figure 9A–C.

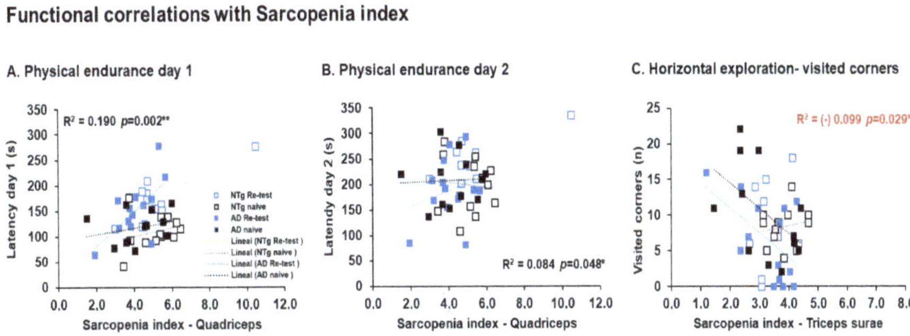

Figure 9. Functional correlations with sarcopenia index. Meaningful, Pearson's correlations analysis of sarcopenia index. Meaningful, Pearson's correlation between sarcopenia index quadriceps and (**A**) physical endurance Day 1, (**B**) physical endurance Day 2. Sarcopenia index, and triceps surae and (**C**) horizontal exploration—visited corners. Statistics: Pearson r^2, $^{**}p < 0.01$, $^{*}p < 0.05$.

On the other hand, males and females had a negative correlation between phenotype score system and functional variables. In the case of males, a negative correlation was detected between stride length and the phenotype scoring system (stride length—phenotype scoring system, $r^2 = (-)\ 0.178$, $p = 0.003$). In females, a negative correlation is observed with physical endurance—total (phenotype scoring system, $r^2 = (-)\ 0.208$, $p = 0.011$), see Figure 10A,B.

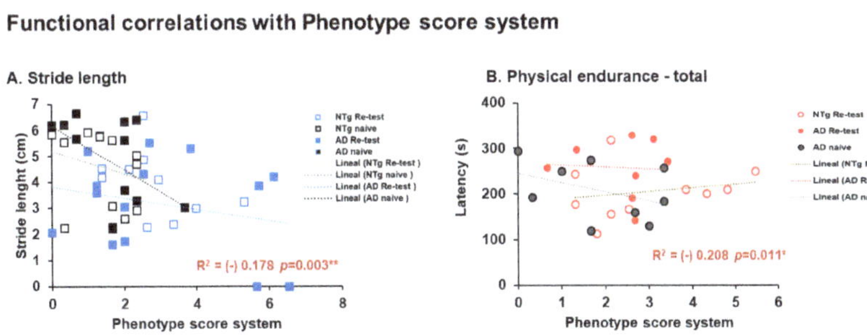

Figure 10. Functional correlations with phenotype score system. Pearson's correlations analysis of phenotype score system. Meaningful, Pearson's correlation between phenotype score system and (**A**) stride length in males, and (**B**) physical endurance—total in females. Statistics: Pearson r^2, $^{**}p < 0.01$, $^{*}p < 0.05$.

There is the summary of results in Table 2.

Table 2. Summary of results.

	Genotype Factor (G)	Sex Factor (S)	Re-Test Factor (R)	Naïve Factor (N)
Phenotype scoring system	↑ deficits 3xTg-AD group ↑ deterioration in 3xTg-AD males in the total score			
Frailty	↑ 3xTg-AD males at 16 m in the re-test			
Kyphosis	↑ 3xTg-AD males increased the severity in the re-test at 16 m			

Table 2. *Cont.*

	Genotype Factor (G)	Sex Factor (S)	Re-Test Factor (R)	Naïve Factor (N)
Quantitative parameters of gait	Speed: ⬆ 3xTg-AD males at 12 m, and ⬇ in the re-test at 16 m ⬇ 16 m naïve NTg and 3xTg-AD Cadence: ⬇ 3xTg-AD males at 12 m and 16 m Re-test ⬇ 3xTg-AD and NTg Re-test group at 12 and 16 m ⬇ Naïve 16 m NTg and 3xTg-AD males had a lower cadence than age-matched re-tests	Speed: ⬆ Re-test and naïve 16 m 3xTg-AD females Variability of stride length: ⬇ Re-test and naïve 16 m 3xTg-AD females	Stride length: ⬇ Re-test 3xTg-AD males at 12 m Cadence: ⬇ Naïve 16 m males 3xTg-AD and NTg ⬇3xTg-AD male in all groups	Stride length: ⬆ Naïve 3xTg-AD and NTg at 16 m
Exploration and neophobia		Exploratory activity (ratio): ⬆ NTg and 3xTg-AD females at 12 m		Freezing: ⬇ Naïve 3xTg-AD and NTg males at 16 m Vertical exploratory activity: ⬆ Naïve 3xTg-AD and NTg males at 16 m Exploratory activity (ratio): ⬆ Naïve 3xTg-AD and NTg males at 16 m ⬆ Naïve 3xTg-AD females at 16 m
Geotaxis		⬆ Naïve 3xTg-AD females at 16 m	⬆ Re-test 3xTg-AD in the re-test group compared to their performance at 12 m.	
Motor learning	⬆ Latency 3xTg-AD males Re-test at 16 m	⬆ Latency and trials females at 12 m in both genotypes. ⬆ Females at 16 m re-test group	⬆ Latency re-test 3xTg-AD males at 16 m ⬆ Latency re-test 3xTg-AD females at 16 m ⬆ N trials among males in re-test group ⬇ N trials among females in re-test group	⬇ Latency naïve 3xTg-AD male and females at 16 m
Physical Endurance	⬇ 3xTg-AD males at 12 m and 16 m in the re-test group. ⬇ Day 2, 3xTg-AD males in all groups ⬇ Day 3, 3xTg-AD males at 12 m	⬆ 3xTg-AD females at 12 m and 16 m ⬆ Day 2–3, 3xTg-AD females at 12 m and 16 m	⬆ NTg re-test males at 16 m ⬆ Re-test at 16 m in all group in 2nd and 3rd training days ⬆ Re-test at 16 m male groups in 1st training day ⬆ Re-test at 16 m female group in 1st and 2nd day	⬆ 16 m naïve 3xTg-AD males than 3xTg-AD Re-test at this age.
HPA axis		⬆ 3xTg-AD re-test at 16 m ⬆ Naïve females at 16 m		⬇ Naïve Re-test males at 16 m ⬆ Naïve females at 16 m
Sarcopenia index		⬇ Triceps surae and sarcopenia index naïve 3xTg-AD females		⬆ Quadriceps and triceps sura muscles naïve males Re-test at 16 m. ⬇ Triceps surae and sarcopenia index naïve 3xTg-AD females re-test females at 16 m
Survival	High mortality, mostly among NTg female mice, rescued in longitudinal designs			
Correlation's interactions	In males, negative correlations between corticosterone and quadriceps, triceps surae; and positive correlations between corticosterone and phenotype score system, frailty score, cadence, and physical endurance Day 1. Females, positives correlated between corticosterone and physical endurance-total, physical endurance Days 2 and 3. Positive correlations in males were detected between sarcopenia index-quadriceps and physical endurance on Days 1 and 2. In females, negative correlations were detected between sarcopenia index–triceps and horizontal activity. Negative correlations in males were identified between phenotype score system and stride length, and in females' phenotype score system and physical endurance—total.			

According to the factors, genotype (G), sex (S), re-test (R) and naïve (N), a summary of the main results of this study is presented. It also includes the correlation's interactions. The symbol ⬆ indicates increase, ⬇ indicates decreases, and m, month.

4. Discussion

Recently, we developed a battery of psychomotor tests that include gait, neophobia and exploration, muscle strength, motor learning, physical resistance, and frailty status [33]. The results, in males, indicated that 3xTg-AD mice exhibit a more significant functional impairment in the quantitative variables of gait and exploratory activity than age-matched NTg counterparts with normal aging. The presence of movement limitations and muscle weakness was determinant for the functional decline related to the stages of severity of the disease that worsened with age. In addition, we detected the presence of signs of physical frailty, which accompany the functional deterioration of these animals. The signs of sarcopenia were present in an advanced stage of AD [31,32]. Therefore, the present study was designed to investigate, for the first time, several aspects: (1) from a gender-medicine perspective, the impact of this functional impairment in 3xTg-AD females as compared to males; (2) the long-term effects of repeated test, either in longitudinal (the same set of animals at 12 and 16 months of age) or transversal (two different sets, pre-tested or naïve, at 16 months of age) designs, both in pathological and normal aging scenarios; (3) to include a phenotype of frailty and physical deterioration that may find a functional correlation with the biological status (HPA axis and sarcopenia), with nuances in male and female animals.

4.1. Survival, Bodyweight, Phenotype Scoring System, Frailty Score, and Kyphosis

4.1.1. Survival

The survival curves on the cohorts of 191 animals allowed us to record higher mortality in females, being the group of NTg females the one that presented the highest number of deaths between 8–12 months of age. Interestingly, only females under the longitudinal design survived and achieved 16 months of age, while the group of naïve NTg females perished before reaching that old age, suggesting that repeated testing might have some protective effects. These results agree with our previous reports in these colonies, where high mortality rates associated with increased frailty were reported in females, and NTg exhibited increased mortality from 12 months of age [42]. In the case of 3xTg-AD mice, females that reached old age were survivors who overcame the disease's advanced neuropathological stages and exhibited lower behavioural differences with their NTg counterparts except for cognitive AD-hallmarks [47]. We have also described that, in male 3xTg-AD mice, an increase of mortality rates is associated with impairment in the neuro-immune-endocrine system compared to their females counterparts or the NTg genotype [48–50]. Noteworthy, we have recently reported survival bias and crosstalk between chronological and behavioral age in an APPswe model, where age- and genotype-sensitivity tests defined behavioral signatures in middle-aged, old, and long-lived mice with normal and AD-associated aging [51]. Therefore, the present work provides further evidence on sex and genotype-dependent differences in life expectancy and supports the key role of frailty and compensatory mechanisms as previously reported by our and other laboratories using different models of AD [29,49–52].

4.1.2. Frailty

In the present work, the frailty results showed genotype differences between males, with NTg being the ones with the highest score. Only 12 of the 30 MCFI parameters were included as the incidence of the other indicators was very low or null. Kane and Brown [29] reported that 3xTg-AD male mice have a higher frailty index (FI) than NTg mice and 3xTg-AD females, and it was associated with their higher mortality ratios. Their study also indicated an increase in the frailty associated with age. On the other hand, in the present work, functional correlations in males found that their corticosterone levels correlated with frailty score and phenotype scoring system, both measures of functional decline. These results could indicate less deficit accumulation or functional capacity at the time of measurement in 3xTg-AD mice [53]. Therefore, it is plausible that other factors contribute to the survival/mortality of animals, and a complex multifactorial scenario be specific for each sex and biological age/stage of disease. In addition, in female C57BL/6 mice, greater frailty from 17 months of age with higher mortality at 26 months has been recently described in contrast to the non-fragile mice that reached 29 months of life [54]. These data have made it possible to identify that the prevalence of frailty in female mice increases throughout life and accurately predicts mortality [54]. Additionally, the animals' bodyweight presented genotype differences that coincide with previous data [33] but the re-test decreased the weight in males, probably due to the training carried out at 12 months of age.

4.1.3. Kyphosis

On the other hand, the severity of kyphosis was differentiated into postural and structural [31,32]. Here, genotype differences between males have been detected that corroborate previous reports, with greater severity in 3xTg-AD mice [31]. In females, here described for the first time, the severity of kyphosis increased with age and was more significant in the 3xTg-AD mice at 16 months in the re-test group, where the structural type predominates. The differences detected in males corroborate our other recent reports [32].

4.1.4. Phenotype Scoring System

Kyphosis is also one of the scores included in the phenotype scoring system [39,40], which has recently been functionally differentiated by a severity classification that allows more information to be collected in contrast to other variables, such as those associated with gait and exploratory activity [32]. Thus, in the phenotype scoring system, we detected that kyphosis at 12 months of age was more significant in NTg of both sexes, a significance that was not reproduced at 16 months in these animals, which corroborates our differentiation of severity in the presence of kyphosis since the postural condition can be positionally modified. In addition, in the gait score, an increase in functional impairment was detected in 3xTg-AD males and females, which appears in the re-test group at 16 months. This variable makes it possible to discriminate a significant impairment of movement and exploratory activity since bizarre behaviours may occur that interfere with movement [31]. The deficits detected in the quantitative parameters of gait will be discussed in the following section.

4.1.5. Clasping

Finally, the presence of increased clasping in naïve 3xTg-AD mice at 16 months can also be highlighted. It was related to a more significant involved or progression of the disease [55,56]. The present results also suggest that repeated tests exerted protective effects in this respect. Lalonde [55] described brain regions and genes affecting limb-clasping responses. In the C57BL/6 strain, age-dependent locomotor deficits, including hindlimb clasping, are associated with a decreased number of dopaminergic neurons in aged mice, with reduced dopamine levels in the striatum [57]. Interestingly, alterations in the dopaminergic system described in 3xTg-AD mice and other AD models may also explain the presence of increased clasping.

4.2. Quantitative Parameters of Gait, and Neophobia and Exploration

4.2.1. Stride Length

Quantitative parameters in the gait analysis indicated that stride length was shorter in re-tested (16-month-old) male mice compared to age-matched naïve animals, and that this variable correlated with the gait phenotype score system. Interestingly, re-tested 3xTg-AD mice had the shortest stride length among the males compared to the naïve. In addition, differences in genotype and sex were observed at 12 and 16 months in the re-test group with greater stride length at 12 months in 3xTg-AD females and re-test in NTg males. In addition, the stride variability in females was lower than that of males, and the 3xTg-AD in all groups had the best performance, so their movement had more homogeneous steps throughout the trajectory. Previously, in our study in male 3xTg-AD mice of 6, 12, and 16 months of age, no differences in stride length or variability were detected, although a trend to increase stride length with age was observed in the case of 3xTg-AD mice while remained stable in the NTg genotype [31]. However, in another study at 6 months of age, increased stride length was reported in 3xTg-AD mice with no sex difference [58]. In addition, at 16 months of age, the gait of 3xTg-AD has been described as normal, without differences in genotype and sex [59,60]. According to the results, we propose that using the variability of the stride can help discriminate the trajectory of the movement during the gait analysis similar to humans where recently the variability was identified as a marker of cortical-cognitive dysfunction in AD patients [61,62].

4.2.2. Speed

A significant decrease in speed in the male 3xTg-AD mice in all groups was observed. This decrease may be associated with a progressive functional decline in the 3xTg-AD male mice and coincides with the findings at 13 months of age we have previously reported [33]. Cadence had a lower performance in the 3xTg-AD males at 12 months of age. However, it increased at 16 months in the re-test group, differing from naïve at this age. Thus, cadence and speed are the variables with the highest sensitivity to discriminate genotypic differences in male mice and differentiate changes in gait attributable to pathological aging in the 3xTg-AD genotype. In the case of 3xTg-AD females, speed in-creases slightly in the 16-months re-test group and was higher than in males in all groups. At the clinical level, the identification of early changes in gait is of great relevance for identifying psychomotor disorders that in the case of AD may be related to the timing of steps and gait speed [63]. Additionally, corticosterone levels were positively correlated with a cadence in males.

4.2.3. Neophobia and Exploration

The neophobia response, expressed as freezing, of 12 and 16-month-old naïve male mice was lower than in re-test mice in both genotypes, and statistically significant when contrasted with 16-month-old naïve mice. In females at 16 months of age, re-tested and naïve, a higher freezing was observed than in 16-month-old naïve females, albeit did not reach the statistical significance.

This neophobia emotional response is a characteristic of the 3xTg-AD model that is ac-companied by reduced immediate exploratory behaviour in a novel environment, as we first described in these animals in the open field test and the corner test already at the early 'premorbid' age of 2.5 months and worsened with the progress of the disease [64]. In addition, it corresponds to more sensitive ethological behaviours of the 3xTg-AD phenotype that has been reported in several other studies [31,33,42]. In addition, the horizontal exploratory activity did not report statistically significant differences.

However, in the vertical exploratory activity (number and latency of rearings), differences between the re-test male mice at 16 months and the naïve of the same age were more statistically significant than the activity in naïve mice. In addition, the ratio (visited corners/rearings) in the re-test male mice of 12 and 16 months increased in the re-test but differed from the females at both ages, being lower in males at 12 months in both genotypes. At 16 months in re-test, NTg male's ratio was high than NTg females, and in 3xTg-AD case, the ratio was increased in females 3xTg-AD. This decrease in activity over time, which is also observed in NTg mice, has been previously described as due to normal aging [64], with 3xTg-AD mice exhibiting less activity in most cases, which is attributed as a pathological trigger similar to BPSD that appear later in NTg mice due to normal aging [64]. In addition, in males was observed that correlated horizontal activity with triceps sural weight.

4.3. Muscular Strength: Forelimb Grip Strength and Muscular Endurance—Hanger Test and Response to Gravity—Geotaxis

4.3.1. Muscular Strength

Muscular strength is associated with global cognitive function in older people [65]. In addition, skeletal muscle mass index and physical performance (timed up and go test and grip strength) have decreased in older adults with AD [66]. Our results have not detected significant differences, although, at 12 months, it seems that females have a superior performance in grip strength and muscular endurance. Previously, we have reported that

13-month-old 3xTg-AD mice in natural isolation have preserved muscular strength [33] and that muscle strength and endurance would be associated with aging [31]. The laboratory of Brown also reported that at 6 months, 3xTg-AD mice have a deficit in grip strength [58], but at 16 months these results are not reproduced [59]. Additionally, the reduction in muscle weight and the appearance of sarcopenia may not yet be evident in the loss of muscle strength and resistance, or aging in this variable has greater importance than the distinction of the effects of the pathology in humans [67–69].

4.3.2. Geotaxis

On the other hand, geotaxis showed differences between the males, with the 3xTg-AD re-test at 16 months being the ones that obtained a worse performance and the 3xTg-AD naïve females at 16 months. In addition, females take longer to pass the test, which is reflected in the differences in GxS in the 16-month-old re-test and naïve group. The usefulness of this test has been previously described [70]. Specifically, the geotaxis has allowed us to differentiate the animals' postural positioning and balance strategies to pass the test and thus detect a possible functional deficit [31,33]. Therefore, 3xTg-AD re-test males and naïve females at 16 months show the most significant deterioration in this task.

4.4. Motor Performance: Learning and Physical Endurance—Rotarod

The motor performance showed superior performance in females of both genotypes. The motor learning tests and the number of trials reached the maximum values of the test in the re-test at 16 months. The increased performance may be due to pretraining done at 12 months, which can produce cognitive improvements with a long-term wheel of activity. In 16-month-old naïve 3xTg-AD males and females, lower latency and high number of trials were observed to achieve motor learning. Male 3xTg-AD mice have the most inferior performance in all tests.

As in motor learning, females have a high physical endurance. The 3xTg-AD females in the re-test group at 16 months achieved the highest performance over the male 3xTg-AD naïve and re-test, and female 3xTg-AD naïve 16-month-old females, and with similar performance to the NTg males of the same age. In addition, all groups increased their performance with training from Day 1 to Day 3, which is evident to a greater extent on the third day of training, and the effect of the re-test is observed at 16 months with an effect on different days for males and females, being in males on the first day of training and in females on the first and second day of training. Additionally, it was possible to distinguish the effect of aging in the naïve male NTg in contrast to the naïve at 12 months and re-test at 16 months. In addition, among the 3xTg-AD group, the sex differences between the 16-month-old re-test mice are distinguished from Day 1 to Day 3 of training. The 3xTg-AD males present the lowest performance among all groups, although with the training in the first day increased de physical endurance at 16 months in re-test group, on the following days, their performance is below 3xTg-AD naïve for 16 months.

The motor performance of 3xTg-AD mice has been reported in different studies. The performance in coordination and motor learning of 3xTg-AD mice has been highlighted over the performance of NTg mice, and these results are observable from 6 months and are reproduced at 16 months [58–60]. It has even been mentioned that 3xTg-AD females perform better than males at these ages [58,59]. In our laboratory, only reproduced the results of Stover et al. and Garvock-de Montbrun et. al. at 13 months, where the 3xTg-AD male mice presented a higher performance than the NTg, but in the latter, the weight factor interfered in the results [33]. Decreased motor function is also associated with aging, as reported in C57BL/6 mice of different ages [71–73]. In addition, we have differentiated the conceptualization of motor performance into motor learning—latency and motor learning—trials learning, since after physical exercise, the animals must manage to stay on a moving wheel in a coordinated manner. Consequently, in the first trials, physical endurance has a workload associated with an anaerobic exercise that progresses to aerobic exercise as the trials and their respective recovery times are replicated. In humans, the decrease in endurance exercise performance and its physiological determinants with aging appear to be mediated mainly by a reduction in the intensity (speed) and volume of exercise performed during training sessions [74]. Under this hypothesis, in their study, Pena et al. reported that 3xTg-AD mice improve their maximum latency in rotarod when subjected to aerobic exercise [75].

These results are accompanied by correlations with corticosterone levels and behave differently between males and females. In the case of males, corticosterone correlates positively with physical endurance on the first day of training, and in the case of females, it correlates positively with total physical endurance and physical endurance on the second and third days. On the other hand, a positive correlation was also detected in males between index-quadriceps sarcopenia and rotarod performance on the first and second days. A negative correlation was also detected between total physical endurance and the phenotype score system in females. Therefore, these interactions could explain the differences in performance between the groups studied.

4.5. Biological Status: HPA Axis and Sarcopenia Index

4.5.1. Corticosterone

Corticosterone levels differed between groups due to sex and re-test factors, but not genotype. Males exhibited lower corticosterone levels in naïve mice of both genotypes, with similar levels between 3xTg-AD and NTg in the re-test group. On the contrary, in females, higher plasma corticosterone levels were observed in the 3xTg-AD re-test, and naïve females had similar levels that exceed the NTg re-test. It is also possible to distinguish that naïve 3xTg-AD females had higher levels than their male counterparts. The results agree with the sexual dimorphism reported by Muntsant et al., with higher plasma corticosterone levels in females [42], and also with plasma levels similar to the intervals described by Giménez-Llort et al. [76]. Additionally, corticosterone levels showed functional correlations with different variables depending on sex. In males, the correlation was inversely associated with the muscle mass of the quadriceps and triceps surae, and positively with frailty and gait cadence indicators. On the other hand, higher corticosterone levels correlated with higher performance on the first day of training in physical endurance. In females, the correlation with corticosterone was related to physical endurance performance with greater significance on the second and third training days. These results could indicate chronic stress if there is a long-term activation of the HPA axis in the case of females [77]. A report suggested that the combination of emotional and physical stress in a period of 5 h of exposure severely affected memory in NTg mice and increased the alterations in 3xTg-AD mice as a consequence of the reduction in the number dendritic spines and increase in the Aβ levels [50]. Additionally, the elevated corticosterone may precede cognitive impairments in genetically vulnerable 3xTg-AD females [78,79] and may, in turn, be related to frailty [80].

4.5.2. Sarcopenia

Furthermore, we have observed that the quadriceps and triceps surae muscles have a greater weight in naïve male mice, whereas in 3xTg-AD females, a lower weight is observed in the triceps surae muscle with significant differences with the group of 3xTg-AD females and re-test and males of this genotype. These differences in naïve 3xTg-AD females are also observed in the sarcopenia index of the triceps surae muscle. In humans, sarcopenia is closely related to dementia, particularly AD, and may be involved in the pathophysiological process of AD [68,81]. On the other hand, poor muscle function but not reduced lean muscle mass drives the association of sarcopenia with cognitive decline in old age [67,82]. Sarcopenia, low grip strength, and slow walking speed were significantly associated with mild cognitive impairment in the community-dwelling elderly [80,83]. Therefore, our results can be helpful to study what occurs in human pathology through a translational approach to motor dysfunction at different levels of disability [31].

Moreover, in the case of males, the weight of the quadriceps and triceps surae muscles negatively correlated with plasma corticosterone levels. A positive correlation of the quadriceps sarcopenia index with physical endurance Days 1 and 2 was also found. In the case of the sural triceps sarcopenia index, it correlated negatively with the number of corners visited in the exploratory activity. These correlations were not found in females.

Finally, the study's limitations were given by the high mortality rate of NTg females that resulted in the lack of 16-month-old naïve group. Therefore, the genotype differences between 3xTg-AD and NTg females could not be contrasted. However, the analyses were carried out to detect the sex differences between the 3xTg-AD group. In future research, it would be interesting to compare the results of this study with NTg females since their functional profile may differ from males in physical or biological variables, such as in 3xTg-AD females.

5. Conclusions

From the results, it is possible to highlight that the high mortality rate in females, and among them that in the NTg group, was prevented in the group of females behaviorally assessed at 12 months of age, and these females were able to reach the age of 16 months completing the longitudinal design. In addition, higher corticosterone levels were detected in females and lower muscle weight of the triceps surae, which could indicate sarcopenia and alteration of the HPAaxis, which was more significant in the naive group at 16 months. Additionally, there were genotype-sensitive variables such as the phenotype scoring system, frailty and kyphosis in which the group of 3xTg-AD males showed physical deterioration. In turn, the motor learning and physical endurance variables were sensitive to re-testing, with 3xTg-AD females achieving the best performance when repeating the behavioral battery at 16 months. In addition, the females exhibited a better performance in gait, where their stride was homogeneous and straight. Additionally, females exhibited less severe scores in physical variables, such as kyphosis, which could explain males' more significant deterioration in some motor tests. On the other hand, males showed deterioration in most of the variables studied. For their part, the correlations could explain the differences obtained between males and females, being positive in females between corticosterone and physical endurance, and the case of males between sarcopenia index and physical endurance as well as corticosterone with physical variables. The present results highlight the complexity of experimental scenarios in neurodegenerative diseases, such as Alzheimer's disease, confirming not only the different impact of factors depending on genotype, sex, and age but their interplay with the methodological approach. They provide evidence that genotype, sex and age-dependent impact of behavioral assessment, as well as the repetition of behavioral tests, should not be underestimated. Conversely, and most importantly, the ability of behavioral assessment and repeated tests to modify the behavioral outputs indicates that they could be considered functional trainings that modify survival, anxiety, and functional profile (physical endurance and motor learning) of old male and female 3xTg-AD mice and also NTg mice counterparts with normal aging.

Supplementary Materials: The following supporting information can be downloaded at: https://www.mdpi.com/article/10.3390/biomedicines10050973/s1, Table S1: Physical performance in males and females Naïve 12-month-old 3xTg-AD and NTg mice; Table S2: Physical performance in males and female 3xTg-AD and NTg after Re-test to 16m; Table S3: Physical performance in males and females Naïve 16-month-old 3xTg-AD and NTg mice; Table S4: Statistics Figure 5C.

Author Contributions: Conceptualization, L.G.-L. and L.C.-M.; behavioral performance, analysis, statistics, L.C.-M.; pathology: L.C.-M.; illustrations: L.C.-M. and L.G.-L. writing—original draft preparation, L.C.-M.; writing—review and editing, L.C.-M. and L.G.-L.; Funding acquisition, L.G.-L. All authors have read and agreed to the published version of the manuscript.

Funding: This work was funded by 2017-SGR-1468 and UAB-GE-260408 to L.G.-L. The colony of 3xTg-AD mice was sustained by ArrestAD H2020 Fet-OPEN-1-2016-2017-737390, European Union's

Horizon 2020 research and innovation program under grant agreement No 737390 to L.G.-L. It also received financial support from Memorial Mercedes Llort Sender 2021/80/09241941.8.

Institutional Review Board Statement: The study was conducted according to the guidelines of the Declaration of Helsinki, and approved by the Ethics Committee of Departament de Medi Ambient i Habitatge, Generalitat de Catalunya (CEEAH 3588/DMAH 9452) on the 8 March 2019.

Informed Consent Statement: Not applicable.

Data Availability Statement: Not applicable.

Acknowledgments: We thank Frank M LaFerla Institute for Memory Impairments and Neurological Disorders, Department of Neurobiology and Behaviour, University of California, Irvine, USA, for kindly providing the progenitors of the Spanish colonies of 3xTg-AD and NTg mice. LC-M is recipient of a CONICYT/BECAS CHILE/72180026 grant.

Conflicts of Interest: The authors declare no conflict of interest. The funders had no role in the study's design, in the collection, analyses, or interpretation of data; in the writing of the manuscript, or in the decision to publish the results.

References

1. Allan, L.M.; Ballard, C.G.; Burn, D.J.; Kenny, R.A. Prevalence and Severity of Gait Disorders in Alzheimer's and Non-Alzheimer's Dementias. *J. Am. Geriatr. Soc.* **2005**, *53*, 1681–1687. [CrossRef] [PubMed]
2. Buchman, A.S.; Wilson, R.S.; Boyle, P.A.; Bienias, J.L.; Bennett, D.A. Change in Motor Function and Risk of Mortality in Older Persons. *J. Am. Geriatr. Soc.* **2007**, *55*, 11–19. [CrossRef] [PubMed]
3. Fried, L.; Tangen, C.M.; Walston, J.; Newman, A.B.; Hirsch, C.; Gottdiener, J.; Seeman, T.; Tracy, R.; Kop, W.J.; Burke, G.; et al. Frailty in Older Adults: Evidence for a Phenotype. *J. Gerontol. Med. Sci.* **2001**, *56*, M146–M156. [CrossRef] [PubMed]
4. Bland, J.S. Age as a Modifiable Risk Factor for Chronic Disease. *Integr. Med. A Clin. J.* **2018**, *17*, 16–19.
5. Lee, D.R.; Santo, E.C.; Lo, J.C.; Ritterman Weintraub, M.L.; Patton, M.; Gordon, N.P. Understanding functional and social risk characteristics of frail older adults: A cross-sectional survey study. *BMC Fam. Pract.* **2018**, *19*, 170. [CrossRef]
6. Beeri, M.S.; Leurgans, S.E.; Bennett, D.A.; Barnes, L.L.; Buchman, A.S. Diverse Motor Performances Are Related to Incident Cognitive Impairment in Community-Dwelling Older Adults. *Front. Aging Neurosci.* **2021**, *13*, 717139. [CrossRef]
7. Geritz, J.; Maetzold, S.; Steffen, M.; Pilotto, A.; Corrà, M.F.; Moscovich, M.; Rizzetti, M.C.; Borroni, B.; Padovani, A.; Alpes, A.; et al. Motor, cognitive and mobility deficits in 1000 geriatric patients: Protocol of a quantitative observational study before and after routine clinical geriatric treatment—The ComOn-study. *BMC Geriatr.* **2020**, *20*, 45. [CrossRef]
8. Liou, W.C.; Chan, L.; Hong, C.T.; Chi, W.C.; Yen, C.F.; Liao, H.F.; Chen, J.H.; Liou, T.H. Hand fine motor skill disability correlates with dementia severity. *Arch. Gerontol. Geriatr.* **2020**, *90*, 104168. [CrossRef]
9. Poirier, G.; Ohayon, A.; Juranville, A.; Mourey, F.; Gaveau, J. Deterioration, Compensation and Motor Control Processes in Healthy Aging, Mild Cognitive Impairment and Alzheimer's Disease. *Geriatrics* **2021**, *6*, 33. [CrossRef]
10. Scarmeas, N.; Hadjigeorgiou, G.M.; Papadimitriou, A.; Dubois, B.; Sarazin, M.; Brandt, J.; Albert, M.; Marder, K.; Bell, K.; Honig, L.S.; et al. Motor signs during the course of Alzheimer disease. *Neurology* **2004**, *63*, 975–982. [CrossRef]
11. Sperling, R.A.; Mormino, E.C.; Schultz, A.P.; Betensky, R.A.; Papp, K.V.; Amariglio, R.E.; Hanseeuw, B.J.; Buckley, R.; Chhatwal, J.; Hedden, T.; et al. The impact of amyloid-beta and tau on prospective cognitive decline in older individuals. *Ann. Neurol.* **2019**, *85*, 181–193. [CrossRef] [PubMed]
12. Morozova, A.; Zorkina, Y.; Abramova, O.; Pavlova, O.; Pavlov, K.; Soloveva, K.; Volkova, M.; Alekseeva, P.; Andryshchenko, A.; Kostyuk, G.; et al. Neurobiological Highlights of Cognitive Impairment in Psychiatric Disorders. *Int. J. Mol. Sci.* **2022**, *23*, 1217. [CrossRef] [PubMed]
13. Dyer, A.H.; Murphy, C.; Lawlor, B.; Kennelly, S.; Segurado, R.; Olde Rikkert, M.G.M.; Howard, R.; Pasquier, F.; Börjesson-Hanson, A.; Tsolaki, M.; et al. Gait speed, cognition and falls in people living with mild-to-moderate Alzheimer disease: Data from NILVAD. *BMC Geriatr.* **2020**, *20*, 117. [CrossRef] [PubMed]
14. You, Z.Z.; You, Z.Z.; Li, Y.; Zhao, S.; Ren, H.; Hu, X. Alzheimer's disease distinction based on gait feature analysis. In Proceedings of the 2020 International Conference on e-health Networking, Applications and Services (HealthCom), Shenzhen, China, 1–2 March 2021; pp. 1–6. [CrossRef]
15. Buchman, A.S.; Bennett, D.A. Loss of motor function in preclinical Alzheimer's disease. *Expert Rev. Neurother.* **2011**, *11*, 665–676. [CrossRef] [PubMed]
16. Wolkowitz, O.W.; Epel, E.S.; Reus, V.I.; Mellon, S.H. Depression gets old fast: Do stress and depression accelerate cell aging? *Depress. Anxiety* **2010**, *27*, 327–338. [CrossRef] [PubMed]
17. Tanaka, M.; Toldi, J.; Vécsei, L. Exploring the Etiological Links behind Neurodegenerative Diseases: Inflammatory Cytokines and Bioactive Kynurenines. *Int. J. Mol. Sci.* **2020**, *21*, 2431. [CrossRef]
18. Chitnis, T.; Weiner, H.L. CNS inflammation and neurodegeneration. *J. Clin. Investig.* **2017**, *127*, 3577. [CrossRef]

19. Battaglia, S.; Garofalo, S.; di Pellegrino, G. Context-dependent extinction of threat memories: Influences of healthy aging. *Sci. Rep.* **2018**, *8*, 12592. [CrossRef]
20. Ferretti, M.T.; Martinkova, J.; Biskup, E.; Benke, T.; Gialdini, G.; Nedelska, Z.; Rauen, K.; Mantua, V.; Religa, D.; Hort, J.; et al. Sex and gender differences in Alzheimer's disease: Current challenges and implications for clinical practice. *Eur. J. Neurol.* **2020**, *27*, 928–943. [CrossRef]
21. Guo, L.; Zhong, M.B.; Zhang, L.; Zhang, B.; Cai, D. Sex Differences in Alzheimer's Disease: Insights From the Multiomics Landscape. *Biol. Psychiatry* **2022**, *91*, 61–71. [CrossRef]
22. Laws, K.R.; Irvine, K.; Gale, T.M. Sex differences in Alzheimer's disease. *Curr. Opin. Psychiatry* **2018**, *31*, 133–139. [CrossRef] [PubMed]
23. Xing, Y.; Tang, Y.; Jia, J. Sex Differences in Neuropsychiatric Symptoms of Alzheimer's Disease: The Modifying Effect of Apolipoprotein e ε 4 Status. *Behav. Neurol.* **2015**, *275256*. [CrossRef] [PubMed]
24. Gabelli, C.; Codemo, A. Gender differences in cognitive decline and Alzheimer's disease. *Ital. J. Gender-Specific Med.* **2015**, *1*, 21–28. [CrossRef]
25. Laws, K.R.; Irvine, K.; Gale, T.M. Sex differences in cognitive impairment in Alzheimer's disease. *World J. Psychiatry* **2016**, *6*, 54–65. [CrossRef]
26. Kirkland, J.L. Translating advances from the basic biology of aging into clinical application. *Exp. Gerontol.* **2013**, *48*, 1–5. [CrossRef]
27. Kirkland, J.L.; Peterson, C. Healthspan, translation, and new outcomes for animal studies of aging. *J. Gerontol. A Biol. Sci. Med. Sci.* **2009**, *64*, 209–212. [CrossRef]
28. Camargo, L.C.; Honold, D.; Bauer, R.; Jon Shah, N.; Langen, K.J.; Willbold, D.; Kutzsche, J.; Willuweit, A.; Schemmert, S. Sex-related motor deficits in the tau-p301l mouse model. *Biomedicines* **2021**, *9*, 1160. [CrossRef]
29. Kane, A.E.; Shin, S.; Wong, A.A.; Fertan, E.; Faustova, N.S.; Howlett, S.E.; Brown, R.E. Sex differences in healthspan predict lifespan in the 3xTg-AD Mouse model of Alzheimer's Disease. *Front. Aging Neurosci.* **2018**, *10*, 172. [CrossRef]
30. O'Leary, T.P.; Robertson, A.; Chipman, P.H.; Rafuse, V.F.; Brown, R.E. Motor function deficits in the 12 month-old female 5xFAD mouse model of Alzheimer's disease. *Behav. Brain Res.* **2018**, *337*, 256–263. [CrossRef]
31. Castillo-Mariqueo, L.; Pérez-García, M.J.; Giménez-Llort, L. Modeling Functional Limitations, Gait Impairments, and Muscle Pathology in Alzheimer's Disease: Studies in the 3xTg-AD Mice. *Biomedicines* **2021**, *9*, 1365. [CrossRef]
32. Castillo-Mariqueo, L.; Giménez-Llort, L. Kyphosis and bizarre patterns impair spontaneous gait performance in end-of-life mice with Alzheimer's disease pathology while gait is preserved in normal aging. *Neurosci. Lett.* **2021**, 136280. [CrossRef] [PubMed]
33. Castillo-Mariqueo, L.; Giménez-Llort, L. Translational Modeling of Psychomotor Function in Normal and AD-Pathological Aging With Special Concerns on the Effects of Social Isolation. *Front. Aging* **2021**, *2*, 648567. [CrossRef]
34. LaFerla, F.M.; Oddo, S. Alzheimer's disease: Abeta, tau and synaptic dysfunction. *Trends Mol. Med.* **2005**, *11*, 170–176. [CrossRef] [PubMed]
35. Oddo, S.; Caccamo, A.; Shepherd, J.D.; Murphy, M.P.; Golde, T.E.; Kayed, R.; Metherate, R.; Mattson, M.P.; Akbari, Y.; LaFerla, F.M. Triple-Transgenic Model of Alzheimer's Disease with Plaques and Tangles: Intracellular Aβ and Synaptic Dysfunction evaluating the efficacy of anti-AD therapies in mitigating. *Neuron* **2003**, *39*, 409–421. [CrossRef]
36. Kilkenny, C.; Browne, W.J.; Cuthill, I.C.; Emerson, M.; Altman, D.G. Improving Bioscience Research Reporting: The ARRIVE Guidelines for Reporting Animal Research. *PLoS Biol.* **2010**, *8*, e1000412. [CrossRef] [PubMed]
37. Ditzler, S.; Stoeck, J.; Leblanc, M.; Kooperberg, C.; Hansen, S.; Olson, J. A Rapid Neurobehavioral Assessment Reveals that FK506 Delays Symptom Onset in R6/2 Huntington's Disease Mice. *Preclinica.* **2003**, *1*, 115–126.
38. Guyenet, S.J.; Furrer, S.A.; Damian, V.M.; Baughan, T.D.; la Spada, A.R.; Garden, G.A. A simple composite phenotype scoring system for evaluating mouse models of cerebellar ataxia. *J. Vis. Exp.* **2010**, 1–3. [CrossRef]
39. Kojic, M.; Gaik, M.; Kiska, B.; Salerno-Kochan, A.; Hunt, S.; Tedoldi, A.; Mureev, S.; Jones, A.; Whittle, B.; Genovesi, L.A.; et al. Elongator mutation in mice induces neurodegeneration and ataxia-like behavior. *Nat. Commun.* **2018**, *9*, 3195. [CrossRef]
40. Ma, Q.L.; Zuo, X.; Yang, F.; Ubeda, O.; Gant, D.; Alaverdyan, M.; Kiosea, N.; Nazari, S.; Chen, P.P.; Nothias, F.; et al. Loss of MAP function leads to hippocampal synapse loss and deficits in the Morris Water Maze with aging. *J. Neurosci.* **2014**, *34*, 7124–7136. [CrossRef]
41. Whitehead, J.C.; Hildebrand, B.A.; Sun, M.; Rockwood, M.R.; Rose, R.A.; Rockwood, K.; Howlett, S.E. A clinical frailty index in aging mice: Comparisons with frailty index data in humans. *J. Gerontol. Ser. A Biol. Sci. Med. Sci.* **2014**, *69*, 621–632. [CrossRef]
42. Muntsant, A.; Jiménez-Altayó, F.; Puertas-Umbert, L.; Jiménez-Xarrie, E.; Vila, E.; Giménez-Llort, L. Sex-dependent end-of-life mental and vascular scenarios for compensatory mechanisms in mice with normal and ad-neurodegenerative aging. *Biomedicines* **2021**, *9*, 111. [CrossRef] [PubMed]
43. Wang, X.; Wang, Q.M.; Meng, Z.; Yin, Z.; Luo, X.; Yu, D. Gait disorder as a predictor of spatial learning and memory impairment in aged mice. *PeerJ* **2017**, *5*, e2854. [CrossRef] [PubMed]
44. Giménez-Llort, L.; García, Y.; Buccieri, K.; Revilla, S.; Suñol, C.; Cristofol, R.; Sanfeliu, C. Gender-Specific Neuroimmunoendocrine Response to Treadmill Exercise in 3xTg-AD Mice. *Int J. Alzheimers Dis.* **2010**, 128354. [CrossRef]
45. Giménez-Llort, L.; Fernández-Teruel, A.; Escorihuela, R.M.; Fredholm, B.B.; Tobeña, A.; Pekny, M.; Johansson, B. Mice lacking the adenosine A1 receptor are anxious and aggressive, but are normal learners with reduced muscle strength and survival rate. *Eur. J. Neurosci.* **2002**, *16*, 547–550. [CrossRef] [PubMed]

46. Edström, E.; Ulfhake, B. Sarcopenia is not due to lack of regenerative drive in senescent skeletal muscle. *Aging Cell* **2005**, *4*, 65–77. [CrossRef]
47. Torres-Lista, V.; Fuente, M.D.; Giménez-Llort, L. Survival Curves and Behavioral Profiles of Female 3xTg-AD Mice Surviving to 18–Months of Age as Compared to Mice with Normal Aging. *J. Alzheimer's Dis. Reports* **2017**, *1*, 47. [CrossRef] [PubMed]
48. Richardson, A.; Fischer, K.E.; Speakman, J.R.; De Cabo, R.; Mitchell, S.J.; Peterson, C.A.; Rabinovitch, P.; Chiao, Y.A.; Taffet, G.; Miller, R.A.; et al. Measures of Healthspan as Indices of Aging in Mice—A Recommendation. *J. Gerontol. Ser. A Biol. Sci. Med. Sci.* **2016**, *71*, 427–430. [CrossRef]
49. Rae, E.A.; Brown, R.E. The problem of genotype and sex differences in life expectancy in transgenic AD mice. *Neurosci. Biobehav. Rev.* **2015**, *57*, 238–251. [CrossRef]
50. Baglietto-Vargas, D.; Chen, Y.; Suh, D.; Ager, R.R.; Rodriguez-Ortiz, C.J.; Mederios, R.; Myczek, K.; Green, K.N.; Baram, T.Z.; LaFerla, F.M. Short-term modern life-like stress exacerbates Aβ-pathology and synapse loss in 3xTg-AD mice. *J. Neurochem.* **2015**, *134*, 915–926. [CrossRef]
51. Giménez-Llort, L.; Marin-Pardo, D.; Marazuela, P.; Del Hernández-Guillamón, M.M. Survival Bias and Crosstalk between Chronological and Behavioral Age: Age- and Genotype-Sensitivity Tests Define Behavioral Signatures in Middle-Aged, Old, and Long-Lived Mice with Normal and AD-Associated Aging. *Biomedicines* **2021**, *9*, 636. [CrossRef]
52. Brown, R.E.; Shin, S.; Woodland, N.; Rae, E.A. Genotype and Sex Differences in Longevity in Transgenic Mouse Models of Alzheimer's Disease. In *Conn's Handbook of Models for Human Aging*; Academic Press: Cambridge, MA, USA, 2018; pp. 563–576. [CrossRef]
53. Seldeen, K.L.; Pang, M.; Troen, B.R. Mouse Models of Frailty: An Emerging Field. *Curr. Osteoporos. Rep.* **2015**, *13*, 280–286. [CrossRef] [PubMed]
54. Kwak, D.; Baumann, C.W.; Thompson, L.D.V. Identifying Characteristics of Frailty in Female Mice Using a Phenotype Assessment Tool. *J. Gerontol. Ser. A.* **2020**, *75*, 640–646. [CrossRef] [PubMed]
55. Lalonde, R.; Strazielle, C. Brain regions and genes affecting limb-clasping responses. *Brain Res. Rev.* **2011**, *67*, 252–259. [CrossRef] [PubMed]
56. Lieu, C.A.; Chinta, S.J.; Rane, A.; Andersen, J.K. Age-Related Behavioral Phenotype of an Astrocytic Monoamine Oxidase-B Transgenic Mouse Model of Parkinson's Disease. *PLoS ONE* **2013**, *8*, e54200. [CrossRef] [PubMed]
57. Noda, S.; Sato, S.; Fukuda, T.; Tada, N.; Hattori, N. Aging-related motor function and dopaminergic neuronal loss in C57BL/6 mice. *Mol. Brain* **2020**, *13*, 46. [CrossRef]
58. Stover, K.R.; Campbell, M.A.; Van Winssen, C.M.; Brown, R.E. Analysis of motor function in 6-month-old male and female 3xTg-AD mice. *Behav. Brain Res.* **2015**, *281*, 16–23. [CrossRef]
59. Garvock-de Montbrun, T.; Fertan, E.; Stover, K.; Brown, R.E. Motor deficits in 16-month-old male and female 3xTg-AD mice. *Behav. Brain Res.* **2019**, *356*, 305–313. [CrossRef]
60. Filali, M.; Lalonde, R.; Theriault, P.; Julien, C.; Calon, F.; Planel, E. Cognitive and non-cognitive behaviors in the triple transgenic mouse model of Alzheimer's disease expressing mutated APP, PS1, and Mapt (3xTg-AD). *Behav. Brain Res.* **2012**, *2*, 334–342. [CrossRef]
61. Pieruccini-Faria, F.; Black, S.E.; Masellis, M.; Smith, E.E.; Almeida, Q.J.; Li, K.Z.H.; Bherer, L.; Camicioli, R.; Montero-Odasso, M. Gait variability across neurodegenerative and cognitive disorders: Results from the Canadian Consortium of Neurodegeneration in Aging (CCNA) and the Gait and Brain Study. *Alzheimers. Dement.* **2021**, *17*, 1317–1328. [CrossRef]
62. Belghali, M.; Chastan, N.; Cignetti, F.; Davenne, D.; Decker, L.M. Loss of gait control assessed by cognitive-motor dual-tasks: Pros and cons in detecting people at risk of developing Alzheimer's and Parkinson's diseases. *GeroScience* **2017**, *39*, 305–329. [CrossRef]
63. Nadkarni, N.K.; Mawji, E.; Mcllroy, W.E.; Black, S.E. Spatial and temporal gait parameters in Alzheimer's disease and aging. *Gait Posture* **2009**, *30*, 452–454. [CrossRef] [PubMed]
64. Roda, A.R.; Villegas, S.; Esquerda-Canals, G.; Martí-Clúa, J. Cognitive Impairment in the 3xTg-AD Mouse Model of Alzheimer's Disease is Affected by A beta-ImmunoTherapy and Cognitive Stimulation. *Pharmaceutics* **2020**, *12*, 944. [CrossRef] [PubMed]
65. Boyle, P.A.; Buchman, A.S.; Wilson, R.S.; Leurgans, S.E.; Bennett, D.A. Association of muscle strength with the risk of Alzheimer disease and the rate of cognitive decline in community-dwelling older persons. *Arch. Neurol.* **2009**, *66*, 1339–1344. [CrossRef] [PubMed]
66. Murata, S.; Ono, R.; Sugimoto, T.; Toba, K.; Sakurai, T. Functional Decline and Body Composition Change in Older Adults With Alzheimer Disease : A Retrospective Cohort Study at a Japanese Memory Clinic. *Alzheimer Dis. Assoc. Disord.* **2021**, *35*, 36–43. [CrossRef]
67. Eeri, M.S.; Leugrans, S.E.; Delbono, O.; Bennett, D.A.; Buchman, A.S. Sarcopenia is associated with incident Alzheimer's dementia, mild cognitive impairment, and cognitive decline. *J. Am. Geriatr. Soc.* **2021**, *69*, 1826–1835. [CrossRef]
68. Ogawa, Y.; Kaneko, Y.; Shimizu, S.; Kanetaka, H.; Hanyu, H. Sarcopenia and Muscle Functions at Various Stages of Alzheimer Disease. *Front. Neurol.* **2018**, *9*, 710. [CrossRef]
69. Larsson, L.; Degens, H.; Li, M.; Salviati, L.; Lee, Y.; Thompson, W.; Kirkland, J.L.; Sandri, M. Sarcopenia: Aging-Related Loss of Muscle Mass and Function. *Physiol. Rev.* **2019**, *99*, 427–511. [CrossRef]
70. Lalonde, R.; Fukuchi, K.I.; Strazielle, C. Neurologic and motor dysfunctions in APP transgenic mice. *Rev. Neurosci.* **2012**, *23*, 363–379. [CrossRef]

71. Graber, T.G.; Maroto, R.; Fry, C.S.; Brightwell, C.R.; Rasmussen, B.B. Measuring Exercise Capacity and Physical Function in Adult and Older Mice. *J. Gerontol. Ser. A Biol. Sci. Med. Sci.* **2021**, *76*, 819–824. [CrossRef]
72. Hamieh, A.M.; Camperos, E.; Hernier, A.M.; Castagné, V. C57BL/6 mice as a preclinical model to study age-related cognitive deficits: Executive functions impairment and inter-individual differences. *Brain Res.* **2021**, *1751*, 147173. [CrossRef]
73. Justice, J.N.; Carter, C.S.; Beck, H.J.; Gioscia-Ryan, R.A.; McQueen, M.; Enoka, R.M.; Seals, D.R. Battery of behavioral tests in mice that models age-associated changes in human motor function. *Age* **2014**, *36*, 583–595. [CrossRef] [PubMed]
74. Tanaka, H.; Seals, D.R. Endurance exercise performance in Masters athletes: Age-associated changes and underlying physiological mechanisms. *J. Physiol.* **2008**, *586*, 55–63. [CrossRef] [PubMed]
75. Pena, G.S.; Paez, H.G.; Johnson, T.K.; Halle, J.L.; Carzoli, J.P.; Visavadiya, N.P.; Zourdos, M.C.; Whitehurst, M.A.; Khamoui, A.V. Hippocampal Growth Factor and Myokine Cathepsin B Expression following Aerobic and Resistance Training in 3xTg-AD Mice. *Int. J. Chronic Dis.* **2020**, *2020*, 5919501. [CrossRef] [PubMed]
76. Giménez-Llort, L.; Arranz, L.; Maté, I.; De la Fuente, M. Gender-specific neuroimmunoendocrine aging in a triple-transgenic 3xTg-AD mouse model for Alzheimer's disease and its relation with longevity. *Neuroimmunomodulation* **2008**, *15*, 331–343. [CrossRef] [PubMed]
77. Stephens, M.A.C.; Wand, G. Stress and the HPA Axis: Role of Glucocorticoids in Alcohol Dependence. *Alcohol Res.* **2012**, *34*, 468–483. [PubMed]
78. Nguyen, E.T.; Selmanovic, D.; Maltry, M.; Morano, R.; Franco-Villanueva, A.; Estrada, C.M.; Solomon, M.B. Endocrine stress responsivity and social memory in 3xTg-AD female and male mice: A tale of two experiments. *Horm. Behav.* **2020**, 126. [CrossRef]
79. Rothman, S.M.; Herdener, N.; Camandola, S.; Texel, S.J.; Mughal, M.R.; Cong, W.N.; Martin, B.; Mattson, M.P. 3xTgAD mice exhibit altered behavior and elevated Aβ after chronic mild social stress. *Neurobiol. Aging* **2012**, *33*, 830.e1–830.e12. [CrossRef]
80. Bai, A.; Xu, W.; Sun, J.; Liu, J.; Deng, X.; Wu, L.; Zou, X.; Zuo, J.; Zou, L.; Liu, Y.; et al. Associations of sarcopenia and its defining components with cognitive function in community-dwelling oldest old. *BMC Geriatr.* **2021**, *21*, 292. [CrossRef]
81. Buchman, A.S.; Schneider, J.A.; Wilson, R.S.; Bienias, J.L.; Bennett, D.A. Body mass index in older persons is associated with Alzheimer disease pathology. *Neurology* **2006**, *67*, 1949–1954. [CrossRef]
82. Buchman, A.S.; Wilson, R.S.; Bienias, J.L.; Shah, R.C.; Evans, D.A.; Bennett, D.A. Change in body mass index and risk of incident Alzheimer disease. *Neurology* **2005**, *65*, 892–897. [CrossRef]
83. Cui, M.; Zhang, S.; Liu, Y.; Gang, X.; Wang, G. Grip Strength and the Risk of Cognitive Decline and Dementia: A Systematic Review and Meta-Analysis of Longitudinal Cohort Studies. *Front. Aging Neurosci.* **2021**, *13*, 625551. [CrossRef] [PubMed]

biomedicines

Article

Inflammation and Rho-Associated Protein Kinase-Induced Brain Changes in Vascular Dementia

Eun Chae Lee [1,2,†], Dong-Yong Hong [1,2,†], Dong-Hun Lee [1,2], Sang-Won Park [1,2], Ji Young Lee [1], Ji Hun Jeong [2], Eun-Young Kim [3], Hyung-Min Chung [3,4], Ki-Sung Hong [3], Se-Pill Park [3,5], Man Ryul Lee [2,*,‡] and Jae Sang Oh [1,2,*,‡]

1 Department of Neurosurgery, College of Medicine, Cheonan Hospital, Soonchunhyang University, Cheonan 31151, Korea; lec9589@gmail.com (E.C.L.); dydehdghd@gmail.com (D.-Y.H.); madeby58@gmail.com (D.-H.L.); ppphilio3@gmail.com (S.-W.P.); applesori82@gmail.com (J.Y.L.)
2 Soonchunhyang Institute of Medi-Bio Science (SIMS), Soon Chun Hyang University, Cheonan 31151, Korea; jihun@sch.ac.kr
3 Mireacellbio Co., Ltd., Seoul 04795, Korea; jlokey@miraecellbio.com (E.-Y.K.); hmchung@kku.ac.kr (H.-M.C.); kshong@miraecellbio.com (K.-S.H.); sppark@jejunu.ac.kr (S.-P.P.)
4 Department of Stem Cell Biology, School of Medicine, Konkuk University, Seoul 05029, Korea
5 Faculty of Biotechnology, College of Applied Life Sciences, Jeju National University, Jeju 63243, Korea
* Correspondence: leeman@sch.ac.kr (M.R.L.); metatron1324@hotmail.com (J.S.O.)
† These authors contributed equally to this work.
‡ These authors contributed equally to this work.

Abstract: Patients with vascular dementia, caused by cerebral ischemia, experience long-term cognitive impairment due to the lack of effective treatment. The mechanisms of and treatments for vascular dementia have been investigated in various animal models; however, the insufficient information on gene expression changes that define pathological conditions hampers progress. To investigate the underlying mechanism of and facilitate treatment development for vascular dementia, we established a mouse model of chronic cerebral hypoperfusion, including bilateral carotid artery stenosis, by using microcoils, and elucidated the molecular pathway underlying vascular dementia development. Rho-associated protein kinase (ROCK) 1/2, which regulates cellular structure, and inflammatory cytokines (IL-1 and IL-6) were upregulated in the vascular dementia model. However, expression of claudin-5, which maintains the blood–brain barrier, and MAP2 as a nerve cell-specific factor, was decreased in the hippocampal region of the vascular dementia model. Thus, we revealed that ROCK pathway activation loosens the tight junction of the blood–brain barrier and increases the influx of inflammatory cytokines into the hippocampal region, leading to neuronal death and causing cognitive and emotional dysfunction. Our vascular dementia model allows effective study of the vascular dementia mechanism. Moreover, the ROCK pathway may be a target for vascular dementia treatment development in the future.

Keywords: animal model; behavior test; biomarker; blood–brain barrier; cognitive dysfunction; inflammation; memory dysfunction; neuronal cell death; Rho-associated protein kinase; vascular dementia

Citation: Lee, E.C.; Hong, D.-Y.; Lee, D.-H.; Park, S.-W.; Lee, J.Y.; Jeong, J.H.; Kim, E.-Y.; Chung, H.-M.; Hong, K.-S.; Park, S.-P.; et al. Inflammation and Rho-Associated Protein Kinase-Induced Brain Changes in Vascular Dementia. *Biomedicines* **2022**, *10*, 446. https://doi.org/10.3390/biomedicines10020446

Academic Editor: Masaru Tanaka

Received: 26 December 2021
Accepted: 11 February 2022
Published: 14 February 2022

1. Introduction

Vascular dementia is the second leading cause of dementia after Alzheimer's disease (AD), and accounts for 30% of dementia cases in Asia. According to TOAST (trial of ORG 10,172 in acute stroke treatment), classifications of major stroke mechanisms, both in the US and Asia, exhibit a higher risk of ischemic stroke and vascular dementia [1–3].

Vascular dementia, unlike dementia caused by AD, is accompanied by extracranial stenosis or intracranial stenosis and it arises from hemodynamic insufficiency in the brain. While cerebral hypoxic damage is considered the main pathogenic factor in vascular dementia, the mechanism of vascular dementia has not been elucidated in prior research [4–6].

Vascular dementia is mediated by several mechanisms, including oxidative stress, altered cytokine and chemokine levels, and mitochondrial dysfunction [7]. The development of bilateral carotid artery stenosis is accompanied by gradual decreases in the cerebral blood flow. Once vascular insufficiency occurs, inflammatory factor levels increase and changes occur in the cytoskeleton [8]. The decrease in cerebral blood flow due to bilateral carotid artery ligation leads to excessive reactive oxygen species (ROS) [9] and inflammatory cytokine production in ischemic blood vessels, leading to antioxidant system inhibition [10], an inflammatory environment [11–13], and a low energy state, resulting in cell damage and mitochondrial dysfunction [14,15]. This was observed as cognitive decline due to nerve damage in the white matter [16], corpus callosum, and hippocampus [17] in both humans and animals. Inflammation is insufficient to explain the pathogenesis of vascular dementia. Additionally, the role of Rho-associated protein kinase (ROCK), an important marker of cytoskeletal changes, has been reported in some ischemia models, but has not been well-studied in vascular dementia.

In the present study, we aimed to elucidate the molecular mechanism underlying vascular dementia development by using an established animal model [18]. The bilateral carotid artery stenosis (BCAS) model is well-known in vascular dementia research and is considered sufficient for representing clinical vascular insufficiency in the brain [19]. In order to implement an accurate disease model, we generated a BCAS model and confirmed, by behavioral analysis, that it represented early vascular dementia. Then, using this model, we investigated the pathogenesis and underlying mechanisms of vascular dementia based on the putative pathways of hypoxia-induced inflammatory blood–brain barrier (BBB) disruption, ROCK-induced cytoskeletal changes caused by vascular insufficiency, cell apoptosis, and structural changes in the cortex, corpus callosum, and hippo-campus.

2. Materials and Methods

2.1. Animals

All experimental procedures were performed at the Experimental Animal Center of the Soonchunhyang Institute of Medi-Bio Science (SIMS, Cheonan, South Korea). All animal experiments were performed in compliance with the Institutional Animal Care and Use Committee of Soon Chun Hyang University (IACUC No. SCH 20-0065) and the Guidelines for the Care and Use of Laboratory Animals specified by the National Research Council.

The experimental mice were housed in room with a 12-h light–dark cycle (7:00 a.m.–7:00 p.m.), with a temperature of 23 °C ± 1–2 °C and with a humidity of 50 ± 5%.

2.2. Experimental Design

Female Balb/c nude mice (nine weeks old) were obtained from Orientbio (Seongnam, South Korea). After a one-week habituation period, we prepared a BCAS model in the 10-week-old mice. We designated the normal type (NT) group as the control group and designated the vascular dementia (VD) group as the experimental group. The experimental design was based on a previously reported study and was performed using microcoil implantation (SWPAO. 08 × 0.18 × 0.5 × 2.5, Samini Spring/Sawane, Shizuoka, Japan) (Figure 1A) [4]. Briefly, the mice were anesthetized with isoflurane (Hana Pharm, Seoul, South Korea). Mice were then fixed on the microscope (in the supine position), and a midline incision was made over the cervical region to expose their common carotid arteries (CCAs), which were then freed from their sheaths. We next carefully affixed microcoils to the carotid artery [20]. Finally, the wound was sutured with 6–0 silk. All processes were performed on a heating pad (25–26 °C). The mice were monitored for weight, body temperature, and paralysis twice weekly after surgery until stabilization occurred. Vascular dementia modeling was confirmed with behavioral analysis when mice were 16 weeks old. Molecular analyses were subsequently performed (Figure 1B).

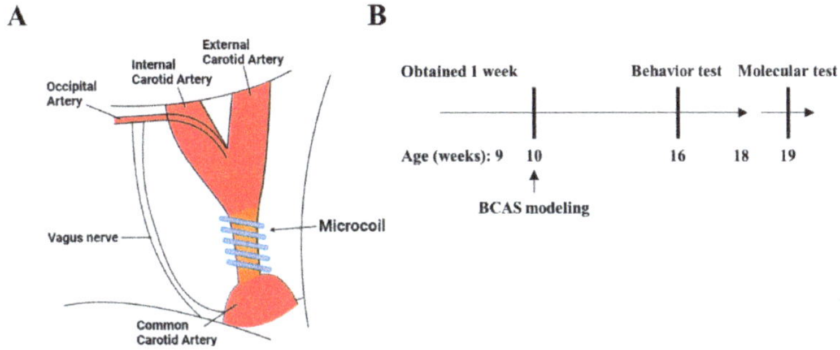

Figure 1. Modeling vascular dementia in a bilateral carotid artery stenosis (BCAS) mouse model. (**A**) The third rotation of the microcoil around the total carotid artery, after which the microcoil was tied. Blood vessel color change due to decreased blood flow due to microcoil ligation. (**B**) Schematic representation of the BCAS surgical strategy.

2.3. Behavior Tests

All behavioral analyses were performed at the Experimental Animal Center of Soonchunhyang Institute of Medi-Bio Science (SIMS, Cheonan, South Korea) and were conducted in a custom-made chamber (Scitech Korea, Seoul, South Korea) to reduce experimental deviation. White noise was present at a level of approximately 60 dB. Additionally, all experimental data (with the exception of the passive avoidance test) were analyzed using Smart v3.0 software (Panlab, Barcelona, Spain). Passive avoidance tests were con-ducted using a shut-avoidance program (Panlab, Barcelona, Spain). Statistically significant differences were confirmed using unpaired t-tests after conducting the experiments in triplicate.

2.3.1. Y-Maze Test

A Y-maze (Gaon-Bio, Yongin, South Korea) was used to assess short-term memory and the locomotor activity index. The experimental time was eight min for each subject. Each mouse was initially placed in arm A (among zones A, B, and C, as well as the center of the maze box) and the correct alteration/total number of entries was recorded. The light intensity was set to 390 lx.

2.3.2. Barnes-Maze Test

The Barnes-maze test (Gaon-Bio, Yongin, South Korea) evaluates learning, memory, and cognitive flexibility. The apparatus for this test was a circular black platform, 90 mm in diameter (18 holes). The experimental design was as follows. Block 1 included a training phase (three minutes to find and enter the escape route). Block 2 included a probe phase (removing the escape box and evaluating the time spent in the quadrant where the escape box had originally been located). Each mouse was placed in the middle of the apparatus. The time spent in each quadrant (i.e., the target zone, the target hole, and the error zone) were recorded. This experiment was repeated every day for four days. The light intensity was set to 390 lx.

2.3.3. Passive Avoidance Test

The passive avoidance test (Harvard Apparatus, Holliston, MA, USA) is a test of long-term memory based on fear. The mouse was placed in a light compartment in the main box and was allowed a search time of 1 min. After 1 min, the door was opened, and the mouse entered a dark compartment. After the mouse entered the dark compartment for 2 s, the door was closed. The mouse was given an electric shock for 5 s. This experiment was repeated for four days. The light intensity in the box was set to 390 lx.

2.3.4. Open Field Test

An open field test (Gaon-Bio, Yongin, South Korea) was used to assess motor activity and anxiety. Specifically, a 45 × 45 × 40-cm square open field was used for this test. The experimental time was 10 min for each subject. Each mouse was placed in the middle of the field. The center and peripheral zones were set to light intensities of 390 lx.

2.3.5. Light and Dark Test

The light and dark test (Domestic) was used to assess locomotor activity and anxiety. The mice were placed in a 45 × 45 × 40 cm diameter square box with a black partition. The experimental time was 10 min for each subject. The large chamber was open and brightly illuminated (390 lx), while the small chamber was closed and dark. Each mouse was placed in the dark box. After 5 s, the door was opened. The experimental zones were maintained with the light and dark zones. The light intensity was set to 390 lx in the light zone.

2.4. Reverse-Transcription Quantitative Real-Time PCR

After being harvested, the frozen left hemisphere of each mouse (200 mg) was prepared and homogenized. To determine the mRNA expression levels of the target genes, total RNA was extracted from the mouse brain tissue using an easy-BLUE™ Total RNA Extraction Kit (iNtRON, Daejeon, Korea) according to the manufacturer's protocol. The concentration and quality of the isolated RNA were determined using a NanoDrop spectrophotometer (NanoDrop Technologies, LLC; Wilmington, DE, USA). Next, cDNA was synthesized using 2 μg total RNA with an All-in-One 5 × First Strand cDNA Master Mix (CellScript, Madison, WI, USA), and quantitative real-time PCR (qRT-PCR) was performed using TOPreal™ qPCR 2X PreMIX (Enzynomics, Daejeon, Korea) according to the manufacturer's protocol. Rock1, Rock2, Occludin, Claudin-5, Il-6, Il-1β, Mcp-1, Ccrr2, and VCAM-1 mRNA transcript levels were detected using the CFX Connect Real-Time PCR Detection System (Bio-Rad, Hercules, CA, USA).

2.5. Immunohistochemical Staining

The paraffin-embedded sections were dewaxed with xylene and dehydrated with a graded alcohol series. Subsequently, sections were incubated in 3% (w/v) H_2O_2 for 2 min and washed with PBS three times for 5 min each. Next, antigens were retrieved with 10 mM sodium citrate buffer. The sections were treated with peroxidase for 10 min in blocking solution to block endogenous peroxidase, and then in 5% goat serum for 10 min to block non-specific antibody binding. Overnight incubation with rabbit anti-alpha smooth muscle actin (α-SMA) polyclonal antibody (1:300; abcam, Boston, MA, USA) or rabbit anti-microtubule-associated protein 2 (MAP2) polyclonal antibody (1:500; GeneTex, Irvine, CA, USA) was performed in humidified boxes at 4 °C. Phosphate-buffered saline (PBS) was used as a negative control. Staining was then developed with a 3,3′-diaminobenzidine (DAB) solution for 3 min. Tissues were rinsed in PBS three times, for 5 min each time, between each step, and then stained with hematoxylin. Sections were subsequently mounted, dehydrated, coverslipped, and examined under a Motic Easyscanone (Houston, TX, USA). Immunohistochemistry was analyzed with an Motic Digital Slide assistant system (Motic China Group Co., Ltd., Xiamen, China).

2.6. Luxol Fast Blue Staining

Luxol fast blue (LFB) staining was performed on brain sections to visualize myelin tracts in the corpus callosum. After rehydration in distilled water, the sections were stained with LFB solution for 2 h at 60 °C followed by differentiation in 0.05% lithium carbonate solution and 70% ethanol for 45 s to 2 min until the gray matter was colorless while the white matter stained blue and was sharply defined. The sections were then washed in distilled water, dehydrated, cleared, and coverslipped.

2.7. Statistical Analysis

Statistical analyses were performed using GraphPad Prism 8 software (GraphPad, Inc., San Diego, CA, USA). Data are presented as means ± standard deviations (SD). For comparisons involving more than two groups, all analyses were performed at least in triplicate and statistical differences were analyzed via unpaired *t*-tests. Two-sided *p*-values of <0.05 were considered statistically significant.

3. Results

3.1. Behavior Testing Results

In the NT group, short-term spatial memory measurements were obtained using the Y-maze test [16,21,22]. However, BCAS mice showed repetitive behavior with memory impairment, entering the same arm repeatedly (Figure 2A). We found that the percentage was lower in the VD group than in the NT group (NT 48.2% vs. VD 34.6%; $p < 0.05$, Figure 2B, Table 1). Moreover, the total number of arm entries during the test was considerably greater in the NT than in the VD group (NT 48.1% vs. VD 34.6%, $p < 0.04$, Figure 2B, Table 1). The higher percentage of alternation triplets in the BCAS model demonstrated a tendency for these mice to explore new environments; thus, our study conclusively confirmed a protocol for building and evaluating a BCAS mouse model [21].

Table 1. Y-maze tests and animal assignments.

	Group	No. of Mice	Mean Value
Y-maze (Alternation triplet)	NT	9	47.22
	VD	9	33.29 *
Y-maze (Total arm entry)	NT	9	48.13
	VD	9	34.61 **

Values are means ± standard deviations. * $p < 0.05$ and ** $p < 0.01$ represent the tendency and significant difference, respectively.

The Barnes-maze test was used to assess spatial learning and memory impairment (Figure 3A) [23,24]. Repeated experiments were conducted over the course of four days to determine if the location of the food was remembered through several instances of repeated learning. In the NT group, the distance and time to find the target was decreased on the last day as compared to the first day, whereas the time to find the target was increased in the VD group (Figure 3B,C, Table 2). During exploratory trials, the VD group animals spent a statistically significant less amount of time in the target quadrant (where the escape box had previously been located; NT 38.84% vs. VD 14.7%, $p < 0.01$, Figure 3D, Table 2). Based on comparison of the time required to find the target hole (NT, 6 s vs. VD, 18.7 s, $p < 0.01$, Figure 3E, Table 2), we concluded that VD group mice found it difficult to locate the target hole, despite repeated training.

Table 2. Barnes-maze tests and animal assignments.

	Group	No. of Mice	Mean Value
Barnes-maze (Time spent in target quadrant)	NT	9	38.84
	VD	8	14.74 **
Barnes-maze (Time to the find target hole)	NT	17	6.060
	VD	9	18.73 ***

Values are means ± standard deviations. ** $p < 0.01$ and *** $p < 0.001$ represent the tendency and significant difference, respectively.

The passive avoidance test was used to evaluate negative learning and long-term memory by repeatedly evoking entrapment. When the mice remembered the stress induced by the electrical shock in the text box, the time spent in the test box differed between the NT and VD groups (Figure 4, Table 3) [16,22,25]. In the VD group, memory was not established, despite repetitive learning, whereas in the NT group, memory was maintained over time.

On day three, we found a statistically significant difference between the VD and NT groups (VD 265.7 s vs. NT 107.4 s). Thus, BCAS modeling could induce mice to step into the electric shock box more frequently, confirming that fear avoidance and hippocampus-dependent contextual memory were degraded in these model mice.

Table 3. Passive avoidance test and animal assignments.

	Group	No. of Mice	Mean Value
Passive avoidance	NT	9	38.84
	VD	8	14.74 **

Values are means ± standard deviations. ** $p < 0.01$ represents the tendency and significant difference.

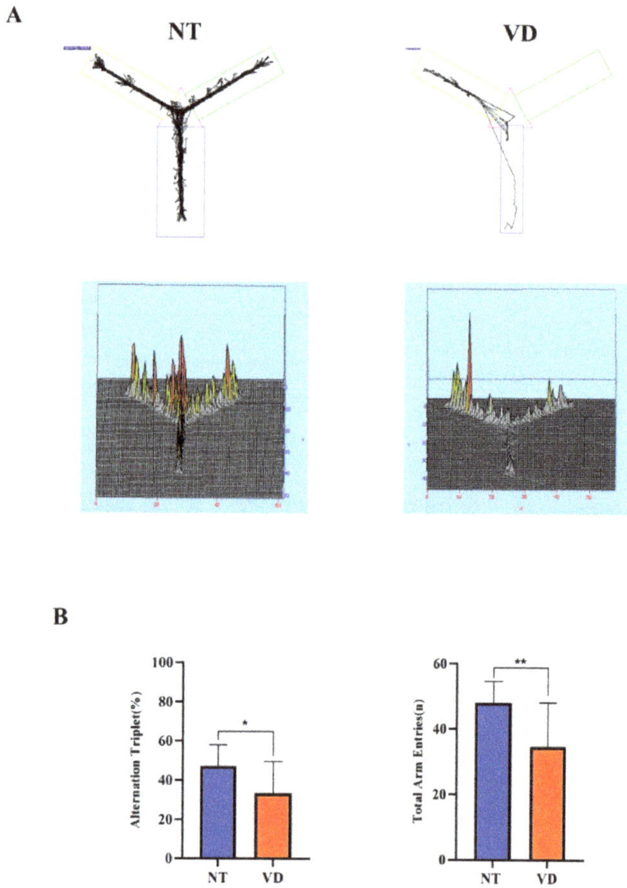

Figure 2. Y-maze test (normal type [NT]: control group and blue color graph, vascular dementia [VD]: BCAS [bilateral carotid artery stenosis] model group and madarin color graph). (**A**) Recorded experimental data. The start zone is the blue box. (**B**) Differences in the alternation triplet percentage between groups (left). Differences in the total number of arm entries between groups (right). Data are expressed as means ± standard deviations (SD). (* $p < 0.05$; ** $p < 0.01$).

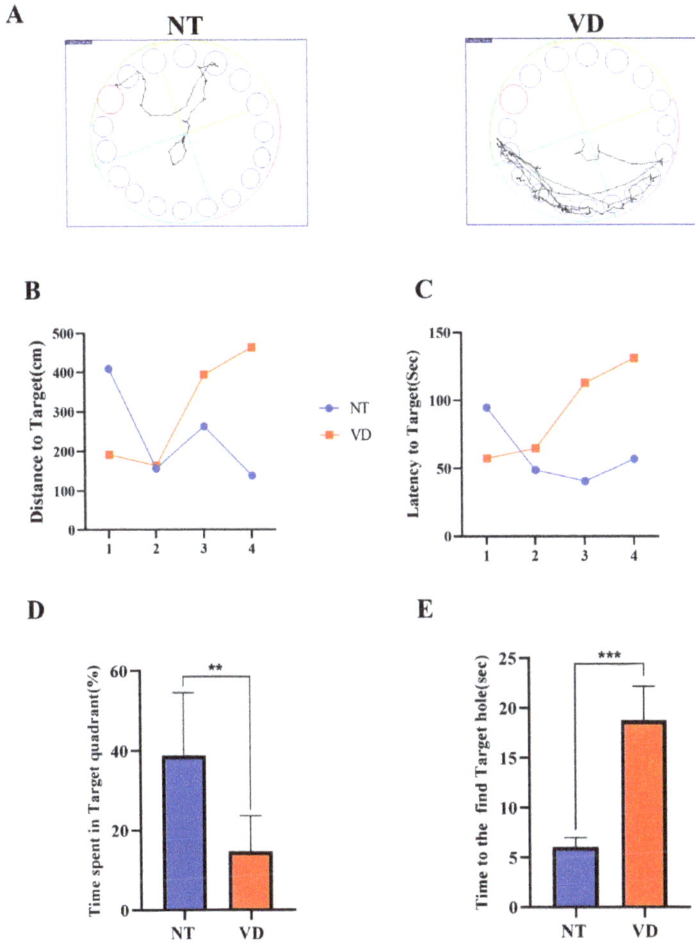

Figure 3. Barnes-maze test (NT [normal type]: control group, VD [vascular dementia]: BCAS [bilateral carotid artery stenosis] model group). (**A**) Recorded experimental data. The target zone was designated via a red circle and the error zone was designated via a blue circle (left: NT, right: VD). (**B**) Differences between groups for the distance to the target (by day). (**C**) Differences between groups for latency to the target (by day). (**D**) Differences between groups in the percentage of time spent in the time quadrant ** $p < 0.01$. (**E**) Differences between groups in the time spent to find the target hole in the time quadrant *** $p < 0.001$. Data are expressed as means ± standard deviations (SD).

In the open field test (an anxiety test for mice), the NT group spent more time in the peripheral area than in the central area (Figure 5A) [26,27]. In the peripheral zone, the VD group moved a shorter distance than did the NT group (Figure 5B, left, Table 4). In the central area, the NT group showed a longer movement distance than did the VD group (Figure 5B, right, Table 4). Total movement distance was only slightly different between the VD and NT groups (Figure 5C, Table 4). The light/dark transition test confirmed that mice in the VD group were less anxious than the NT mice, given that mice demonstrate more anxiety in bright light (Figure 5D, Table 4) [28,29] (NT 22.1 vs. VD 12.5, $p < 0.0113$).

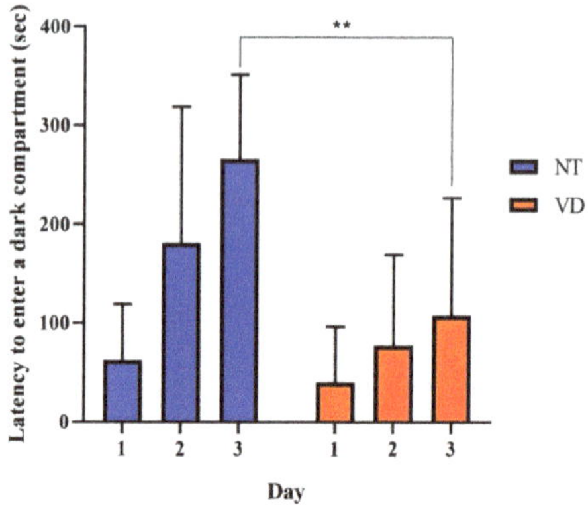

Figure 4. Passive avoidance test. Negative memory was evaluated based on the mean latency time (s) to enter the electric shock box. (NT [normal type]: control group, VD [vascular dementia]: BCAS [bilateral carotid artery stenosis] model group). Data are expressed as means ± standard deviations (SD), ** $p < 0.01$.

Table 4. Open field, light and dark test, and animal assignments.

	Group	No. of Mice	Mean Value
Open field (Distance in periphery zone)	NT VD	9 8	3192 3050
Open field (Distance in center zone)	NT VD	11 10	477.6 504.8
Open field (Total distance)	NT VD	12 9	NS
Light and dark (Transition)	NT VD	13 7	22.15 12.57 *

Values are means ± standard deviations * $p < 0.05$ represents the tendency and significant difference.

These behavioral analyses confirmed that the BCAS animal model demonstrated clinical characteristics of human vascular dementia.

3.2. Increases in ROCK Expression in the Brains of VD Model Mice

Next, to identify the specific mechanism associated with induced vascular dementia, we isolated the brains of the VD model mice and used RT-qPCR to determine mRNA transcription levels of ROCK in the NT and VD groups to identify the mechanisms causing ischemic brain injury in VD mice. ROCK regulates actin cytoskeletal reorganization and interaction with tight junction (TJ) proteins in endothelial cells. ROCK mRNA levels were higher in the VD group than in the NT group (Rock1: 1.00 [NT] vs. 17.48 [VD], $p = 0.0003$; Figure 6A, Table 5; Rock2: 1.00 [NT] vs. 15.01 [VD], $p = 0.0006$, Figure 6B, Table 5). Therefore, BCAS statistically significantly increased Rock expression, suggesting that TJ protein redistribution occurred in BCAS-induced brain injury.

Table 5. List of the experimental groups (Rock1/2).

	Group	No. of Mice	Mean Value
Rock1	NT VD	9 9	1 17.48 ***
Rock2	NT VD	9 9	1 15.01 ***

Values are means ± standard deviations. *** $p < 0.001$ represents the tendency and significant difference.

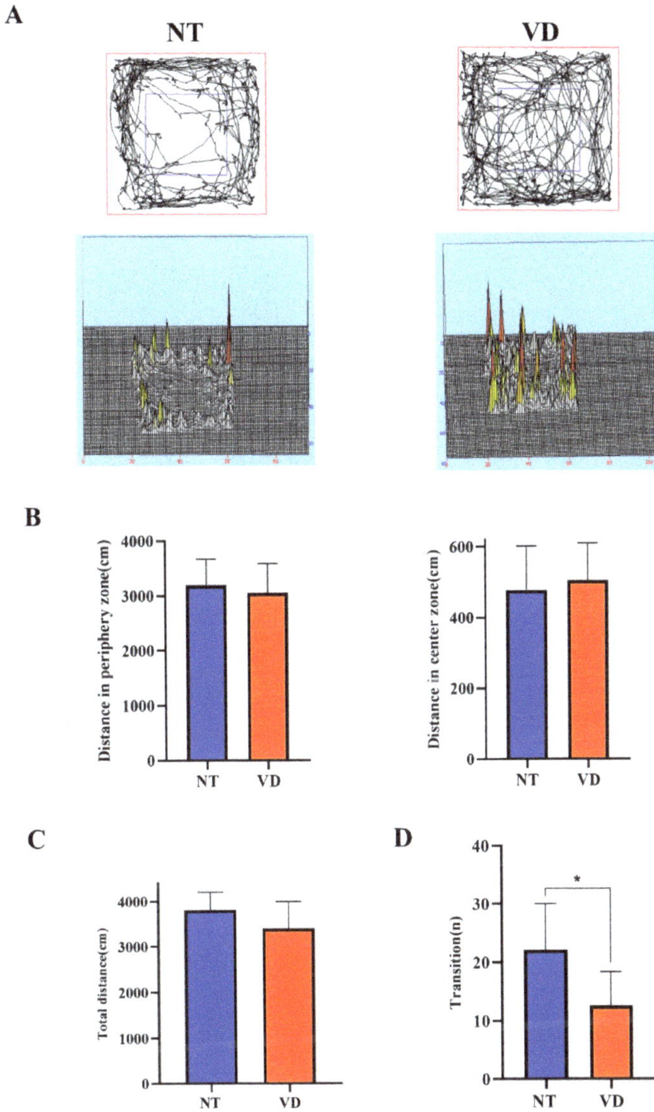

Figure 5. A depiction of the open field test and the light and dark test (NT [normal type]: control group, VD [vascular dementia]: BCAS [bilateral carotid artery stenosis] model group). (**A**) Smart 3.0 analysis program data (left: NT, right: VD). (**B**) Differences in the distance moved between the peripheral zone (NT, 3192.1 cm; VD, 3050.2 cm) and the central zone (NT, 483 cm; VD, 521.8 cm) (**C**) Differences between groups in the total distance moved in the open field test. (**D**) Differences between groups in the number of transitions in the light/dark transition test, * $p < 0.05$. Data are expressed as means ± standard deviations (SD).

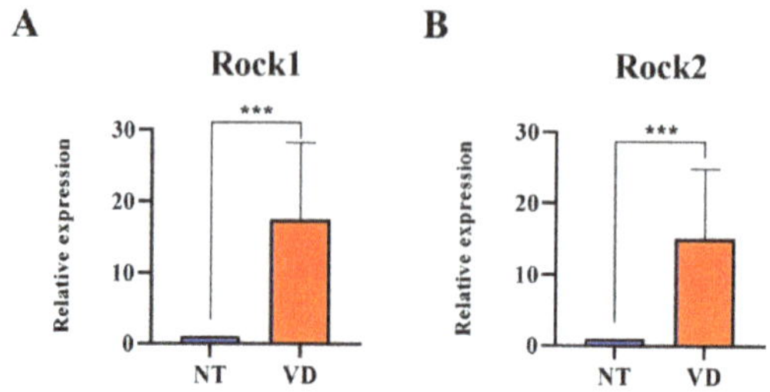

Figure 6. Rock mRNA expression in the brain of bilateral carotid artery stenosis (BCAS) mice. (NT [normal type]: control group, VD [vascular dementia]: BCAS [bilateral carotid artery stenosis] model group). (**A**,**B**) mRNA expression of ROCK1/2 was determined by quantitative real-time polymerase chain reaction in the two groups (NT, VD) after BCAS. *** $p < 0.001$. The results are expressed as mean values and the error bars represent standard deviations.

3.3. Reduction in TJ Protein Expression in the Brain of VD Model Mice

Increased expression of ROCK in VD mice indicated a decrease in TJ-related proteins. In brain vascular endothelial cells, TJs form barriers that limit cell permeability. After BCAS, the mRNA expression levels of Occludin and Claudin-5, which encode proteins in-volved in TJs, were statistically significantly reduced in the BCAS group as compared to the NT group (Occludin: 1.00 [NT] vs. 0.69 [VD], $p = 0.0745$, Figure 7A, Table 6; Claudin-5: 1.00 [NT] vs. 0.58 [VD], $p = 0.0300$, Figure 7B, Table 6). BCAS disrupted the BBB through decreased endothelial adhesion junction protein expression and increased ROCK expression. The decrease in the expression of Occludin and Claudin-5 indicates the collapse of the BBB structure, which is likely to increase inflammatory reactions.

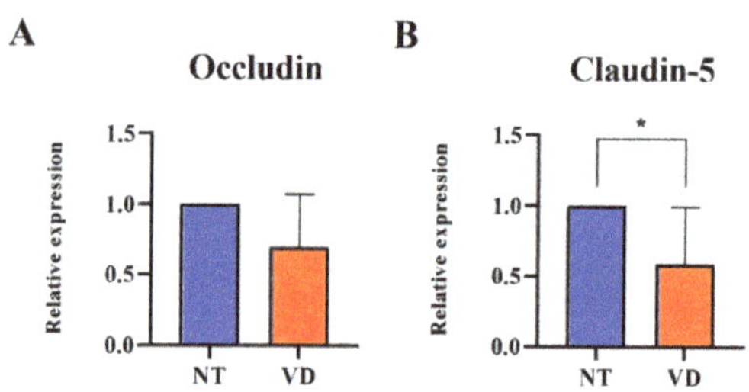

Figure 7. Quantitative real-time polymerase chain reaction analysis revealed that bilateral carotid artery stenosis (BCAS) induced decreased mRNA levels of Occludin and Claudin-5 in the VD group. (NT [normal type]: control group, VD [vascular dementia]: BCAS [bilateral carotid artery stenosis] model group). (**A**,**B**) Relative mRNA expressioin levels of Occludin and Claudin-5. * $p < 0.05$. The results are represented as mean values and the error bars represent standard deviations.

Table 6. Occludin and Claudin-5.

	Group	No. of Mice	Mean Value
Occludin	NT VD	9 9	1 0.69
Claudin-5	NT VD	9 9	1 0.58 *

Values are means ± standard deviations. * $p < 0.05$ represents the tendency and significant difference.

3.4. Increased Expression of Adhesion Molecules and Pro-Inflammatory Cytokines in VD Mice

Vascular cell attachment molecules-1 (VCAM-1) control the occurrence and amplification of tissue inflammation during ischemic brain damage. Many inflammatory factors are elevated in brain diseases when the BBB is damaged. Inflammatory factors bound to white blood cell ligands by cell adhesion molecules migrate to the injured brain tissue [30–33]. In this study, the change in mRNA expression in the pro-inflammatory milieu of the BCAS model was confirmed by RT-qPCR. VCAM-1, Il-6, Il-1β, Mcp-1, and Ccr2 were statistically significantly higher in the VD group than in the NT group (VCAM-1: 1.00 [NT] vs. 2.82 [VD], $p < 0.0001$, Figure 8E, Table 7; Il-6: 1.00 [NT] vs. 116.7 [VD], $p < 0.0007$, Figure 8A, Table 7; Il-1β: 1.00 [NT] vs. 20.08 [VD], $p < 0.0058$, Figure 8B, Table 7; Mcp-1: 1.00 [NT] vs. 4.12 [VD], $p < 0.0635$, Figure 8C, Table 7; Ccr2: 1.00 [NT] vs. 1.69 [VD], $p = 0.3846$, Figure 8D, Table 7). These results suggested that increased inflammatory reactions occur through the expression of high levels of adhesion molecules and pro-inflammatory cytokines associated with pathological conditions in the VD group.

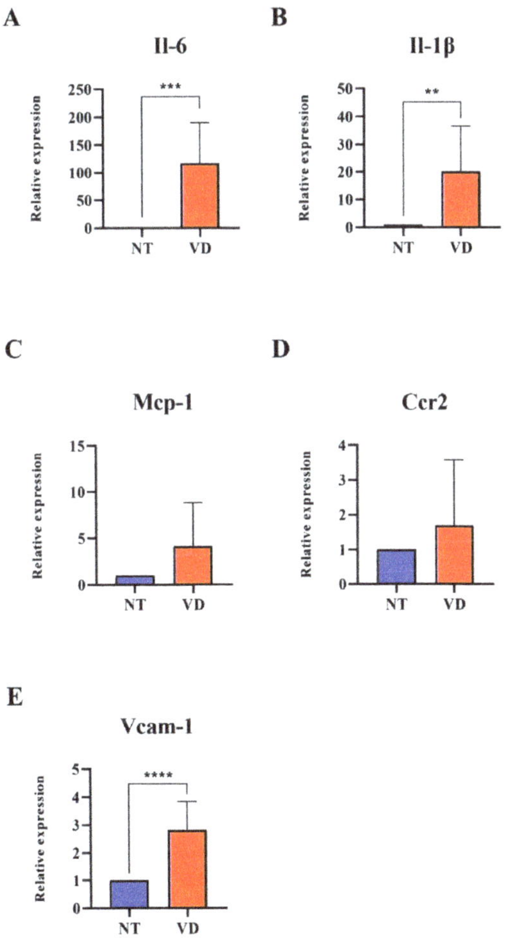

Figure 8. Upregulated expression of adhesion molecules and pro-inflammatory cytokines after BCAS (NT [normal type]: control group, VD [vascular dementia]: BCAS [bilateral carotid artery stenosis] model group) (**A–E**) Relative mRNA expression levels of IL-6, IL-1β, Mcp-1, Ccr2, and VCAM-1. ** $p < 0.01$, *** $p < 0.001$, and **** $p < 0.001$. The results are presented as mean values and the error bars standard deviations.

Table 7. Pro-inflammatory cytokines.

	Group	No. of Mice	Mean Value
Il-6	NT VD	9 9	1 116.7 ***
Il-1β	NT VD	9 9	1 20.08 **
Mcp-1	NT VD	9 9	1 4.12
Ccr2	NT VD	9 9	1 1.69
Vcam-1	NT VD	9 9	1 2.82 ****

Values are means ± standard deviations. ** $p < 0.01$, *** $p < 0.001$, and **** $p < 0.0001$ represent the tendency and significant difference, respectively.

3.5. Vasoconstriction and Apoptosis in the VD Group

α-SMA induces chronic angiopathy in obstructive vascular diseases, including ischemic stroke. The terminal deoxynucleotidyl transferase dUTP nick end labeling (TUNEL) assay detects DNA fragments generated during cell apoptosis. In the VD mouse brains, α-SMA and TUNEL were confirmed by immunohistochemistry (IHC). The VD group showed statistically significantly higher α-SMA (Figure 9A, Table 8) and TUNEL (Figure 9B, Table 8) staining than the NT group. These results suggest that BCAS can induce brain damage by increasing α-SMA expression in the hippocampus, as well as by inducing an increase in vasoconstriction and apoptosis.

Table 8. α-SMA and TUNEL.

	Group	No. of Mice	Mean Value
α-SMA	NT VD	3 1	0 0.165
TUNEL	NT VD	1 1	0.187 0.451

Values are means ± standard deviations.

3.6. Changes in Brain Structure in the VD Group

The cerebral cortex is a collection of neurons located on the surface of the cerebrum. The corpus callosum consists of thick bundles of nerve fibers that connect to the cerebral hemispheres, allowing interhemispheric conduction of signals [34,35]. In the VD group, irregularities in cortical arrangement (Figure 10A,B) and decreased MAP2-positive neurons (Figure 10C,D) in the cornu ammonis (CA1) region of the hippocampus were confirmed. LFB staining appeared uniformly throughout the corpus callosum in the NT group, but was not uniformly found in the VD group (Figure 10E,F, Table 9) [36]. The corpus callosum thickness was reduced in the VD group as compared to the NT group [37]. These results suggest increased cortical, hippocampal, and corpus callosum damage in the VD group, due to decreased cerebral blood flow.

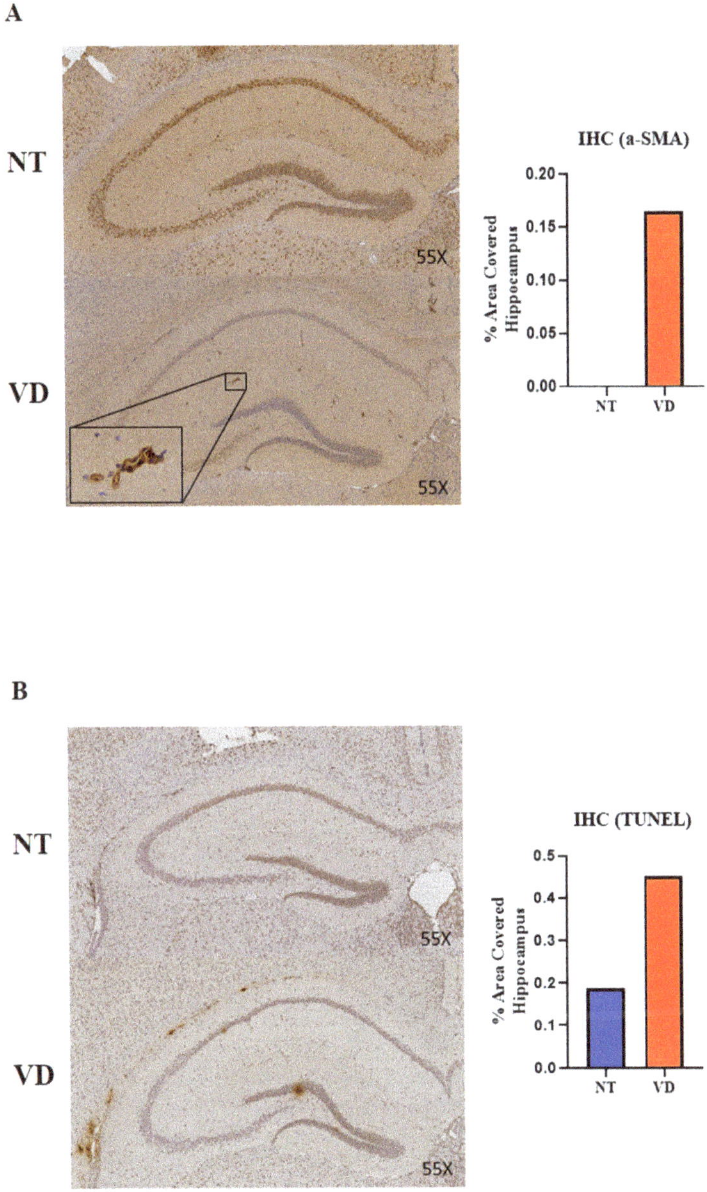

Figure 9. Immunoreactivity of alpha smooth muscle actin (α-SMA) and results of a terminal deoxynucleotidyl transferase dUTP nick end labeling (TUNEL) assay in the hippocampus in the NT and VD groups (NT [normal type]: control group, VD [vascular dementia]: BCAS [bilateral carotid artery stenosis] model group). (**A**,**B**) Left: representative photomicrographs of α-SMA in TUNEL immunoreactive cells. Right: quantification of α-SMA through TUNEL immunoreactivity.

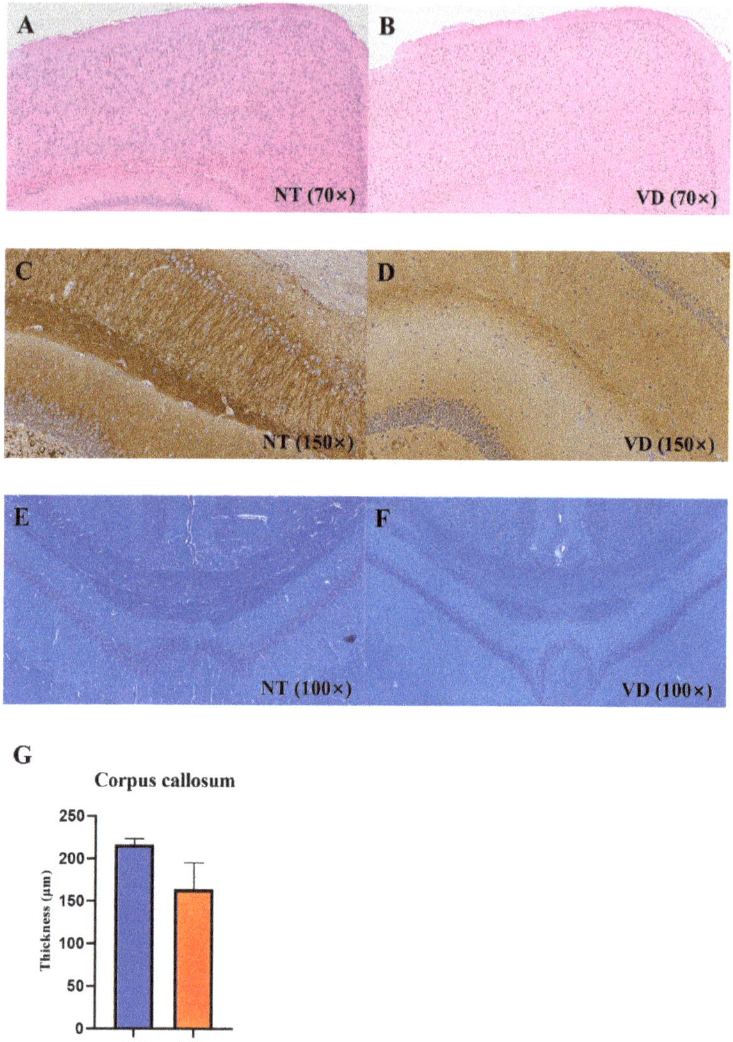

Figure 10. Hematoxylin and eosin (H&E), immunohistochemistry (IHC; MAP2), and Luxol fast blue staining in the brains of the VD group. NT [normal type]: control group, VD [vascular dementia]: BCAS [bilateral carotid artery stenosis] model group). (**A**,**B**) H&E staining in the NT and VD groups. (**C**,**D**) MAP2 IHC in the NT and VD groups (hippocampal cornu ammonis [CA1] region). (**E**,**F**) Myelin staining. Coronal sections of paraffin-embedded brains from the NT and VD groups were stained with Luxol fast blue. All images are of the cerebral cortex (left) and the hippocampus (right). (**G**) Thickness of the corpus callosum in NT and in VD mouse tissue, obtained using Image J software.

Table 9. Corpus callosum.

	Group	No. of Mice	Mean Value
Corpus callosum	NT	3	216.2
	VD	2	163.9

Values are means ± standard deviations.

4. Discussion

Chronic hypoperfusion has two effects. First, a hypoxic injury phenomenon is induced, which can cause BBB collapse, which results in inflammation and cytokine changes. It is already established that an ischemic dementia model can elucidate the mechanisms of neuronal death and dysfunction after ischemia. In the present study, we established a vascular insufficiency model (a BCAS model) using a microcoil [38–40]. The low ischemia was induced by occlusion of the common carotid and vertebral arteries, resulting in inflammation and BBB disruption in the absence of motor weakness. Results from our study identified behavioral deficits in the VD model. The results of the Y-maze and Barnes-maze confirmed that spatial learning, short-term memory, spatial cognitive ability, and cognitive ability were adversely affected by BCAS in the VD group [41–44]. As a confirmation of early vascular dementia, we found that cell changes in CA1 levels in the hippocampus occurred at 6 weeks post-BCAS. Changes in the nucleus and cell rearrangement in the brain cortex, corpus callosum, and white matter tract were similarly confirmed [16,45]. We then investigated the pathogenesis and mechanisms for vascular dementia according to the putative pathways of hypoxia-induced inflammatory BBB disruption: ROCK-induced cytoskeletal changes due to vascular insufficiency, apoptosis, and structural changes in the cortex, corpus callosum, and hippocampus (Figure 11), and showed gene expression changes that reflected these events. BBB disruption is a pathological hallmark of ischemic brain injury [46]. However, the mechanism underlying this process remains unclear. In our study, we found that increased Rock and inflammatory factors accompanied BBB disruption (Figures 6–8). Our findings suggest that ROCK, adhesion molecules, and pro-inflammatory cytokines are important physiological and pathological modulators.

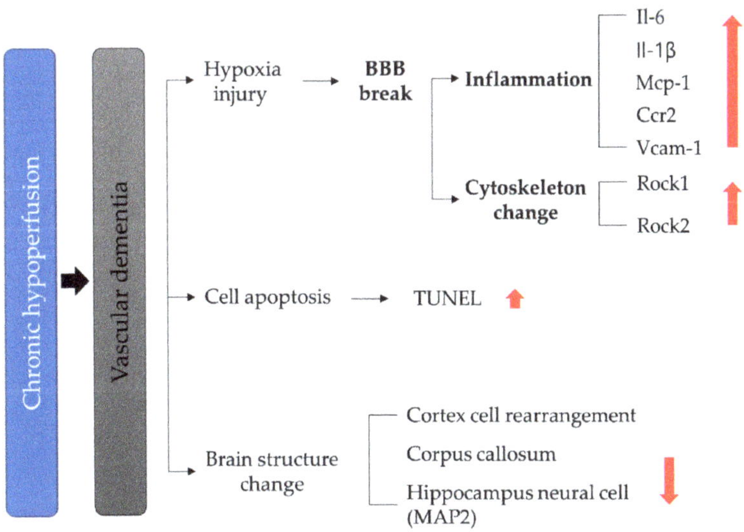

Figure 11. Schematic representation of vascular dementia.

Ischemic brain injury is accompanied by increased inflammation as well as increased BBB permeability [47]. In the ischemic brain, inflammatory mediators stimulate cerebral endothelial cells to induce inflammatory responses [48,49]. Expression of the VCAM-1 adhesion molecule has been comprehensively studied as an indicator of inflammation in models of cerebral ischemia [50]. Our results indicated an increase in VCAM-1 levels after the BCAS group. Additionally, the major pro-inflammatory cytokines evaluated in this study were Il1, Il6, and Mcp1 [47,51]. These cytokines are initiators of the inflammatory response and promote the expression of adhesion molecules [52], suggesting that pro-inflammatory cytokines upregulated adhesion molecules and aggravated brain injury in the VD mice in our study [53].

The BBB is required for the structural stabilization of TJ proteins as structural components that maintain cerebrovascular integrity and BBB function [54,55]. Activated ROCK and pro-inflammatory cytokines correspond to vascular endothelial damage [51,56]. We found an inflammatory response that was upregulated by higher vascular permeability in the ischemic-injured brains of the VD group (Figure 8A–E).

The cerebral cortex is the largest site of neural integration in the central nervous sys-tem, and plays an important role in memory, language, and consciousness. When the blood supply to the brain is reduced due to narrowing of the brain arteries, the brain tissue suffers ischemic damage. [41,44,57]. In the BCAS group, we confirmed that the cortical cell arrangement was altered and demonstrated irregular cell shapes. These results suggested damage to the cortex, which is responsible for cognitive function (Figure 10A,B).

MAP2, a cytoskeletal microtubule-associated protein distributed in the hippocampal region which is responsible for learning and memory processes, plays an important regulatory role in maintaining neuronal plasticity and differentiated neuron morphology. The statistically significant decrease in MAP2-dependent neuronal plasticity and structural integrity in the hippocampal CA1 region of the VD group seen in this study suggests a detrimental effect on the ability to learn new facts and store memory (Figure 10C,D).

The corpus callosum is a myelinated structure that acts as a bridge between the brain hemispheres and is responsible for signal transmission. Damage to the corpus callosum disrupts contact between the two hemispheres, leading to various impairments (e.g., language and cognitive functions). Myelin staining of the corpus callosum was decreased in the VD group and was not uniform, as compared with the NT group. The corpus callosum thickness was also decreased in the VD group, suggesting a decrease in the corpus callosum myelin and cognitive decline in the VD model group [58] (Figure 10E,F).

Many previous studies of cognitive disorders used a model of acute ischemic conditions, such as middle cerebral artery occlusion. This model focused on acute neuronal injury and death after an abrupt decrease in cerebral blood flow or complete cessation of cerebral perfusion. Occlusion of the cerebral arteries quickly induced the neuronal cell loss in the hippocampus, directly resulting in cognitive impairment. However, this model cannot represent patients with other causes of VD, such as large artery atherosclerosis, an etiology more common than acute cerebral ischemia. Our study used one of the models of chronic progressive hypoperfusion of the brain. Many previous studies investigating novel treatments for VD failed because the pathogenesis of VD was unclear and appropriate animal models had not yet been developed. Our study reveals the parallel effect of the ROCK pathway and inflammation on VD development, confirmed through behavioral tests. Our results demonstrated the potential of ROCK, pro-inflammatory cytokines, and the BBB status to be early markers of vascular dementia. Moreover, the potential improvement in vascular pathology through ROCK inhibitors or stem cell treatment warrants further investigation. Thus, our findings indicate directions for further research into early- and later-stage vascular dementia research and may ultimately inform medical guidelines.

5. Conclusions

Vascular dementia is chronic, presenting with persistent hypoperfusion injury [59]. Chronic hypoperfusion injury causes a long-term decrease in blood flow, resulting in cognitive impairment rather than in severe neurological impairment in the brain. We found that the BCAS VD mouse model established in this study reflects clinical characteristics of the vascular dementia disease course. More specifically, we confirmed the underlying molecular mechanism of vascular dementia to be as follows: In vascular dementia, an in-crease in ROCK levels leads to a decrease in TJ proteins (Occludin, Claudin-5) that form part of the BBB, which regulates vascular permeability, by inducing restructuring of the cytoskeleton. This induces neuroinflammation through the BBB, with increased vascular permeability, and an inflammatory environment in which pro-inflammatory cytokines and chemokine levels (e.g., VCAM-1, IL-6, IL-1β, MCP-1, and CCR2) are increased. This causes damage to the (1) hippocampus, which is responsible for learning and memory; (2) the cerebral cortex, which is responsible for long-term memory; and (3) the corpus callosum, which functions in interhemispheric integration, which explains the decrease in cognitive function and memory in the BCAS group. Our study showed pathological changes leading to early vascular dementia and causing it to become chronic. This can mimic the pathological phenomenon seen in patients with early vascular dementia.

Author Contributions: Conceptualization, J.S.O., M.R.L., E.-Y.K. and H.-M.C.; methodology, E.C.L., D.-Y.H., D.-H.L., J.Y.L., J.H.J., J.S.O., M.R.L. and K.-S.H.; software, J.S.O., S.-W.P.; validation, M.R.L. and J.S.O.; formal analysis, E.C.L. and D.-Y.H.; investigation, E.-Y.K., H.-M.C., K.-S.H. and S.-P.P.; resources, E.C.L., D.-Y.H., J.S.O. and M.R.L.; data curation, E.C.L., D.-Y.H., D.-H.L., J.S.O. and M.R.L.; writing—original draft preparation, E.C.L., D.-Y.H., J.S.O. and M.R.L.; writing—review and editing, E.C.L., D.-Y.H., J.S.O. and M.R.L.; visualization, E.C.L., D.-Y.H., D.-H.L., J.S.O. and M.R.L.; supervision, J.S.O., M.R.L., H.-M.C. and S.-P.P.; project administration, J.S.O., M.R.L., E.-Y.K., H.-M.C., K.-S.H. and S.-P.P.; funding acquisition, J.S.O., M.R.L., E.-Y.K., H.-M.C., K.-S.H. and S.-P.P. All authors have read and agreed to the published version of the manuscript.

Funding: This research was supported by a grant from the Jeollanam-do Science and Technology R&D Project (Development of stem cell-derived new drug), funded by the Jeollanam-do, Korea. This research was supported by the Soonchunhyang University Fund. by the Bio & Medical Technology Development Program of the National Research Foundation funded by the Korean government (NRF-2019M3E5D1A02069061, NRF-2020R1F1A1066362), and by the Korea Medical Device Development Fund grant funded by the Korea government (the Ministry of Science and ICT, the Ministry of Trade, Industry and Energy, the Ministry of Health & Welfare, Republic of Kore (202015 × 17).

Institutional Review Board Statement: All animal experiments were performed in compliance with the Institutional Animal Care and Use Committee of Soon Chun Hyang University (IACUC No. SCH 20-0065) and the Guidelines for the Care and Use of Laboratory Animals specified by the National Research Council.

Informed Consent Statement: Not applicable.

Data Availability Statement: No new data were created or analyzed in this study. Data sharing is not applicable to this article.

Conflicts of Interest: The authors declare that they have no conflicts of interest.

References

1. White, H.; Boden-Albala, B.; Wang, C.; Elkind, M.S.; Rundek, T.; Wright, C.B.; Sacco, R.L. Ischemic stroke subtype incidence among whites, blacks, and Hispanics: The Northern Manhattan Study. *Circulation* **2005**, *111*, 1327–1331. [CrossRef] [PubMed]
2. Stewart, J.A.; Dundas, R.; Howard, R.S.; Rudd, A.G.; Wolfe, C.D.A. Ethnic differences in incidence of stroke: Prospective study with stroke register. *BMJ* **1999**, *318*, 967–971. [CrossRef]
3. Yu, K.H.; Bae, H.J.; Kwon, S.U.; Kang, D.W.; Hong, K.S.; Lee, Y.S.; Rha, J.H.; Koo, J.S.; Kim, J.S.; Kim, J.H.; et al. Analysis of 10,811 cases with acute ischemic stroke from Korean Stroke Registry: Hospital-based multicenter prospective registration study. *J. Korean Neurol. Assoc.* **2006**, *24*, 535–543.
4. Wolters, F.J.; Ikram, M.A. Epidemiology of Vascular Dementia. *Arterioscler. Thromb. Vasc. Biol.* **2019**, *39*, 1542–1549. [CrossRef]
5. Smith, E.E. Clinical presentations and epidemiology of vascular dementia. *Clin. Sci.* **2017**, *131*, 1059–1068. [CrossRef]
6. Kalaria, R.N.; Ballard, C. Overlap between pathology of Alzheimer disease and vascular dementia. In *Alzheimer Disease and Associated Disorders*; Lippincott Williams & Wilkins, Inc.: Philadelphia, PA, USA, 1999.
7. Du, S.Q.; Wang, X.R.; Xiao, L.Y.; Tu, J.F.; Zhu, W.; He, T.; Liu, C.Z. Molecular Mechanisms of Vascular Dementia: What Can Be Learned from Animal Models of Chronic Cerebral Hypoperfusion? *Mol. Neurobiol.* **2017**, *54*, 3670–3682. [CrossRef]
8. Bink, D.I.; Ritz, K.; Aronica, E.; Van Der Weerd, L.; Daemen, M.J. Mouse models to study the effect of cardiovascular risk factors on brain structure and cognition. *J. Cereb. Blood Flow Metab.* **2013**, *33*, 1666–1684. [CrossRef] [PubMed]
9. Zhang, X.; Wu, B.; Nie, K.; Jia, Y.; Yu, J. Effects of acupuncture on declined cerebral blood flow, impaired mitochondrial respiratory function and oxidative stress in multi-infarct dementia rats. *Neurochem. Int.* **2014**, *65*, 23–29. [CrossRef]
10. Chen, H.; Yoshioka, H.; Kim, G.S.; Jung, J.E.; Okami, N.; Sakata, H.; Maier, C.M.; Narasimhan, P.; Goeders, C.E.; Chan, P.H. Oxidative stress in ischemic brain damage: Mechanisms of cell death and potential molecular targets for neuroprotection. *Antioxid. Redox. Signal.* **2011**, *14*, 1505–1517. [CrossRef]

11. Kim, M.S.; Bang, J.H.; Lee, J.; Han, J.S.; Kang, H.W.; Jeon, W.K. Fructus mume Ethanol Extract Prevents Inflammation and Normalizes the Septohippocampal Cholinergic System in a Rat Model of Chronic Cerebral Hypoperfusion. *J. Med. Food* **2016**, *19*, 196–204. [CrossRef]
12. Tanaka, M.; Toldi, J.; Vecsei, L. Exploring the Etiological Links behind Neurodegenerative Diseases: Inflammatory Cytokines and Bioactive Kynurenines. *Int. J. Mol. Sci.* **2020**, *21*, 2431. [CrossRef]
13. Garcia-Lara, E.; Aguirre, S.; Clotet, N.; Sawkulycz, X.; Bartra, C.; Almenara-Fuentes, L.; Sunol, C.; Corpas, R.; Olah, P.; Tripon, F.; et al. Antibody Protection against Long-Term Memory Loss Induced by Monomeric C-Reactive Protein in a Mouse Model of Dementia. *Biomedicines* **2021**, *9*, 828. [CrossRef]
14. Benkhalifa, M.; Ferreira, Y.J.; Chahine, H.; Louanjli, N.; Miron, P.; Merviel, P.; Copin, H. Mitochondria: Participation to infertility as source of energy and cause of senescence. *Int. J. Biochem. Cell Biol.* **2014**, *55*, 60–64. [CrossRef]
15. Brunetti, D.; Catania, A.; Viscomi, C.; Deleidi, M.; Bindoff, L.A.; Ghezzi, D.; Zeviani, M. Role of PITRM1 in Mitochondrial Dysfunction and Neurodegeneration. *Biomedicines* **2021**, *9*, 833. [CrossRef]
16. Jiwa, N.S.; Garrard, P.; Hainsworth, A.H. Experimental models of vascular dementia and vascular cognitive impairment: A systematic review. *J. Neurochem.* **2010**, *115*, 814–828. [CrossRef] [PubMed]
17. Farkas, E.; Luiten, P.G.; Bari, F. Permanent, bilateral common carotid artery occlusion in the rat: A model for chronic cerebral hypoperfusion-related neurodegenerative diseases. *Brain Res. Rev.* **2007**, *54*, 162–180. [CrossRef] [PubMed]
18. Ihara, M.; Tomimoto, H. Lessons from a mouse model characterizing features of vascular cognitive impairment with white matter changes. *J. Aging Res.* **2011**, *2011*, 978761. [CrossRef] [PubMed]
19. Tuo, Q.Z.; Zou, J.J.; Lei, P. Rodent Models of Vascular Cognitive Impairment. *J. Mol. Neurosci.* **2021**, *71*, 1–12. [CrossRef]
20. Shibata, M.; Ohtani, R.; Ihara, M.; Tomimoto, H. White matter lesions and glial activation in a novel mouse model of chronic cerebral hypoperfusion. *Stroke* **2004**, *35*, 2598–2603. [CrossRef]
21. Gudapati, K.; Singh, A.; Clarkson-Townsend, D.; Feola, A.J.; Allen, R.S. Behavioral assessment of visual function via optomotor response and cognitive function via Y-maze in diabetic rats. *JoVE J. Vis. Exp.* **2020**, *164*, e61806. [CrossRef]
22. Kang, S.; Ha, S.; Park, H.; Nam, E.; Suh, W.H.; Suh, Y.H.; Chang, K.A. Effects of a dehydroevodiamine-derivative on synaptic destabilization and memory impairment in the 5xFAD, Alzheimer's disease mouse model. *Front. Behav. Neurosci.* **2018**, *12*, 273. [CrossRef]
23. Doze, V.A.; Papay, R.S.; Goldenstein, B.L.; Gupta, M.K.; Collette, K.M.; Nelson, B.W.; Lyons, M.J.; Davis, B.A.; Luger, E.J.; Wood, S.G.; et al. Long-term α1A-adrenergic receptor stimulation improves synaptic plasticity, cognitive function, mood, and longevity. *Mol. Pharmacol.* **2011**, *80*, 747–758. [CrossRef] [PubMed]
24. Wu, C.; Yang, L.; Tucker, D.; Dong, Y.A.N.; Zhu, L.; Duan, R.U.I.; Liu, T.C.; Zhang, Q. Beneficial effects of exercise pretreatment in a sporadic Alzheimer's rat model. *Med. Sci. Sports Exerc.* **2018**, *50*, 945. [CrossRef] [PubMed]
25. Lian, W.; Fang, J.; Xu, L.; Zhou, W.; Kang, D.; Xiong, W.; Jia, H.; Liu, A.L.; Du, G.H. DL0410 Ameliorates Memory and Cognitive Impairments Induced by Scopolamine via Increasing Cholinergic Neurotransmission in Mice. *Molecules* **2017**, *22*, 410. [CrossRef] [PubMed]
26. Seibenhener, M.L.; Wooten, M.C. Use of the open field maze to measure locomotor and anxiety-like behavior in mice. *JoVE J. Vis. Exp.* **2015**, *96*, e52434. [CrossRef]
27. de Lombares, C.; Heude, E.; Alfama, G.; Fontaine, A.; Hassouna, R.; Vernochet, C.; de Chaumont, F.; Olivo-Marin, C.; Ey, E.; Parnaudeau, S.; et al. Dlx5 and Dlx6 expression in GABAergic neurons controls behavior, metabolism, healthy aging and lifespan. *Aging* **2019**, *11*, 6638–6656. [CrossRef]
28. Shimada, T.; Matsumoto, K.; Osanai, M.; Matsuda, H.; Terasawa, K.; Watanabe, H. The modified light/dark transition test in mice: Evaluation of classic and putative anxiolytic and anxiogenic drugs. *Gen. Pharmacol.* **1995**, *26*, 205–210. [CrossRef]
29. Kulesskaya, N.; Voikar, V. Assessment of mouse anxiety-like behavior in the light-dark box and open-field arena: Role of equipment and procedure. *Physiol. Behav.* **2014**, *133*, 30–38. [CrossRef]
30. Supanc, V.; Biloglav, Z.; Kes, V.B.; Demarin, V. Role of cell adhesion molecules in acute ischemic stroke. *Ann. Saudi Med.* **2011**, *31*, 365–370. [CrossRef]
31. Eidson, L.N.; Gao, Q.; Qu, H.; Kikuchi, D.S.; Campos, A.C.P.; Faidley, E.A.; Sun, Y.Y.; Kuan, C.Y.; Pagano, R.L.; Lassègue, B. Poldip2 controls leukocyte infiltration into the ischemic brain by regulating focal adhesion kinase-mediated VCAM-1 induction. *Sci. Rep.* **2021**, *11*, 5533. [CrossRef]
32. Fang, W.; Sha, L.; Kodithuwakku, N.D.; Wei, J.; Zhang, R.; Han, D.; Mao, L.; Li, Y. Attenuated blood-brain barrier dysfunction by XQ-1H following ischemic stroke in hyperlipidemic rats. *Mol. Neurobiol.* **2015**, *52*, 162–175. [CrossRef]
33. Hosoki, S.; Tanaka, T.; Ihara, M. Diagnostic and prognostic blood biomarkers in vascular dementia: From the viewpoint of ischemic stroke. *Neurochem. Int.* **2021**, *146*, 105015. [CrossRef]
34. Schüz, A.; Preiβl, H. Basic connectivity of the cerebral cortex and some considerations on the corpus callosum. *Neurosci. Biobehav. Rev.* **1996**, *20*, 567–570. [CrossRef]
35. Westerhausen, R.; Luders, E.; Specht, K.; Ofte, S.H.; Toga, A.W.; Thompson, P.M.; Helland, T.; Hugdahl, K. Structural and functional reorganization of the corpus callosum between the age of 6 and 8 years. *Cereb. Cortex* **2011**, *21*, 1012–1017. [CrossRef]
36. Rosenberg, G.A.; Sullivan, N.; Esiri, M.M. White matter damage is associated with matrix metalloproteinases in vascular dementia. *Stroke* **2001**, *32*, 1162–1167. [CrossRef] [PubMed]

37. Choi, B.R.; Kim, D.H.; Back, D.B.; Kang, C.H.; Moon, W.J.; Han, J.S.; Choi, D.H.; Kwon, K.J.; Shin, C.Y.; Kim, B.R.; et al. Characterization of White Matter Injury in a Rat Model of Chronic Cerebral Hypoperfusion. *Stroke* **2016**, *47*, 542–547. [CrossRef] [PubMed]
38. Hase, Y.; Craggs, L.; Hase, M.; Stevenson, W.; Slade, J.; Lopez, D.; Mehta, R.; Chen, A.; Liang, D.; Oakley, A.; et al. Effects of environmental enrichment on white matter glial responses in a mouse model of chronic cerebral hypoperfusion. *J. Neuroinflammation* **2017**, *14*, 81. [CrossRef]
39. Zhang, S.H.; Si, W.; Yu, Q.; Wang, Y.; Wu, Y. Therapeutic effects of combination environmental enrichment with necrostatin-1 on cognition following vascular cognitive impairment in mice. *Eur. J. Inflamm.* **2019**, *17*, 2058739219834832. [CrossRef]
40. Bannai, T.; Mano, T.; Chen, X.; Ohtomo, G.; Ohtomo, R.; Tsuchida, T.; Koshi-Mano, K.; Hashimoto, T.; Okazawa, H.; Iwatsubo, T.; et al. Chronic cerebral hypoperfusion shifts the equilibrium of amyloid beta oligomers to aggregation-prone species with higher molecular weight. *Sci. Rep.* **2019**, *9*, 2827. [CrossRef]
41. Hattori, Y.; Enmi, J.; Kitamura, A.; Yamamoto, Y.; Saito, S.; Takahashi, Y.; Iguchi, S.; Tsuji, M.; Yamahara, K.; Nagatsuka, K.; et al. A Novel Mouse Model of Subcortical Infarcts with Dementia. *J. Neurosci.* **2015**, *35*, 3915–3928. [CrossRef]
42. Hattori, Y.; Kitamura, A.; Tsuji, M.; Nagatsuka, K.; Ihara, M. Motor and cognitive impairment in a mouse model of ischemic carotid artery disease. *Neurosci. Lett.* **2014**, *581*, 1–6. [CrossRef]
43. Toyama, K.; Spin, J.M.; Deng, A.C.; Huang, T.T.; Wei, K.; Wagenhauser, M.U.; Yoshino, T.; Nguyen, H.; Mulorz, J.; Kundu, S.; et al. MicroRNA-Mediated Therapy Modulating Blood-Brain Barrier Disruption Improves Vascular Cognitive Impairment. *Arter. Thromb. Vasc. Biol.* **2018**, *38*, 1392–1406. [CrossRef] [PubMed]
44. Madureira, S.; Verdelho, A.; Pantoni, L.; Scheltens, P. White matter changes: New perspectives on imaging, clinical aspects, and intervention. *J. Aging Res.* **2011**, *2011*, 841913. [CrossRef] [PubMed]
45. Shibata, M.; Yamasaki, N.; Miyakawa, T.; Kalaria, R.N.; Fujita, Y.; Ohtani, R.; Ihara, M.; Takahashi, R.; Tomimoto, H. Selective impairment of working memory in a mouse model of chronic cerebral hypoperfusion. *Stroke* **2007**, *38*, 2826–2832. [CrossRef] [PubMed]
46. Roberts, J.M.; Maniskas, M.E.; Bix, G.J. Bilateral carotid artery stenosis causes unexpected early changes in brain extracellular matrix and blood-brain barrier integrity in mice. *PLoS ONE* **2018**, *13*, e0195765. [CrossRef]
47. Pawluk, H.; Wozniak, A.; Grzesk, G.; Kolodziejska, R.; Kozakiewicz, M.; Kopkowska, E.; Grzechowiak, E.; Kozera, G. The Role of Selected Pro-Inflammatory Cytokines in Pathogenesis of Ischemic Stroke. *Clin. Interv. Aging* **2020**, *15*, 469–484. [CrossRef]
48. Amantea, D.; Nappi, G.; Bernardi, G.; Bagetta, G.; Corasaniti, M.T. Post-ischemic brain damage: Pathophysiology and role of inflammatory mediators. *FEBS J.* **2009**, *276*, 13–26. [CrossRef]
49. Doyle, K.P.; Simon, R.P.; Stenzel-Poore, M.P. Mechanisms of ischemic brain damage. *Neuropharmacology* **2008**, *55*, 310–318. [CrossRef]
50. Frijns, C.J.; Kappelle, L.J. Inflammatory cell adhesion molecules in ischemic cerebrovascular disease. *Stroke* **2002**, *33*, 2115–2122. [CrossRef]
51. Stamatovic, S.M.; Keep, R.F.; Kunkel, S.L.; Andjelkovic, A.V. Potential role of MCP-1 in endothelial cell tight junction 'opening': Signaling via Rho and Rho kinase. *J. Cell Sci.* **2003**, *116*, 4615–4628. [CrossRef]
52. Nourshargh, S.; Alon, R. Leukocyte migration into inflamed tissues. *Immunity* **2014**, *41*, 694–707. [CrossRef]
53. Lloyd, E.; Somera-Molina, K.; Van Eldik, L.J.; Watterson, D.M.; Wainwright, M.S. Suppression of acute proinflammatory cytokine and chemokine upregulation by post-injury administration of a novel small molecule improves long-term neurologic outcome in a mouse model of traumatic brain injury. *J. Neuroinflammation* **2008**, *5*, 28. [CrossRef] [PubMed]
54. Almutairi, M.M.; Gong, C.; Xu, Y.G.; Chang, Y.; Shi, H. Factors controlling permeability of the blood-brain barrier. *Cell Mol. Life Sci.* **2016**, *73*, 57–77. [CrossRef] [PubMed]
55. Hussain, B.; Fang, C.; Chang, J. Blood-Brain Barrier Breakdown: An Emerging Biomarker of Cognitive Impairment in Normal Aging and Dementia. *Front. Neurosci.* **2021**, *15*, 688090. [CrossRef]
56. Kim, Y.; Lee, S.; Zhang, H.; Lee, S.; Kim, H.; Kim, Y.; Won, M.H.; Kim, Y.M.; Kwon, Y.G. CLEC14A deficiency exacerbates neuronal loss by increasing blood-brain barrier permeability and inflammation. *J. Neuroinflammation* **2020**, *17*, 48. [CrossRef]
57. Huang, L.; He, Z.; Guo, L.; Wang, H. Improvement of cognitive deficit and neuronal damage in rats with chronic cerebral ischemia via relative long-term inhibition of rho-kinase. *Cell Mol. Neurobiol.* **2008**, *28*, 757–768. [CrossRef]
58. An, L.; Shen, Y.; Chopp, M.; Zacharek, A.; Venkat, P.; Chen, Z.; Li, W.; Qian, Y.; Landschoot-Ward, J.; Chen, J. Deficiency of Endothelial Nitric Oxide Synthase (eNOS) Exacerbates Brain Damage and Cognitive Deficit in A Mouse Model of Vascular Dementia. *Aging Dis.* **2021**, *12*, 732–746. [CrossRef] [PubMed]
59. Roman, G.C. Brain hypoperfusion: A critical factor in vascular dementia. *Neurol. Res.* **2004**, *26*, 454–458. [CrossRef]

biomedicines

MDPI

Article

Tryptophan Metabolites, Cytokines, and Fatty Acid Binding Protein 2 in Myalgic Encephalomyelitis/Chronic Fatigue Syndrome

Manuela Simonato [1], Stefano Dall'Acqua [2], Caterina Zilli [3], Stefania Sut [2], Romano Tenconi [4], Nicoletta Gallo [5], Paolo Sfriso [4], Leonardo Sartori [4], Francesco Cavallin [6], Ugo Fiocco [4], Paola Cogo [7], Paolo Agostinis [8], Anna Aldovini [9,10], Daniela Bruttomesso [4], Renzo Marcolongo [4], Stefano Comai [2,11,12,13,*,†] and Aldo Baritussio [4,†]

1 PCare Laboratory, Fondazione Istituto di Ricerca Pediatrica, Citta' della Speranza, 35127 Padova, Italy; m.simonato@irpcds.org
2 Department of Pharmaceutical and Pharmacological Sciences, University of Padua, 35131 Padua, Italy; stefano.dallacqua@unipd.it (S.D.); stefania.sut@unipd.it (S.S.)
3 Pediatrician, Via Galvani 6, 35020 Padua, Italy; zillicat@gmail.com
4 Department of Medicine, University of Padova, 35128 Padova, Italy; romano.tenconi@unipd.it (R.T.); paolo.sfriso@unipd.it (P.S.); leonardo.sartori@unipd.it (L.S.); ugo.fiocco@unipd.it (U.F.); daniela.bruttomesso@unipd.it (D.B.); renzo.marcolongo@aopd.veneto.it (R.M.); aldo.baritussio@unipd.it (A.B.)
5 Department of Laboratory Medicine, Policlinico Azienda Ospedaliera di Padova, 35128 Padova, Italy; nicoletta.gallo@aopd.veneto.it
6 Independent Statistician, 36020 Solagna, Italy; cescocava@libero.it
7 Department of Medicine, University Hospital Santa Maria della Misericordia, University of Udine, 33100 Udine, Italy; paola.cogo@uniud.it
8 Department of Medicine, Ospedale Sant'Antonio Abate, Azienda Sanitaria del Friuli Centrale, 33100 Udine, Italy; agostinispaolo@gmail.com
9 Department of Medicine, Boston Children's Hospital, Boston, MA 02115, USA; anna.aldovini@childrens.harvard.edu
10 Department of Pediatrics, Harvard Medical School, Boston, MA 02115, USA
11 Department of Biomedical Sciences, University of Padua, 35121 Padua, Italy
12 Department of Psychiatry, McGill University, Montreal, QC H4H 1R3, Canada
13 Division of Neuroscience, IRCSS San Raffaele Scientific Institute, 20132 Milan, Italy
* Correspondence: stefano.comai@unipd.it; Tel.: +39-049-827-5098
† These authors contributed equally to this work.

Citation: Simonato, M.; Dall'Acqua, S.; Zilli, C.; Sut, S.; Tenconi, R.; Gallo, N.; Sfriso, P.; Sartori, L.; Cavallin, F.; Fiocco, U.; et al. Tryptophan Metabolites, Cytokines, and Fatty Acid Binding Protein 2 in Myalgic Encephalomyelitis/Chronic Fatigue Syndrome. *Biomedicines* **2021**, *9*, 1724. https://doi.org/10.3390/biomedicines9111724

Academic Editors: Masaru Tanaka and Nóra Török

Received: 16 October 2021
Accepted: 15 November 2021
Published: 19 November 2021

Abstract: Patients with Myalgic Encephalomyelitis/Chronic Fatigue Syndrome (ME/CFS) differ for triggers, mode of start, associated symptoms, evolution, and biochemical traits. Therefore, serious attempts are underway to partition them into subgroups useful for a personalized medicine approach to the disease. Here, we investigated clinical and biochemical traits in 40 ME/CFS patients and 40 sex- and age-matched healthy controls. Particularly, we analyzed serum levels of some cytokines, Fatty Acid Binding Protein 2 (FAPB-2), tryptophan, and some of its metabolites via serotonin and kynurenine. ME/CFS patients were heterogeneous for genetic background, trigger, start mode, symptoms, and evolution. ME/CFS patients had higher levels of IL-17A ($p = 0.018$), FABP-2 ($p = 0.002$), and 3-hydroxykynurenine ($p = 0.037$) and lower levels of kynurenine ($p = 0.012$) and serotonin ($p = 0.045$) than controls. Changes in kynurenine and 3-hydroxykynurenine were associated with increased kynurenic acid/kynurenine and 3-hydroxykynurenine/kynurenine ratios, indirect measures of kynurenine aminotransferases and kynurenine 3-monooxygenase enzymatic activities, respectively. No correlation was found among cytokines, FABP-2, and tryptophan metabolites, suggesting that inflammation, anomalies of the intestinal barrier, and changes of tryptophan metabolism may be independently associated with the pathogenesis of the disease. Interestingly, patients with the start of the disease after infection showed lower levels of kynurenine ($p = 0.034$) than those not starting after an infection. Changes in tryptophan metabolites and increased IL-17A levels in ME/CFS could both be compatible with anomalies in the sphere of energy metabolism. Overall, clinical traits together with serum biomarkers related to inflammation, intestine function, and tryptophan metabolism deserve to be further considered for the development of personalized medicine strategies for ME/CFS.

Keywords: ME/CFS heterogeneity; cytokines; intestinal permeability; tryptophan metabolism; kynurenine pathway; 3-hydroxykynurenine; kynurenine; serotonin; biomarkers; personalized medicine

1. Introduction

Myalgic Encephalomyelitis/Chronic Fatigue Syndrome (ME/CFS) is a multisystem condition characterized by chronic fatigue, post-exertional malaise, unrefreshing sleep, cognitive changes, autonomic disturbances, flu-like symptoms, abdominal complaints, and intolerance to stress, noise, light, heat, or cold. Females are more frequently affected, and over half of cases happen after infection [1].

Several pathogenetic mechanisms have been proposed. Some disease manifestations, such as flu-like symptoms, indicate an inflammatory/immune basis [2]. An immune basis for ME/CFS is also suggested by evidence showing increased cytokine levels in plasma and cerebrospinal fluid and T-cell dysfunction and by imaging data pointing to an involvement of the microglia [3,4]. Furthermore, studies on the intestinal microbiome have found loss of microbial diversity and signs of increased bacterial translocation across the intestinal barrier that could also contribute to systemic inflammation [5,6].

Other disease manifestations like low exercise tolerance or the propensity to produce an excess of lactic acid during exercise hint at a metabolic basis for ME/CFS, as is also suggested by the presence of mitochondrial abnormalities [7,8].

Joining the realm of immunity with that of energy production, it has been recently shown that subsets of T cells isolated from patients with ME/CFS are unable to redirect energy metabolism towards aerobic glycolysis during activation [9]. Along the same line, poor performance during exercise could be linked to sub-optimal venous return caused by immune-mediated autonomic dis-regulation of small vessels [10].

A large body of research, based on neuroimaging, has addressed brain changes in patients with ME/CFS. The most consistent findings have been the recruitment of additional brain regions during cognitive tasks, brain stem anomalies suggestive of inflammation, and a reduction of fluorodeoxyglucose uptake, indicative of hypometabolism (reviewed by Shan et al. [11]). Brain serotonin status has also been considered, but results have been discordant, with some studies demonstrating activation of this system [3,12], while others indicate inhibition [13]. Serum levels of tryptophan, precursor and direct determinant of brain serotonin [14], have also been studied, but the results are again contrasting with some authors showing higher levels in ME/CFS [15], while others found no change [16]. Interest in tryptophan metabolism in ME/CFS is justified by the fact that tryptophan metabolites along both the serotonin and the kynurenine pathways have a role in depression [14], sleep regulation [17] and Irritable Bowel Syndrome (IBS), frequent comorbidities in patients with ME/CFS [18]. Measurements of tryptophan to kynurenine metabolites and their ratios seem thus promising in the current growing interest of developing clinically useful biomarkers of several diseases [14,19].

Patients diagnosed with ME/CFS, while displaying a platform of shared symptoms, may differ for triggers, mode of start, associated symptoms, disease evolution, and biochemical traits [15,16,20,21]. For this reason, attempts are underway to partition them into different phenotypes, most recently looking at metabolic peculiarities [22], the first stage of developing possible personalized strategies for treatment.

The scope of this work was to study clinical and biochemical traits of a cohort of patients from North-East Italy and to compare them with a group of healthy volunteers. In detail, we examined clinical data and measured serum levels of some cytokines, of a group of tryptophan metabolites via serotonin and kynurenine and of an index of altered intestinal permeability in 40 patients with ME/CFS and in 40 sex- and age-matched healthy controls.

ME/CFS is emerging as a significant health issue worldwide, with an estimated prevalence of 0.8% [23], undefined pathogenesis, and no acknowledged treatment. We thought that combining clinical information with the measurement of variables reflecting different pathogenetic mechanisms could help to identify subgroups and facilitate a personalized approach to patient care.

2. Materials and Methods

2.1. Patients

From 1 January 2017 to 31 June 2018, 70 consecutive patients with unexplained fatigue were seen at the site of a charitable health care center near Padova (Italy) (Table S1). At visit 1, information was collected about diseases in the family, medical history, medication, menarche, menstrual cycle, bowel habits, smoking, alcohol consumption, use of contraceptives, duration of illness, and level of physical activity using the Bell scale [24]. Fatigue and associated symptoms were then investigated using the Canadian Clinical Criteria [25], and patients were asked to grade symptom intensity on a scale from 0 (no symptom) to 6 (maximum intensity). Patients received a physical examination. The evidence thus obtained was discussed by an internist, a pediatrician, and a geneticist, and a decision was made about the diagnosis of ME/CFS, following accepted exclusion criteria [1]. Forty-five patients were diagnosed with ME/CFS.

Afterward, contact with patients was maintained through periodic visits and, after the start of the COVID-19 pandemic, through phone calls or e-mail.

2.2. Case-Control Study

Patients were asked to take part in an investigation with the scope of studying serum levels of some cytokines, tryptophan metabolites, and a marker of increased intestinal permeability in ME/CFS. Forty patients were accepted. Of the five who did not, a 67-year-old female, with 22 years of disease duration, died of pancreatic cancer during recruitment, one patient declined to participate, and 3 patients could not be contacted. Forty healthy controls, matched for sex and age (26 females and 14 males; median age 33 years with interquartile range 22–46 years), were recruited among patient's friends, school companions, medical students, and other hospital personnel. Inclusion criteria for the healthy control group were the absence of any current or past psychiatric, neurological, or other known medical conditions. Informed consent was obtained from patients and controls, and approval for the study was obtained from the Ethics Committee of Policlinico Universitario, Padova, Italy (Protocol Number 4776/AO/19). Experiments were conducted in accordance with the Declaration of Helsinki.

Patient blood samples, collected after an overnight fast, were allowed to clot at room temperature for 45 min and then were centrifuged for 10 min at 3500× g. Serum was aliquoted and stored at −80 °C. Aliquots were used just once after thawing. Blood samples from healthy controls were obtained within 2 weeks of the respective patient and processed in the same way. Blood collection was terminated by 1 December 2019.

2.3. Follow-Up

After blood sample collection, contact with patients was maintained through periodic visits and, after the start of the COVID-19 pandemic, through phone calls or e-mail. During May 2021, patients were requested to answer a questionnaire with both multiple choice and open questions concerning their feelings about their current condition and prevailing symptoms. When needed, patients were also contacted by phone. During 2021, we also checked by phone the health status of the controls used in this study.

2.4. Biochemical Assays

Serum cytokines were measured with ELISA. To obviate the variability between lots, sera from patients and controls were tested using the same kit [2]. ELISA kits were from Thermo Scientific, Monza, Italy (IL-4, IL-10, IL-17A, IL-18, IFN-γ) and RayBiotech,

Peachtree Corner, GA, USA (IL-18). The above cytokines were chosen based on existing evidence and on the fact that for all patients' serum levels of IL-1α, IL-1β, IL-2, IL2R, IL-6, IL-8, TNF-α, and TGF1β had already been measured at the EU-certified Central Laboratory of Padova University Hospital.

Fatty Acid Binding Protein 2 (FABP-2), an index of increased intestinal permeability [5], was measured by ELISA (myBioSource, Dan Diego, CA, USA).

The serum concentration of tryptophan and tryptophan metabolites pertaining to the Kynurenine Pathway (kynurenine, 3-hydroxykynurenine, kynurenic acid, quinolinic acid) and the Serotonin Pathway (serotonin and melatonin) were studied (Figure 1). Tryptophan, serotonin, and kynurenine were determined using a standard method in the lab [26,27] consisting of an HPLC system coupled with fluorometric and UV-Vis detectors. 3-hydroxykynurenine, kynurenic acid, quinolinic acid, and melatonin were quantified by LC-MS/MS on a Varian system composed of a binary Prostar pump, 410 autosampler, and MS320 triple quadrupole mass spectrometer equipped with Electro Spray ion source. The instrument was operating in multiple reaction monitoring modes, working in positive ion mode except for the quinolinic acid that was analyzed in negative mode. LC analysis was performed using an Agilent Eclipse XDB C8 column (3 $\times$ 150 mm, 3.5 μm) and a gradient elution with (A) water 1% formic acid and (B) Acetonitrile (0 min: 95% A; 5 min: 30% A; 8.3 min: 10% A; 10 min: 10% A; 11 min: 95% A; 15 min: 95% A) at a flow rate of 400 μL/min. The quantification of the kynurenines was computed using alfa-methyl tryptophan as an internal standard. The following ratios were used as indirect indexes of the activity of the enzymes involved in the different metabolic steps of the kynurenine pathway: kynurenine/tryptophan as an index of tryptophan 2,3-dioxygenase (TDO) and indoleamine 2,3-dioxygenase (IDO) activity; 3-hydroxykynurenine/kynurenine as an index of kynurenine 3-monooxygenase (KMO) activity; kynurenic acid/3-hydroxykynurenine as an index of the kynurenine aminotransferase (KAT) activity. Finally, the ratio kynurenic acid/quinolinic acid was calculated as an index of neuroprotection [14].

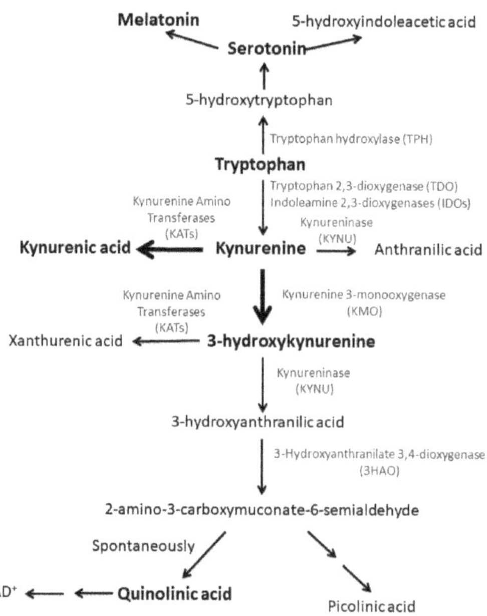

Figure 1. Schematic representation of the metabolism of tryptophan through the serotonin and kynurenine pathways. Enzymes involved in the different biochemical steps are indicated next to the arrow. Metabolites analyzed in this study are in bold.

2.5. Statistical Analysis

Data were reported as median and interquartile range (IQR, for continuous data), or frequency and percentage (categorical data). Among patients, comparisons between two groups were performed using Mann–Whitney test (continuous data) and chi-square test or Fisher's test (categorical data). In the matched case-control analysis, serum cytokines, FABP2, and tryptophan metabolites were compared between cases and controls or post-infection and non-post-infection cases using Quade's rank analysis of covariance with BMI, sex, and age as covariates. Correlation between continuous variables was assessed using Spearman rank correlation coefficient. Adjustment for multiple testing was not performed due to the exploratory purpose of this study. All tests were two-sided, and a p-value less than 0.05 was considered significant. Statistical analysis was performed using R 4.1 (R Foundation for Statistical Computing, Vienna, Austria) and SPSS 27 (Chicago, IL, USA).

3. Results

3.1. Patients

The analysis included 40 patients with ME/CFS (14 males and 26 females, median age 33 years, disease duration 6 years) (Table 1). Thirty-one patients had already received a diagnosis of ME/CFS from other colleagues. For nine patients, ME/CFS was a new diagnosis.

Table 1. ME/CFS patient characteristics.

Variable	All (n = 40)
Age, years [a]	32 (23–46)
Males	14 (35%)
Disease duration, years [a,b]	6 (3–12)
Symptom start:	
Slow (months)	18/40 (45%)
Fast (weeks)	22/40 (55%)
ME/CFS, fatigue, or fibromyalgia in the family	13/38 [d] (34%)
Immune diseases in the family	17/38 [d] (44%)
Symptom score (0–6): [a]	
Fatigue	6 (5–6)
PEM	5 (5–6)
Unrefreshing sleep	4 (4–5)
Pain	4 (3–5)
Cognitive anomalies	5 (4–5)
OI/POTS	4 (4–5)
GI abnormalities	4 (3–4)
Flu-like symptoms	4 (3–5)
Bell scale score (0–100%) [a,c]	30 (25–50)
Bowel habit: [a]	
Normal	23/38 [d] (61%)
Styptic	10/38 [d] (26%)
Diarrheic	5/38 [d] (13%)
Abdominal pain—IBS [e]	23/40 (58%)

Data expressed as n (%) or [a] median (IQR). PEM—post-exertional malaise; OI—orthostatic intolerance; POTS: postural orthostatic tachycardia syndrome; GI—gastro-intestine; IBS—irritable bowel syndrome. Data were not available in [b] 1, [c] 4, and [d] 2 patients; [e] diagnosed according to the Rome IV criteria [28].

Nine patients had severe ME/CFS with a Bell score $\leq$ 25%. The other patients had a serious disease with a Bell score of 26–65% (Table 1).

ME/CFS started with an infection in 19 patients (47.5%). Infections mostly regarded the upper airways. Three patients developed ME/CFS after Lyme disease and one patient after acute giardiasis during a trip to a tropical country.

All patients fulfilled the criteria for the diagnosis of ME/CFS; some of them, however, presented peculiarities that could not be discounted. These rare manifestations included differences in the way ME/CFS started, the presence of symptoms suggestive of immune disease (dry eyes, oral aphthae), neurological anomalies (jerks, paresthesias, hypersomnia), signs suggestive of autonomic dysregulation (livedo reticularis, acrocyanosis) and hyperlaxity (Table 2). Some patients presented anomalies at the muscle biopsy that could not be attributed to known diseases (Table 2). Finally, some presented genetic abnormalities whose importance is unclear (Table 2).

Table 2. Symptoms, laboratory data, and genetic abnormalities present in a minority of patients.

Variable	Number of Patients (%)	Notes
Disease start		
After a neoplasia	2 (5)	Meningioma, Hodgkin lymphoma
After a vaccine	1 (2)	
Symptoms, signs, and laboratory data		
Skin hyperlaxity	4 (10)	
Livedo reticularis	2 (5)	
Dry eyes/mouth	2 (5)	
Oral aphthae	2 (5)	
Paresthesias	3 (7)	
Jerks	2 (5)	
Hypersomnia	2 (5)	
Bouts of fever, flu-like symptoms, increase in CRP and serum amyloid A	2 (5)	Response to colchicine, canakinumab
Muscle biopsy anomalies	1 (2)	Thickened basal membrane of small vessels, glycogen accumulation within myocytes
Serum cytokines above normal *		
IL-1α	2 (5)	
IL-2	9 (22)	
IL-6	2 (5)	
IL-8	1 (2)	
TNF-α	7 (17)	
TGF-β	13 (32)	
Genetic abnormalities		
CASQ1 gene mutation	1 (2)	N227I, heterozygous. Muscle biopsy: thickened vessel basal membrane, fibrils of unknown nature around myocytes.
15q13.3 duplication (340 BP)	1 (2)	
Ehlers–Danlos syndrome	1 (2)	
Myotonia congenita	1 (2)	

BP—base pairs; CRP—C reactive protein; * measured in 39 patients.

3.2. Follow-Up

Median follow-up was 41 months (IQR 32–47) (Table 3). Most patients (57%) reported worsening of symptoms during follow-up, with fatigue (49%) and cognitive problems (28%) as the prevailing symptom (Table 3). For 18% of patients' symptoms remained unchanged. Twenty-two percent of patients reported improvement. No differences were found during follow-up between patients starting or not starting with an infection.

Table 3. Follow-up clinical information of the 40 ME/CFS patients.

Follow-Up, Months [a]	41 (32–47)
Symptom evolution during follow up:	
Unchanged	8/40 (20%)
Worsened	21/40 (52%)
Improved	11/40 (28%)
Prevailing symptoms during follow-up:	
Fatigue	20 (50%)
PEM	7 (17%)
Unrefreshing sleep	2 (5%)
Pain	6 (15%)
Cognitive anomalies	12 (30%)
OI/POTS	1 (2%)
Abdominal pain/IBS [b]	1 (2%)
Flu-like	1 (2%)

Data expressed as *n* (%) or [a] median (IQR). PEM—post-exertional malaise; OI—orthostatic intolerance; POTS—postural orthostatic tachycardia syndrome; IBS—irritable bowel syndrome. [b]: diagnosed according to the Rome IV criteria [28].

Two of the patients who improved (17 and 21 years old, both females, disease duration 1 and 8 years) had recurrent bouts of fever, muscle pain, and flu-like symptoms. During such periods, serum levels of C reactive protein (CRP) and amyloid A increased slightly. Patients also had modest increases of IL-4, TNF-α, IL-17A, and IFN-γ. IL-1β, IL-18, and IL-33 were within normal limits or undetectable, and no mutations were found in genes related to the pathogenesis of autoinflammatory syndromes (MEFV, MVK, TNFRSF1A, NLRP3, and NLRP12). One patient responded rapidly to colchicine, the Bell scale grading increasing from 30 to 100% in a few days. The other, who responded partially to colchicine, was treated with monthly canakinumab (IL-1β antagonist), with dramatic results (Bell scale grading went from 20 to 90% within hours after the first dose, post-exertional malaise and brain fog disappeared, and orthostatic intolerance improved markedly). Since no alternative diagnosis emerged, we have retained these patients in the ME/CFS cohort. Both patients have continued treatment, and the improvement is still persisting after 2 years.

3.3. *Case-Control Study*

3.3.1. Intestinal Permeability

In the case-control analysis (Figure 2), serum levels of FABP-2 were significantly higher in ME/CFS patients than in controls ($F_{1,72} = 24.022$, $p < 0.001$, $\eta_p^2 = 0.255$). No correlation was found between FABP-2 levels and bowl habits or intestinal complaints.

3.3.2. Cytokines

Thirty-nine patients had baseline measurements of several serum cytokines. In most cases, cytokine concentrations were within normal limits. The cytokines more frequently increased were TGF-β, IL-2, and TNF-α (Table 2).

In the case-control analysis (Figure 2), serum levels of IL-17 were higher in ME/CFS patients than in controls ($F_{1,73} = 5.901$, $p = 0.018$, $\eta_p^2 = 0.075$), while no differences between ME-CFS patients and controls was found concerning IL-4, IL-10, IL-18, and IFN-γ. In both ME/CFS patients and controls, serum cytokines were not correlated with clinical characteristics nor with any of the other variables measured in this study (data not shown).

3.3.3. Tryptophan Metabolites

As shown in Figure 1, tryptophan can be metabolized through the kynurenine (95%) and the serotonin pathways (2%). With respect to controls, ME/CFS patients had differences in the serum concentration of metabolites pertaining to both pathways when controlling for the possible confounding effect of age, sex, and BMI (Figure 3).

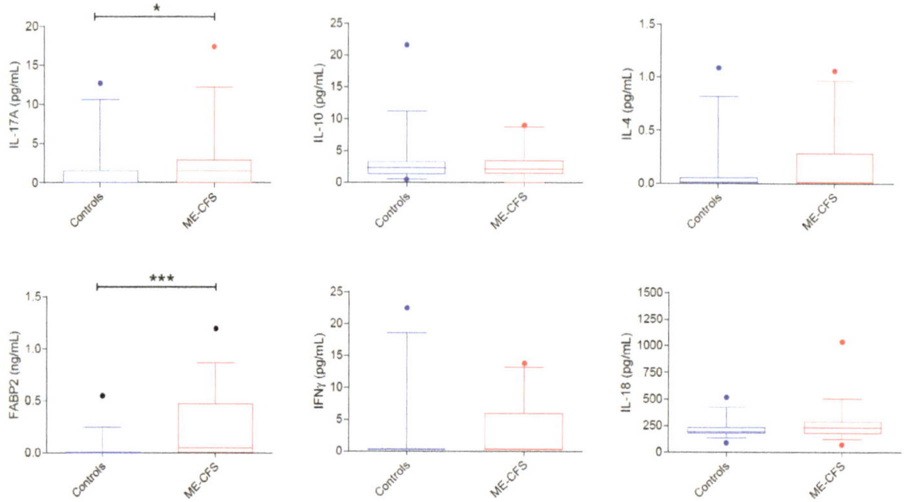

Figure 2. Case-control comparison of serum cytokines and FABP2 (n = 9). Serum IL-17A and FABP2 levels are higher in ME/CFS patients than in controls. Data are presented as boxplots with median and interquartile ranges and 5–95 percentiles. Dots represent data outside the 5–95 percentiles. * $p < 0.05$ and *** $p < 0.001$; Quade's rank analysis of covariance with BMI, sex, and age as covariates.

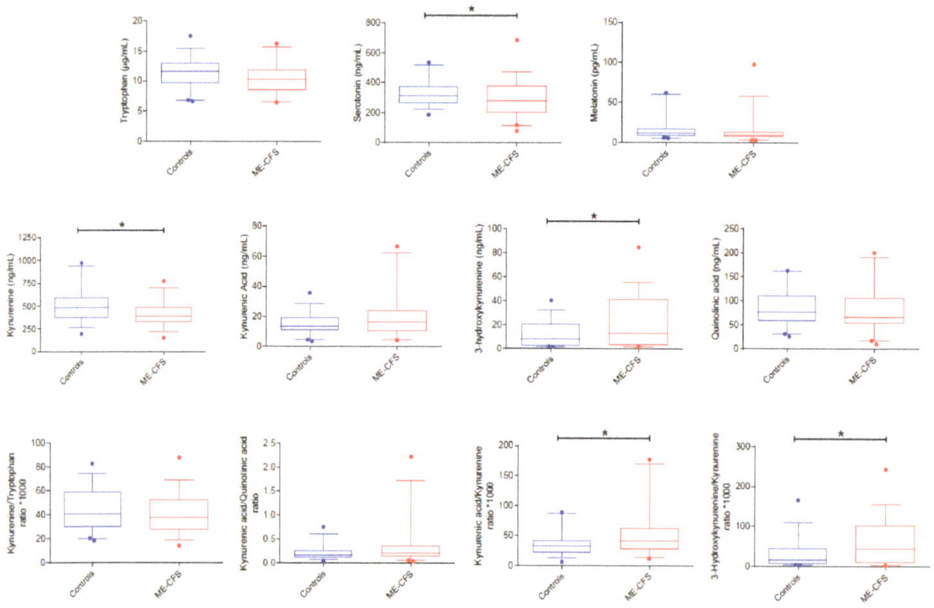

Figure 3. Case-control comparison of tryptophan metabolites via serotonin and kynurenine (n = 39). Serum levels of serotonin and kynurenine are lower and those of 3-hydroxykynurenine higher in ME-CFS patients than in controls. The kynurenic acid/kynurenine and 3-hydroxykynurenine/kynurenine ratios, indirect measures of kynurenine aminotransferases and kynurenine 3-monooxygenase enzymatic activities, respectively, are higher in ME-CFS patients than in controls. Data are presented as boxplots with median and interquartile ranges and 5–95 percentiles. Dots represent data outside the 5–95 percentiles. * $p < 0.05$; Quade's rank analysis of covariance with BMI, sex, and age as covariates.

Serum levels of tryptophan tended to be lower in ME/CFS patients than in controls ($F_{1,75} = 3.979$, $p = 0.05$, $\eta_p^2 = 0.050$). Concerning the serotonin pathway, serum levels of serotonin were lower in ME/CFS patients ($F_{1,75} = 4.169$, $p = 0.045$, $\eta_p^2 = 0.053$), while no difference was seen for melatonin (Figure 3). Concerning the kynurenine pathway, ME/CFS patients had lower serum levels of kynurenine ($F_{1,75} = 6.657$, $p = 0.012$, $\eta_p^2 = 0.082$) and higher levels of 3-hydroxy-kynurenine ($F_{1,74} = 4.499$, $p = 0.037$, $\eta_p^2 = 0.057$) (Figure 3). No differences were seen for quinolinic and kynurenic acids.

Considering the kynurenine/tryptophan ratio, no difference was found between ME/CFS patients and controls. In contrast, patients with ME/CFS had higher 3-hydroxykynurenine/kynurenine ($F_{1,75} = 6.025$, $p = 0.016$, $\eta_p^2 = 0.074$) and kynurenic acid/kynurenine ($F_{1,75} = 6.072$, $p = 0.016$, $\eta_p^2 = 0.075$) ratios (Figure 3).

No differences were observed between ME/CFS patients and controls for the neuroprotective ratio kynurenic acid/quinolinic acid (Figure 3; $F_{1,75} = 2.967$, $p = 0.089$, $\eta_p^2 = 0.038$).

Mode of symptom onset (infectious vs. non-infectious), the evolution of the clinical picture (improved, unchanged, worsened), symptom frequency, and intensity did not correlate with any of the measured biomarkers (data not shown).

3.4. Comparisons between Post-Infectious and Non-Post-Infectious ME/CFS Patients

Patients with post-infectious ME/CFS reported more frequently a fast start ($p < 0.0001$) and a higher Bell score ($p = 0.02$), and a tendency to be older ($p = 0.05$) than patients with non-post-infection ME/CFS (Table 4). Starting with or without infection was not associated with differences in symptom scores, bowel habit, abdominal pain, the diagnosis of irritable bowel syndrome, or with the presence of CFS/fatigue/fibromyalgia or immune diseases in the family (Table 4). Concerning circulating levels of cytokines, FABP-2 and tryptophan metabolites, after controlling for sex, age, and BMI, we found a tendency to lower serum levels of IL-18 ($p = 0.068$), lower kynurenine ($p = 0.026$), and lower kynurenine/tryptophan ratio ($p = 0.015$) in post-infection than in non-post-infection ME/CFS patients (Table 5). No differences between the two groups were seen for the other cytokines, FABP-2, and other tryptophan metabolites (Table 5).

Table 4. Clinical characteristics of post-infectious ($n = 19$) and non-post-infections ($n = 21$) ME/CFS patients.

Variable	ME/CFS Did Not Start after an Infection ($n = 21$)	ME/CFS Started after an Infection ($n = 19$)	Statistics
Age, years [a]	30 (20–44)	35 (28–48)	U = 261.5, $p = 0.093$
Males	8 (38%)	6 (32%)	$\chi^2 = 0.186$, $p = 0.66$
Disease duration, years [a,b]	8 (3–13)	5 (3–11)	U = 169.5, $p = 0.59$
Symptom start:			
Slow (months)	17/21 (81%)	1/19 (5%)	$\chi^2 = 23.089$, $p < 0.0001$
Fast (weeks)	4/21 (19%)	18/19 (95%)	
ME/CFS, fatigue or fibromyalgia in the family	7/19 [d] (37%)	6/19 (31%)	$\chi^2 = 0.000$, 0.99
Immune diseases in the family	9/19 [d] (47%)	8/19 (42%)	$\chi^2 = 0.010$, 0.92
Symptom score (0–6): [a]			
Fatigue	6 (5–6)	6 (5–6)	
PEM	5 (5–6)	5 (5–6)	U = 193.0, $p = 0.84$ U = 211.0
Unrefreshing sleep	5 (4–5)	4 (4–5)	$p = 0.74$ U = 214.0,
Pain	4 (3–5)	4 (3–6)	$p = 0.69$ U = 212.0,
Cognitive anomalies	5 (4–5)	5 (4–5)	$p = 0.73$ U = 179.0
OI/POTS	4 (4–5)	4 (4–5)	$p = 0.55$ U = 249.0,
GI abnormalities	4 (0–4)	4 (3–5)	$p = 0.17$ U = 250.0,
Flu-like symptoms	4 (3–4)	5 (3–5)	$p = 0.16$ U = 242.0, $p = 0.24$

Table 4. *Cont.*

Variable	ME/CFS Did Not Start after an Infection (n = 21)	ME/CFS Started after an Infection (n = 19)	Statistics
Bell scale score (0–100%) [a,c]	30 (22–41)	43 (30–50)	U = 236.0, p = 0.02
Bowel habit: [a]			
Normal [d]	11/20 (55%)	12/18 (67%)	χ^2 = 5.353, p = 0.07
Styptic [d]	8/20 (40%)	2/18 (11%)	
Diarrheic [d]	1/20 (5%)	4/18 (22%)	
Abdominal pain—IBS [e]	13/21 (62%)	10/19 (53%)	χ^2 = 0.351, p = 0.55

Data expressed as n (%) or [a] median (IQR). PEM—post-exertional malaise; OI—orthostatic intolerance; POTS—postural orthostatic tachycardia syndrome; GI—gastro-intestine; IBS—irritable bowel syndrome. Data were not available in [b] 1, [c] 4, and [d] 2 patients; [e] diagnosed according to the Rome IV criteria [28].

Table 5. Serum levels of cytokines, FABP-2, and tryptophan metabolites along the serotonin and kynurenine pathways in post-infection (n = 19) and non-post-infection (n = 21) ME/CFS patients.

	ME/CFS Did Not Start after an Infection (n = 21)	ME/CFS Started after an Infection (n = 19)	Statistics
Cytokines			
IL-17A (pg/mL)	1.6 (0.2–5.3)	1.6 (0.0–2.8)	$F_{1,36}$ = 0.073, p = 0.789, η_p^2 = 0.002
IL-10 (pg/mL)	2.2 (1.7–4.2)	2.0 (1.3–2.7)	$F_{1,36}$ = 1.311, p = 0.260, η_p^2 = 0.035
IL-4 (pg/mL)	0.0 (0.0–0.5)	0.0 (0.0–0.3)	$F_{1,36}$ = 0.503, p = 0.485, η_p^2 = 0.021
IFN-γ (pg/mL)	0.3 (0.3–8.2)	0.3 (0.3–4.5)	$F_{1,36}$ = 0.205, p = 0.654 η_p^2 = 0.006
IL-18 (pg/mL)	255.3 (195.9–303.4)	196.9 (155.6–250.1)	$F_{1,36}$ = 4.521, p = 0.068, η_p^2 = 0.091
FABP-2 (ng/mL)	0.0 (0.0–0.5)	0.13 (0.0–0.5)	$F_{1,34}$ = 0.492 p = 0.488, η_p^2 = 0.015
Kynurenine pathway			
Tryptophan (μg/mL)	9.36 (8.26–12.01)	10.68 (9.56–11.99)	$F_{1,37}$ = 1.640, p = 0.208, η_p^2 = 0.042
Kynurenine (ng/mL)	413.4 (339.2–539.6)	347.6 (260.1–397.9)	$F_{1,37}$ = 5.410, p = 0.026, η_p^2 = 0.128
3-hydroxykynurenine (ng/mL)	12.3 (3.3–41.7)	17.5 (5.9–39.6)	$F_{1,37}$ = 1.102, p = 0.301, η_p^2 = 0.029
Kynurenic acid (ng/mL)	16.6 (11.0–24.1)	14.2 (9.1–35.8)	$F_{1,37}$ = 0.216, p = 0.645, η_p^2 = 0.006
Quinolinic acid (ng/mL)	59.6 (40.9–102.6)	67.2 (59.6–111.6)	$F_{1,37}$ = 0.298, p = 0.588, η_p^2 = 0.008
Kynurenine/tryptophan ratio * 1000	44.1 (32.9–57.9)	33.2 (24.8–38.8)	$F_{1,37}$ = 6.525, p = 0.015, η_p^2 = 0.150
3-hydroxykynurenine/kynurenine ratio * 1000	42.4 (7.8–97.9)	80.6 (19.0–107.7)	$F_{1,37}$ = 0.499, p = 0.485, η_p^2 = 0.013
Kynurenic acid/kynurenine ratio	39.6 (26.5–59.7)	50.6 (27.6–84.1)	$F_{1,37}$ = 0.313, p = 0.579, η_p^2 = 0.008
Kynurenic acid/quinolinic acid ratio	0.2 (0.1–0.4)	0.2 (0.1–0.3)	$F_{1,37}$ = 0.131, p = 0.719, η_p^2 = 0.004
Serotonin pathway			
Serotonin (ng/mL)	301.4 (218.3–382.4)	258.8 (180.4–377.4)	$F_{1,37}$ = 1.261, p = 0.269, η_p^2 = 0.033
Melatonin (pg/mL)	9.8 (6.3–20.2)	10.2 (8.1–13.7)	$F_{1,37}$ = 0.076, p = 0.784, η_p^2 = 0.002

Data are median (IQR). Comparisons have been computed using Quade's rank analysis of covariance with BMI, sex, and age as covariates.

4. Discussion

Our results indicate that ME/CFS patients differ from control healthy subjects for several serum biomarkers, including FABP-2, IL-17A, and tryptophan metabolites, such as kynurenine, serotonin, 3-hydroxykynurenine, and the ratios kynurenic acid/quinolinic acid and 3-hydroxykynurenine/kynurenine. Moreover, a difference in serum levels of kynurenine and the ratio of kynurenine/tryptophan is also present within ME/CFS patients according to whether the disease started after an infection or not.

4.1. Study Population

Our patients fulfilled the criteria of the Canadian Consensus Criteria for the diagnosis of ME/CFS, and for the majority of them, the diagnosis of ME/CFS was also made by independent colleagues. It is clear, however, that they were a heterogeneous group of individuals with differences in disease start, symptoms, laboratory data, and genetic background. Some of the rarer aspects of our patients, such as jerks, hyperlaxity, and livedo reticularis, are long known [29,30], while others, including disturbances in glycogen metabolism, have just been reported [31]. Some clinical and basal laboratory characteristics of our cohort, however, seem novel. Two patients had bouts of low-grade fever and increased serum levels of CRP and amyloid A, as found in auto-inflammatory syndromes [32]. We thus decided to subject them to a trial of drugs used in autoinflammatory syndromes, such as colchicine or the anti-IL1-β monoclonal antibody canakinumab [33], with lasting benefit. Auto-inflammatory syndromes are due to the inappropriate activation of the inflammasome with the production of cytokines of the IL-1β family that mostly act locally so that their serum levels usually remain within normal limits [32]. Although fever and inflammation of the skin, mucosae, serosal surfaces, and osteoarticular structures are cardinal manifestations of these syndromes, fatigue is emerging as an important symptom [34]. We could not attribute these cases to a defined autoinflammatory syndrome, but they clearly responded to the abovementioned treatments, suggesting that it might be convenient to add auto-inflammatory syndromes to the list of differential diagnoses when considering patients with suspected ME/CFS.

One of our patients had a micro-duplication on chromosome 15 (15q13.3), a rare chromosomal disorder that may present with developmental delay, behavioral and psychiatric abnormalities, feeding problems, sleep disturbances, decreased muscle tone, and seizures [35]. The duplication involves the locus of the gene CHRNA7, which codes for the α7 nicotinic acetylcholine receptor (a member of the cholinergic anti-inflammatory pathway) and of the gene CHRFAM7A that acts as a dominant negative inhibitor of the CHRNA7 gene [36–38]. At present, we do not know the significance of this anomaly for our patients.

We conclude that our patients had differences in genetic background, disease start, symptoms, basal laboratory data, response to treatment, and evolution.

4.2. Intestinal Permeability

ME/CFS patients had increased serum levels of FABP-2, a low molecular weight protein involved in the intracellular traffic of fatty acids, which comprises 4–6% of enterocyte cytosolic proteins, is undetectable or present in very low concentrations in the serum of healthy persons and is used as a marker of increased intestinal permeability [39]. Our observation partially agrees with evidence obtained by Giloteaux et al. [5], who found in a larger cohort of patients increased serum levels of Lipopolysaccharide Binding Protein, another index of increased intestinal permeability, while FABP-2 was increased but not significantly.

The mechanism leading to increased intestinal permeability remains unclear. Intestinal complaints are frequent among patients with ME/CFS, and a recent paper examining fecal bacterial metagenomics in a cohort of patients with ME/CFS concluded that IBS comorbidity was the strongest factor driving separation of data into topological networks [40].

Components of the normal intestinal flora regulate the barrier function of the intestine and exert anti-infective and anti-inflammatory activity [41]. An imbalance in the composition of the intestinal microbiome, well documented in patients with ME/CFS [5,6], could thus contribute to the genesis of the intestinal barrier dysfunction.

4.3. Cytokines

In agreement with the literature, no specific cytokine profile could be identified in our patients [2,42].

In the case-control study, the only cytokine with a serum concentration different from controls was IL-17A, which was modestly but significantly increased in ME/CFS patients.

IL-17A is a cytokine produced by multiple cell types ($CD4^+$ T cells, $CD8^+$ T cells, $\gamma\delta$ T cells, invariant natural T cells, innate lymphoid cells, and lung memory T lymphocytes) that can be either pro-inflammatory (in the skin) or protective (in the airways and the intestine) [43]. In the intestine, IL-17A regulates the formation of tight junctions, increases the release of secretory IgA, and favors the production of antibacterial peptides; thus, its increase in our patients might represent a response to a local noxa [43]. On the other side, Th17 polarization and increased production of IL-17A have recently been linked to an increased extracellular concentration of lactate [44]. Considering that in patients with ME/CFS, the intestinal microbiome has an increased ability to produce lactate [45], and that tissue hypoperfusion due to anomalies of peripheral blood flow auto-regulation has been proposed as a possible pathogenetic mechanism of ME/CFS [22], the relationship between energy metabolism and Th17 polarization may merit further scrutiny. Finally, it has been recently suggested that IL-17A may play a role in depression associated with psoriasis and obesity [46]. The present data suggest that it might be worthwhile to see if a relationship exists between IL-17A serum levels and ME/CFS-associated depression.

4.4. Tryptophan and Kynurenine Metabolites

Changes in peripheral circulating levels of tryptophan and some of its metabolites via serotonin and kynurenine are considered good biomarkers of their changes in the brain [14,47]. Indeed, most of the brain kynurenine is derived from tryptophan outside the central nervous system. Kynurenine then crosses the blood-brain barrier and is metabolized to kynurenic acid, xanthurenic acid, or 3-hydroxykynurenine [14,48]. 3-hydroxykynurenine is further metabolized to quinolinic acid (Figure 1). Interestingly, among kynurenine metabolites, 3-hydroxykynurenine crosses the blood–brain barrier readily, while kynurenic acid and quinolinic acid, due to high polarity, do not [48].

Metabolites of the kynurenine pathway play a significant role in the homeostasis of the central nervous system, playing both neuroprotective and neurotoxic effects [14,49]. In fact, kynurenine exerts anti-inflammatory activity by binding to aryl hydrocarbon receptor and stimulating the production of regulatory T cells [50]. On the other hand, 3-hydroxykynurenine is neurotoxic since it undergoes oxidation in physiological conditions, producing highly reactive hydroxyl radicals [51]. Kynurenic acid, on the opposite, is neuroprotective since it inhibits all excitatory amino acid receptors (NMDA, kainate, AMPA), inhibits the 7α acetylcholine receptor, binds to aryl hydrocarbon receptor and G-protein coupled receptor 35 (GPR35), inhibits the circuit IL-23/IL-17, and acts as an oxy-radical scavenger [14,48,52,53]. Quinolinic acid is neurotoxic since it stimulates NMDA receptors in specific brain regions, favors lipid peroxidation, inhibits gluconeogenesis, and inhibits mitochondrial monoamine oxidase activity [48].

In ME/CFS, blood tryptophan concentration has been found increased by some authors [15] and unchanged by others [16,54]. In our cohort of patients, serum tryptophan concentration was not different from controls, although patients tended to present lower values (p = 0.05). Patients had, instead, lower levels of kynurenine, higher levels of 3-hydroxykynurenine, and an increase in the ratios kynurenic acid/kynurenine (indirect index of KAT activity) and 3-hydroxykynurenine/kynurenine (indirect index of KMO activity).

The mechanisms leading to low serum levels of kynurenine remain undefined, the change being compatible with the decreased transformation of tryptophan into kynurenine and/or, more likely, the increased transformation of kynurenine into kynurenic acid and 3-hydroxykynurenine as we found an increase in the ratios of kynurenic acid/kynurenine and 3-hydroxykynurenine/kynurenine. It is also unclear why patients with a post-infectious start had lower levels of kynurenine than patients not starting with an infection.

In ME/CFS patients, we found increased serum levels of 3-hydroxykynurenine but normal levels of its product quinolinic acid. Since 3-hydroxykynurenine crosses the blood–

brain barrier freely [48], increased blood levels of 3-hydroxykynurenine could translate into increased transfer of this toxic molecule to the brain.

Our findings differ from those of Groven et al. [54], who, in a group of patients with ME/CFS, found decreased plasma levels of anthranilic acid, a neuroprotective kynurenine derivative not considered in this study, and a decrease in the ratio kynurenic acid/quinolinic acid, while tryptophan, kynurenine, kynurenic acid, and 3-hydroxykynurenine were not different from controls. On the other side, our data agree in part with evidence recently presented by Hoel et al. [22], who reported lower levels of kynurenine and kynurenic acid and normal levels of tryptophan and serotonin in ME/CFS patients. These discrepancies could be due to differences between the populations studied, given the high heterogeneity within ME/CFS patients. For this reason, we here also included a nosological description of our study population so that it could be used for comparisons with future studies in the field. A further and important point that may explain possible discrepancies between our and the abovementioned studies is the fact that serum samples in Groven et al. [54] and Hoel et al. [22] were collected without restrictions about the feeding state, which is an important factor in determining circulating levels of tryptophan and its metabolites [14]. Of interest, changes in tryptophan biomarkers similar to those found in our patients (low tryptophan, kynurenine, and serotonin and high 3-hydroxykynurenine) have been observed in diabetic ketoacidosis [55,56]. Thus, it is possible that part of the discrepancy between our findings and those of Groven et al. [54] and Hoel et al. [22] may rely on a particular response to fasting by patients with ME/CFS, who present an increased expression of enzymes involved in ketone body metabolism [57] and, for their energy needs, may depend on fatty acid β–oxidation more than healthy controls [8]).

In ME/CFS patients, we also found low serum levels of serotonin, which is over 90% produced by intestinal enterochromaffin cells and is mostly associated with platelet granules [14]. Our findings bear similarities with the observation that circulating serotonin is low in patients with irritable bowel syndrome with constipation [58], a condition characterized by low serotonin concentration in the intestinal wall [59].

4.5. Relevance of the Present Findings for the Explanation of ME/CFS Pathogenesis

Overall, we found no significant correlation among cytokines, FABP2, and tryptophan metabolites, likely indicating that inflammation, anomalies of the intestinal barrier, and changes of tryptophan metabolism may be independently associated with the establishment of disease. Despite clear differences among patients, however, our findings remain compatible with the view that persons with ME/CFS may have common or largely shared pathogenetic mechanisms. Indeed, in the present study, changes in tryptophan metabolites and increased IL-17A levels are both compatible with anomalies in the sphere of energy metabolism.

4.6. Limitations

This study has several limitations: first, the small sample size; second, its essentially exploratory nature; third, the use of ELISA methods for cytokine measurement that were not of the highest sensitivity, an aspect important for cytokines normally present in blood at very low concentrations; fourth, the lack of deep knowledge about patient diet, supplements, vitamins, and probiotics could have influenced the gut status and tryptophan metabolism; fifth, uncertainty about the extent to which serum levels of tryptophan metabolites reflect changes occurring in the central nervous system; sixth, the presence of control subjects with serum levels of some biomarkers outside the 5–95 percentile (see Figures 2 and 3) is possibly due to undiagnosed underlying disease; however, even if these potential outliers were excluded, the differences observed in the case-control analyses would remain significant; seventh, we did not investigate the physical activity of healthy controls, a factor known to influence serum levels of inflammatory cytokines and tryptophan metabolites [60]. Therefore, the possible confounding effect of exercise in the case-control study was not considered.

5. Conclusions

We found substantial heterogeneity among patients with ME/CFS; however, in spite of many differences, patients shared traits of possible significance for the explanation of their symptoms. Our data suggest that clinical aspects and serum biomarkers related to inflammation, intestinal function, and tryptophan metabolism deserve to be further investigated, both for the identification of ME/CFS subtypes and as a way towards a personalized patient care approach. This implies, on one side, the use of larger patient samples and, on the other side, the use of all modern medical tools for the diagnosis and treatment of individual cases.

Supplementary Materials: The following are available online at https://www.mdpi.com/article/10.3390/biomedicines9111724/s1, Table S1: Study design.

Author Contributions: Conceptualization, U.F., A.A., R.M., S.C. and A.B.; data curation, M.S. and S.C.; formal analysis, F.C.; investigation, M.S., S.D., C.Z., S.S., N.G., P.S., L.S., U.F., P.C., P.A., A.A., D.B., R.M., S.C. and A.B.; methodology, R.T.; resources, C.Z. and D.B.; supervision, A.B.; writing—original draft, M.S., A.A., S.C. and A.B. All authors have read and agreed to the published version of the manuscript.

Funding: This research did not receive any specific grant from funding agencies in the public, commercial, or not-for-profit sectors.

Institutional Review Board Statement: The study was conducted according to the guidelines of the Declaration of Helsinki and approved by the Institutional Review Board Ethics Committee of Policlinico Universitario, Padova, Italy (Protocol Number 4776/AO/19).

Informed Consent Statement: Informed consent was obtained from all subjects involved in the study.

Data Availability Statement: The data sets analyzed during the current study are available from the corresponding author on reasonable request.

Acknowledgments: We thank our patients for their efforts to make this project possible. We also thank Chiara Sacchetto and Girolamo Carollo for their help and enthusiasm and Claudio Masello for generous support.

Conflicts of Interest: The authors declare no conflict of interest.

References

1. Shepherd, D.C.; Chaudhuri, D.A. *ME/CFS/PVFS: An Exploration of the Key Clinical Issues*; ME Association: Gawcott, UK, 2019.
2. VanElzakker, M.B.; Brumfield, S.A.; Lara Mejia, P.S. Neuroinflammation and Cytokines in Myalgic Encephalomyelitis/Chronic Fatigue Syndrome (ME/CFS): A Critical Review of Research Methods. *Front. Neurol.* **2018**, *9*, 1033. [CrossRef]
3. Yamamoto, S.; Ouchi, Y.; Onoe, H.; Yoshikawa, E.; Tsukada, H.; Takahashi, H.; Iwase, M.; Yamaguti, K.; Kuratsune, H.; Watanabe, Y. Reduction of serotonin transporters of patients with chronic fatigue syndrome. *Neuroreport* **2004**, *15*, 2571–2574. [CrossRef]
4. Noda, M.; Ifuku, M.; Hossain, M.S.; Katafuchi, T. Glial Activation and Expression of the Serotonin Transporter in Chronic Fatigue Syndrome. *Front. Psychiatry* **2018**, *9*, 589. [CrossRef] [PubMed]
5. Giloteaux, L.; Goodrich, J.K.; Walters, W.A.; Levine, S.M.; Ley, R.E.; Hanson, M.R. Reduced diversity and altered composition of the gut microbiome in individuals with myalgic encephalomyelitis/chronic fatigue syndrome. *Microbiome* **2016**, *4*, 30. [CrossRef] [PubMed]
6. Lupo, G.F.D.; Rocchetti, G.; Lucini, L.; Lorusso, L.; Manara, E.; Bertelli, M.; Puglisi, E.; Capelli, E. Potential role of microbiome in Chronic Fatigue Syndrome/Myalgic Encephalomyelits (CFS/ME). *Sci. Rep.* **2021**, *11*, 7043. [CrossRef] [PubMed]
7. Tomas, C.; Brown, A.; Strassheim, V.; Elson, J.L.; Newton, J.; Manning, P. Cellular bioenergetics is impaired in patients with chronic fatigue syndrome. *PLoS ONE* **2017**, *12*, e0186802. [CrossRef] [PubMed]
8. Missailidis, D.; Sanislav, O.; Allan, C.Y.; Smith, P.K.; Annesley, S.J.; Fisher, P.R. Dysregulated Provision of Oxidisable Substrates to the Mitochondria in ME/CFS Lymphoblasts. *Int. J. Mol. Sci.* **2021**, *22*, 2046. [CrossRef]
9. Mandarano, A.H.; Maya, J.; Giloteaux, L.; Peterson, D.L.; Maynard, M.; Gottschalk, C.G.; Hanson, M.R. Myalgic encephalomyelitis/chronic fatigue syndrome patients exhibit altered T cell metabolism and cytokine associations. *J. Clin. Investig.* **2020**, *130*, 1491–1505. [CrossRef]
10. Joseph, P.; Arevalo, C.; Oliveira, R.K.F.; Faria-Urbina, M.; Felsenstein, D.; Oaklander, A.L.; Systrom, D.M. Insights From Invasive Cardiopulmonary Exercise Testing of Patients With Myalgic Encephalomyelitis/Chronic Fatigue Syndrome. *Chest* **2021**, *160*, 642–651. [CrossRef]

11. Shan, Z.Y.; Barnden, L.R.; Kwiatek, R.A.; Bhuta, S.; Hermens, D.F.; Lagopoulos, J. Neuroimaging characteristics of myalgic encephalomyelitis/chronic fatigue syndrome (ME/CFS): A systematic review. *J. Transl. Med.* **2020**, *18*, 335. [CrossRef]
12. Cleare, A.J.; Messa, C.; Rabiner, E.A.; Grasby, P.M. Brain 5-HT1A receptor binding in chronic fatigue syndrome measured using positron emission tomography and [11C]WAY-100635. *Biol. Psychiatry* **2005**, *57*, 239–246. [CrossRef] [PubMed]
13. Nakatomi, Y.; Mizuno, K.; Ishii, A.; Wada, Y.; Tanaka, M.; Tazawa, S.; Onoe, K.; Fukuda, S.; Kawabe, J.; Takahashi, K.; et al. Neuroinflammation in Patients with Chronic Fatigue Syndrome/Myalgic Encephalomyelitis: An ^{11}C-(R)-PK11195 PET Study. *J. Nucl. Med.* **2014**, *55*, 945–950. [CrossRef] [PubMed]
14. Comai, S.; Bertazzo, A.; Brughera, M.; Crotti, S. Tryptophan in health and disease. *Adv. Clin. Chem.* **2020**, *95*, 165–218. [CrossRef] [PubMed]
15. Badawy, A.A.; Morgan, C.J.; Llewelyn, M.B.; Albuquerque, S.R.; Farmer, A. Heterogeneity of serum tryptophan concentration and availability to the brain in patients with the chronic fatigue syndrome. *J. Psychopharmacol.* **2005**, *19*, 385–391. [CrossRef]
16. Georgiades, E.; Behan, W.M.; Kilduff, L.P.; Hadjicharalambous, M.; Mackie, E.E.; Wilson, J.; Ward, S.A.; Pitsiladis, Y.P. Chronic fatigue syndrome: New evidence for a central fatigue disorder. *Clin. Sci.* **2003**, *105*, 213–218. [CrossRef]
17. Branchi, I.; Poggini, S.; Capuron, L.; Benedetti, F.; Poletti, S.; Tamouza, R.; Drexhage, H.A.; Penninx, B.W.; Pariante, C.M. Brain-immune crosstalk in the treatment of major depressive disorder. *Eur. Neuropsychopharmacol.* **2021**, *45*, 89–107. [CrossRef]
18. Gheorghe, C.E.; Martin, J.A.; Manriquez, F.V.; Dinan, T.G.; Cryan, J.F.; Clarke, G. Focus on the essentials: Tryptophan metabolism and the microbiome-gut-brain axis. *Curr. Opin. Pharmacol.* **2019**, *48*, 137–145. [CrossRef]
19. Tanaka, M.; Vécsei, L. Monitoring the kynurenine system: Concentrations, ratios or what else? *Adv. Clin. Exp. Med.* **2021**, *30*, 775–778. [CrossRef]
20. Hornig, M.; Montoya, J.G.; Klimas, N.G.; Levine, S.; Felsenstein, D.; Bateman, L.; Peterson, D.L.; Gottschalk, C.G.; Schultz, A.F.; Che, X.; et al. Distinct plasma immune signatures in ME/CFS are present early in the course of illness. *Sci. Adv.* **2015**, *1*, e1400121. [CrossRef]
21. White, P.D. Chronic fatigue syndrome: Is it one discrete syndrome or many? Implications for the "one vs. many" functional somatic syndromes debate. *J. Psychosom. Res.* **2010**, *68*, 455–459. [CrossRef]
22. Hoel, F.; Hoel, A.; Pettersen, I.K.; Rekeland, I.G.; Risa, K.; Alme, K.; Sørland, K.; Fosså, A.; Lien, K.; Herder, I.; et al. A map of metabolic phenotypes in patients with myalgic encephalomyelitis/chronic fatigue syndrome. *JCI Insight* **2021**, *6*, e149217. [CrossRef] [PubMed]
23. Lim, E.-J.; Ahn, Y.-C.; Jang, E.-S.; Lee, S.-W.; Lee, S.-H.; Son, C.-G. Systematic review and meta-analysis of the prevalence of chronic fatigue syndrome/myalgic encephalomyelitis (CFS/ME). *J. Transl. Med.* **2020**, *18*, 100. [CrossRef] [PubMed]
24. Bell, D.S. *The Doctor's Guide to Chronic Fatigue Syndrome: Understanding, Treating, and Living with CFIDS*; Da Capo Press: Cambridge, MA, USA, 1994.
25. Carruthers, B.M.; Jain, A.K.; De Meirleir, K.L.; Peterson, D.L.; Klimas, N.G.; Lerner, A.M.; Bested, A.C.; Flor-Henry, P.; Joshi, P.; Powles, A.P. Myalgic encephalomyelitis/chronic fatigue syndrome: Clinical working case definition, diagnostic and treatment protocols. *J. Chronic Fatigue Syndr.* **2003**, *11*, 7–115. [CrossRef]
26. Messaoud, A.; Mensi, R.; Douki, W.; Neffati, F.; Najjar, M.F.; Gobbi, G.; Valtorta, F.; Gaha, L.; Comai, S. Reduced peripheral availability of tryptophan and increased activation of the kynurenine pathway and cortisol correlate with major depression and suicide. *World J. Biol. Psychiatry* **2019**, *20*, 703–711. [CrossRef] [PubMed]
27. Nazzari, S.; Molteni, M.; Valtorta, F.; Comai, S.; Frigerio, A. Prenatal IL-6 levels and activation of the tryptophan to kynurenine pathway are associated with depressive but not anxiety symptoms across the perinatal and the post-partum period in a low-risk sample. *Brain Behav. Immun.* **2020**, *89*, 175–183. [CrossRef]
28. Drossman, D.A. The Rome IV Committees editor. History of functional gastrointestinal symptoms and disorders and chronicle of the Rome Foundation. In *Rome IV Functional Gastrointestinal Disorders of Gut-Brain Interaction*; Drossman, D.A., Chang, L.C., Kellow, W.J., Tack, J., Whitehead, W.E., Eds.; The Rome Foundation: Raleigh, NC, USA, 2016; pp. 549–576.
29. Chu, L.; Valencia, I.J.; Garvert, D.W.; Montoya, J.G. Onset Patterns and Course of Myalgic Encephalomyelitis/Chronic Fatigue Syndrome. *Front. Pediatrics* **2019**, *7*, 12. [CrossRef]
30. Martín-Martínez, E.; Martín-Martínez, M. Varied Presentation of Myalgic Encephalomyelitis/Chronic Fatigue Syndrome and the Needs for Classification and Clinician Education: A Case Series. *Clin. Ther.* **2019**, *41*, 619–624. [CrossRef] [PubMed]
31. Brown, D.; Birch, C.; Younger, J.; Worthey, E. ME/CFS: Whole genome sequencing uncovers a misclassified case of glycogen storage disease type 13 previously diagnosed as ME/CFS. *Mol. Genet. Metab.* **2021**, *132*, S194–S195. [CrossRef]
32. Goldbach-Mansky, R.; Dailey, N.J.; Canna, S.W.; Gelabert, A.; Jones, J.; Rubin, B.I.; Kim, H.J.; Brewer, C.; Zalewski, C.; Wiggs, E.; et al. Neonatal-onset multisystem inflammatory disease responsive to interleukin-1beta inhibition. *N. Engl. J. Med.* **2006**, *355*, 581–592. [CrossRef]
33. De Benedetti, F.; Gattorno, M.; Anton, J.; Ben-Chetrit, E.; Frenkel, J.; Hoffman, H.M.; Koné-Paut, I.; Lachmann, H.J.; Ozen, S.; Simon, A.; et al. Canakinumab for the Treatment of Autoinflammatory Recurrent Fever Syndromes. *N. Engl. J. Med.* **2018**, *378*, 1908–1919. [CrossRef]
34. Yadlapati, S.; Efthimiou, P. Impact of IL-1 inhibition on fatigue associated with autoinflammatory syndromes. *Mod. Rheumatol.* **2016**, *26*, 3–8. [CrossRef] [PubMed]

35. Van Bon, B.W.; Mefford, H.C.; Menten, B.; Koolen, D.A.; Sharp, A.J.; Nillesen, W.M.; Innis, J.W.; de Ravel, T.J.; Mercer, C.L.; Fichera, M.; et al. Further delineation of the 15q13 microdeletion and duplication syndromes: A clinical spectrum varying from non-pathogenic to a severe outcome. *J. Med. Genet.* **2009**, *46*, 511–523. [CrossRef] [PubMed]
36. Murray, K.; Reardon, C. The cholinergic anti-inflammatory pathway revisited. *Neurogastroenterol. Motil.* **2018**, *30*, e13288. [CrossRef] [PubMed]
37. Chang, E.H.; Chavan, S.S.; Pavlov, V.A. Cholinergic Control of Inflammation, Metabolic Dysfunction, and Cognitive Impairment in Obesity-Associated Disorders: Mechanisms and Novel Therapeutic Opportunities. *Front. Neurosci.* **2019**, *13*, 263. [CrossRef] [PubMed]
38. Benfante, R.; Antonini, R.A.; De Pizzol, M.; Gotti, C.; Clementi, F.; Locati, M.; Fornasari, D. Expression of the α7 nAChR subunit duplicate form (CHRFAM7A) is down-regulated in the monocytic cell line THP-1 on treatment with LPS. *J. Neuroimmunol.* **2011**, *230*, 74–84. [CrossRef] [PubMed]
39. Cifarelli, V.; Abumrad, N.A. Enterocyte Fatty Acid Handling Proteins and Chylomicron Formation. In *Physiology of the Gastrointestinal Tract*; Elsevier: Amsterdam, The Netherlands, 2018; pp. 1087–1107.
40. Nagy-Szakal, D.; Barupal, D.K.; Lee, B.; Che, X.; Williams, B.L.; Kahn, E.J.R.; Ukaigwe, J.E.; Bateman, L.; Klimas, N.G.; Komaroff, A.L.; et al. Insights into myalgic encephalomyelitis/chronic fatigue syndrome phenotypes through comprehensive metabolomics. *Sci. Rep.* **2018**, *8*, 10056. [CrossRef]
41. Ling, X.; Linglong, P.; Weixia, D.; Hong, W. Protective Effects of Bifidobacterium on Intestinal Barrier Function in LPS-Induced Enterocyte Barrier Injury of Caco-2 Monolayers and in a Rat NEC Model. *PLoS ONE* **2016**, *11*, e0161635. [CrossRef]
42. Corbitt, M.; Eaton-Fitch, N.; Staines, D.; Cabanas, H.; Marshall-Gradisnik, S. A systematic review of cytokines in chronic fatigue syndrome/myalgic encephalomyelitis/systemic exertion intolerance disease (CFS/ME/SEID). *BMC Neurol.* **2019**, *19*, 207. [CrossRef]
43. Friedrich, M.; Pohin, M.; Powrie, F. Cytokine Networks in the Pathophysiology of Inflammatory Bowel Disease. *Immunity* **2019**, *50*, 992–1006. [CrossRef]
44. Pucino, V.; Certo, M.; Bulusu, V.; Cucchi, D.; Goldmann, K.; Pontarini, E.; Haas, R.; Smith, J.; Headland, S.E.; Blighe, K.; et al. Lactate Buildup at the Site of Chronic Inflammation Promotes Disease by Inducing $CD4^+$ T Cell Metabolic Rewiring. *Cell Metab.* **2019**, *30*, 1055–1074.e8. [CrossRef]
45. Guo, C.; Che, X.; Briese, T.; Allicock, O.; Yates, R.A.; Cheng, A.; Ranjan, A.; March, D.; Hornig, M.; Komaroff, A.L.; et al. Deficient butyrate-producing capacity in the gut microbiome of Myalgic Encephalomyelitis/Chronic Fatigue Syndrome patients is associated with fatigue symptoms. *medRxiv* **2021**. [CrossRef]
46. Zafiriou, E.; Daponte, A.I.; Siokas, V.; Tsigalou, C.; Dardiotis, E.; Bogdanos, D.P. Depression and Obesity in Patients With Psoriasis and Psoriatic Arthritis: Is IL-17-Mediated Immune Dysregulation the Connecting Link? *Front. Immunol.* **2021**, *12*. [CrossRef] [PubMed]
47. Török, N.; Tanaka, M.; Vécsei, L. Searching for Peripheral Biomarkers in Neurodegenerative Diseases: The Tryptophan-Kynurenine Metabolic Pathway. *Int. J. Mol. Sci.* **2020**, *21*, 9338. [CrossRef]
48. Schwarcz, R.; Bruno, J.P.; Muchowski, P.J.; Wu, H.Q. Kynurenines in the mammalian brain: When physiology meets pathology. *Nat. Rev. Neurosci.* **2012**, *13*, 465–477. [CrossRef] [PubMed]
49. Tanaka, M.; Tóth, F.; Polyák, H.; Szabó, A.; Mándi, Y.; Vécsei, L. Immune Influencers in Action: Metabolites and Enzymes of the Tryptophan-Kynurenine Metabolic Pathway. *Biomedicines* **2021**, *9*, 734. [CrossRef] [PubMed]
50. Sekine, H.; Mimura, J.; Oshima, M.; Okawa, H.; Kanno, J.; Igarashi, K.; Gonzalez, F.J.; Ikuta, T.; Kawajiri, K.; Fujii-Kuriyama, Y. Hypersensitivity of aryl hydrocarbon receptor-deficient mice to lipopolysaccharide-induced septic shock. *Mol. Cell. Biol.* **2009**, *29*, 6391–6400. [CrossRef]
51. Goldstein, L.E.; Leopold, M.C.; Huang, X.; Atwood, C.S.; Saunders, A.J.; Hartshorn, M.; Lim, J.T.; Faget, K.Y.; Muffat, J.A.; Scarpa, R.C.; et al. 3-Hydroxykynurenine and 3-hydroxyanthranilic acid generate hydrogen peroxide and promote alpha-crystallin cross-linking by metal ion reduction. *Biochemistry* **2000**, *39*, 7266–7275. [CrossRef]
52. Wirthgen, E.; Hoeflich, A.; Rebl, A.; Günther, J. Kynurenic Acid: The Janus-Faced Role of an Immunomodulatory Tryptophan Metabolite and Its Link to Pathological Conditions. *Front. Immunol.* **2017**, *8*, 1957. [CrossRef]
53. Kim, Y.K.; Jeon, S.W. Neuroinflammation and the Immune-Kynurenine Pathway in Anxiety Disorders. *Curr. Neuropharmacol.* **2018**, *16*, 574–582. [CrossRef]
54. Groven, N.; Reitan, S.K.; Fors, E.A.; Guzey, I.C. Kynurenine metabolites and ratios differ between Chronic Fatigue Syndrome, Fibromyalgia, and healthy controls. *Psychoneuroendocrinology* **2021**, *131*, 105287. [CrossRef]
55. Carl, G.F.; Hoffman, W.H.; Blankenship, P.R.; Litaker, M.S.; Hoffman, M.G.; Mabe, P.A. Diabetic ketoacidosis depletes plasma tryptophan. *Endocr. Res.* **2002**, *28*, 91–102. [CrossRef] [PubMed]
56. Hoffman, W.H.; Whelan, S.A.; Lee, N. Tryptophan, kynurenine pathway, and diabetic ketoacidosis in type 1 diabetes. *PLoS ONE* **2021**, *16*, e0254116. [CrossRef] [PubMed]
57. Sweetman, E.; Kleffmann, T.; Edgar, C.; de Lange, M.; Vallings, R.; Tate, W. A SWATH-MS analysis of Myalgic Encephalomyelitis/Chronic Fatigue Syndrome peripheral blood mononuclear cell proteomes reveals mitochondrial dysfunction. *J. Transl. Med.* **2020**, *18*, 365. [CrossRef] [PubMed]
58. Chojnacki, C.; Błońska, A.; Kaczka, A.; Chojnacki, J.; Stępień, A.; Gąsiorowska, A. Evaluation of serotonin and dopamine secretion and metabolism in patients with irritable bowel syndrome. *Pol. Arch. Intern. Med.* **2018**, *128*, 711–713. [CrossRef] [PubMed]

59. Manocha, M.; Khan, W.I. Serotonin and GI Disorders: An Update on Clinical and Experimental Studies. *Clin. Transl. Gastroenterol.* **2012**, *3*, e13. [CrossRef]
60. Martin, K.S.; Azzolini, M.; Lira Ruas, J. The kynurenine connection: How exercise shifts muscle tryptophan metabolism and affects energy homeostasis, the immune system, and the brain. *Am. J. Physiol. Cell Physiol.* **2020**, *318*, C818–C830. [CrossRef] [PubMed]

biomedicines

MDPI

Article

Chronic Lithium Treatment Affects Anxious Behaviors and theExpression of Serotonergic Genes in Midbrain Raphe Nuclei of Defeated Male Mice

Dmitry A. Smagin [1], Irina L. Kovalenko [1], Anna G. Galyamina [1], Irina V. Belozertseva [2], Nikolay V. Tamkovich [3], Konstantin O. Baranov [4] and Natalia N. Kudryavtseva [1,5,6,*]

1 FRC Institute of Cytology and Genetics, Siberian Branch of Russian Academy of Sciences, 630090 Novosibirsk, Russia; smagin@bionet.nsc.ru (D.A.S.); koir@bionet.nsc.ru (I.L.K.); galyamina@bionet.nsc.ru (A.G.G.)
2 Valdman Institute of Pharmacology, First Pavlov State Medical University of St. Petersburg, 197022 St. Petersburg, Russia; beloiz@spmu.rssi.ru
3 Biolabmix, 630090 Novosibirsk, Russia; nv_tamk@niboch.nsc.ru
4 Institute of Molecular and Cellular Biology, Siberian Branch of Russian Academy of Sciences, 630090 Novosibirsk, Russia; baranov@mcb.nsc.ru
5 Pavlov Institute of Physiology, Russian Academy of Sciences, 188680 St. Petersburg, Russia
6 Head of Neuropathology Modeling Laboratory, Institute of Cytology and Genetics SB RAS, pr. Ac. Lavrentjev, 10, 630090 Novosibirsk, Russia
* Correspondence: natnik@bionet.nsc.ru; Tel.: +7-(383)-363-49-65

Citation: Smagin, D.A.; Kovalenko, I.L.; Galyamina, A.G.; Belozertseva, I.V.; Tamkovich, N.V.; Baranov, K.O.; Kudryavtseva, N.N. Chronic Lithium Treatment Affects Anxious Behaviors and theExpression of Serotonergic Genes in Midbrain Raphe Nuclei of Defeated Male Mice. *Biomedicines* **2021**, 9, 1293. https://doi.org/10.3390/biomedicines9101293

Academic Editor: Masaru Tanaka

Received: 29 June 2021
Accepted: 17 September 2021
Published: 22 September 2021

Publisher's Note: MDPI stays neutral with regard to jurisdictional claims in published maps and institutional affiliations.

Abstract: There is experimental evidence that chronic social defeat stress is accompanied by the development of an anxiety, development of a depression-like state, and downregulation of serotonergic genes in midbrain raphe nuclei of male mice. Our study was aimed at investigating the effects of chronic lithium chloride (LiCl) administration on anxiety behavior and the expression of serotonergic genes in midbrain raphe nuclei of the affected mice. A pronounced anxiety-like state in male mice was induced by chronic social defeat stress in daily agonistic interactions. After 6 days of this stress, defeated mice were chronically treated with saline or LiCl (100 mg/kg, i.p., 2 weeks) during the continuing agonistic interactions. Anxiety was assessed by behavioral tests. RT-PCR was used to determine *Tph2*, *Htr1a*, *Htr5b*, and *Slc6a4* mRNA expression. The results revealed anxiolytic-like effects of LiCl on social communication in the partition test and anxiogenic-like effects in both elevated plus-maze and social interaction tests. Chronic LiCl treatment upregulated serotonergic genes in midbrain raphe nuclei. Thus, LiCl effects depend on the treatment mode, psycho-emotional state of the animal, and experimental context (tests). It is assumed that increased expression of serotonergic genes is accompanied by serotonergic system activation and, as a side effect, by higher anxiety.

Keywords: chronic social defeat stress; anxiety; depression; lithium chloride; mice

1. Introduction

Lithium salts are widely used in psychiatric practice in monotherapy regimens as mood stabilizers [1–4], in the supportive therapy of psycho-emotional disorders [5], and in the prevention of suicidal behaviors in patients [6–8]. Lithium is also used at the onset of the depressive phase in bipolar disorders and for the prevention of mood disorders [3,9–12] or relapses in schizophrenia with aggressive or suicidal behavior, convulsions, and other health problems [13–16]. Nevertheless, according to these studies, in clinical practice, patients with bipolar disorder demonstrate two types of lithium responsiveness: they are either good or poor responders. Lithium as monotherapy or in combination with other drugs is effective in 60% of chronically treated patients, but the treatment response remains heterogeneous and a large number of patients require a change in treatment after several weeks or months.

Lithium is obviously a multitarget drug and, as a consequence, with multiple mechanisms of action [17,18], and this property complicates the elucidation of its mechanism of action in a given context. The latest findings revealed numerous genes associated with a lithium response in bipolar disorder [18–22]. Therefore, there is a substantial need for tools that can guide clinicians in selecting a correct treatment strategy and that can aid in understanding individual differences in the response to lithium in clinical practice. We agree that important questions regarding the mechanism of lithium action on anxiety and depression remain open [17,18], despite much practical application.

In our previous study, a lithium-based enterosorbent called "Noolit" had obvious anxiolytic and antidepressant effects in adult defeated male mice [23]. In the present study, we provide experimental data on the impact of chronic treatment with lithium chloride (LiCl) on the anxiety-like state caused by chronic social defeat stress that leads to a mixed anxiety/depression-like state in male mice [24–26]. Obvious similarities in symptoms (general behavioral deficits, helplessness, anxiety, and decreased communication), etiology, sensitivity to antidepressants and anxiolytics (imipramine, fluoxetine, and diazepam), and serotonergic changes in the brain were demonstrated here between mice with clinical manifestations and patients. Our current results will be compared with the effects of the chronic lithium treatment seen in similar previous experiments on male mice with repeated experiences of aggression in daily agonistic interactions, which are accompanied by the development of a whole range of changes in behavior and a psycho-emotional state. Chronically aggressive male mice are known to demonstrate an increased number of stereotypical behaviors including enhanced anxiety, hyperactivity, and strong aggressive motivation, which, along with other signs, indicate the development of psychosis-like behavior [27,28].

There is evidence that therapeutic action of lithium is due to the effects on serotonergic neurotransmission [29,30]. Studies on humans have demonstrated that the effects of lithium on the serotonergic system depend on tryptophan hydroxylase variants [11] and that lithium may act through 5-HT_{1B} receptors, as shown in animal models [31]. Regular administration of lithium increases the density of the serotonin uptake site in cortical regions, suggesting an increase in the number of serotonin transporters in the brain regions containing nerve terminals of serotonergic neurons [32].

In the present study, we took into account many of the recently obtained data on the existence of lithium-sensitive genes that may be involved in the development of affective and neurodegenerative disorders [19–22,33,34]. Our previous experiments [35] revealed the downregulation of serotonergic gene expression in midbrain raphe nuclei of male mice with defeated experience in daily agonistic interactions, which induced the development of anxiety and depression-like states. The aim of the current work was to study the effect of chronic administration of LiCl on anxiety-like behaviors and expressions of serotonergic genes in this brain region. Considering lithium is used at the initial stage of the depressive phase of bipolar disorder and for the prevention of mood diseases in patients [10–12], in our experiment, we administered LiCl during the period of repeated agonistic interactions, which are accompanied by the development of an anxiety-like state from the first day of experiencing defeats.

2. Methods

2.1. Animals

Adult C57BL/6 male mice were obtained from the Animal Breeding Facility, a branch of the Institute of Bioorganic Chemistry, RAS (Pushchino, Moscow region, Russia). The animals were housed under standard conditions (12:12 h light/dark cycle, lights on at 8.00 a.m.; food (pellets) and water were available ad libitum). The mice were weaned at 1 month of age and housed in groups of 8–10 in plastic cages (36 × 23 × 12 cm). All procedures were carried out in compliance with the international regulations for animal experiments (Directive 2010/63/EU of the European Parliament and of the Council on the Protection of Animals Used for Scientific Purposes). The protocol for the study was approved by Scientific Council No. 9 of the Institute of Cytology and Genetics, SB RAS, of 24 March 2010, N 613 (Novosibirsk).

2.2. *Chronic Social Defeat Stress and LiCl Treatment*

Prolonged exposure to chronic social defeat stress that is accompanied by a strong anxiety-like state in male mice was induced in accordance with the sensory contact model [24,28]. Pairs of weight-matched animals were each placed in a cage (28 × 14 × 10 cm) bisected by a perforated transparent partition, allowing the animals to see, hear, and smell each other but preventing physical contact. The animals were left undisturbed for 3 days to adapt to the new housing conditions and sensory contact before they were subjected to an encounter. Then, every afternoon (2:00–5:00 p.m., local time), the cage lid was replaced by a transparent one, and 5 min later (the period necessary to stimulate mouse activity), the partition was removed for 10 min to encourage agonistic interactions. The superiority of one of the mice was firmly established within two or three encounters with the same opponent. The superior aggressive mouse was attacking, biting, and chasing the other mouse, who was displaying only defensive behavior (upright postures, sideways postures, freezing or withdrawal, and lying on the back). As a rule, the agonistic interactions between the two males were discontinued by lowering the partition if the aggression lasted for 3 min or in some cases even less. Each defeated mouse (loser) was exposed to the same aggressive mouse (winner) for 3 days. Afterwards, each loser was placed once a day after the fight in an unfamiliar cage with an unfamiliar aggressive mouse behind the partition. Each winning mouse remained in its original cage. This procedure was performed once a day and yielded equal numbers of winners and losers.

To investigate the effect of LiCl on anxiety-like behavior, we employed an experimental approach that is used for the screening of psychotropic drugs in settings mimicking clinical conditions [36,37]. This pharmacological approach makes it possible to study protective properties of drugs used in the preventive mode (Figure 1) and their therapeutic properties in animals having a behavioral pathology.

LiCl was administered during the period of the repeated agonistic interactions and we expected to see its protective effects. For this purpose, after 6 days of the agonistic interactions accompanied by chronic social defeat stress, the defeated mice were treated with either saline or LiCl (Merck, Germany) at a dose of 100 mg/kg intraperitoneally once a day in the morning (9.00–10.00 a.m., local time). Three groups of animals were used in the behavioral experiment (Figure 1): (i) controls, i.e., mice without consecutive experiences of agonistic interactions; (ii) defeated males chronically treated with saline (Sal-treated losers); and (iii) defeated males chronically treated with LiCl (LiCl-treated losers). After 2 weeks of the LiCl or saline injections against the background of agonistic interactions, the behavior of the animals was evaluated in behavioral tests (one test per day), which were used for quantifying the anxiety-like state in different experimental conditions.

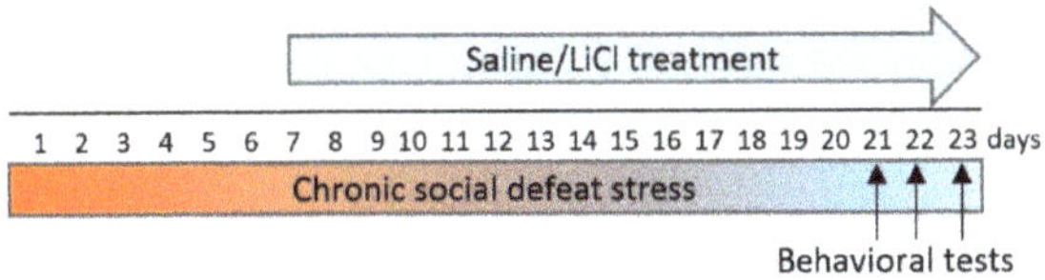

Figure 1. An outline of the experiment: chronic LiCl and/or saline treatment of defeated mice in preventive mode starting from the 7th day of the agonistic interactions in order to study the possible protective effect of LiCl on the development of behavioral pathology. Behavioral tests: day 21, the partition test; day 22, the elevated plus-maze test; and day 23, the social interaction test.

2.3. *Behavioral Tests*

2.3.1. The Partition Test

This test can be utilized for the estimation of a mouse behavioral reaction to a conspecific behind the transparent perforated partition dividing the experimental cage into equal parts [38]. The number of approaches to the partition and the total time spent near it (e.g., moving near the partition, smelling and touching it with the nose or with one or two paws, and sticking the nose into the holes) were scored during 5 min as indices of reacting to the partner. The duration of a sideways position or "turning away" near the partition was not included in the total time of the test. The experimental procedure was as follows: the pair of mice resided together in a cage with a partition. On the testing day, the lid of the cage was replaced by a transparent one; 5 min later (period of activation), behavioral responses of the losers and controls toward the unfamiliar partner were recorded for 5 min. This test is used in the research on communicativeness (sociability) and anxiety: it has been shown that a decrease of partition parameters correlates with indices of anxiety-like behavior, estimated in the elevated plus-maze test [38].

2.3.2. The Elevated Plus-Maze Test

The elevated plus-maze consisted of two open arms (25 × 5 cm) and two closed arms (25 × 5 × 15 cm), and was placed in a dimly lit room. The two arms of each type were opposite to each other and extended from a central platform (5 × 5 cm). The maze was elevated by 50 cm above the room floor [39].

The cover of the experimental cage with a mouse was replaced by a transparent lid in the same room 5 min before placement in the plus-maze. The mouse was placed on the central platform with the nose to the closed arm. The following measures were recorded for 5 min: (1) total entries; (2) open arm entries (four paws in an open arm), closed arm entries (four paws in a closed arm), and central platform entries; (3) time spent in open arms, closed arms, and the central platform (center); (4) the number of passages from one closed arm to another; (5) the number of head dips (looking down on the floor below the plus-maze); and (6) the number of peeping-out instances when the mouse was in closed arms. Indices 2 and 3 are considered measures of the level of anxiety, indices 1 and 4 are related to locomotor activity, and indices 5 and 6 quantify the risk assessment behavior. The time spent in closed arms and open arms, and on the central platform (center) was calculated as percentages of the total testing time. The elevated plus-maze was thoroughly cleaned between the sessions.

2.3.3. Exploratory Activity and Social Interaction Tests

An open field (36 × 23 cm) was used with a perforated container (an inverted pencil holder made of metal wire, bottom diameter: 10.5 cm) in one of the cage corners. Each mouse was placed individually in the corner opposite to the pencil holder for 5 min. This test allows to estimate the exploratory behavior of mice under novel conditions with an unfamiliar object, namely the pencil holder [40]. This test is thought to cause pronounced stress. Then, an unfamiliar male from the housed group was placed under the pencil holder for 5 min to study the reaction of the male mouse to the conspecific animal in a familiar situation (social interaction test).

The EthoVision XT software (version 11.0; Noldus Information Technology, Wageningen, The Netherlands) automatically registered the tracking score (distance) during the testing time with differentiation of the place near the pencil holder (5 cm around it) in the cage as well as the total time spent in the corner opposite to the pencil holder.

Manual registration with Observer XT (version 7.0; Noldus Information Technology, the Netherlands) of the following behavioral indicators of communicativeness was carried out: the number and/or duration of (1) rearings (exploratory activity); (2) groomings (self-oriented behavior: licking of the fur on the flanks or abdomen and washing over the head from an ear to snout); and (3) approaches to the pencil holder and total time (s) spent near it (moving near the pencil holder, smelling and touching it with the nose or with one or more paws). The duration of a sideways position or "turning away" near the pencil holder was not included in the total time. After each test, the open field and pencil holder were thoroughly washed and dried off with napkins.

Preliminary analysis of LiCl-treated losers' behavior in the exploratory activity test clearly stratified the animals into two groups: LiCl-sensitive - $LiCl^+$-treated and LiCl-less-sensitive - $LiCl^-$-treated losers in relation to the chronic LiCl treatment. As a behavioral parameter for the division into groups, we employed avoidance of a novel object (pencil holder): $LiCl^+$-treated losers did not approach the pencil holder at all, sat in the corner only, and did not explore the cage. Among the controls as well as the Sal-treated and $LiCl^-$-treated losers, we observed a natural exploratory activity under the novel conditions.

2.4. Real-Time Polymerase Chain Reaction (RT-PCR)

To understand the possible effect of LiCl on the behavior of the experimental animals, we conducted an additional experiment that, we hoped, would explain the effect of LiCl (150 mg/kg) on the expression of serotonergic genes in midbrain raphe nuclei, which contain bodies of serotonergic neurons. The expression of the following genes was analyzed: *Tph2*, encoding tryptophan hydroxylase, which is a rate-limiting enzyme of serotonin synthesis; *Slc6a4*, encoding a serotonin transporter; and genes *Htr1a* and *Htr5b*, encoding serotonin receptors. To measure mRNA levels of serotonergic genes in midbrain raphe nuclei, we studied the 21-day losers after chronic LiCl or saline injections at 24 h after the last agonistic interaction, alongside the controls.

The determination of serotonin-related gene expression in midbrain raphe nuclei by RT-PCR was done at the Biolabmix Company (https://biolabmix.ru (accessed on 17 March 2020), Novosibirsk, Russia). The measurement data were provided by the Bio-Rad Amplifier software (Berkeley, CA, USA). RNA was isolated using the TRIzol reagent (Invitrogen, Waltham, MA, USA). To remove DNA impurities, the obtained RNA samples were treated with DNase I (Fermentas) for 1 h at 37 °C according to the manufacturer's protocol and the enzyme was inhibited by adding EDTA and heating at 65 °C for 10 min. The quality of the isolated RNA was checked spectrophotometrically and its integrity by electrophoretic mobility in a 2% agarose gel. The absence of genomic DNA was confirmed for each sample by PCR. The cDNA was prepared from each RNA sample in two parallel reactions in a volume of 20 μL using the M-MuLV–RH First Strand cDNA Synthesis Kit (Biolabmix, Novosibirsk, Russia). RNA (1 μg), 100 U of MuMLV reverse transcriptase (murine leukemia virus reverse transcriptase), and 0.3 μM random hexoprimer were used in the reaction. The reaction was carried out according to the manufacturer's protocol. The level of RNA expression in the samples was assessed by RT-PCR with fluorescent probes. For this purpose, primers specific to the four functional genes under study (*Tph2, Slc6a4, Htr1a,* and *Htr5b*) were used (Table S1).

PCR was conducted in a 25 μL reaction solution containing 2× BioMaster HS-qPCR (2×) reaction mixture (Biolabmix, Novosibirsk, Russia), an aliquot of the reaction mixture after reverse transcription, 300 nM forward and reverse primers, and 200 nM fluorescent probe. The amplification was performed on the Real-Time CFX96 Touch (Bio-Rad, Berkeley, CA, USA) according to the following program: 1st cycle consisted of 5 min at 95 °C; 45 cycles consisted of 20 s at 95 °C and 60 s at 60 °C". Each sample was amplified in triplicates.

In animals of all experimental groups after quick decapitation, the midbrain raphe nuclei area was dissected according to the map presented in the Allen Mouse Brain Atlas http://mouse.brain-map.org/static/atlas (accessed on 24 April 2005). Dissection of the brain region was made by the same experimenter. The brain regions were removed and chilled rapidly on ice. All biological samples were encrypted, rapidly frozen in liquid nitrogen, and stored at −70 °C until use.

2.5. Statistical Analysis

The analysis of the behavioral data was performed by either one-way ANOVA for parametric variables or by the Kruskal–Wallis test. The Kruskal–Wallis test was conducted with "group" as a factor (controls, Sal-treated losers, $LiCl^-$-treated losers, and $LiCl^+$-treated losers) for the social interaction test and with "group" as a factor (controls, Sal-treated losers, and LiCl-treated losers) for both the partition and elevated plus-maze tests, which were followed by either Tukey's multiple-comparison post hoc test for parametric variables or by Dunn's multiple-comparison post hoc test if the parametric criteria were not met. To display the variance of the values, the data are presented as a box-whisker plot showing means (*plus sign*), medians (*solid lines*), and 25%/75% quartiles, with whiskers indicating 10th and 90th percentiles. All statistical analyses were performed using the XLStat software (Addinsoft, www.xlstat.com (accessed on 31 March 2016)). For the parameter "number of entries" (four paws in open arms) in the elevated plus-maze test, the chi-square test was used.

3. Results

3.1. Experiment 1. Effects of Chronic LiCl Treatment on Anxious Behavior of Defeated Mice

3.1.1. Effects of Chronic LiCl Treatment on the Behavior of Defeated Mice in the Partition Test

One-way ANOVA revealed an influence of the "group" factor on the numbers of approaches (F(2,33) = 6.619, p = 0.0038) and rearings (F(2,33) = 3.293, p = 0.0496). The Kruskal–Wallis test uncovered an impact of the "group" factor on the total time spent near the partition (H = 9.816, p = 0.0074). According to either Tukey or Dunn's multiple-comparison post hoc test, significant differences between the Sal-treated losers and controls were found in the number of approaches (p = 0.0027), in the total time spent near the partition (p = 0.0053), and in the number of rearings (p = 0.0390) (Figure 2).

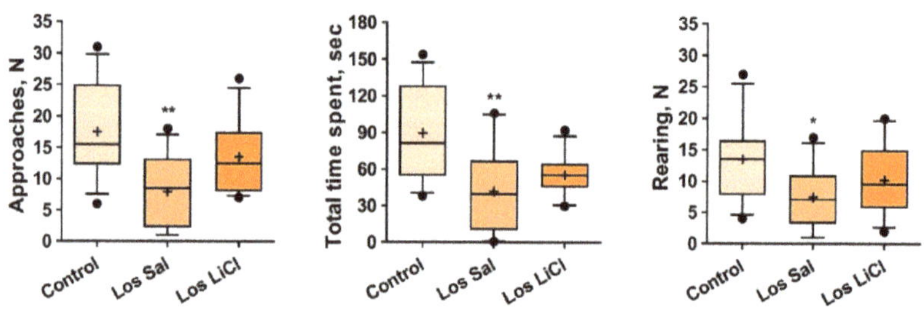

Figure 2. Effects of chronic LiCl treatment on the behavior of defeated mice in the partition test. Note: Los Sal-Sal-treated losers; and Los LiCl-LiCl-treated losers. Data are presented as means (*plus sign*), medians (solid lines), and 25%/75% quartiles in the box-whisker plot, with whiskers indicating the 10th and 90th percentiles. * $p < 0.05$ and ** $p < 0.01$ vs. controls; n = 12 for each group.

Thus, in comparison with the control, Sal-treated losers demonstrated lower behavioral activity (communication and sociability), as evidenced by the number of approaches to and total time spent near the partition as a reaction to the partner in the neighboring compartment as well as by the decreased exploratory activity, estimated as the number of rearings. After the LiCl treatment, these parameters did not differ significantly from the control. We can assume that LiCl had slight anxiolytic effects on the losers.

3.1.2. Effects of Chronic LiCl Treatment on the Behavior of Defeated Mice in the Elevated Plus-Maze Test

One-way ANOVA revealed a significant influence of "group" (controls, Sal-treated losers, and LiCl-treated losers) on the numbers of central platform entries (F(2,31) = 4.130, p = 0.0257), closed arm entries (F(2,31) = 4.661, p = 0.0170), passages (F(2,31) = 4.717, p = 0.0163), head dips (F(2,31) = 3.590, p = 0.0396), and total entries (F(2,31) = 4.552, p = 0.0185). Tukey's multiple-comparison *post hoc* test detected differences between the LiCl-treated and control mice in the numbers of central platform entries (p = 0.0277), closed arm entries (p = 0.0185), passages (p = 0.0166), head dips (p = 0.0403), and total entries (p = 0.0192) (Figure 3). The chi-square test did not reveal differences between experimental groups in the parameter "number of entries" (four paws in open arms).

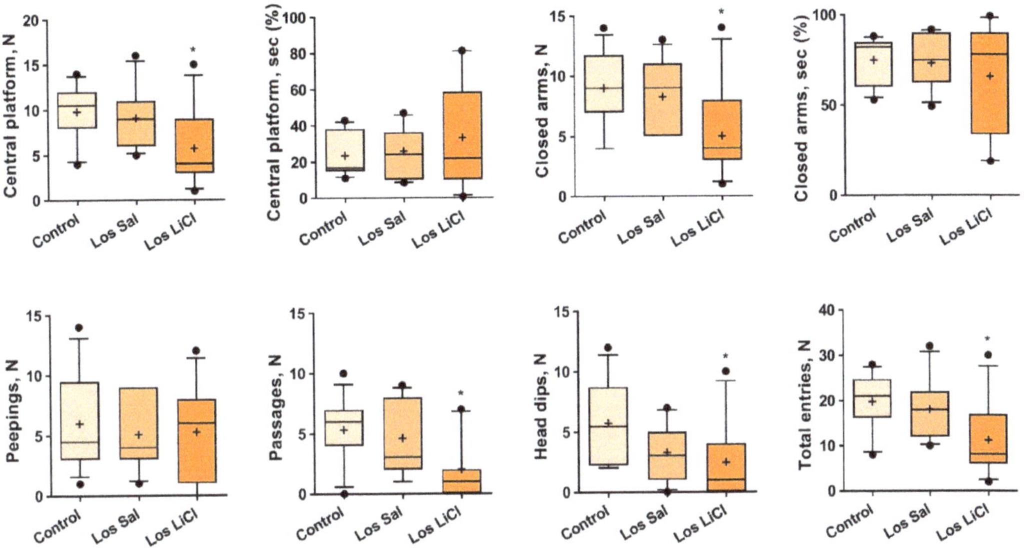

Figure 3. Effects of chronic LiCl treatment on the behavior of defeated mice in the elevated plus-maze test. Note: Los Sal-Sal-treated losers; and Los LiCl-LiCl-treated losers. * $p < 0.05$ vs. controls, Tukey's multiple-comparison post hoc test ($n = 12$ for each group). The presented values are means (plus sign), medians (solid lines), and 25%/75% quartiles in the box-whisker plot, with whiskers indicating the 10th and 90th percentiles.

Therefore, LiCl caused a decrease in all parameters of locomotor activity; this effect can be easily explained by the general behavioral deficit that develops within a depression-like state in mice [24–26]. This effect of LiCl may also be considered pro-depressive in this experimental context.

Previously, it has been repeatedly reported that well-pronounced anxiety-like behavior develops in the losers after 20-day social defeat stress, as estimated by the elevated plus-maze test [26,36]. During the chronic saline treatment in our study, these negative changes were less pronounced. It can be cautiously concluded that saline has a protective effect when administered as chronic injections. By contrast, the general decrease in locomotor activity during our chronic treatment with LiCl can be regarded as an anxiogenic effect.

3.1.3. Effects of Chronic LiCl Treatment on the Exploratory Activity of Defeated Mice with Different Sensitivities to LiCl in the Novel Situation toward the Unfamiliar Object (Empty Pencil Holder)

According to the level of pencil holder avoidance (see the description in Materials and Methods), we subdivided the losers after LiCl injections into two subgroups: $LiCl^{+}$-treated and $LiCl^{-}$-treated losers. One-way ANOVA revealed an impact of the factor "group" (controls or Sal-treated, $LiCl^{-}$-treated, or $LiCl^{+}$-treated losers) on the total tracking score (cm; $F(3,29) = 26.50$, $p < 0.0001$). Tukey's multiple-comparison test showed significant differences between the Controls and Sal-treated ($p = 0.0003$), $LiCl^{-}$-treated ($p < 0.0001$), or $LiCl^{+}$-treated losers ($p < 0.0001$), as well as between $LiCl^{+}$-treated and Sal-treated losers ($p = 0.0013$). The Kruskal–Wallis test detected an influence of the "group" factor on the time spent in the corner ($H = 18.03$, $p = 0.0004$) and near the pencil holder ($H = 17.56$, $p = 0.0005$). Dunn's multiple-comparison test detected differences in the following parameters: the time (s) spent in the corner of Controls vs. $LiCl^{+}$-treated losers ($p = 0.0027$); Sal-treated losers vs. $LiCl^{+}$-treated losers ($p = 0.0012$)] and time (s) spent near the pencil holder (Controls vs. $LiCl^{+}$ treated losers ($p = 0.0040$)); and Sal-treated losers vs. $LiCl^{+}$-treated losers ($p = 0.0010$)] (Figure 4).

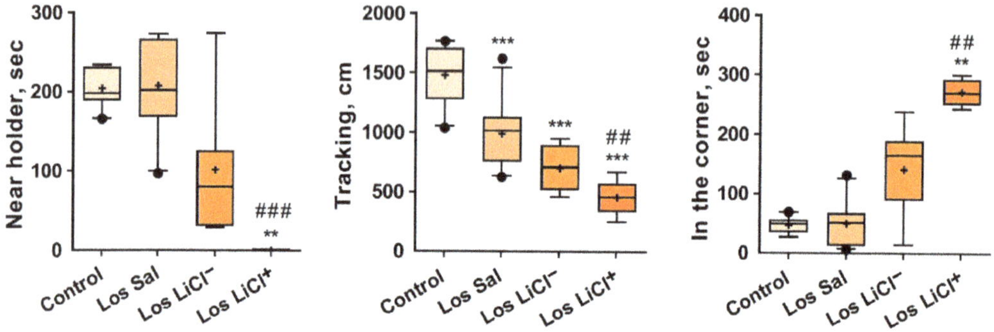

Figure 4. Effects of LiCl on the exploratory behavior of defeated mice in the novel environment and towards the novel object (pencil holder). Note: Control (n = 9); Los Sal-Sal-treated losers (n = 11); Los LiCl-LiCl-treated losers (n = 7); Los $LiCl^+$-$LiCl^+$-treated losers (n = 5). The values are means (plus sign), medians (solid lines), and 25%/75% quartiles in the box-whisker plot, with whiskers indicating the 10th and 90th percentiles. ** $p < 0.01$, *** $p < 0.01$ vs. controls; ## $p < 0.01$, and ### $p < 0.001$ vs. Sal-treated losers (Tukey's multiple-comparison post hoc test).

The $LiCl^+$-treated losers were more sensitive to LiCl and exhibited lower exploratory activity, as estimated by the total tracking time. They spent most of the time in the corner and were never near the pencil holder. Together with the behavior in the plus-maze and partition tests, these data are suggestive of decreased exploratory activity and an enhanced anxiety-like state after chronic LiCl treatment.

3.1.4. The Impact of Chronic LiCl Treatment on the Reaction of Mice to an Unfamiliar Partner in the Social Interaction Test

One-way ANOVA indicated a significant influence of the factor "group" (controls or Sal-treated, $LiCl^-$-treated, or $LiCl^+$-treated losers) on the number of approaches to a partner ($F(3,31) = 11.35$, $p < 0.0001$) and on the total time spent near the pencil holder (approaches; $F(3,31) = 20.98$, $p < 0.0001$). The Kruskal–Wallis test uncovered an impact of the "group" factor on the duration of self-grooming ($H = 9.816$, $p = 0.0212$). Tukey's multiple-comparison test was applied to the following behavioral parameters (Figure 5): approaches (n (controls vs. $LiCl^+$-treated losers [$p < 0.0001$]; Sal-treated losers vs. $LiCl^+$-treated losers [$p = 0.0008$]; and $LiCl^-$-treated vs. $LiCl^+$-treated losers [$p = 0.0020$])) and approaches (sec (controls vs. Sal-treated losers [$p < 0.0001$], $LiCl^-$-treated losers [$p = 0.0017$], or $LiCl^+$-treated losers [$p < 0.0001$]; Sal-treated losers vs. $LiCl^+$-treated losers [$p = 0.0083$]; and $LiCl^-$-treated losers vs. $LiCl^+$-treated losers [$p = 0.0073$])). Dunn's multiple-comparison test was applied to the duration (sec) of self-grooming (controls vs. Sal-treated losers ($p < 0.0133$)) (Figure 5).

We believe that this test measures the level of communicativeness towards an unfamiliar partner under the conditions that have already become familiar during the 5 min before the introduction of the partner. During the preceding 5 min, the mouse realized that it was not in danger and soon began to examine the cage.

Chronic LiCl treatment had a strong anxiogenic effect on $LiCl^+$-treated losers in comparison with the controls and Sal-treated losers, as evidenced by the decreased number of approaches to and total time spent near the pencil holder containing a partner (approaches, sec). Their time spent in corners was significantly longer in comparison with all other groups. The anxiogenic effects were significantly less different between the $LiCl^-$ -treated losers and control mice.

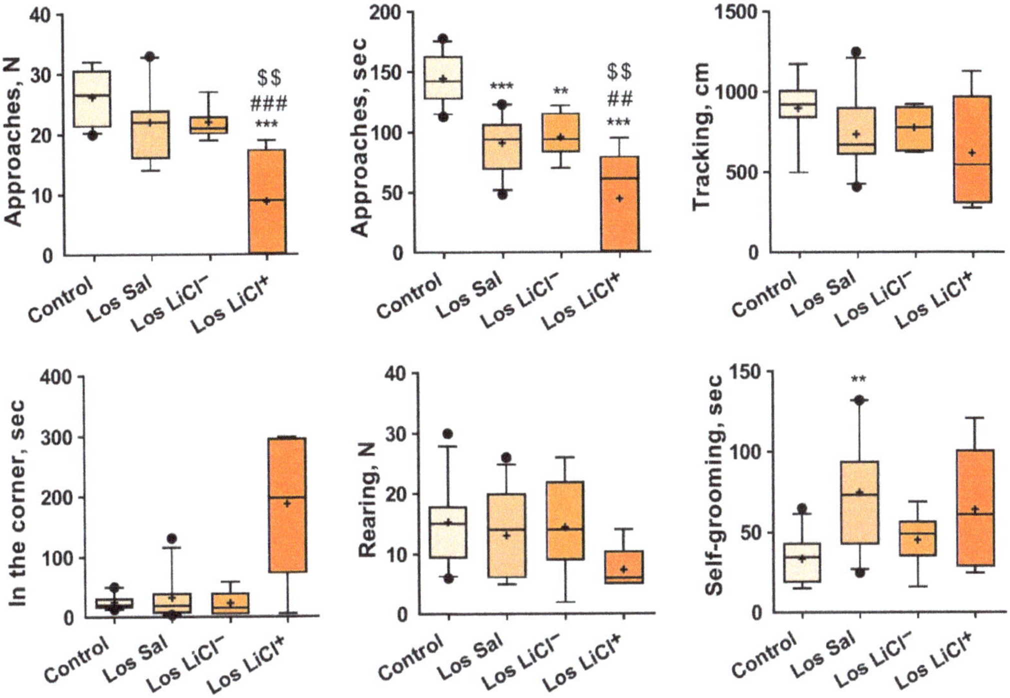

Figure 5. Effects of LiCl on the behavior of defeated mice in the social interaction test as a reaction to the partner under the pencil holder. Note: Control (n = 9); Los Sal-Sal-treated losers (n = 11); Los $LiCl^-$-$LiCl^-$-treated losers (n = 7); Los $LiCl^+$-$LiCl^+$-treated losers (n = 5). The data are shown as means (plus sign), medians (solid lines), and 25%/75% quartiles in the box-whisker plot, with whiskers indicating the 10th and 90th percentiles. ** $p < 0.01$, *** $p < 0.001$ vs. controls; ## $p < 0.01$, and ### $p < 0.001$ vs. Sal-treated losers; $$ $p < 0.01$ vs. $LiCl^-$-treated losers.

3.2. Experiment 2. Effects of the Chronic LiCl Treatment on the Expression of Serotonergic Genes in the Midbrain Raphe Nuclei of Defeated Mice

In comparison with the controls and Sal-treated losers, chronic LiCl treatment induced overexpression of the *Tph2* gene ($p < 0.01$ for both), *Slc6a4* gene ($p < 0.05$ and $p < 0.01$), *Htr1a* gene ($p < 0.01$ for both), and *Htr5b* gene ($p < 0.01$ and $p < 0.05$) in the midbrain raphe nuclei of defeated mice (Figure 6).

Some discrepancy between the data obtained earlier [35] and our current results can be explained by slight experimental differences. In the earlier study, we did not chronically administer saline to the losers but we did in the present experiment. There is also the possibility that saline may have a protective impact, similar to those in the elevated plus-maze test, with chronic injections attenuating the adverse effects of chronic social defeat stress.

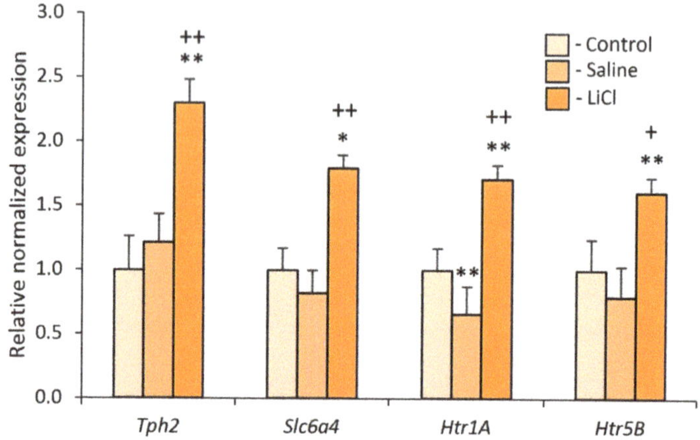

Figure 6. The influence of chronic LiCl treatment on serotonergic gene expression in midbrain raphe nuclei of defeated mice. The measurement data were processed in the Bio-Rad Amplifier software (USA). Bars: the control ($n = 9$); Saline - Sal-treated losers ($n = 7$); LiCl - LiCl-treated losers ($n = 9$). * $p < 0.05$ and ** $p < 0.01$ vs. controls, and + $p < 0.05$ and ++ $p < 0.01$ vs. Sal-treated losers according to Student's t-test. The data are presented as mean ± SEM.

4. Discussion

An important finding here is the varied sensitivity to a drug in mice of the same group, in particular regarding LiCl in this work. When evaluating the behavior of aggressive [41] and defeated male mice (this study) in the social interaction test, we found that mice of one group can be subdivided into subgroups according to differential sensitivity to LiCl: only 40% of chronically aggressive and defeated males were sensitive to chronic lithium treatment. Naturally, a question arises: why did the group of inbred mice split into groups of sensitive and less sensitive to the drug under obviously identical experimental conditions? One plausible reason, as supposed in References [42,43], concerns the differences in prenatal and early postnatal development, which have been overlooked in the standardized experimental setting. In our opinion, however, a more likely assumption is that baseline psycho-emotional states were different among the experimental animals raised under the group housing conditions at the animal facility. Mice are known to form a despotic dominance hierarchy with one male being dominant and others being subordinate [44]. Social status leaves an imprint on the behavior and brain neurochemistry of mice. In this study, we obtained additional evidence that the effect of a drug may depend on the psycho-emotional state of an individual. In other words, the neurochemical background can modify the effect of a drug, sometimes yielding the opposite of the expected influence.

Moreover, some effects of a drug can be detectable in one situation (test) and undetectable in another. Apparently, the reason for this is that the predominant motivation that develops under the experimental conditions underlies many (but not all) types of behavior. Sometimes, there is a struggle between two opposite motivations (ambivalence), for example, fear and communicativeness (the test of social interactions) or anxiety and exploratory activity (the elevated plus-maze test). The balance between major motivations depends on a context, is reflected in the psycho-emotional state, and logically is influenced by the underlying neurochemical background, which may affect the biological activities of the drug. The subdivision of the defeated male mice into the subgroups—susceptible or resistant to chronic social defeat stress—has also been observed by other researchers in numerous studies [45–47].

In behavioral tests, chronic LiCl injections into unstressed (intact) male mice for 2 weeks were found to have anxiolytic effects in our previous study: the anxiety-like state decreased as estimated by the elevated plus-maze and social interaction tests [41]. In the present study, during preventive treatment of defeated male mice experiencing a severe anxiety-like state, the effect of LiCl correlated with the behavioral scores in various tests. Slight anxiolytic effects were observed in the partition test and decreased exploratory activities were noted in the elevated plus-maze test. Apparent anxiogenic effects of LiCl on the losers in the social interaction test may be a consequence of the frightening situation. In the group of defeated mice, LiCl had strong and varied effects: ~40% of the $LiCl^+$-treated losers manifested pronounced anxiety-like behaviors in the novel environment toward the novel object and toward an unfamiliar partner under the pencil holder.

Earlier in similar experiments, LiCl has been administered preventively to male mice with repeated aggression during daily agonistic interactions accompanied by wins, as well as therapeutically to males subjected to a 20-day aggression experience with treatment in the subsequent 2-week period without agonistic interactions [41]. In that study, the preventive chronic LiCl injections into the winners were found to have well-pronounced anxiogenic effects, similar to those in the losers: LiCl further enhanced the anxiety-like state, as reported earlier for male mice, with repeated aggression in the partition test and elevated plus-maze test [41,48]. In the social interaction test, ~40% of aggressive mice demonstrated pronounced anxiety-like behavior after LiCl treatment, along with a decrease of communicativeness and exploratory activity as compared with the controls. Therefore, the anxiogenic effect of LiCl is likely to be a consequence of the stress that accompanies agonistic interactions common for aggressive and defeated mice.

During the therapeutic intervention in the no-fight period, the anxiolytic effect of LiCl became evident in the social interaction test performed on winners and was characterized by increased interest in the partner placed under the pencil holder [41]. Nevertheless, in the elevated plus-maze and partition tests, no effects of LiCl were detectable. In a study on the effects of diazepam, similar data were obtained in a slightly different experimental context: acute administration of the drug to mice with a short-term aggression experience had an anxiogenic impact, whereas in the males with a long-term experience of aggression, diazepam had an anxiolytic effect [49]. Similar results were also obtained in another work: the effects of anxiolytic chlordiazepoxide on aggressive behavior differed between animals of different social status [50].

Accordingly, the effects of chronic LiCl treatment can depend on the mode of treatment (preventive or therapeutic), on the psycho-emotional state developing during a positive or negative social experience of animals (intact, aggressive, or defeated), and on the experimental context (tests), and the effects can be anxiogenic, anxiolytic, or undetectable, as shown in our study (Table 1).

Table 1. Effects of chronic LiCl treatment on the anxiety-like behavior of mice with opposite social experiences.

Tests	Preventive Treatment of the Losers	Preventive Treatment of the Winners [41]	Therapeutic Treatment of the Winners [41]	Intact Males [41]
Partition	Anxiolytic effects	Anxiogenic effects	No effects	-
Plus-maze	Anxiogenic effects	Anxiogenic effects	No effects	Anxiolytic effects
Social interactions	Anxiogenic effects (40% of mice)	Anxiogenic effects (40% of mice)	Anxiolytic effects	Anxiolytic effects

Moreover, the response to new conditions and to anxiolytics differs among different strains of mice; this phenomenon may be explained by features of the hereditarily determined anxiety (state or trait) [51–53] that develops in behavioral tests. In our experiments, male mice of the C57BL/6J strain with hereditarily determined enhanced "trait" anxiety [53,54] have been used. Our data may be useful for understanding individual differences in the response to lithium in clinical practice, as reported in many studies [12,14,17].

The central role of the brain serotonergic system in the mechanisms of stress, anxiety, depression, bipolar disorder [55–57], and in neural plasticity [58–62] has been proven in numerous studies. It is widely believed that a serotonergic imbalance is a key pathophysiological mechanism of major depression. We have put forward [26] the idea that effects of LiCl treatment depend on brain serotonergic activity, which can change from day to day during the daily agonistic interactions in mice. We have previously documented an interaction between (1) a developing anxiety and depression-like state, and (2) dynamic changes in brain serotonergic activity that progress in the affected mice [26]. It was shown in that study that social defeat stress induces strong anxiety, starting from the first days of the agonistic interactions, which are accompanied by the activation of the serotonergic system. After 20 days of chronic social stress, downregulation of serotonergic genes in depressive mice is seen in midbrain raphe nuclei [35,63], which contain serotonergic neuron bodies. These data indicate links among the duration of stress, serotonergic activity, and both anxiety and depression-like states, also shown in other research on animals and humans [58–62]. These observations also suggest that chronic preventive administration of LiCl before and during severe stress and anxiety in animals with an experience of aggression or social defeat produces an anxiogenic effect.

In this article, we present our data on the upregulation of serotonergic genes *Tph2, Slc6a4, Htr1a,* and *Htr5b* in the midbrain raphe nuclei after preventive LiCl treatment; supposedly, these changes may lead to the activation of the serotonergic system and, as a consequence, to the development of anxiety as a side effect of LiCl. Our data are consistent with other pharmacogenomic studies which have identified candidate genes that may be sensitive to antidepressants and mood stabilizers (in particular, to lithium) including, for example, serotonergic genes *Htr2a, Htr1a, Slc6a4, Maoa,* and *Tph;* for more detail, review [33]. These results may be useful for clarifying the mechanisms of psychotropic LiCl action through the increased serotonergic gene expression and thereby serotonergic activity. Conversely, it is necessary to take into consideration that numerous other genes associated both with lithium exposure and bipolar disorder have been identified [21,22,33,64,65], and differential expression of these genes in brain tissue samples from patients and healthy controls has been investigated [66]: lithium exposure significantly affected 1108 genes, 702 of which were upregulated and 406 downregulated. Our neurogenomic data obtained in recent years by transcriptomic analysis also revealed changes in the expression of mitochondrial [67], ribosomal [68,69], monoaminergic [70–73], or autism-associated [74] genes under chronic social defeat stress. In addition, alterations in the expression of neurotrophic and transcription factors' genes [75,76] and collagen genes [77] specific for brain regions in mice with a mixed anxiety/depression-like state have been revealed. These observations confirm that there are various mechanisms that may mediate the effects of lithium [78–80] at neurochemical, cellular, and genomic levels. It is becoming apparent that the research on molecular mechanisms of neuroplasticity is most promising for elucidating the pathogenesis of chronic anxiety and depression, and the efficacy of anxiolytics and antidepressants. Our behavioral approach can help to understand the effects of lithium in order to study in detail the neurogenomic mechanisms of drug action in psycho-emotional disorders.

5. Conclusions

The use of a pharmacological approach for screening psychotropic drugs in settings mimicking clinical conditions [36,37] allowed us to study the impact of chronic LiCl administration on anxiety-like behavior in male mice with long-term social experience of daily agonistic interactions. As shown in our study, chronic treatment with LiCl can have anxiogenic, anxiolytic, or undetectable effects, and may depend on the mode of treatment (preventive or therapeutic), on the psycho-emotional state that develops as a result of a positive or negative social experience of the animals (intact, aggressive, or defeated), and on the experimental context (tests). Our experiments suggest that preventive chronic administration of LiCl to defeated male mice under these social conditions can be accompanied by an increased expression of serotonergic genes in the midbrain raphe nuclei. Our data can clarify the individual differences in the response to lithium that are seen in clinical practice.

The limitations of this study include the following:

One should keep in mind that according to our previous neurogenomic studies, the expression of many genes in various brain regions changes under the influence of chronic agonistic interactions. Moreover, as other authors have shown, there are many genes that are sensitive to lithium. Accordingly, our results on the changes in the expression of serotonergic genes in the midbrain raphe nuclei obtained in this pharmacological study may be valid for the mixed anxiety/depression-like disorder in mice within the framework of the experimental model used. This is just the beginning of research regarding the effects of lithium treatment on the psycho-emotional state, on the one hand, and on the expression of serotonergic genes, on the other hand. Additional neurogenomic studies on the effects of lithium are needed to identify a link between the transcription of other candidate genes and anxious behaviors in mice.

Another goal is to better understand the neurogenomic mechanisms of lithium action on the expression of serotonergic and other genes, at least in the midbrain raphe nuclei, depending on the psycho-emotional state of the person, as well as the severity of the disease. It follows from this study that lithium should be given concomitantly with anxiolytics for beneficial effects; in doing so, its positive effect on the depressive state may be more pronounced. We hope that our experimental approach to studying the protective and therapeutic effects of drugs will open up new ways to more effectively treat anxiety and depressive symptoms.

Supplementary Materials: The Supplement 1 is available online at https://www.mdpi.com/article/10.3390/biomedicines9101293/s1, Table S1: Primer sequences.

Author Contributions: D.A.S. obtained the behavioral and brain data, analyzed and processed the data statistically, and wrote the manuscript text. I.L.K. contributed to the behavioral data acquisition and collected the brain samples. A.G.G. contributed to the behavioral data acquisition. I.V.B. organized the experiments and critically revised both the statistical analysis and the text of the manuscript. N.V.T. determined the gene expression by RT-PCR and together with K.O.B. analyzed the data. N.N.K. designed the study, analyzed and interpreted the data, and wrote the main manuscript text. All the authors gave final approval. All authors have read and agreed to the published version of the manuscript.

Funding: This research study was funded by the Russian Science Foundation (grant number No 19-15-00026 to NNK). Preparation and maintenance of experimental animals was carried out in the Conventional vivarium of the Institute of Cytology and Genetics, SB RAS and was funded under Budget Project (number 0259-2021-0016). The funding body had no role in the design of the study; in the collection, analysis, and interpretation of the data; and in the writing of the manuscript.

Institutional Review Board Statement: All procedures were carried out in compliance with international regulations for animal experiments (Directive 2010/63/EU of the European Parliament and of the Council on the Protection of Animals Used for Scientific Purposes). The protocol for the experiments was approved by Scientific Council No. 9 of the Institute of Cytology and Genetics SD RAS of March 24, 2010, N 613 (Novosibirsk).

Informed Consent Statement: Study are available from the corresponding author upon reasonable request.

Data Availability Statement: The statistics of the obtained data used to support the findings of this.

Acknowledgments: We are grateful to V.N. Babenko and O.E. Redina for the helpful discussions, and to O.A. Kharlamova for the correction of the manuscript text. The English language was corrected and certified by shevchuk-editing.com.

Conflicts of Interest: The authors declare no conflict of interest.

References

1. Shastry, B.S. On the functions of lithium: The mood stabilizer. *Bioassays* **1997**, *19*, 199–200. [CrossRef]
2. Shelton, R.C. Mood-stabilizing drugs in depression. *J. Clin. Psychiatry* **1999**, *60*, 37–40.
3. Post, R.M. The new news about lithium: An underutilized treatment in the United States. *Neuropsychopharmacology* **2018**, *43*, 1174–1179. [CrossRef]
4. Nolen, W.A.; Bloemkolk, D. Treatment of bipolar depression, a review of the literature and a suggestion for an algorithm. *Neuropsychobiology* **2000**, *42*, 11–17. [CrossRef]
5. Blacker, D. Maintenance treatment of major depression: A review of the literature. *Harv. Rev. Psychiatry* **1996**, *4*, 1–9. [CrossRef]
6. Sanghvi, I.; Gershon, S. Rubidium and lithium: Evaluation as antidepressant and anti-manic agents. *Res. Commun. Chem. Pathol. Pharmacol.* **1973**, *6*, 293–300.
7. Rosenthal, N.E.; Goodwin, F.K. The role of the lithium ion in medicine. *Annu. Rev. Med.* **1982**, *33*, 555–568. [CrossRef] [PubMed]
8. Baldessarini, R.J.; Tondo, L.; Davis, P.; Pompili, M.; Goodwin, F.K.; Hennen, J. Decreased risk of suicides and attempts during long-term lithium treatment: A meta-analytic review. *Bipolar. Disord.* **2006**, *8*, 625–639. [CrossRef] [PubMed]
9. Denicoff, K.D.; Smith-Jackson, E.E.; Disney, E.R.; Ali, S.O.; Leverich, G.S.; Post, R.M. Comparative prophylactic efficacy of lithium, carbamazepine, and the combination in bipolar disorder. *J. Clin. Psychiatry* **1997**, *58*, 470–478. [CrossRef] [PubMed]
10. Bowden, C.L. Efficacy of lithium in mania and maintenance therapy of bipolar disorder. *J. Clin. Psychiatry* **2000**, *61*, 35–40. [PubMed]
11. Serretti, A.; Lattuada, E.; Franchini, L.; Smeraldi, E. Melancholic features and response to lithium prophylaxis in mood disorders. *Depress. Anxiety* **2000**, *11*, 73–79. [CrossRef]
12. Compton, M.T.; Nemeroff, C.B. The treatment of bipolar depression. *J. Clin. Psychiatry* **2000**, *61*, 57–67. [PubMed]
13. Müller-Oerlinghausen, B.; Lewitzka, U. Lithium reduces pathological aggression and suicidality: A mini-review. *Neuropsychobiology* **2010**, *62*, 43–49. [CrossRef]
14. Jones, R.M.; Arlidge, J.; Gillham, R.; Reagu, S.; van den Bree, M.; Taylor, P.J. Efficacy of mood stabilisers in the treatment of impulsive or repetitive aggression: Systematic review and meta-analysis. *Br. J. Psychiatry* **2011**, *198*, 93–98. [CrossRef]
15. Comai, S.; Tau, M.; Pavlovic, Z.; Gobbi, G. The psychopharmacology of aggressive behavior: A translational approach: Part 2: Clinical studies using atypical antipsychotics, anticonvulsants, and lithium. *J. Clin. Psychopharmacol.* **2012**, *32*, 237–260. [CrossRef] [PubMed]
16. Cipriani, A.; Hawton, K.; Stockton, S.; Geddes, J.R. Lithium in the prevention of suicide in mood disorders: Updated systematic review and meta-analysis. *BMJ* **2013**, *346*, 3646. [CrossRef] [PubMed]
17. Vosahlikova, M.; Svobod, P. Lithium—Therapeutic tool endowed with multiple beneficiary effects caused by multiple mechanisms. *Acta. Neurobiol. Exp.* **2016**, *76*, 1–19. [CrossRef]
18. Bellivier, F.; Marie-Claire, C. Molecular signatures of lithium treatment: Current knowledge. *Pharmacopsychiatry* **2018**, *51*, 212–219. [CrossRef] [PubMed]
19. Miranda, A.; Shekhtman, T.; McCarthy, M.; DeModena, A.; Leckband, S.G.; Kelsoe, J.R. Study of 45 candidate genes suggests CACNG2 may be associated with lithium response in bipolar disorder. *J. Affect. Disord.* **2019**, *248*, 175–179. [CrossRef]
20. Pisanu, C.; Heilbronner, U.; Squassina, A. The role of pharmacogenomics in bipolar disorder: Moving towards precision medicine. *Mol. Diagn. Ther.* **2018**, *22*, 409–420. [CrossRef]
21. Oedegaard, K.J.; Alda, M.; Anand, A.; Andreassen, O.A.; Balaraman, Y.; Berrettini, W.H.; Bhattacharjee, A.; Brennand, K.J.; Burdick, K.E.; Calabrese, J.R.; et al. The pharmacogenomics of bipolar disorder study (PGBD): Identification of genes for lithium response in a prospective sample. *BMC Psychiatry* **2016**, *16*, 129. [CrossRef] [PubMed]
22. Song, J.; Bergen, S.E.; Di Florio, A.; Karlsson, R.; Charney, A.; Ruderfer, D.M.; Stahl, E.A.; Members of the International Cohort Collection for Bipolar Disorder (ICCBD); Chambert, K.D.; Moran, J.L.; et al. Genome-wide association study identifies SESTD1 as a novel risk gene for lithium-responsive bipolar disorder. *Mol. Psychiatry* **2016**, *21*, 1290–1297. [CrossRef]
23. Borodin, J.I.; Kudryavtseva, N.N.; Tenditnik, M.V.; Rachkovskaya, L.N.; Shurlygina, A.V.; Trufakin, V.A. Behavioral effects of novel enterosorbent Noolit on mice with mixed depression/anxiety-like state. *Pharmacol. Biochem. Behav.* **2002**, *72*, 131–141. [CrossRef]
24. Kudryavtseva, N.N.; Bakshtanovskaya, I.V.; Koryakina, L.A. Social model of depression in mice of C57BL/6J strain. *Pharmacol. Biochem. Behav.* **1991**, *2*, 315–320. [CrossRef]
25. Kudryavtseva, N.N.; Avgustinovich, D.F. Behavioral and physiological markers of experimental depression induced by social conflicts (DISC). *Aggress. Behav.* **1998**, *24*, 271–286. [CrossRef]
26. Avgustinovich, D.F.; Alekseyenko, O.V.; Bakshtanovskaya, I.V.; Koryakina, L.A.; Lipina, T.V.; Kudryavtseva, N.N. Dynamic changes of brain serotonergic and dopaminergic activities during development of anxious depression: Experimental study. *Uspekhi Fiziol. Nauk.* **2004**, *35*, 19–40.
27. Kudryavtseva, N.N. Psychopathology of repeated aggression: A neurobiological aspect. In *Perspectives on the Psychology of Aggression*; Morgan, J.P., Ed.; NOVA Science Publishers Inc.: New York, NY, USA, 2006; pp. 35–64.
28. Kudryavtseva, N.N.; Smagin, D.A.; Kovalenko, I.L.; Vishnivetskaya, G.B. Repeated positive fighting experience in male inbred mice. *Nat. Prot.* **2014**, *9*, 2705–2717. [CrossRef] [PubMed]

29. Serretti, A.; Malitas, P.N.; Mandelli, L.; Lorenzi, C.; Ploia, C.; Alevizos, B.; Nikolaou, C.; Boufidou, F.; Christodoulou, G.N.; Smeraldi, E. Further evidence for a possible association between serotonin transporter gene and lithium prophylaxis in mood disorders. *Pharmacogenomics J.* **2004**, *4*, 267–273. [CrossRef]
30. Delgado, P.L. Depression: The case for a monoamine deficiency. *J. Clin. Psychiatry* **2000**, *61* (Suppl. 6), 7–11.
31. Redrobe, J.P.; Bourin, M. The effect of lithium administration in animal models of depression: A short review. Fundam. *Clin. Pharmacol.* **1999**, *13*, 293–299. [CrossRef]
32. Carli, M.; Reader, T.A. Regulation of central serotonin transporters by chronic lithium: An autoradiographic study. *Synapse* **1997**, *27*, 83–89. [CrossRef]
33. Amare, A.T.; Schubert, K.O.; Baune, B.T. Pharmacogenomics in the treatment of mood disorders: Strategies and opportunities for personalized psychiatry. *EPMA J.* **2017**, *8*, 211–227. [CrossRef] [PubMed]
34. Budde, M.; Degner, D.; Brockmöller, J.; Schulze, T.G. Pharmacogenomic aspects of bipolar disorder: An update. *Eur. Neuropsychopharmacol.* **2017**, *27*, 599–609. [CrossRef]
35. Boyarskikh, U.A.; Bondar, N.P.; Filipenko, M.L.; Kudryavtseva, N.N. Downregulation of serotonergic genes expression in the raphe nuclei of midbrain under chronic social defeat stress in male mice. *Mol. Neurobiol.* **2013**, *48*, 13–21. [CrossRef] [PubMed]
36. Kudryavtseva, N.N.; Avgustinovich, D.F.; Bondar, N.P.; Tenditnik, M.V.; Kovalenko, I.L. An experimental approach for the study of psychotropic drug effects under simulated clinical conditions. *Curr. Drug. Metab.* **2008**, *9*, 352–360. [CrossRef]
37. Kudryavtseva, N.N.; Avgustinovich, D.F.; Bondar, N.P.; Tenditnik, M.V.; Kovalenko, I.L. Method for screening drugs with supposed psychotropic actions. Patent RU2006140591; 200611116, 6 December 2007.
38. Kudryavtseva, N.N. Use of the "partition" test in behavioral and pharmacological experiments. *Neurosci. Behav. Physiol.* **2003**, *33*, 461–471. [CrossRef]
39. Rodgers, R.J.; Cole, J.C. The elevated plus-maze: Pharmacology, methodology and ethology. In *Ethology and Psychopharmacology*; Cooper, S.J., Hendrie, C.A., Eds.; John Wiley & Sons Ltd.: Chichester, UK, 1994; pp. 9–44.
40. Kovalenko, I.L.; Galyamina, A.G.; Smagin, D.A.; Michurina, T.V.; Kudryavtseva, N.N.; Enikolopov, G. Extended effect of chronic social defeat stress in childhood on the behaviors in adulthood. *PLoS ONE* **2014**, *9*, e91762. [CrossRef] [PubMed]
41. Smagin, D.A.; Kudryavtseva, N.N. Anxiogenic and anxiolytic effects of lithium chloride under preventive and therapeutic treatments of male mice with repeated experience of aggression. *Zhurnal Vyss. Nervn. Deiatelnosti Im. IP Pavlov.* **2014**, *64*, 646–659.
42. Wong, A.H.; Gottesman, I.I.; Petronis, A. Phenotypic differences in genetically identical organisms: The epigenetic perspective. *Hum. Mol. Genet.* **2005**, *14*, 11–18. [CrossRef]
43. Peaston, A.E.; Whitelaw, E. Epigenetics and phenotypic variation in mammals. *Mamm. Genome* **2006**, *17*, 365–374. [CrossRef]
44. Mondragon, R.; Mayagoitia, L.; Lopez-Lujan, A.; Diaz, J.-L. Social structure features in three inbred strains of mice, C57Bl/6J, Balb/cj, and NIH: A comparative study. *Behav. Neur. Biol.* **1987**, *47*, 384–391. [CrossRef]
45. Krishnan, V.; Han, M.H.; Graham, D.L.; Berton, O.; Renthal, W.; Russo, S.J.; Laplant, Q.; Graham, A.; Lutter, M.; Lagace, D.C.; et al. Molecular adaptations underlying susceptibility and resistance to social defeat in brain reward regions. *Cell* **2007**, *131*, 391–404. [CrossRef]
46. Cao, J.L.; Covington, H.E., 3rd; Friedman, A.K.; Wilkinson, M.B.; Walsh, J.J.; Cooper, D.C.; Nestler, E.J.; Han, M.H. Mesolimbic dopamine neurons in the brain reward circuit mediate susceptibility to social defeat and antidepressant action. *J. Neurosci.* **2010**, *30*, 16453–16458. [CrossRef] [PubMed]
47. Golden, S.A.; Covington, H.E., 3rd; Berton, O.; Russo, S.J. A standardized protocol for repeated social defeat stress in mice. *Nat. Prot.* **2011**, *6*, 1183–1991. [CrossRef] [PubMed]
48. Kudryavtseva, N.N.; Bondar, N.P.; Avgustinovich, D.F. Association between repeated experience of aggression and anxiety in male mice. *Behav. Brain Res.* **2002**, *133*, 83–93. [CrossRef]
49. Kudryavtseva, N.N.; Bondar, N.P. Anxiolytic and anxiogenic effects of diazepam in male mice with different experience of aggression. *Bull. Exp. Biol. Med.* **2002**, *133*, 372–376. [CrossRef]
50. Ferrari, P.F.; Parmigiani, S.; Rodgers, R.J.; Palanza, P. Differential effects of chlordiazepoxide on aggressive behavior in male mice: The influence of social factors. *Psychopharmacology* **1997**, *134*, 258–265. [CrossRef]
51. Griebel, G. 5-hydroxytryptamine-interacting drugs in animal models of anxiety disorders: More than 30 years of research. *Pharmacol. Ther.* **1995**, *65*, 319–395. [CrossRef]
52. Griebel, G.; Belzung, C.; Misslin, R.; Vogel, E. The free exploratory paradigm, an effective method for measuring neophobic behavior in mice and testing potential neophobia reducing drugs. *Behav. Pharmacol.* **1993**, *4*, 637–644.
53. Avgustinovich, D.F.; Lipina, T.V.; Bondar, N.P.; Alekseyenko, O.V.; Kudryavtseva, N.N. Features of the genetically defined anxiety in mice. *Behav. Genet.* **2000**, *30*, 101–109. [CrossRef] [PubMed]
54. Kudryavtseva, N.N.; Avgustinovich, D.F.; Bakshtanovskaya, I.V.; Koryakina, L.A.; Alekseyenko, O.V.; Lipina., T.V.; Bondar, N.P. Experimental studies of hereditary predisposition to the development of depression. In *Animal Models of Biological Psychiatry*; Chapter 5; Kalueff, A., Ed.; Nova Science Publichers: New York, NY, USA, 2006; pp. 75–95.
55. Ressler, K.J.; Nemeroff, C.B. Role of serotonergic and noradrenergic systems in the pathophysiology of depression and anxiety disorders. *Depress. Anxiety* **2000**, *12*, 2–19. [CrossRef]
56. Carr, G.V.; Lucki, I. The role of serotonin receptor subtypes in treating depression: A review of animal studies. *Psychopharmacology* **2011**, *213*, 265–287. [CrossRef] [PubMed]

57. Challis, C.; Berton, O. Top-Down control of serotonin systems by the prefrontal cortex: A path toward restored socioemotional function in depression. *ACS Chem. Neurosci.* **2015**, *6*, 1040–1054. [CrossRef] [PubMed]
58. Liu, B.; Liu, J.; Wang, M.; Zhang, Y.; Li, L. From serotonin to neuroplasticity: Evolvement of theories for major depressive disorder. *Front. Cell Neurosci.* **2017**, *11*, 305. [CrossRef] [PubMed]
59. Kraus, C.; Castrén, E.; Kasper, S.; Lanzenberger, R. Serotonin and neuroplasticity—Links between molecular, functional and structural pathophysiology in depression. *Neurosci. Biobehav. Rev.* **2017**, *77*, 317–326. [CrossRef] [PubMed]
60. Azmitia, E.C. Serotonin neurons, neuroplasticity, and homeostasis of neural tissue. *Neuropsychopharmacology* **1999**, *21*, 33–45. [CrossRef]
61. Crispino, M.; Volpicelli, F.; Perrone-Capano, C. Role of the serotonin receptor 7 in brain plasticity: From development to disease. *Int. J. Mol. Sci.* **2020**, *21*, 505. [CrossRef]
62. Tanaka, M.; Bohár, Z.; Martos, D.; Telegdy, G.; Vécsei, L. Antidepressant-like effects of kynurenic acid in a modified forced swim test. *Pharmacol. Rep.* **2020**, *72*, 449–455. [CrossRef]
63. Kudryavtseva, N.N.; Smagin, D.A.; Kovalenko, I.L.; Galyamina, A.G.; Vishnivetskaya, G.B.; Babenko, V.N.; Orlov, Y.L. Serotonergic genes in the development of anxiety/depression-like state and pathology of aggressive behavior in male mice: RNA-seq data. *Mol. Biol.* **2017**, *51*, 251–262. [CrossRef]
64. Pickard, B.S. Genomics of lithium action and response. *Neurotherapeutics* **2017**, *14*, 582–587. [CrossRef]
65. Ge, W.; Jakobsson, E. Systems biology understanding of the effects of lithium on affective and neurodegenerative disorders. *Front. Neurosci.* **2018**, *12*, 933. [CrossRef] [PubMed]
66. Akkouh, I.A.; Skrede, S.; Holmgren, A.; Ersland, K.M.; Hansson, L.; Bahrami, S.; Andreassen, O.A.; Steen, V.M.; Djurovic, S.; Hughes, T. Exploring lithium's transcriptional mechanisms of action in bipolar disorder: A multi-step study. *Neuropsychopharmacology* **2020**, *45*, 947–955. [CrossRef]
67. Babenko, V.N.; Smagin, D.A.; Galyamina, A.G.; Kovalenko, I.L.; Kudryavtseva, N.N. Altered *Slc25* family gene expression as markers of mitochondrial dysfunction in brain regions under experimental mixed anxiety/depression-like disorder. *BMC Neurosci.* **2018**, *19*, 79. [CrossRef] [PubMed]
68. Smagin, D.A.; Kovalenko, I.L.; Galyamina, A.G.; Bragin, A.O.; Orlov, Y.L.; Kudryavtseva, N.N. Dysfunction in ribosomal gene expression in the hypothalamus and hippocampus following chronic social defeat stress in male mice as revealed by RNA-seq. *Neural Plast.* **2016**, *2016*, 3289187. [CrossRef]
69. Smagin, D.A.; Kovalenko, I.L.; Galyamina, A.G.; Orlov, Y.L.; Babenko, V.N.; Kudtyavtseva, N.N. Heterogeneity of brain ribosomal genes expression following repeated experience of aggression in male mice as revealed by RNA-seq. *Mol. Neurobiol.* **2018**, *55*, 390–401. [CrossRef]
70. Kudryavtseva, N.N.; Filipenko, M.L.; Bakshtanovskaya, I.V.; Avgustinovich, D.F.; Alekseenko, O.V.; Beilina, A.G. Changes in the expression of monoaminergic genes under the influence of repeated experience of agonistic interactions: From behavior to gene. *Russ. J. Genet.* **2004**, *40*, 590–604. [CrossRef]
71. Filipenko, M.L.; Beilina, A.G.; Alekseyenko, O.V.; Dolgov, V.V.; Kudryavtseva, N.N. Increase in expression of brain serotonin transporter and monoamine oxidase a genes induced by repeated experience of social defeats in male mice. *Biochemistry* **2002**, *67*, 451–455.
72. Kovalenko, I.L.; Smagin, D.A.; Galyamina, A.G.; Orlov, Y.L.; Kudryavtseva, N.N. Changes in the expression of dopaminergic genes in brain structures of male mice exposed to chronic social defeat stress: An RNA-seq study. *Mol. Biol.* **2016**, *50*, 184–187. [CrossRef]
73. Babenko, V.N.; Smagin, D.A.; Galyamina, A.G.; Kovalenko, I.L.; Kudryavtseva, N.N. Differentially expressed genes of the *Slc6a* family as markers of altered brain neurotransmitter system function in pathological states in mice. *Neurosci. Behav. Physiol.* **2020**, *50*, 199–209. [CrossRef]
74. Kudryavtseva, N.N.; Kovalenko, I.L.; Smagin, D.A.; Galyamina, A.G.; Babenko, V.N. Abnormal social behaviors and dysfunction of autism-related genes associated with daily agonistic interactions in mice. In *Molecular-Genetic and Statistical Techniques for Behavioral and Neural Research*; Gerlai, R.T., Ed.; Academic Press: San Diego, CA, USA, 2018; Volume 14, pp. 309–344.
75. Berton, O.; McClung, C.A.; Dileone, R.J.; Krishnan, V.; Renthal, W.; Russo, S.J.; Graham, D.; Tsankova, N.M.; Bolanos, C.A.; Rios, M.; et al. Essential role of BDNF in the mesolimbic dopamine pathway in social defeat stress. *Science* **2006**, *311*, 864–868. [CrossRef]
76. Kudryavtseva, N.N.; Bondar, N.P.; Boyarskikh, U.A.; Filipenko, M.L. *Snca* and *Bdnf* gene expression in the VTA and raphe nuclei of midbrain in chronically victorious and defeated male mice. *PLoS One* **2010**, *5*, e14089. [CrossRef] [PubMed]
77. Smagin, D.A.; Galyamina, A.G.; Kovalenko, I.L.; Babenko, V.N.; Kudryavtseva, N.N. Aberrant expression of collagen gene family in the brain regions of male mice with behavioral psychopathologies induced by chronic agonistic interactions. *BioMed. Res. Int.* **2019**, *2019*, 7276389. [CrossRef]
78. Mota de Freitas, D.; Leverson, B.D.; Goossens, J.L. Lithium in medicine: Mechanisms of action. *Met. Ions Life Sci.* **2016**, *16*, 557–584. [PubMed]
79. Machado-Vieira, R. Lithium, stress, and resilience in bipolar disorder: Deciphering this key homeostatic synaptic plasticity regulator. *J. Affect. Disord.* **2018**, *233*, 92–99. [CrossRef] [PubMed]
80. Ng, Q.X.; Yeo, W.S.; Sivalingam, V. Lithium-associated renal dysfunction: To stop or not to stop? *Bipolar Disord.* **2020**, *22*, 91–92. [CrossRef]

biomedicines

Review

Co-Players in Chronic Pain: Neuroinflammation and the Tryptophan-Kynurenine Metabolic Pathway

Masaru Tanaka [1,2], Nóra Török [1,2], Fanni Tóth [1], Ágnes Szabó [2] and László Vécsei [1,2,*]

1 MTA-SZTE, Neuroscience Research Group, Semmelweis u. 6, H-6725 Szeged, Hungary; tanaka.masaru.1@med.u-szeged.hu (M.T.); toroknora85@gmail.com (N.T.); toth.fanni@med.u-szeged.hu (F.T.)
2 Interdisciplinary Excellence Centre, Department of Neurology, Faculty of Medicine, University of Szeged, H-6725 Szeged, Hungary; szabo.agnes.4@med.u-szeged.hu
* Correspondence: vecsei.laszlo@med.u-szeged.hu; Tel.: +36-62-545-351

Citation: Tanaka, M.; Török, N.; Tóth, F.; Szabó, Á.; Vécsei, L. Co-Players in Chronic Pain: Neuroinflammation and the Tryptophan-Kynurenine Metabolic Pathway. *Biomedicines* **2021**, *9*, 897. https://doi.org/10.3390/biomedicines9080897

Academic Editor: Rosanna Di Paola

Received: 3 June 2021
Accepted: 19 July 2021
Published: 26 July 2021

Abstract: Chronic pain is an unpleasant sensory and emotional experience that persists or recurs more than three months and may extend beyond the expected time of healing. Recently, nociplastic pain has been introduced as a descriptor of the mechanism of pain, which is due to the disturbance of neural processing without actual or potential tissue damage, appearing to replace a concept of psychogenic pain. An interdisciplinary task force of the International Association for the Study of Pain (IASP) compiled a systematic classification of clinical conditions associated with chronic pain, which was published in 2018 and will officially come into effect in 2022 in the 11th revision of the International Statistical Classification of Diseases and Related Health Problems (ICD-11) by the World Health Organization. ICD-11 offers the option for recording the presence of psychological or social factors in chronic pain; however, cognitive, emotional, and social dimensions in the pathogenesis of chronic pain are missing. Earlier pain disorder was defined as a condition with chronic pain associated with psychological factors, but it was replaced with somatic symptom disorder with predominant pain in the Diagnostic and Statistical Manual of Mental Disorders, 5th Edition (DSM-5) in 2013. Recently clinical nosology is trending toward highlighting neurological pathology of chronic pain, discounting psychological or social factors in the pathogenesis of pain. This review article discusses components of the pain pathway, the component-based mechanisms of pain, central and peripheral sensitization, roles of chronic inflammation, and the involvement of tryptophan-kynurenine pathway metabolites, exploring the participation of psychosocial and behavioral factors in central sensitization of diseases progressing into the development of chronic pain, comorbid diseases that commonly present a symptom of chronic pain, and psychiatric disorders that manifest chronic pain without obvious actual or potential tissue damage.

Keywords: chronic pain; nociceptive pain; neuropathic pain; nociplastic pain; psychogenic pain; neuroinflammation; kynurenine

1. Introduction

Chronic pain is an unpleasant sensory and emotional experience that persists or recurs more than three months and may extend beyond the expected time of healing [1,2]. Chronic pain occurs as a part of symptoms due to an underlying medical condition or remains despite successful treatment of the condition that originally caused it [3]. Chronic pain frequently becomes the sole or predominant clinical complaint [4]. The prevalence of chronic pain estimates as much as 20%, and the incidence reaches about 10% every year of the world adult population [5]. Nearly 10% of individuals with chronic pain was found to suffer from moderate to severe debilitating pain [6]. Furthermore, individuals with severe chronic pain are twice more likely to die of respiratory disease or heart disease than those with mild pain or without pain [5]. The Global Burden of Disease Research ranked low back pain and migraine first and second place of Years Lived with Disability (YLD), respectively, and thus, chronic pain imposes a substantial socioeconomic burden directly and indirectly on society [7].

The International Classification of Diseases, Eleventh Revision (ICD-11), classifies chronic pain into primary and secondary. Primary chronic pain is fibromyalgia or low-back pain; the secondary chronic pain occurs secondary to an underlying medical condition subcategorizing into cancer-related, post-trauma, neuropathic, headache and orofacial, visceral, and musculoskeletal pain. ICD-11 offers minimal options for recording psychological or social factors in chronic pain [8]. Meanwhile, the Diagnostic and Statistical Manual of Mental Disorders, 5th Edition (DSM-5) recognizes chronic pain in the diagnosis of somatic symptom disorder (SSD), having replaced pain disorder, a condition with chronic pain due to psychological factors [9]. SSD is caused by somatosensory amplification, which is associated with fibromyalgia [10]. The trend toward a neurological explanation obviously discounts cognitive, emotional, and social dimensions in the pathomechanism of chronic pain. Hyperalgesia is a condition of abnormally increased sensitivity to pain caused by injury to tissues or nerves. Nociceptive sensation is also caused by exposure to opioids used for pain treatment, which paradoxically makes individuals more sensitive to certain stimuli. Hyperalgesia is a challenging issue for pain specialists who treat patients at terminal care [11]. Chronic pain is often elicited by stimuli that previously did not provoke discomfort sensation. It is called allodynia. Allodynia is commonly observed in patients with neuropathies, fibromyalgia, migraine, complex regional pain syndrome, and postherpetic neuralgia [12]. Chronic pain may proceed to clinical conditions accompanied often by mood alterations, such as depression, anxiety, anger, cognitive disturbance including memory impairment, sleep disturbances, fatigue, loss of libido, and/or disability, called chronic pain syndrome (CPS). CPS appears to be linked to the dysfunction of the hypothalamic–pituitary–adrenal axis and the central nervous system (CNS), but exact mechanisms remain unknown [13].

Neuroinflammation has been intricately linked to the pathogenesis of chronic pain. Chronic pain was proposed to be caused by the disturbance of peripheral nociception, neuropathy in the somatosensory system, motor system, central and peripheral nociplasticity, and/or psychosocial system [14]. Increasing evidence suggests that chronic inflammation is strongly tied to aberration in each mechanism of chronic pain. Furthermore, the tryptophan (TRP)–kynurenine (KYN) pathway and its metabolites were observed to play an important role in neuroinflammation and chronic pain [15]. This review article presents the components of the pain pathway; mechanisms of chronic pain based on the components; the development of chronic pain through peripheral and central sensitization; evidence of the presence of chronic neuroinflammation in each pain mechanism; the involvement of the TRP–KYN metabolic pathway; and the need of a psychogenic component in the pathogenesis of chronic pain.

2. The Pain Pathway, Mechanisms, Neuroinflammation, and Tryptophan Metabolism

Pain perception is signaling through the pain pathway, whose components consist of transduction, conduction, transmission, modulation, and perception. Transduction is the process by which noxious or potentially damaging stimuli activate the nociceptors to convert to neural signals. Transmission refers to the signal transfer from the peripheral neurons to the second-order neurons in the spinal cord, which wire the signals to the thalamus and brain stem in the brain. Pain modulation takes place by inhibition of pain signaling in the spinal cord and the activation of the descending inhibitory fibers. The third-order neurons project to the somatosensory cortex, enabling the perception of pain. Perception is the subjective awareness in connection with arousal, physiological, and behavioral brain centers, involving the integration of psychological processes such as attention, expectation, and interpretation [16–18] (Figure 1).

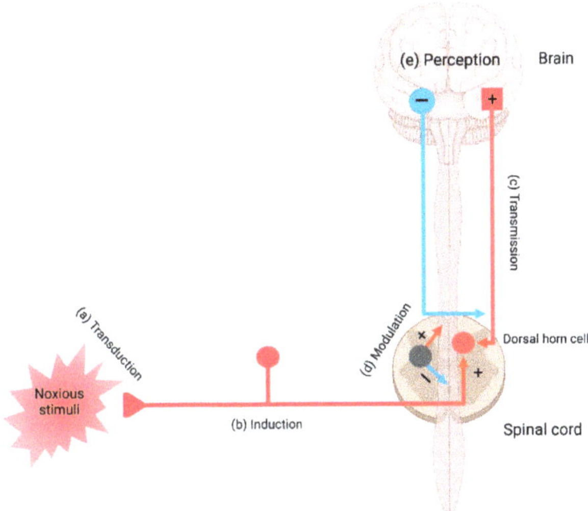

Figure 1. The main components in the pain pathway: (**a**) transduction, (**b**) induction, (**c**) transmission, (**d**) modulation, and (**e**) perception. Created with BioRender.com.

Pain is a complex and intricate process attributable to nocicептic, neuropathic, and/or neuroplastic mechanisms. The most common type of pain is nociceptive pain caused by damage or potentially harmful to peripheral tissues involving nociceptors responsible for transduction. Neuropathic pain is caused by lesions or diseases affecting the somatosensory nervous system responsible for the transmission of peripheral to central pain signals. Nociplastic pain refers to the condition caused by altered nociceptive processing without actual or potentially harmful tissue damage activating peripheral nociceptors (nociceptive pain) or without lesions or diseases of the somatosensory nervous system (neuropathic pain). Cortical perception is one of the main components in the pain pathway; however, the ICD-11 excludes psychogenic pain [19] (Figure 2). Thus, participation of cortical perception in chronic pain mechanisms remains ambiguous.

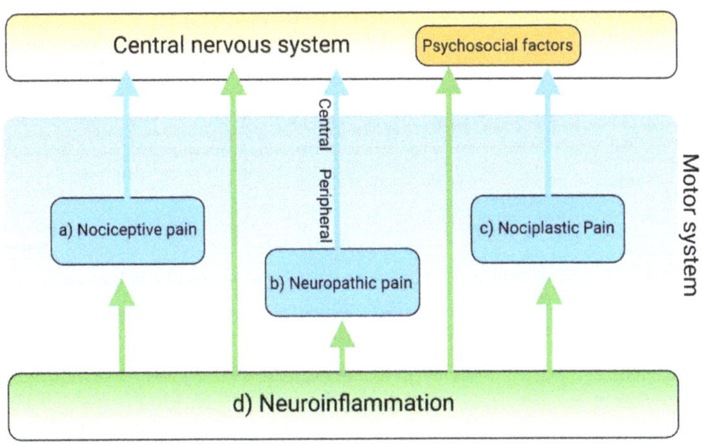

Figure 2. The main mechanisms of pain and the involvement of neuroinflammation. The mechanisms of pain are classified into (**a**) nociceptive, (**b**) neuropathic, and (**c**) nociplastic pain. Neuroinflammation (**d**) is involved in each pain mechanism. Created with BioRender.com.

Inflammation is generally involved in the pathogenesis of various diseases and plays a key role in diseases that cause chronic pain [20]. Resident and recruited immune cells release inflammatory mediators at peripheral nerve innervating damaged or inflammatory tissue to trigger action potentials in sensor neurons or sensitize neurons by increasing transduction and excitability. Inflammatory mediators also act directly on peripheral nerves to damage peripheral transmission [21]. Immune cells infiltrate the spinal cord and the dorsal root ganglia to damage the central transmission and/or modulate pain sensitivity [22]. Activated immune cells release inflammatory cytokines, chemokines, and other factors that influence cognition, mood, and behaviors through immune-to-CNS signaling [16,23]. Accumulating evidence suggests that chronic dysregulation of the immune response is involved in the pathogenesis of psychiatric disorders such as mood disorders, substance abuse disorders, psychotic disorders, attention-deficit disorders, and autism spectrum disorders [24–26] (Figure 2).

Inflammation is invariably linked to the activation of TRP metabolism [27,28]. The essential amino acid TRP is a precursor to serotonin, melatonin, and nicotinamide adenine dinucleotide (NAD^+), among others. More than 95% of TRP is metabolized through the TRP–KYN pathway, synthesizing various bioactive metabolites such as neuroprotective antioxidants and neuroprotectants, toxic oxidants and neurotoxins, as well as immunomodulators. The disturbance of KYN metabolites has been linked to immune disorders, cancers, neurodegenerative diseases, and psychiatric disorders [29]. Furthermore, TRP–KYN metabolites are under extensive research in search of peripheral biomarkers as well as novel drug prototypes for a wide range of diseases [30–36]. Inflammation activates the TRP–KYN pathway, elevating the levels of oxidative compounds or neurotoxic ligands to receptors of the excitatory glutamatergic nervous system, which damage the peripheral nervous system or CNS through the broken blood–nerve or blood–brain barrier, respectively [16]. Furthermore, immunomodulators are known to trigger the shift of acute inflammatory status toward tolerogenic and chronic inflammation, perpetuating low-grade inflammation [28,37]. KYN is synthesized from TRP by the tryptophan 2,3-dioxygenase (TDO) in the liver and the indoleamine 2,3-dioxygenases (IDOs) in the brain and the immune system, which are induced by cortisol, and interferon (IFN)-α, IFN-γ, and tumor necrosis factor (TNF)-α, respectively [38]. Anthranilic acid (AA), 3-hydroxykynurenine (3-HK), or kynurenic acid (KYNA) are produced from KYN by the kynureninase (KYNU), the KYN-3-monooxygenase (KMO), or the kynurenine aminotransferases (KATs), respectively. The KATs also convert 3-HK to xanthurenic acid (XA). XA converts into cinnabarinic acid by autoxidation. AA and 3-HK convert into 3-hydroxyanthranilic acid (3-HAA) and then into picolinic acid and quinolinic acid (QA). QA converts into NADH, which is a feedback inhibitor of TDO [31] (Figure 3). Generally, 3-HK and QA are described as neurotoxic, while KYNA is considered to be neuroprotective. The 3-HK/KYNA ratio is often applied as an indicator of neurotoxicity. However, emerging evidence suggests that some metabolites of the TRP–KYN pathway possess Janus-face properties, depending on the dose or the situation. For example, KYNA is excitatory in lower concentrations but inhibitory in higher concentrations at α-amino-3-hydroxy-5-methyl-4-isoxazole propionic acid (AMPA) receptors. 3-HK is known to be an oxidant but observed to be an antioxidant in certain conditions [27,39].

The stress hormone cortisol, the strong immune activator lipopolysaccharide, proinflammatory cytokines, positive feedback loops, diminished levels of antioxidant system enzyme superoxide dismutase, and anti-inflammatory cytokines all lead to the potentiation of the TRP–KYN pathway [28]. Furthermore, the action of the KYN enzymes and metabolites are complicated by the interactions with adjacent biosystems such as the oxidative stress complex, the antioxidant enzyme systems, the serotonin neurotransmission, the glutamate neurotransmission, the tetrahydrobiopterin pathway, the cannabinoid system, and the aryl hydrocarbon receptor signaling [28,39].

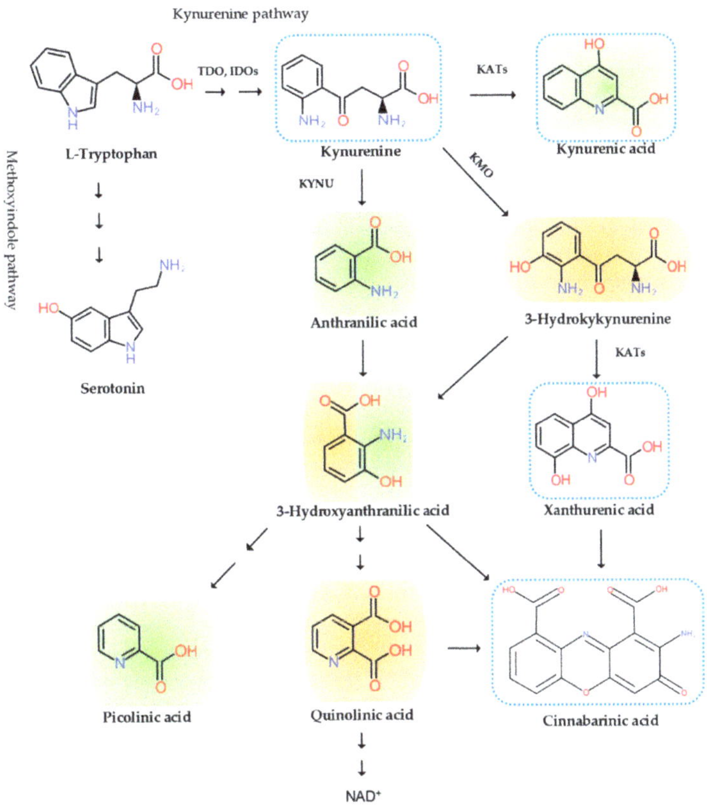

Figure 3. The tryptophan (TRP)–kynurenine (KYN) metabolic pathway and its metabolites. The pathway varies from the type of cells. Some enzyme is missing in some cells, not producing some metabolites. The TRP–KYN metabolic pathway synthesizes various metabolites, including oxidants (**orange color**), antioxidants (**green color**), and immunomodulators (**blue dotted line**). TDO: tryptophan 2,3-dioxygenase; IDO: indoleamine 2, 3-dioxygenase; KYNU: kynureninase; KMO: kynurenine-3-monooxygenase; KATs: kynurenine aminotransferases.

3. Transduction and Nociceptive Pain

The transduction of the pain sensation takes place when noxious stimuli depolarize the afferent terminal of nociceptive myelinated A-beta (Aß) and A-delta (Aδ) fibers and unmyelinated C fibers through the terminal membrane proteins and voltage-gated ion channels converting them into electric signals in the neurons (Figure 1a).

Nociceptive pain is the most common pain that originates from a tissue injury or inflammation in which the nociceptor of peripheral sensory nerves detects noxious or potentially harmful stimuli [40]. In chronic pain, the peripheral nociceptors continue to transmit painful stimuli even after the original injury has healed [41]. Osteoarthritis is a classical nociceptive pain condition when abnormal loading of a damaged joint opens mechanogated ion channels on nociceptive nerve endings [42]. Overextending or tearing a ligament sensitizes nociceptors, which causes acute nociceptive pain, such as in the case of an ankle sprain. In addition to mechanical irritation or physical injury, the primary cells of the epidermis, keratinocytes, induce pain by releasing endogenous mediators, such as adenosine triphosphate (ATP), Interleukin (IL)-1 beta (β), prostaglandin E2, endothelin, and nerve growth factor. However, keratinocytes act in a dual matter in pain sensation: They release β–endorphin that help pleasurable feeling during modest sun-bathing but activate transient receptor potential cation channel subfamily V member 4 (TRPV4) and release pro-inflammatory cytokines, eliciting the pain sensation of a sunburn [43,44] (Figure 2a and Table 1).

Table 1. Pain pathway components, pain mechanisms, and representative diseases.

Pain Pathway Components	Pain Mechanisms	Diseases, Disorders, and Injuries
Transduction	Nociceptive pain	Ankle sprain and osteoarthritis
Conduction transmission	Neuropathic pain	Diabetic neuropathy, shingles, nutritional deficiencies, toxins, cancer, Guillain-Barre syndrome, amyloidosis, Fabry's disease, and nerve trunk injuries
Modulation	Nociplastic pain	Fibromyalgia temporomandibular disorders, and nonspecific back pain
Perception	Psychogenic pain	Depression, anxiety, and cognitive impairment

Inflammation also activates nociceptors in the nerve endings. Inflammatory mediators bind to their receptors on nociceptive sensory neurons in the peripheral nervous system, resulting in pain [20]. Pro-inflammatory factors including TNF-γ and IL-1β secreted by monocytes and macrophages at the site of a peripheral injury facilitate pain transduction and conduction by modifying ion channels including transient receptor potential cation channel subfamily A member 1 (TRPA1), transient receptor potential cation channel subfamily V member 1 (TRPV1), and Nav1.7–1.9. However, those cells secret anti-inflammatory factors such as IL-10 and/or pro-resolution mediators, including resolvins, protectins, and maresins, to reduce nociception in the resolution phase of acute inflammation. Different phenotypes of macrophages, such as pro-inflammatory M1 and anti-inflammatory M2, contribute to the induction and resolution of pain, respectively [45]. Schwann cells of the peripheral nervous system also secret TNF-γ and IL-1β to sensitize nociceptors at axons in neuronal injury. Activated Schwann cells secrete matrix metalloprotease (MMP) 9 that help open the blood–nerve barrier, resulting in the recruitment of immune cells that release inflammatory cytokines [22,46]. Furthermore, nociceptive afferent sensory neurons directly modulate inflammation by releasing inflammatory mediators, such as substance P, calcitonin gene-related peptide (CGRP), neurokinin A, and endothelin-3. The process is called neurogenic inflammation (Figure 2d).

The disturbance of TRP metabolism is observed in neurogenic inflammation. The increased levels of the stress hormone cortisol and inflammatory cytokines such as IFN-α, IFN-γ, and TNF-α activate the TRP–KYN pathway producing higher levels of oxidant KYN metabolites which leak into the peripheral nervous system through the damaged gap junction following the immune reaction. The oxidative KYN metabolites 3-HK, 3-HA, and QA are harmful compounds to nerve endings of the afferent sensory neurons (Figure 3).

4. Conduction, Transmission, and Neuropathic Pain

In conduction, the electrical signals are conducted from the peripheral neurons to the central neurons where a network of interneurons facilitates or inhibits transmission to the second-order neurons in the dorsal horn [47]. The presynaptic terminals of C fibers release glutamate, substance P, and CGRP, which activate postsynaptic AMPA receptors, NK1 receptors, and CGRP receptors, respectively [48] (Figure 1b). In transmission, the activation of the postsynaptic receptors generates an action potential of the second-order neurons and interneurons, which relay signals through the contralateral spinothalamic tract to the thalamus; or the spinoreticular and spinomesencephalic tracts to the medulla and brain stem; or the spinohypothalamic tract to the hypothalamus [49] (Figure 1c).

Neuropathic pain originates from lesions or diseases of the somatosensory nervous system made up of peripheral and central components. Peripheral neuropathic pain is commonly caused by diabetic neuropathy, metabolic disorders, shingles, HIV-related distal symmetrical neuropathies, nutritional deficiencies, toxins such as arsenic and thallium, a paraneoplastic manifestation of cancer, immune-mediated inflammatory diseases such as Guillain-Barre syndrome, amyloidosis, Fabry's disease, and nerve trunk injuries [50]. Presumably, burning and poorly localized pain is transmitted by C fibers, while sharp and lancinating pain is relayed by Aδ fibers [51]. Diabetic neuropathy is the most common neuropathy associated with severe pain, which presents a distal symmetrical polyneuropathy with numbness and loss of sensation in the distal extremities, often accompanied by peripheral vascular diseases, leading to infection and ultimately amputation [52]. Neuropathic pain is also caused by direct invasion to peripheral nerves by tumor, side effects of chemotherapy, radiation injury, or surgery [53] (Figure 2b and Table 1). Central neuropathic pain is a common sequela to injury to the CNS such as vascular accidents, including ischemic and hemorrhagic stroke, infections, including abscess, encephalitis, and myelitis, demyelinating diseases, including multiple sclerosis, tumors, and brain or spinal cord [54–56] (Figure 2b and Table 1). Mixed pain is a term never formally defined, but it indicates pain caused by a combination of nociceptive and neuropathic mechanisms observed in patients who suffer from osteoarthritis, sciatica, and cancer.

Neuropathic pain is often manifested as a part of the symptoms of psychological disorders. The lifetime and current prevalence of psychiatric disorders in patients with chronic peripheral pain were 39% and 20%, respectively [57]. Diseases that cause neuropathic pain include diabetes, herpes zoster infection, nerve compression, nerve trauma, channelopathies, and autoimmune diseases. The most common psychiatric disorders were generalized anxiety disorders and mood disorders [57]. Furthermore, antidepressants showed efficacy for neuropathic pain in patients with depression, suggesting neuropathic pain and depression have a bidirectional relationship [58]. Individuals with chronic neuropathic pain were associated with substance abuse or suicide ideation [59] (Figure 2b and Table 1).

Inflammation plays an important role in neuropathic pain. Around afferent peripheral nerves, monocytes and macrophages release pro-inflammatory factors, including TNF-γ and IL-1β, while they secrete anti-inflammatory factor IL-10 and pro-resolving lipid mediators at the resolution of acute inflammation [60]. T lymphocytes (T-cells) play an important role in neuropathic pain. T-cells secret a pro-inflammatory cytokine IL-17 and accumulate in the dorsal root ganglion (DRG) to release pro-analgesic leukocyte elastase, inducing mechanical allodynia. In the resolution phase, T-cells secrete anti-inflammatory cytokines IL-4 and IL-10. In response to noxious stimuli, the satellite glial cells (SGCs) are activated and proliferated at DRG to release pro-inflammatory cytokines TNF and IL-1β and a nociceptive neurotransmitter ATP signaling through P2 receptors [61]. SGCs also release MMPs that open the blood–nerve barriers, allowing entry of immune cells [62]. Bone marrow stem cells trigger analgesic actions by secreting anti-inflammatory cytokine-transforming growth factor-beta 1 by suppressing glial activation induced by nerve injury and migrating to DRG via a (C-X-C motif) chemokine ligand (CXCL) 12 chemotactic signal after intrathecal injection [63].

Spinal cord microglia play major roles in pathological pain. Following peripheral injury, ATP, colony-stimulating factor 1, chemokines including (C-C motif) chemokine ligand (CCL) 2 and fractalkine (CX3CL1), and proteases activate spinal microglia [64]. Meanwhile, the expression of the receptors for ATP and CX3CL1 increases, converging an intracellular signaling cascade, leading to the phosphorylation of p38 mitogen-activated protein (MAP) kinase, which, in turn, elevates production and release of TNF-γ, IL-1β, IL-18, brain-derived growth factor (BDNF), and prostaglandin E2. TNF-γ and Il-1β increase synaptic transmission and decrease inhibitory synaptic transmission of lamina II spinal cord neurons [22]. BDNF suppressed gamma-aminobutyric acid inhibitory synaptic transmission in projection to lamina I spinal cord neurons. Microglia release anti-inflammatory cytokine IL-10 in the resolution phase of inflammation [65].

An astrocyte is in contact with more than one million synapses, and thus, chronic pain in astrocyte activation is more persistent [66]. Astrocytes communicate with neurons through gap junction mediated by connexin-43 (Cx43). Cx43 is upregulated in astrocytes after nerve injury, serving as a paracrine modulator. The paracrine modulation results in elevating the release of glutamate, ATP, MMP2 and chemokines, including CCL2 and CXCL1. The chemokines function as neuromodulators that potentiate excitatory synaptic transmission. Meanwhile, following nerve injury, spinal cord neurons upregulate CXCL13 that activates astrocytes via C-C chemokine receptor type 5 to sustain neuropathic pain [67]. The spinal cord and cortical astrocytes upregulate thrombospondin 4 that leads to new synapsis formation and subsequent somatosensory cortical circuit rewiring, causing neuropathic pain [68]. Astrocytes cause neuronal hyperexcitability resulting from disturbance of homeostasis of extracellular potassium and glutamate. IFN-α produced by astrocytes inhibits nociceptive transmission in the spinal cord [66].

Oligodendrocytes form myelin sheath insulating axons in the CNS [69]. Little is known about their roles in pain. IL-33 produced from oligodendrocytes contributes to pain sensitivity via MAP kinases and nuclear factor kappa-light-chain-enhancer of activated B cells in chronic constriction injury model of nerve injury-induced neuropathic pain [70]. Diphtheria toxin ablation of oligodendrocytes leads to neuropathic pain, suggesting analgesic roles of the cells. Following nerve injury, T-cells infiltrate the spinal cord, contributing to the development of mechanical sensitivity. T-cells release pro-inflammatory cytokine TNF-γ, they secrete anti-inflammatory cytokines IL-4 and IL-10 in the resolution phase of inflammation [71]. Following chemotherapy, intrathecal injection of cytotoxic T-cells enhanced neuropathic pain, while the injection of regulatory T-cells diminished neuropathic pain [72] (Figure 2d).

The involvement of the TRP–KYN pathway was reported in inflammation-induced neuropathic pain. The enzyme activities of the TRP–KYN pathway were studied in a lipopolysaccharide-stimulated chronic constriction injury at the spinal cord and DRG levels of rats. The intrathecal administration of L-KYN and the intraperitoneal injection of L-KYN and an organic anion transport inhibitor probenecid significantly reversed tactile allodynia in L5-L6 spinal nerve root-ligated rats, suggesting that the N-methyl-D-aspartate (NMDA) receptor, an organic anion transport inhibitor agonist KYNA, mediates relieving the allodynia [73]. The increased ratio of QA/KYN and the mRNA expression of KMO, KYNU, and 3-hydroxyanthranilate dioxygenase (HAOO) was elevated in neuronal nuclear antigen-positive neurons of the contralateral hippocampal dentate gyrus in a neuropathic mouse model [74]. TDOIDO1 and 2, KMO, KYNU, and HAOO were found to be derived from cerebral microglial cells, and mRNA expression of IDO2, KMO, and HAOO were upregulated at the spinal cord after one week. Microglia inhibitor, minocycline, decreased the levels of IDO2 and KMO enzymes and tactile and thermal hypersensitivity; furthermore, IDO2 inhibitor 1-methyl-d-tryptophan and KMO inhibitor UPF 648 significantly decreased mechanical and thermal hypersensitivity [75]. This suggests the participation of IDO2 and KMO enzymes in the pathogenesis of neuropathic pain. The intracerebroventricular administration of KMO inhibitor Ro 61-8048 alleviated spared nerve injury-induced depressive-like behavior, and the intrathecal injection of Ro 61-8048 attenuated both the depressive-like behavior and mechanical allodynia in rats [76]. The NMDA receptor seems to play a major role in neuropathic pain and in the development of opioid tolerance. Dextromethorphan is an NMDA antagonist at high doses. Both animal and human studies showed that NMDA antagonist ketamine was beneficial for analgesics [77] (Figure 3).

5. Modulation and Nociplastic Pain

Modulation of pain transmission occurs at all levels of the pain pathway from peripheral to the brain, as well as from upward-to-downward pain regulations, involving both excitatory and inhibitory mechanisms that facilitate or suppress the responses of second-order neurons, respectively [48]. Peripheral pain modulation is achieved through local growth factor, hormonal, and peptide release, which alters signaling through neurotransmitter, ion, or receptor-based mechanisms. The pain modulation takes place neuronal signaling through corticospinal, corticoperiheral, and intraspinal pathways and neuroplasticity regulation [78] (Figures 1d and 4).

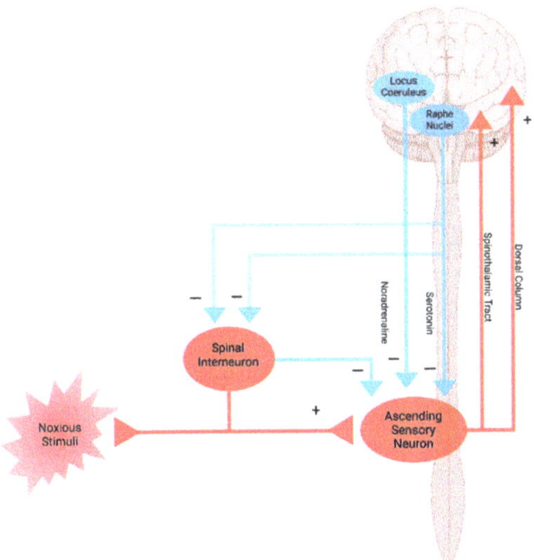

Figure 4. Pain pathway and pain modulation. Nociplastic pain is caused by the disturbance of central pain processing mechanisms, such as elevated excitability of ascending and descending pain facilitatory pathways and/or reduced inhibition of the descending anti-nociceptive pathway. Created with BioRender.com.

Nociplastic pain is defined as pain that arises from altered nociception despite no clear evidence of actual or threatened tissue damage causing the activation of peripheral nociceptors or no clear evidence of diseased lesions of the somatosensory nervous system causing the pain [79,80]. Nociplastic pain is generally chronic and widespread and is caused by the disturbance of central pain processing mechanisms, such as elevated excitability of ascending and descending pain facilitatory pathways and/or reduced inhibition of the descending anti-nociceptive pathway [14,81,82] (Figure 4). The condition refers to central sensitization in which pain is elicited by innocuous stimuli or different kinds of stimuli, resulting in central hyperalgesia or allodynia, respectively [83]. The process involves increased activity of the insula, anterior cingulate cortex, and the prefrontal cortex, which becomes active during acute pain sensation as well as of the brain stem nuclei, dorsolateral frontal cortex, and parietal cortex, which do not participate during acute pain sensation [84] (Figure 4). Fatigue, negative affect, unrefreshing sleep, and cognitive dysfunction are common accompanying findings in centralized nociplastic pain [85]. This typical pattern of nociplastic pain is observed in fibromyalgia, a medical condition of unknown cause but known to be involved in genetic and environmental factors [86]. Temporomandibular disorder and nonspecific back pain are also characterized by central sensitization (Figure 2c and Table 1).

The inflammatory response is remarkable in nociplastic pain. The levels of proinflammatory cytokines including IL-6 and IL-8 were observed to be higher, while anti-inflammatory cytokines IL-1 receptor antagonist was higher and IL-4 was lower in patients with fibromyalgia. Several chemokine levels were elevated in fibromyalgia patients. They were monocyte recruiting such as protein eotaxin (CCL11), TARC (CCL17), and MDC (CCL22) and neutrophil chemoattractant MIG (CXCL9) and I-TAC (CXCL11) [87]. Furthermore, the disruption of the proinflammatory and anti-inflammatory cytokine network was considered to play a key role in the pathogenesis of central sensitization in fibromyalgia. Chronic inflammation has been considered to induce central pain in rheumatoid arthritis [88]. Thus, inflammation certainly contributes to the development of nociplastic pain, as in fibromyalgia (Figure 2d).

The alteration of TRP metabolism has been linked to nociplastic pain such as the temporomandibular disorders myalgia and fibromyalgia. The levels of TRP were observed to be significantly lower in the plasma of fibromyalgia patients compared to control, and the KYN/TRP ratio was negatively correlated with anxiety levels. The plasma TRP levels were negatively correlated with the wrist pain intensity, whereas the KYN/TRP ratio was positively correlated with the average and wrist pain intensity in temporomandibular disorders [89]. TRP depletion appears to be involved in the pathogenesis of fibromyalgia and temporomandibular disorders; however, little is known about the roles of NMDA receptor agonists 3-HK and QA and NMDA receptor antagonist KYNA. Furthermore, the direct link between KYNs and nociplastic pain has not been reported (Figure 3).

6. Cortical Perception and Psychogenic Pain

The perception of pain is processed in the brain and the spinal cord. The thalamus, sensorimotor cortex, insular cortex, and anterior cingulate decode signals of unpleasant sensation carried through ascending spinothalamic tract, whereas the amygdala and hypothalamus decode signals of urgency and intensity brought through ascending the spinobulbar tract. The third-order neurons transfer signals and communicate with the cortex centers. Overall, the integration of sensations, emotions, and cognition in the brain lead to the perception of pain [90] (Figure 1e). Psychogenic pain is pain without relevant anatomic tissue injury or inconsistent with functional causes in distribution and is considered to be caused by psychological factors such as depression, anxiety, and emotion [91]. Depression, anxiety, and cognitive disturbance are common symptoms that manifest in a wide range of diseases and comorbidity [92]. Individuals with depression and anxiety often experience psychogenic pain all over their bodies without any relevant physical cause [93,94]. Other psychiatric disorders frequently observed in individuals with chronic pain include substance abuse, somatoform disorder, and panic disorders [95]. Furthermore, chronic pain is associated with the disturbance of cognitive functions such as attention, working memory, reasoning ability, information processing, and verbal communication [96,97].

Inflammation is obviously involved in psychiatric disorders such as depression and anxiety. Meta-analyses reported strong evidence of significantly increased levels of c-reactive protein (CRP), IL-1, IL-6, TNF-α and soluble IL-2 receptor in the serum of major depressive disorder (MDD) patients [98–102]. A higher concentration of CCL2/MCP-1 was also reported in patients with MDD. CRP levels in blood, serum or plasma samples was significantly raised in generalized anxiety disorder (GAD) patients by meta-analysis, and IFN-γ and TNF-α levels were significantly increased in at least two or more studies [103]. Lower levels of IL-10 and higher ratios of TNF-α/IL-10, TNF-α/IL-4, IFN-γ/IL-10, and IFN-γ/IL-4 were observed in the serum of GAD patients, showing significantly increased pro- to anti-inflammatory cytokine ratios, which suggests a distinct cytokine imbalance [104] (Figure 2d).

Similarly, activation of the TRP–KYN pathway has been reported in depression and anxiety. Meta-analyses reported decreased TRP levels in plasma and decreased levels of KYN and KYNA in MDD patients, while antidepressant-free patients showed an increased level of QA. The postmortem brain tissues from patients with MDD showed the increased QA immunoreactivity in the prefrontal cortex and hippocampus [105,106]. Magnetic resonance spectroscopy suggested a higher turnover of cells with KYN and the 3-HAA/KYN ratio in adolescent depression. Those findings are in accordance with the activation of the TRP-KYN pathway toward 3-HK and QA branches by pro-inflammatory cytokines activating IDOs, and KMO, resulting in higher neurotoxic 3-HK and QA levels [107]. Decreased plasma KYN levels were observed in endogenous anxiety and normalized after treatment [108]. The alteration of the TRP-KYN pathway by stress or inflammation may cause serotonin and melatonin deficiency, making an individual more susceptible to anxiety (Figure 3).

7. Conclusions and Future Perspective

The pain pathway, pain mechanisms, inflammation, KYN metabolites and enzymes of the TRP–KYN pathway, and diseases associated with chronic pain are overviewed in this review article. Pain sensation can be attributed to damage and/or potential harm in various components of the pain pathway and corresponding pain mechanisms, involving inflammation and alteration of the TRP–KYN pathway [109]. Chronic inflammation triggers not only nociceptive pain but induces other pain mechanisms, including psychogenic pain. Thus, a search for unique inflammatory signatures and various interventional targets in chronic inflammation is currently under extensive research [110–113]. Intervention through the TRP–KYN pathway is under comprehensive research to alleviate oxidative stress and excitotoxicity in various illnesses [114–121]. Meanwhile, the effectiveness of motor cortex stimulation and spinal cord stimulation to alleviate chronic pain caused by various underlying conditions is under evaluation [122,123].

Chronic pain arises through a complex pathogenic process involving more components and developing into the pain continuum. Central sensitization, peripheral sensitization, and somatization are pathogenic processes of pain development in the pain continuum spanning components of the pain pathway and the pain mechanism, which is hardly understood without the presence of the cortical perception (Figure 5). The nociplastic mechanism of pain attempts to delineate pain without relevant cause or lesions of the somatosensory nervous system, such as altered perception of nociception. Chronic pain presented in fibromyalgia syndrome, chronic back pain, and complex regional pain syndrome is best understood in the framework of pain perception, including cognitive, emotional, and social components. Chronic pain experienced in psychiatric conditions, in particular, is not fully explainable in the view of the nociplastic pain mechanism. Pain sensation is developed through complex interactions with higher cortical centers governing mood, emotion, and cognition.

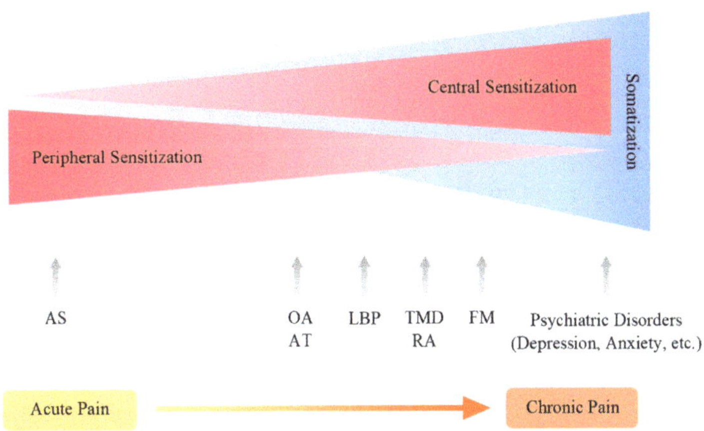

Figure 5. The continuum of pain sensitization and somatization. Chronic pain arises through a complex pathogenic process involving more components and developing into the pain continuum. Central sensitization, peripheral sensitization, and somatization are pathogenic processes of pain development spanning components of the pain pathway and the pain mechanism, which is hardly understood without the presence of the cortical perception. Acute pain may develop into chronic pain. AS: ankle sprain, OA: osteoarthritis, AT; Achilles tendinopathy; LBT: low back pain, TMD: temporomandibular joint disorder, FM: fibromyalgia.

Animal studies are one of the most important arenas for pain research. The endothelin receptor mediates the alteration of astrocyte functions, leading to the alleviation of neuropathic pain [124]. The dissociative anesthetics ketamine induces analgesic effects in models of acute pain and relieves thermal and mechanical allodynia in a chronic neuropathic pain model [125]. The involvement of the serotonergic neurotransmission in analgesic actions has been studied using neuropathic pain models in rats [126]. The gender difference in pain sensation and emotional domain has been reported using the transgenic mouse model of Alzheimer's disease [127].

More and more emerging findings shed light on the relationship between psychiatric symptoms and networks of the brain centers in neuropsychiatric disorders [128–130]. Stimulus-evoked functional magnetic resonance imaging (fMRI), task-free fMRI, and perfusion MRI revealed that chronic pains arise from pre-existing vulnerabilities and sustained abnormal input [131]. Neuroimaging techniques, including fMRI and positron emission tomography, may open the gate to understanding underlying mechanisms in signaling to the third-order neurons to the cortex in chronic pain sensation [132–134]. Pain relief can be achieved through accompanying symptoms such as cognition, mood, and sleep by pharmacotherapy and/or psychotherapy [132,135–137]. Therefore, psychogenic components of pain play an essential role in understanding the pathomechanism of chronic pain unless the nociplastic pain mechanism can sufficiently elucidate the reciprocal interaction with third-order neurons in the pathogenesis of chronic pain.

Author Contributions: Conceptualization, M.T. and L.V.; writing—original draft preparation, M.T.; writing—review and editing, M.T., N.T., F.T., Á.S. and L.V.; visualization, M.T. and Á.S.; supervision, L.V.; project administration, L.V.; funding acquisition, L.V. All authors have read and agreed to the published version of the manuscript.

Funding: This research was funded by GINOP 2.3.2-15-2016-00034, GINOP 2.3.2-15-2016-00048, TUDFO/47138-1/2019-ITM, and TKP2020 Thematic Excellence Programme 2020—The APC was funded by the University of Szeged Open Access Fund (4942).

Institutional Review Board Statement: Not applicable.

Informed Consent Statement: Not applicable.

Data Availability Statement: Not applicable.

Acknowledgments: The authors are grateful to Eleonóra Spekker for the technical assistance of graphic design.

Conflicts of Interest: The authors declare no conflict of interest.

Abbreviations

AA	anthranilic acid
Aß fiber	A-beta fiber
Aδ fiber	A-delta fiber
AMPA	α-amino-3-hydroxy-5-methyl-4-isoxazole propionic acid
AS	ankle sprain
AT	Achilles tendinopathy
ATP	Adenosine triphosphate
BDNF	brain-derived growth factor
CCL	(C-C motif) chemokine ligand
CGRP	calcitonin gene-related peptide
CNS	central nervous system
CPS	chronic pain syndrome
CX3CL1	fractalkine
Cx43	connexin-43
CXCL	(C-X-C motif) chemokine ligand
DRG	dorsal root ganglion
DSM-5	Diagnostic and Statistical Manual of Mental Disorders, 5th Edition

FM	fibromyalgia
fMRI	functional magnetic resonance imaging
GAD	generalized anxiety disorder
3-HAA	3-hydroxyanthranilic acid
3-HK	3-hydroxykynurenine
HAOO	3-hydroxyanthranilate dioxygenase
ICD-11	11th revision of the International Statistical Classification of Diseases and Related Health Problems
IDO	indolamine 2,3-dioxygenase
IFN	interferon
IL	interleukin
KAT	kynurenine aminotransferase
KMO	kynurenine 3-monooxygenase
KYN	kynurenine
KYNA	kynurenic acid
KYNU	kynureninase
LBP	low back pain
MAP	mitogen-activated
MDD	major depressive disorder
MMP	matrix metalloprotease
NAD^+	nicotinamide adenine dinucleotide
NMDA	N-methyl-D-aspartate
OA	osteoarthritis
QA	quinolinic acid
SGCs	satellite glial cells
SSD	somatic symptom disorder
T-cells	T lymphocytes
TDO	tryptophan 2,3-dioxygenase
TMD	temporomandibular joint disorder
TNF-γ	tumor necrosis factor gamma
TRP	tryptophan
TRPA1	transient receptor potential cation channel, subfamily A member 1
TRPV1	transient receptor potential cation channel subfamily V member 1
TRPV4	transient receptor potential cation channel subfamily V member 4
XA	xanthurenic acid

References

1. IASP. Definitions of Chronic Pain Syndromes. Available online: https://www.iasp-pain.org/Advocacy/icd.aspx?ItemNumber=5354#chronicpain (accessed on 18 December 2020).
2. Di Lernia, D.; Lacerenza, M.; Ainley, V.; Riva, G. Altered Interoceptive Perception and the Effects of Interoceptive Analgesia in Musculoskeletal, Primary, and Neuropathic Chronic Pain Conditions. *J. Pers. Med.* **2020**, *10*, 201. [CrossRef]
3. Medicina. Special Issue "Chronic Pain Management". Available online: https://www.mdpi.com/journal/medicina/special_issues/chronic_pain_management (accessed on 18 December 2020).
4. Mäntyselkä, P.; Kumpusalo, E.; Ahonen, R.; Kumpusalo, A.; Kauhanen, J.; Viinamäki, H.; Halonen, P.; Takala, J. Pain as a reason to visit the doctor: A study in Finnish primary health care. *Pain* **2001**, *89*, 175–180. [CrossRef]
5. Mills, S.; Nicolson, K.P.; Smith, B.H. Chronic pain: A review of its epidemiology and associated factors in population-based studies. *Br. J. Anaesth.* **2019**, *123*, e273–e283. [CrossRef] [PubMed]
6. Johnson, M.I. The Landscape of Chronic Pain: Broader Perspectives. *Medicina* **2019**, *55*, 182. [CrossRef] [PubMed]
7. GBD 2016 Disease and Injury Incidence and Prevalence Collaborators. Global, regional, and national incidence, prevalence, and years lived with disability for 328 diseases and injuries for 195 countries, 1990–2016: A systematic analysis for the Global Burden of Disease Study 2016. *Lancet* **2017**, *390*, 1211–1259. [CrossRef]
8. Treede, R.D.; Rief, W.; Barke, A.; Aziz, Q.; Bennett, M.I.; Benoliel, R.; Cohen, M.; Evers, S.; Finnerup, N.B.; First, M.B.; et al. Chronic pain as a symptom or a disease: The IASP Classification of Chronic Pain for the International Classification of Diseases (ICD-11). *Pain* **2019**, *160*, 19–27. [CrossRef]
9. American Psychiatric Association. Diagnostic and Statistical Manual of Mental Disorders, 5th ed. Available online: https://doi.org/10.1176/appi.books.9780890425596 (accessed on 27 December 2020).
10. Ciaramella, A.; Silvestri, S.; Pozzolini, V.; Federici, M.; Carli, G. A retrospective observational study comparing somatosensory amplification in fibromyalgia, chronic pain, psychiatric disorders and healthy subjects. *Scand. J. Pain* **2020**. [CrossRef]

11. Rivat, C.; Ballantyne, J. The dark side of opioids in pain management: Basic science explains clinical observation. *Pain Rep.* **2016**, *1*, e570. [CrossRef]
12. He, Y.; Kim, P.Y. Allodynia. In *StatPearls*; StatPearls Publishing: Treasure Island, FL, USA, 2020. Available online: https://www.ncbi.nlm.nih.gov/books/NBK537129/ (accessed on 27 December 2020).
13. Yasaei, R.; Peterson, E.; Saadabadi, A. Chronic Pain Syndrome. In *StatPearls*; StatPearls Publishing: Treasure Island, FL, USA. Available online: https://www.ncbi.nlm.nih.gov/books/NBK470523/ (accessed on 18 December 2020).
14. Chimenti, R.L.; Frey-Law, L.A.; Sluka, K.A. A Mechanism-Based Approach to Physical Therapist Management of Pain. *Phys. Ther.* **2018**, *98*, 302–314. [CrossRef]
15. Jovanovic, F.; Candido, K.D.; Knezevic, N.N. The Role of the Kynurenine Signaling Pathway in Different Chronic Pain Conditions and Potential Use of Therapeutic Agents. *Int. J. Mol. Sci.* **2020**, *21*, 6045. [CrossRef]
16. Dantzer, R.; O'Connor, J.C.; Freund, G.G.; Johnson, R.W.; Kelley, K.W. From inflammation to sickness and depression: When the immune system subjugates the brain. *Nat. Rev. Neurosci.* **2008**, *9*, 46–56. [CrossRef]
17. Lovelace, M.D.; Varney, B.; Sundaram, G.; Franco, N.F.; Ng, M.L.; Pai, S.; Lim, C.K.; Guillemin, G.J.; Brew, B.J. Current Evidence for a Role of the Kynurenine Pathway of Tryptophan Metabolism in Multiple Sclerosis. *Front. Immunolog.* **2016**, *7*, 246. [CrossRef] [PubMed]
18. Ong, W.Y.; Stohler, C.S.; Herr, D.R. Role of the Prefrontal Cortex in Pain Processing. *Mol. Neurobiol.* **2019**, *56*, 1137–1166. [CrossRef] [PubMed]
19. Trouvin, A.P.; Perrot, S. New concepts of pain. *Best Pract. Res. Clin. Rheumatol.* **2019**, *33*, 101415. [CrossRef] [PubMed]
20. Pinho-Ribeiro, F.A.; Verri, W.A.; Chiu, I.M. Nociceptor Sensory Neuron-Immune Interactions in Pain and Inflammation. *Trends Immunol.* **2017**, *38*, 5–19. [CrossRef] [PubMed]
21. Gonçalves dos Santos, G.; Delay, L.; Yaksh, T.L.; Corr, M. Neuraxial Cytokines in Pain States. *Front Immunol.* **2020**, *10*, 3061. [CrossRef]
22. Ji, R.R.; Chamessian, A.; Zhang, Y.Q. Pain regulation by non-neuronal cells and inflammation. *Science* **2016**, *354*, 572–577. [CrossRef] [PubMed]
23. Matsuda, M.; Huh, Y.; Ji, R.-R. Roles of Inflammation, Neurogenic inflammation, and Neuroinflammation in Pain. *J. Anesth.* **2019**, *33*, 131–139. [CrossRef]
24. Misiak, B.; Frydecka, D.; Stanczykiewicz, B.; Samochowiec, J. Editorial: Peripheral Markers of Immune Response in Major Psychiatric Disorders: Where Are We Now and Where Do We Want to Be? *Front. Psychiatry* **2019**, *10*, 5. [CrossRef]
25. Verlaet, A.A.J.; Maasakkers, C.M.; Hermans, N.; Savelkoul, H.F.J. Rationale for Dietary Antioxidant Treatment of ADHD. *Nutrients* **2018**, *10*, 405. [CrossRef]
26. Fung, T.C.; Olson, C.A.; Hsiao, E.Y. Interactions between the microbiota, immune and nervous systems in health and disease. *Nat. Neurosci.* **2017**, *20*, 145–155. [CrossRef] [PubMed]
27. Encyclopedia. The Tryptophan-Kynurenine Metabolic Pathway. Available online: https://encyclopedia.pub/8633 (accessed on 13 April 2021).
28. Tanaka, M.; Tóth, F.; Polyák, H.; Szabó, Á.; Mándi, Y.; Vécsei, L. Immune Influencers in Action: Metabolites and Enzymes of the Tryptophan-Kynurenine Metabolic Pathway. *Biomedicines* **2021**, *9*, 734. [CrossRef] [PubMed]
29. Tanaka, M.; Bohár, Z.; Vécsei, L. Are Kynurenines Accomplices or Principal Villains in Dementia? Maintenance of Kynurenine Metabolism. *Molecules* **2020**, *25*, 564. [CrossRef] [PubMed]
30. Dezsi, L.; Tuka, B.; Martos, D.; Vecsei, L. Alzheimer's disease, astrocytes and kynurenines. *Curr. Alzheimer Res.* **2015**, *12*, 462–480. [CrossRef]
31. Török, N.; Tanaka, M.; Vécsei, L. Searching for Peripheral Biomarkers in Neurodegenerative Diseases: The Tryptophan-Kynurenine Metabolic Pathway. *Int. J. Mol. Sci.* **2020**, *21*, 9338. [CrossRef] [PubMed]
32. Erabi, H.; Okada, G.; Shibasaki, C.; Setoyama, D.; Kang, D.; Takamura, M.; Yoshino, A.; Fuchikami, M.; Kurata, A.; Kato, T.A.; et al. Kynurenic acid is a potential overlapped biomarker between diagnosis and treatment response for depression from metabolome analysis. *Sci. Rep.* **2020**, *10*, 16822. [CrossRef]
33. Carrillo-Mora, P.; Pérez-De la Cruz, V.; Estrada-Cortés, B.; Toussaint-González, P.; Martínez-Cortéz, J.A.; Rodríguez-Barragán, M.; Quinzaños-Fresnedo, J.; Rangel-Caballero, F.; Gamboa-Coria, G.; Sánchez-Vázquez, I.; et al. Serum Kynurenines Correlate with Depressive Symptoms and Disability in Poststroke Patients: A Cross-sectional Study. *Neurorehabilit. Neural Repair* **2020**, *34*, 936–944. [CrossRef]
34. Tanaka, M.; Török, N.; Vécsei, L. Novel Pharmaceutical Approaches in Dementia. In *NeuroPsychopharmacotherapy*; Riederer, P., Laux, G., Nagatsu, T., Le, W., Riederer, C., Eds.; Springer: Cham, Switzerland, 2021. Available online: https://doi.org/10.1007/978-3-319-56015-1_444-1 (accessed on 1 June 2021).
35. Ulivieri, M.; Wierońska, J.M.; Lionetto, L.; Martinello, K.; Cieslik, P.; Chocyk, A.; Curto, M.; Di Menna, L.; Iacovelli, L.; Traficante, A.; et al. The Trace Kynurenine, Cinnabarinic Acid, Displays Potent Antipsychotic-Like Activity in Mice and Its Levels Are Reduced in the Prefrontal Cortex of Individuals Affected by Schizophrenia. *Schizophr. Bull.* **2020**, *46*, 1471–1481. [CrossRef]
36. Tanaka, M.; Vécsei, L. Monitoring the Redox Status in Multiple Sclerosis. *Biomedicines* **2020**, *8*, 406. [CrossRef] [PubMed]
37. Tanaka, M.; Toldi, J.; Vécsei, L. Exploring the Etiological Links behind Neurodegenerative Diseases: Inflammatory Cytokines and Bioactive Kynurenines. *Int. J. Mol. Sci.* **2020**, *21*, 2431. [CrossRef] [PubMed]

38. Török, N.; Maszlag-Török, R.; Molnár, K.; Szolnoki, Z.; Somogyvári, F.; Boda, K.; Tanaka, M.; Klivényi, P.; Vécsei, L. Single Nucleotide Polymorphisms of Indoleamine 2,3-Dioxygenase 1 Influenced the Age Onset of Parkinson's Disease. *Preprints* **2020**. [CrossRef]
39. Tanaka, M.; Vécsei, L. Monitoring the Kynurenine System in Neurodegenerative and Psychiatric Illnesses: Concentrations, Ratios, or What Else? *Adv. Clin. Exp. Med* **2021**, *30*. in press.
40. Armstrong, S.A.; Herr, M.J. Physiology, Nociception. In *StatPearls*; StatPearls Publishing: Treasure Island, FL, USA, 2020. Available online: https://www.ncbi.nlm.nih.gov/books/NBK551562/ (accessed on 27 December 2020).
41. Tompkins, D.A.; Hobelmann, J.G.; Compton, P. Providing chronic pain management in the "Fifth Vital Sign" Era: Historical and treatment perspectives on a modern-day medical dilemma. *Drug Alcohol Depend.* **2017**, *173* (Suppl. 1), S11–S21. [CrossRef]
42. Fu, K.; Robbins, S.R.; McDougall, J.J. Osteoarthritis: The genesis of pain. *Rheumatology* **2018**, *57* (Suppl. 4), iv43–iv50. [CrossRef]
43. Talagas, M.; Lebonvallet, N.; Berthod, F.; Misery, L. Lifting the veil on the keratinocyte contribution to cutaneous nociception. *Protein Cell* **2020**, *11*, 239–250. [CrossRef] [PubMed]
44. Moore, C.; Cevikbas, F.; Pasolli, H.A.; Chen, Y.; Kong, W.; Kempkes, C.; Parekh, P.; Lee, S.H.; Kontchou, N.A.; Yeh, I.; et al. UVB radiation generates sunburn pain and affects skin by activating epidermal TRPV4 ion channels and triggering endothelin-1 signaling. *Proc. Natl. Acad. Sci. USA* **2013**, *110*, E3225–E3234. [CrossRef]
45. Hwang, S.-M.; Chung, G.; Kim, Y.H.; Park, C.-K. The Role of Maresins in Inflammatory Pain: Function of Macrophages in Wound Regeneration. *Int. J. Mol. Sci.* **2019**, *20*, 5849. [CrossRef]
46. Calvo, M.; Dawes, J.M.; Bennett, D.L. The role of the immune system in the generation of neuropathic pain. *Lancet Neurol.* **2012**, *11*, 629–642. [CrossRef]
47. Dubin, A.E.; Patapoutian, A. Nociceptors: The sensors of the pain pathway. *J. Clin. Investig.* **2010**, *120*, 3760–3772. [CrossRef] [PubMed]
48. Yam, M.F.; Loh, Y.C.; Tan, C.S.; Khadijah Adam, S.; Abdul Manan, N.; Basir, R. General Pathways of Pain Sensation and the Major Neurotransmitters Involved in Pain Regulation. *Int. J. Mol. Sci.* **2018**, *19*, 2164. [CrossRef]
49. Raney, E.B.; Thankam, F.G.; Dilisio, M.F.; Agrawal, D.K. Pain and the pathogenesis of biceps tendinopathy. *Am. J. Transl. Res.* **2017**, *9*, 2668–2683.
50. Barohn, R.J.; Amato, A.A. Pattern-recognition approach to neuropathy and neuronopathy. *Neurol. Clin.* **2013**, *31*, 343–361. [CrossRef] [PubMed]
51. Bourne, S.; Machado, A.G.; Nagel, S.J. Basic anatomy and physiology of pain pathways. *Neurosurg. Clin. N. Am.* **2014**, *25*, 629–638. [CrossRef] [PubMed]
52. Zakin, E.; Abrams, R.; Simpson, D.M. Diabetic Neuropathy. *Semin. Neurol.* **2019**, *39*, 560–569. [CrossRef]
53. Macone, A.; Otis, J.A.D. Neuropathic Pain. *Semin. Neurol.* **2018**, *38*, 644–653.
54. Meacham, K.; Shepherd, A.; Mohapatra, D.P.; Haroutounian, S. Neuropathic Pain: Central vs. Peripheral Mechanisms. *Curr. Pain. Headache Rep.* **2017**, *21*, 28. [CrossRef] [PubMed]
55. Watson, J.C.; Sandroni, P. Central Neuropathic Pain Syndromes. *Mayo Clin. Proc.* **2016**, *91*, 372–385. [CrossRef] [PubMed]
56. Yoon, S.Y.; Oh, J. Neuropathic cancer pain: Prevalence, pathophysiology, and management. *Korean J. Intern. Med.* **2018**, *33*, 1058–1069. [CrossRef]
57. Radat, F.; Margot-Duclot, A.; Attal, N. Psychiatric co-morbidities in patients with chronic peripheral neuropathic pain: A multicentre cohort study. *Eur. J. Pain* **2013**, *17*, 1547–1557. [CrossRef]
58. Obata, H. Analgesic Mechanisms of Antidepressants for Neuropathic Pain. *Int. J. Mol. Sci.* **2017**, *18*, 2483. [CrossRef]
59. Hooten, W.M. Chronic Pain and Mental Health Disorders: Shared Neural Mechanisms, Epidemiology, and Treatment. *Mayo Clin. Proc.* **2016**, *91*, 955–970. [CrossRef]
60. Liu, J.A.; Yu, J.; Cheung, C.W. Immune Actions on the Peripheral Nervous System in Pain. *Int. J. Mol. Sci.* **2021**, *22*, 1448. [CrossRef]
61. Inoue, K.; Tsuda, M. Nociceptive signaling mediated by P2X3, P2X4 and P2X7 receptors. *Biochem. Pharmacol.* **2020**, 114309. [CrossRef]
62. Rempe, R.G.; Hartz, A.; Bauer, B. Matrix metalloproteinases in the brain and blood-brain barrier: Versatile breakers and makers. *J. Cereb. Blood. Flow Metab.* **2016**, *36*, 1481–1507. [CrossRef]
63. Huh, Y.; Ji, R.R.; Chen, G. Neuroinflammation, Bone Marrow Stem Cells, and Chronic Pain. *Front. Immunol.* **2017**, *21*, 1014. [CrossRef]
64. Ji, R.R.; Nackley, A.; Huh, Y.; Terrando, N.; Maixner, W. Neuroinflammation and Central Sensitization in Chronic and Widespread Pain. *Anesthesiology* **2018**, *129*, 343–366. [CrossRef]
65. Chen, G.; Zhang, Y.Q.; Qadri, Y.J.; Serhan, C.N.; Ji, R.R. Microglia in Pain: Detrimental and Protective Roles in Pathogenesis and Resolution of Pain. *Neuron* **2018**, *100*, 1292–1311. [CrossRef]
66. Ji, R.R.; Donnelly, C.R.; Nedergaard, M. Astrocytes in chronic pain and itch. *Nat. Rev. Neurosc.* **2019**, *20*, 667–685. [CrossRef]
67. Jiang, B.C.; Cao, D.L.; Zhang, X.; Zhang, Z.J.; He, L.N.; Li, C.H.; Zhang, W.W.; Wu, X.B.; Berta, T.; Ji, R.R.; et al. CXCL13 drives spinal astrocyte activation and neuropathic pain via CXCR5. *J. Clin. Investig.* **2016**, *126*, 745–761. [CrossRef] [PubMed]
68. Kim, S.K.; Hayashi, H.; Ishikawa, T.; Shibata, K.; Shigetomi, E.; Shinozaki, Y.; Inada, H.; Roh, S.E.; Kim, S.J.; Lee, G.; et al. Cortical astrocytes rewire somatosensory cortical circuits for peripheral neuropathic pain. *J. Clinvinvest.* **2016**, *126*, 1983–1997. [CrossRef] [PubMed]

69. Malta, I.; Moraes, T.; Rodrigues, G.; Franco, P.; Galdino, G. The role of oligodendrocytes in chronic pain: Cellular and molecular mechanisms. *J. Physiol. Pharmacol.* **2019**, *70*. [CrossRef]
70. Popiolek-Barczyk, K.; Mika, J. Targeting the Microglial Signaling Pathways: New Insights in the Modulation of Neuropathic Pain. *Curr. Med. Chem.* **2016**, *23*, 2908–2928. [CrossRef] [PubMed]
71. Kany, S.; Vollrath, J.T.; Relja, B. Cytokines in Inflammatory Disease. *Int. J. Mol. Sci.* **2019**, *20*, 6008. [CrossRef]
72. Starobova, H.; Vetter, I. Pathophysiology of Chemotherapy-Induced Peripheral Neuropathy. *Front. Mol. Neurosci.* **2017**, *10*, 174. [CrossRef] [PubMed]
73. Pineda-Farias, J.B.; Perez-Severiano, F.; Gonzalez-Esquivel, D.F.; Barragan-Iglesias, P.; Bravo-Hernandez, M.; Cervantes-Duran, C.; Aguilera, P.; Ríos, C.; Granados-Soto, V. The L-kynurenine-probenecid combination reduces neuropathic pain in rats. *Eur. J. Pain* **2013**, *17*, 1365–1373. [CrossRef] [PubMed]
74. Laumet, G.; Zhou, W.; Dantzer, R.; Edralin, J.D.; Huo, X.; Budac, D.P.; O'Connor, J.C.; Lee, A.W.; Heijnen, C.J.; Kavelaars, A. Upregulation of neuronal kynurenine 3-monooxygenase mediates depression-like behavior in a mouse model of neuropathic pain. *Brain Behav. Immun.* **2017**, *66*, 94–102. [CrossRef] [PubMed]
75. Rojewska, E.; Ciapała, K.; Piotrowska, A.; Makuch, W.; Mika, J. Pharmacological Inhibition of Indoleamine 2,3-Dioxygenase-2 and Kynurenine 3-Monooxygenase, Enzymes of the Kynurenine Pathway, Significantly Diminishes Neuropathic Pain in a Rat Model. *Front. Pharmacol.* **2018**, *9*, 724. [CrossRef]
76. Rojewska, E.; Piotrowska, A.; Makuch, W.; Przewlocka, B.; Mika, J. Pharmacological kynurenine 3-monooxygenase enzyme inhibition significantly reduces neuropathic pain in a rat model. *Neuropharmacology* **2016**, *102*, 80–91. [CrossRef]
77. Aiyer, R.; Mehta, N.; Gungor, S.; Gulati, A. A Systematic Review of NMDA Receptor Antagonists for Treatment of Neuropathic Pain in Clinical Practice. *Clin. J. Pain* **2018**, *34*, 450–467. [CrossRef]
78. Zheng, H.; Lim, J.Y.; Seong, J.Y.; Hwang, S.W. The Role of Corticotropin-Releasing Hormone at Peripheral Nociceptors: Implications for Pain Modulation. *Biomedicines* **2020**, *8*, 623. [CrossRef]
79. IASP. IASP Terminology. Available online: https://www.iasp-pain.org/Education/Content.aspx?ItemNumber=1698#Nociplasticpain (accessed on 27 December 2020).
80. Aydede, M.; Shriver, A. Recently introduced definition of "nociplastic pain" by the International Association for the Study of Pain needs better formulation. *Pain* **2018**, *159*, 1176–1177. [CrossRef]
81. Meeus, M.; Nijs, J. Central sensitization: A biopsychosocial explanation for chronic widespread pain in patients with fibromyalgia and chronic fatigue syndrome. *Clin. Rheumatol.* **2007**, *26*, 465–473. [CrossRef] [PubMed]
82. Meeus, M.; Nijs, J.; Van de Wauwer, N.; Toeback, L.; Truijen, S. Diffuse noxious inhibitory control is delayed in chronic fatigue syndrome: An experimental study. *Pain* **2008**, *139*, 439–448. [CrossRef] [PubMed]
83. Shin, H.-J.; Na, H.-S.; Do, S.-H. Magnesium and Pain. *Nutrients* **2020**, *12*, 2184. [CrossRef] [PubMed]
84. Seifert, F.; Maihöfner, C. Central mechanisms of experimental and chronic neuropathic pain: Findings from functional imaging studies. *Cell. Mol. Life Sci.* **2009**, *66*, 375. [CrossRef] [PubMed]
85. Schrepf, A.; Williams, D.A.; Gallop, R.; Naliboff, B.D.; Basu, N.; Kaplan, C.; Harper, D.E.; Landis, J.R.; Clemens, J.Q.; Strachan, E.; et al. Sensory sensitivity and symptom severity represent unique dimensions of chronic pain: A MAPP Research Network study. *Pain* **2018**, *159*, 2002–2011. [CrossRef] [PubMed]
86. Journal of Clinical Medicine. Special Issue "New Frontiers in the Diagnosis, Prediction, Prevention, and Management of Fibromyalgia". Available online: https://www.mdpi.com/journal/jcm/special_issues/NF_Fibromyalgia (accessed on 27 December 2020).
87. Rodriguez-Pintó, I.; Agmon-Levin, N.; Howard, A.; Shoenfeld, Y. Fibromyalgia and cytokines. *Immunol. Lett.* **2014**, *161*, 200–203. [CrossRef]
88. Hong, J.I.; Park, I.Y.; Kim, H.A. Understanding the Molecular Mechanisms Underlying the Pathogenesis of Arthritis Pain Using Animal Models. *Int. J. Mol. Sci.* **2020**, *21*, 533. [CrossRef]
89. Barjandi, G.; Louca Jounger, S.; Löfgren, M.; Bileviciute-Ljungar, I.; Kosek, E.; Ernberg, M. Plasma tryptophan and kynurenine in females with temporomandibular disorders and fibromyalgia-An exploratory pilot study. *J. Oral Rehabil.* **2020**, *47*, 150–157. [CrossRef]
90. Bushnell, M.C.; Ceko, M.; Low, L.A. Cognitive and emotional control of pain and its disruption in chronic pain. *Nat. Rev. Neurosci.* **2013**, *14*, 502–511. [CrossRef]
91. Yao, Z.F.; Hsieh, S. Neurocognitive Mechanism of Human Resilience: A Conceptual Framework and Empirical Review. *Int. J. Environ. Res. Public Health* **2019**, *16*, 5123. [CrossRef] [PubMed]
92. Tanaka, M.; Vécsei, L. Editorial of Special Issue "Crosstalk between Depression, Anxiety, and Dementia: Comorbidity in Behavioral Neurology and Neuropsychiatry". *Biomedicines* **2021**, *9*, 517. [CrossRef] [PubMed]
93. Bransfield, R.C.; Friedman, K.J. Differentiating Psychosomatic, Somatopsychic, Multisystem Illnesses, and Medical Uncertainty. *Healthcare* **2019**, *7*, 114. [CrossRef]
94. Defrin, R.; Amanzio, M.; de Tommaso, M.; Dimova, V.; Filipovic, S.; Finn, D.P.; Gimenez-Llort, L.; Invitto, S.; Jensen-Dahm, C.; Lautenbacher, S.; et al. Experimental pain processing in individuals with cognitive impairment: Current state of the science. *Pain* **2015**, *156*, 1396–1408. [CrossRef] [PubMed]
95. Fu, X.; Zhang, F.; Liu, F.; Yan, C.; Guo, W. Editorial: Brain and Somatization Symptoms in Psychiatric Disorders. *Front. Psychiatry* **2019**, *10*, 146. [CrossRef]

96. Jacobsen, H.B.; Stiles, T.C.; Stubhaug, A.; Landrø, N.I.; Hansson, P. Comparing objective cognitive impairments in patients with peripheral neuropathic pain or fibromyalgia. *Sci. Rep.* **2021**, *11*, 673. [CrossRef]
97. Gimenez-Llort, L.; Serrano, A.; Roquer, A.; Moriana, I.; Pajuelos, L.; Monllau, A.; Sanchez, M. Loose Verbal Communication of Pain in the Elderly People with Dementia. *Int. Psychogeriatr.* **2019**, *31*, 31.
98. Howren, M.B.; Lamkin, D.M.; Suls, J. Associations of depression with C-reactive protein, IL-1, and IL-6: A meta-analysis. *Psychosom. Med.* **2009**, *71*, 171–186. [CrossRef]
99. Dowlati, Y.; Herrmann, N.; Swardfager, W.; Liu, H.; Sham, L.; Reim, E.K.; Lanctôt, K.L. A meta-analysis of cytokines in major depression. *Biol. Psychiatry* **2010**, *67*, 446–457. [CrossRef]
100. Liu, Y.; Ho, R.C.; Mak, A. Interleukin (IL)-6, tumour necrosis factor alpha (TNF-α) and soluble interleukin-2 receptors (sIL-2R) are elevated in patients with major depressive disorder: A meta-analysis and meta-regression. *J. Affec. Disord.* **2012**, *139*, 230–239. [CrossRef]
101. Valkanova, V.; Ebmeier, K.P.; Allan, C.L. CRP, IL-6 and depression: A systematic review and meta-analysis of longitudinal studies. *J. Affect. Disord.* **2013**, *150*, 736–744. [CrossRef] [PubMed]
102. Haapakoski, R.; Mathieu, J.; Ebmeier, K.P.; Alenius, H.; Kivimäki, M. Cumulative meta-analysis of interleukins 6 and 1β, tumour necrosis factor α and C-reactive protein in patients with major depressive disorder. *Brain Behav. Immun.* **2015**, *49*, 206–215. [CrossRef] [PubMed]
103. Costello, H.; Gould, R.L.; Abrol, E.; Howard, R. Systematic review and meta-analysis of the association between peripheral inflammatory cytokines and generalized anxiety disorder. *BMJ Open* **2019**, *9*, e027925. [CrossRef]
104. Hou, R.; Garne, M.; Holmes, C.; Osmond, C.; Teeling, J.; Lau, L.; Baldwin, D.S. Peripheral inflammatory cytokines and immune balance in Generalised Anxiety Disorder: Case-controlled study. *Brain Behav. Immun.* **2017**, *62*, 212–218. [CrossRef]
105. Ogawa, S.; Fujii, T.; Koga, N.; Hori, H.; Teraishi, T.; Hattori, K.; Noda, T.; Higuchi, T.; Motohashi, N.; Kunugi, H. Plasma L-tryptophan concentration in major depressive disorder: New data and meta-analysis. *J. Clin. Psychiatry* **2014**, *75*, e906-15. [CrossRef]
106. Ogyu, K.; Kubo, K.; Noda, Y.; Iwata, Y.; Tsugawa, S.; Omura, Y.; Wada, M.; Tarumi, R.; Plitman, E.; Moriguchi, S.; et al. Kynurenine pathway in depression: A systematic review and meta-analysis. *Neurosci. Biobehav. Rev.* **2018**, *90*, 16–25. [CrossRef]
107. Réus, G.; Jansen, K.; Titus, S.; Carvalho, A.F.; Gabbay, V.; Quevedo, J. Kynurenine pathway dysfunction in the pathophysiology and treatment of depression: Evidences from animal and human studies. *J. Psychiatric Res.* **2015**, *68*, 316–328. [CrossRef] [PubMed]
108. Orlikov, A.B.; Prakhye, I.B.; Ryzov, I.V. Kynurenine in blood plasma and DST in patients with endogenous anxiety and endogenous depression. *Biol. Psychiatry* **1994**, *36*, 97–102. [CrossRef]
109. Tanaka, M.; Török, N.; Vécsei, L. Editorial: Are 5-HT1 receptor agonists effective anti-migraine drugs? *Opin. Pharmacother.* **2021**, *12*, 1–5.
110. González-Sanmiguel, J.; Schuh, C.M.A.P.; Muñoz-Montesino, C.; Contreras-Kallens, P.; Aguayo, L.G.; Aguayo, S. Complex Interaction between Resident Microbiota and Misfolded Proteins: Role in Neuroinflammation and Neurodegeneration. *Cells* **2020**, *9*, 2476. [CrossRef]
111. Diez-Iriepa, D.; Chamorro, B.; Talaván, M.; Chioua, M.; Iriepa, I.; Hadjipavlou-Litina, D.; López-Muñoz, F.; Marco-Contelles, J.; Oset-Gasque, M.J. Homo-Tris-Nitrones Derived from α-Phenyl-N-tert-butylnitrone: Synthesis, Neuroprotection and Antioxidant Properties. *Int. J. Mol. Sci.* **2020**, *21*, 7949. [CrossRef] [PubMed]
112. Hunt, C.; Macedo e Cordeiro, T.; Suchting, R.; de Dios, C.; Cuellar Leal, V.A.; Soares, J.C.; Dantzer, R.; Teixeira, A.L.; Selvaraj, S. Effect of immune activation on the kynurenine pathway and depression symptoms—A systematic review and meta-analysis. *Neurosci. Biobeha. Rev.* **2020**, *118*, 514. [CrossRef] [PubMed]
113. Pérez-Pérez, A.; Sánchez-Jiménez, F.; Vilariño-García, T.; Sánchez-Margalet, V. Role of Leptin in Inflammation and Vice Versa. *Int. J Mol. Sci.* **2020**, *21*, 5887. [CrossRef]
114. Jiménez-Jiménez, F.J.; Alonso-Navarro, H.; García-Martín, E.; Agúndez, J.A.G. Anti-Inflammatory Effects of Amantadine and Memantine: Possible Therapeutics for the Treatment of Covid-19? *J. Pers. Med.* **2020**, *10*, 217. [CrossRef] [PubMed]
115. Abdul Aziz, N.U.; Chiroma, S.M.; Mohd Moklas, M.A.; Adenan, M.I.; Ismail, A.; Hidayat Baharuldin, M.T. Antidepressant-Like Properties of Fish Oil on Postpartum Depression-Like Rats Model: Involvement of Serotonergic System. *Brain Sci.* **2020**, *10*, 733. [CrossRef]
116. Zhang, Y.; Li, L.; Zhang, J. Curcumin in antidepressant treatments: An overview of potential mechanisms, pre-clinical/clinical trials and ongoing challenges. *Basic Clin. Pharmacol. Toxicol.* **2020**. [CrossRef]
117. Leonel Javeres, M.N.; Habib, R.; Judith, N.; Iqbal, M.; Nepovimova, E.; Kuca, K.; Batool, S.; Nurulain, S.M. Analysis of PON1 gene polymorphisms (rs662 and rs854560) and inflammatory markers in organophosphate pesticides exposed cohorts from two distinct populations. *Environ. Res.* **2020**, *191*, 110210. [CrossRef]
118. Małgorzata, P.; Paweł, K.; Iwona, M.L.; Brzostek, T.; Andrzej, P. Glutamatergic dysregulation in mood disorders: Opportunities for the discovery of novel drug targets. *Expert Opin. Ther. Targets* **2020**, *24*, 1187–1209. [CrossRef] [PubMed]
119. Koola, M.M. Galantamine-Memantine combination in the treatment of Alzheimer's disease and beyond. *Psychiatry Res.* **2020**, *293*, 113409. [CrossRef]
120. Tanaka, M.; Bohár, Z.; Martos, D.; Telegdy, G.; Vécsei, L. Antidepressant-like effects of kynurenic acid in a modified forced swim test. *Pharmacol. Rep.* **2020**, *72*, 449–455. [CrossRef]
121. Negro, A.; Martelletti, P. Novel synthetic treatment options for migraine. *Expert Opin. Pharmacother.* **2020**, *28*, 1–16.

122. Sokal, P.; Harat, M.; Zieliński, P.; Furtak, J.; Paczkowski, D.; Rusinek, M. Motor cortex stimulation in patients with chronic central pain. *Adv. Clin. Exp. Med.* **2015**, *24*, 289–296. [CrossRef]
123. Harat, A.; Sokal, P.; Zieliński, P.; Harat, M.; Rusicka, T.; Herbowski, L. Assessment of economic effectiveness in treatment of neuropathic pain and refractory angina pectoris using spinal cord stimulation. *Adv. Clin. Exp. Med.* **2012**, *21*, 653–663.
124. Koyama, Y. Endothelin ET_B Receptor-Mediated Astrocytic Activation: Pathological Roles in Brain Disorders. *Int. J. Mol. Sci.* **2021**, *22*, 4333. [CrossRef]
125. Doncheva, N.D.; Vasileva, L.; Saracheva, K.; Dimitrova, D.; Getova, D. Study of antinociceptive effect of ketamine in acute and neuropathic pain models in rats. *Adv. Clin. Exp. Med.* **2019**, *28*, 573–579. [CrossRef]
126. Muchacki, R.; Szkilnik, R.; Malinowska-Borowska, J.; Żelazko, A.; Lewkowicz, Ł.; Nowak, P.G. Impairment in Pain Perception in Adult Rats Lesioned as Neonates with 5.7-Dihydroxytryptamine. *Adv. Clin. Exp. Med.* **2015**, *24*, 419–427. [CrossRef] [PubMed]
127. Cañete, T.; Gimenez-Llort, L. Preserved thermal pain in 3xTg-AD mice with increased sensory-discriminative pain sensitivity in females but affective-emotional dimension in males as early sex-specific AD. *Front. Aging Neurosci.* **2021**, *13*, 323. [CrossRef]
128. Kowalska, K.; Krzywoszański, Ł.; Droś, J.; Pasińska, P.; Wilk, A.; Klimkowicz-Mrowiec, A. Early Depression Independently of Other Neuropsychiatric Conditions, Influences Disability and Mortality after Stroke (Research Study—Part of PROPOLIS Study). *Biomedicines* **2020**, *8*, 509. [CrossRef]
129. Cantón-Habas, V.; Rich-Ruiz, M.; Romero-Saldaña, M.; Carrera-González, M.P. Depression as a Risk Factor for Dementia and Alzheimer's Disease. *Biomedicines* **2020**, *8*, 457. [CrossRef] [PubMed]
130. Park, S.; Bak, A.; Kim, S.; Nam, Y.; Kim, H.; Yoo, D.-H.; Moon, M. Animal-Assisted and Pet-Robot Interventions for Ameliorating Behavioral and Psychological Symptoms of Dementia: A Systematic Review and Meta-Analysis. *Biomedicines* **2020**, *8*, 150. [CrossRef] [PubMed]
131. Davis, K.D.; Moayedi, M. Central mechanisms of pain revealed through functional and structural MRI. *J. Neuroimmune Pharmacol.* **2013**, *8*, 518–534. [CrossRef] [PubMed]
132. Balogh, L.; Tanaka, M.; Török, N.; Vécsei, L.; Taguchi, S. Crosstalk between Existential Phenomenological Psychotherapy and Neurological Sciences in Mood and Anxiety Disorders. *Biomedicines* **2021**, *9*, 340. [CrossRef]
133. Kim, J.; Kim, Y.-K. Crosstalk between Depression and Dementia with Resting-State fMRI Studies and Its Relationship with Cognitive Functioning. *Biomedicines* **2021**, *9*, 82. [CrossRef]
134. Komatsu, H.; Watanabe, E.; Fukuchi, M. Psychiatric Neural Networks and Precision Therapeutics by Machine Learning. *Biomedicines* **2021**, *9*, 403. [CrossRef] [PubMed]
135. Bannister, K.; Kucharczyk, M.; Dickenson, A.H. Hopes for the future of pain control. *Pain Ther.* **2017**, *6*, 117–128. [CrossRef] [PubMed]
136. Kordestani-Moghadam, P.; Assari, S.; Nouriyengejeh, S.; Mohammadipour, F.; Pourabbasi, A. Cognitive impairments and associated structural brain changes in metabolic syndrome and implications of neurocognitive intervention. *J. Obes. Metab. Syndr.* **2021**, *29*, 174–179. [CrossRef] [PubMed]
137. Kordestani-Moghadam, P.; Nasehi, M.; Vaseghi, S.; Khodagholi, F.; Zarrindast, M.R. The role of sleep disturbances in depressive-like behavior with emphasis on α-ketoglutarate dehydrogenase activity in rats. *Physiol. Behav.* **2020**, *224*, 113023. [CrossRef] [PubMed]

biomedicines

MDPI

Article

The Oscillatory Profile Induced by the Anxiogenic Drug FG-7142 in the Amygdala–Hippocampal Network Is Reversed by Infralimbic Deep Brain Stimulation: Relevance for Mood Disorders

Hanna Vila-Merkle [1,†], Alicia González-Martínez [1,†], Rut Campos-Jiménez [1], Joana Martínez-Ricós [1,*], Vicent Teruel-Martí [1], Arantxa Blasco-Serra [2], Ana Lloret [3,4], Pau Celada [5,6,7] and Ana Cervera-Ferri [1,*]

1 Neuronal Circuits Laboratory, Department of Human Anatomy and Embryology, University of Valencia, 46010 Valencia, Spain; hanna.vila@uv.es (H.V.-M.); gonmara3@alumni.uv.es (A.G.-M.); rutcj97@gmail.com (R.C.-J.); vicent.teruel@uv.es (V.T.-M.)
2 GESADA Laboratory, Department of Human Anatomy and Embryology, University of Valencia, 46010 Valencia, Spain; arantxa.blasco@uv.es
3 Department of Physiology, Faculty of Medicine, University of Valencia, 46010 Valencia, Spain; ana.lloret@uv.es
4 Health Research Institute INCLIVA, 46010 Valencia, Spain
5 Department of Neurochemistry and Neuropharmacology, CSIC-Institut d'Investigacions Biomèdiques de Barcelona (IIBB-CSIC), 08036 Barcelona, Spain; pau.celada@iibb.csic.es
6 Institut d'Investigacions Biomèdiques August Pi i Sunyer (IDIBAPS), 08036 Barcelona, Spain
7 Centro de Investigación Biomédica en Red de Salud Mental (CIBERSAM), 08036 Barcelona, Spain
* Correspondence: joana.martinez@uv.es (J.M.-R.); ana.cervera-ferri@uv.es (A.C.-F.)
† H. Vila-Merkle and A. González-Martínez contributed equally to this work.

Citation: Vila-Merkle, H.; González-Martínez, A.; Campos-Jiménez, R.; Martínez-Ricós, J.; Teruel-Martí, V.; Blasco-Serra, A.; Lloret, A.; Celada, P.; Cervera-Ferri, A. The Oscillatory Profile Induced by the Anxiogenic Drug FG-7142 in the Amygdala–Hippocampal Network Is Reversed by Infralimbic Deep Brain Stimulation: Relevance for Mood Disorders. *Biomedicines* **2021**, *9*, 783. https://doi.org/10.3390/biomedicines9070783

Academic Editors: Masaru Tanaka and Nóra Török

Received: 21 May 2021
Accepted: 29 June 2021
Published: 6 July 2021

Abstract: Anxiety and depression exhibit high comorbidity and share the alteration of the amygdala–hippocampal–prefrontal network, playing different roles in the ventral and dorsal hippocampi. Deep brain stimulation of the infralimbic cortex in rodents or the human equivalent—the subgenual cingulate cortex—constitutes a fast antidepressant treatment. The aim of this work was: (1) to describe the oscillatory profile in a rodent model of anxiety, and (2) to deepen the therapeutic basis of infralimbic deep brain stimulation in mood disorders. First, the anxiogenic drug FG-7142 was administered to anaesthetized rats to characterize neural oscillations within the amygdala and the dorsoventral axis of the hippocampus. Next, deep brain stimulation was applied. FG-7142 administration drastically reduced the slow waves, increasing delta, low theta, and beta oscillations in the network. Moreover, FG-7142 altered communication in these bands in selective subnetworks. Deep brain stimulation of the infralimbic cortex reversed most of these FG-7142 effects. Cross-frequency coupling was also inversely modified by FG-7142 and by deep brain stimulation. Our study demonstrates that the hyperactivated amygdala–hippocampal network associated with the anxiogenic drug exhibits an oscillatory fingerprint. The study contributes to comprehending the neurobiological basis of anxiety and the effects of infralimbic deep brain stimulation.

Keywords: oscillations; anxiety; deep brain stimulation; electrophysiology; prefrontal; hippocampus; amygdala

1. Introduction

The present paper analyzes the effects of an anxiogenic drug, *N*-methyl-β-carboline-3-carboxamide (FG-7142), on the oscillatory activity of the prefrontal–amygdala–hippocampal network, which is altered in both anxiety and depression. Furthermore, this study explores whether anxiogenic-induced changes in the network can be reversed by deep brain stimulation (DBS) of the infralimbic cortex (IL-DBS) in urethane-anaesthetized rats. With this preclinical study, we aimed to contribute to the understanding of the neurobiological basis of anxiety, and to assess whether the IL-DBS could modify an aberrant connectivity in this network.

1.1. Depression and Anxiety as Comorbid Disorders

Depression and anxiety are among the most prevalent mental disorders considered "common" mental disorders, and they could be classified as part of an emergent pandemic of mood disorders [1]. According to the World Health Organization's (WHO) Global Health Estimates [2], more than 320 million people worldwide suffer from depression, with a growing global prevalence to 4.4% in 2015. Regarding its prevalence, anxiety is the second most common mental disorder, affecting 264 million people globally (3.6%). Both disorders are among the most significant contributors to non-fatal health loss, measured as years lived with a disability. In addition, mental disorders are stronger predictors of suicidal behavior, which is a leading cause of death worldwide, causing almost 800,000 deaths every year. While major depressive disorder is the strongest predictor of suicidal ideation, comorbidity with anxiety increases the possibility of suicide plans or attempts [3,4].

According to the Diagnostic and Statistical Manual of the American Psychiatric Association (DSM-V), major depressive disorder (MDD) is a syndrome that includes episodes of persistent negative mood or anhedonia, together with additional emotional, psychological, and somatic symptoms [5]. To be considered MDD, these symptoms must persist for at least two weeks and not be secondary to any substance, medical condition, or other psychiatric disorder; nor can the symptoms be better explained by normal grief. On the other hand, clinical anxiety involves a maladaptative "marked, persistent, and excessive or unreasonable fear", which significantly interferes with everyday life.

Anxiety and depression are often comorbid and, when they occur together, the pathology presents a diminished clinical outcome and quality of life [6]. Indeed, according to epidemiological data of The Netherlands Study of Depression and Anxiety [7], 67% of individuals suffering from depressive disorder had a current anxiety disorder and 75% had a lifetime comorbid anxiety disorder. On the other hand, 63% of patients with a current anxiety disorder had a simultaneous depressive disorder, and 81% had a lifetime depressive disorder. Usually, anxiety symptoms precede depression. Additionally, patients presenting comorbidity of both pathologies present higher symptom severity, which is the prognosis for comorbid anxiety and depression that is worse than either condition alone. Thus, there is an alternative proposal for a continuum model for anxiety syndromes including mild, moderate, and severe/psychotic depression [1,8].

A significant problem is finding fast-acting treatments that reverse aberrant neural activity. Despite the high incidence and relevance of depression, to date, antidepressant therapies are not helpful for all patients, and one-third of people suffering MDD are not responders [9]. The failure of usual antidepressant treatments may be due to a lack of understanding of the precise neurobiological basis of MDD and the constellations of symptoms included in the syndrome [10]. According to Holtzheimer and Mayberg, the goal of antidepressant therapy should be to maintain normal mood regulation over time instead of an acute resolution of the symptoms.

1.2. Prefrontal Deep Brain Stimulation in the Treatment of Depression

However, DBS in different targets has generated promising results in various mental disorders. Its success resides in manipulating the precise malfunctioning circuits in a broad range of disorders, including psychiatric conditions [11,12]. Thus, it is a different therapeutic approach and a powerful tool to study altered brain networks. Nevertheless, the underlying mechanisms require further research.

In depression, DBS has proven to induce immediate positive subjective experiences in patients [13], with sustained effects on mood, anxiety, sleep, and somatic symptoms after months of stimulation [13–16]. Additionally, following DBS, a reduction in anxiety in seconds to minutes, followed by mood changes in timing from hours to days, has been reported [17,18]. Since 2005, different targets have been used in clinical studies for treatment-resistant depression, with electrodes targeting regions altered in the pathology, such as the subcallosal or subgenual anterior cingulate cortex (sACC), the equivalent Brodmann area 25/24 [13,15,19,20], ventral striatum [19,20], and medial forebrain bundle [21].

Regional cerebral blood flow in sACC increases in depression [22] and anticipatory anxiety [23], and is related to negative affect in healthy subjects [24]. Based on this hyperactivity in negative affect, Mayberg and colleagues targeted sACC for DBS for the first time in MDD patients [13]. In this seminal work, the patients showed acute and short-term beneficial effects of the DBS, time-locked with the stimulation and without effects elicited by sham stimulation. Together with the antidepressant response, the regional cerebral blood flow in the sACC decreased. Puigdemont et al. also reported an early response, with a high response and remission rate at 1 week and lasting effects, with a remission rate of 50% after 1 year of treatment [25]. According to the meta-analysis conducted by Zhou et al., sACC DBS significantly alleviates depressive symptoms [26]. Khairuddin and colleagues [27] wrote a recent review of subcallosal DBS for treating depression that reported long-lasting maintenance of an antidepressant response, reducing the occurrence of recurrent depressive episodes; this treatment was usually well tolerated. From 39 clinical studies, they found that response rate increased with treatment duration from 63.8% at $\leq$6 months to 76% at $\geq$24 months, and a remission rate ranging from 36.5% to 62.5%. Recently, an 8-year follow-up study from Mayberg's group with 28 patients reported response and remission rates of 50% and 30%, respectively. However, there is not a conclusive consensus regarding whether DBS for depression, and likely for anxiety, is effective, since a multisite, randomized, sham-controlled trial also detected positive effects in sham-operated patients [28]. The authors suggested that these controversial effects could be due to a placebo effect, clinical features of the patient population, or suboptimal electrode placement. Nevertheless, systematic reviews and meta-analyses following standard protocols [29], such as PRISMA (Preferred Reporting Items for Systematic Reviews and Meta-analyses), on DBS effects are needed to confirm its efficacy and optimize this surgical intervention. Additionally, further clinical and preclinical studies are needed to gain a better understanding of DBS mechanisms.

Given the involvement of the prefrontal cortex in psychiatric disorders, analyzing its activity in animal models is of interest. However, the homology between human and rodent prefrontal cortex [30], or even the existence of prefrontal cortex in non-primate mammals [31,32], is controversial. The divergence primarily refers to the absence of a granular layer and the lack of exact rodent correlation to the dorsolateral prefrontal cortex. However, comparing cortical areas of distant species based on cytoarchitectonic criteria has been questioned [31], and there is evidence of a rodent behavioral and connectional homology of the medial prefrontal cortex (mPFC) [30]. The rat mPFC can be subdivided into a dorsal and a ventral component based on several anatomical and functional criteria. The latter includes the ventral prelimbic, infralimbic (IL), and medial orbital areas [33].

A recent study compared rat, marmoset, and human brain functional connectivity in the resting-state by functional magnetic resonance imaging (fMRI). The authors found that area 25 was most similar in all three species, unlike other medial prefrontal regions, which showed a higher divergence between rats and primates [34]. Indeed, they found robust functional connectivity between area 25 and amygdala in rats and primates, which is relevant for its involvement in mood disorders. In the rodent brain, area 25 corresponds to the IL region of the mPFC [34–36] Tracing studies also report similar connectivity between the IL and the sACC, with the most robust connections found for the hypothalamus, nucleus accumbens, the fornix, and the medial temporal lobe, including the amygdala, insula, and anterior hippocampus in human, or the ventral hippocampus [35,36], which is the equivalent in a rodent brain [37]. Moreover, the IL region is susceptible to stressful or anxiogenic stimuli, and its lesioning induces anxiolytic responses in the elevated plus-maze test [34] and decreases plasma corticosterone levels in response to acute restraint [38].

Additionally, in rats, IL-DBS has fast antidepressant-like and anxiolytic-like effects [39–41]: the use of 1 h of IL-DBS reduces immobility time and increases climbing behavior in the forced swimming test; it also reduces the latency in feeding in the novelty-suppressed feeding test. Neurochemically, IL-DBS delivered for one hour increases the release of glutamate, serotonin, dopamine, and noradrenaline in the mPFC [40,41]. Although DBS's neurochemical and behavioral effects have been examined, less attention has been paid to the influence of DBS on the network dynamics between different brain areas. To date, no previous study has investigated the effects of IL-DBS in a pharmacological model of anxiety. Thus, research on neural systems involved in anxiety and depression could improve our understanding of mood disorders' neurobiology and help design better targets for intervention.

1.3. The Amygdala–Hippocampal–Prefrontal Network in Depression and Anxiety

Mood disorders present an alteration in the amygdala–hippocampal–prefrontal network. Within the control network of emotional processing, the mPFC plays a key role. Dysfunction of this circuitry is one of the hallmarks of depression and anxiety [42].

In humans, imaging studies have displayed a decreased hippocampal volume in clinical anxiety [43] and depression [44,45], as well as in hippocampal microstructure abnormalities in comorbid anxiety and depression, which are associated with exacerbated threat processing [46]. Rodent studies have also evidenced alterations in the hippocampus in clinical anxiety [47], with a stronger association with anxiety than depression-like behavior [48]. In addition, hypersecretion of glucocorticoids involved in the acute and chronic stress response induces alterations in neuroplasticity in the hippocampus, leading to atrophy and neuronal loss in depression [49,50]. However, the involvement of the hippocampus in mood disorders is not fully understood.

The hippocampus is anatomically, neurochemically, and functionally subdivided along the septotemporal axis into dorsal, intermediate, and ventral regions [51–54]. While the dorsal hippocampus (dHPC) is mainly related to cortical regions and involved in cognitive processing, the ventral hippocampus (vHPC) has reciprocal projections to the amygdala and hypothalamus, and processes emotional and stress-related behaviors. However, Strange and colleagues suggested a gradient of functional hippocampal domains instead of precise distributed functions [37]. In addition, the neurochemical organization of the hippocampal formation evidences a high density of adrenergic receptors in the ventral region [54], which is relevant in stress response and depression and their links with decreased neurogenesis.

On the other hand, the amygdala is pivotal in normal emotional processing [55,56] and changes in its activity are related to anxiety and depression. In rodents, chronic stress induces hyperexcitability [57] and maladaptive stress leading to anxiety induces plastic changes in the amygdala [58,59]. An over-reactive amygdala has also been evidenced both in anxiety-prone humans [60] and in depressed patients by imaging studies [61]. Antidepressants can reverse this altered activity, as can gene expression [62–64]. Finally, lesion studies highlight that the amygdala plays a significant role not only in the establishment of depression-like behaviors but also in hippocampal atrophy [65]. Under normal conditions, the stress response of the amygdala is under control of the ventromedial prefrontal cortex, while the disruption of the prefrontal control is found in mental illnesses [66].

In a previous study, we demonstrated that IL-DBS improves communication and functional connectivity in the amygdala–hippocampal network in normal anaesthetized rats [67]. However, its effect on anxious animals has not yet been analyzed. Modelling psychiatric disorders is not a straightforward question and a spectrum of experimental models of anxiety is available; however, these models' validity has faced criticism [68,69]. In the present paper, we have chosen a proven anxiogenic drug to study the amygdala–hippocampal network and its modulation by IL-DBS.

1.4. FG-7142 as an Anxiogenic Drug

β-carbolines are stress-sensitive compounds present in the rat brain that are excreted in urine and act as benzodiazepine inhibitors [70]. The β-carboline FG-7142 acts as a partial inverse agonist at the benzodiazepine allosteric site of the GABAA receptor, with the highest affinity for the α1-subunit [71].

There is a growing body of evidence that this drug elicits anxious behaviors, both in freely moving rodents [72–74] and in humans [71], as well as activating neural networks underlying the anxious response [75]. Studies over the past five decades have provided information about the anxiogenic-like effects of FG-7142 in a variety of species, including mice, rats, cats, monkeys, and humans. Experimental testing in humans reported severe anxiogenic and panic-like responses following administration of β-carboline, which has been the reason for stopping human research with the drug [76,77]. Given the large body of literature reports on the behavioral effects of FG-7142 as a pharmacological model of anxiety, our study was conducted under anesthesia to exclude other confounding factors, i.e., motor activity. However, we are aware that the lack of behavioral correlates and the anesthesia itself could be considered limitations, as we will discuss further.

Evans and Lowry performed a detailed compilation of FG-7142 effects in many experimental paradigms [71]. In rats, FG-7142 induces an increase of nonambulatory motor activity, which is related to increased arousal and vigilance [78]. Additionally, its administration exerts a proconflicting action, enhances shock-induced drinking suppression [79], reduces exploratory behavior in both mice and rats [80,81], enhances behavioral suppression in response to safety signal withdrawal [82], and impairs fear extinction [83]. In the elevated plus-maze, many rodent studies found that FG-7142 reduces the exploration time spent in the open arms and increases the time spent in the closed arms [71]. Several authors have also described a reduction in social interaction in rodents [84,85].

In accordance with its behavioral effects, FG-7142 increases corticosterone in the plasma levels of rats [86,87]. Additionally, there are reports, both in monkey and in cats, of FG-7142 actions on behavioral agitation and autonomic responses, including increases in heart rate and blood pressure and rises in plasma cortisol, corticosterone, and catecholamines [88,89]. In cats, FG-7142 also generates a state of elevated arousal and fearfulness [90]. In rats and mice, at similar doses, the drug increases c-fos expression in a widespread network involved in stress, anxiety, and fear-related behavioral and autonomic responses. This network includes forebrain structures such as the amygdala, ventral hippocampus, bed nucleus of the stria terminalis, cingulate, prelimbic and IL cortices, and brainstem nuclei of the reticular ascending arousal system, including locus coeruleus, periaqueductal grey, nucleus incertus, and dorsal raphe nucleus [74,75,78,91–93]. In addition, noradrenergic neurons in the locus coeruleus and serotonergic neurons in the dorsal raphe nucleus [74] are activated by FG-7142.

1.5. Brain Oscillations as a Measure of Network Dynamics

Network dynamics and information coding are reflected in brain oscillations [94]. These neural signals reflect the activity of distributed populations of neurons and can be recorded by means of surface electrodes aimed at the skull (electroencephalogram, EEG signals) or at the brain surface (electrocorticogram), or as local field potentials (LFPs) using intracranial electrodes inserted directly in the recorded area. LFPs emerge as the result of the interaction of local electrical activity (i.e., neuronal discharges) with postsynaptic potentials generated by the inputs from interconnected brain areas. Given their biophysical properties, there is an inverse relationship between the frequency of the oscillations and the extent of the network involved: while fast oscillations are influenced more by local neuronal activity, lower frequencies allow for communication among more distant areas [95]. Additionally, an increase in synchronization is usually assumed to reflect an increase in communication in the network [96]. Therefore, measuring oscillatory changes and isolating the relevant signals are useful for inferring the function of neural networks in normal conditions and mental disorders [97,98].

In this paper, we first analyze the oscillatory activity of the amygdala–hippocampal network in anaesthetized rats in basal conditions and after FG-7142 administration. LFPs were recorded in the dorsal, intermediate, and ventral subregions of the hippocampus and the basolateral amygdala. Next, we applied IL-DBS on the same animals to deepen the knowledge of the mechanisms of this therapeutic approach, focusing on its effects on the modulation of the amygdala–hippocampal network.

In brief, our work showed that the anxiogenic drug FG-7142 induces a characteristic oscillatory profile in the amygdala–hippocampal circuit. Furthermore, 1 h of IL-DBS reverses most of the altered oscillations induced by FG-7142. Thus, the study suggests possible anxiety-related biomarkers and helps us understand the effects of IL-DBS on mood disorders.

2. Materials and Methods

2.1. Animal Model and Surgical Procedures

To minimize the number of animals used and their suffering, behavioral experiments to evidence the anxious state were not replicated. However, we used FG-7142 doses, which have been extensively evidenced in the bibliography to induce anxious responses in rats [71], as well as an IL-DBS protocol that has already proved to have antidepressant and anxiolytic-like effects [40]. A total number of 24 male Wistar rats (250–350 g; Charles River Company, Barcelona, Spain) were used. Animals were housed in the Central Research Unit at the University of Valencia (Spain) under a 12 h/12 h light–dark cycle and a controlled temperature of 22 ± 2 °C and humidity (55 ± 10%). Food and water were available ad libitum. All the experimental protocols were followed according to the Animal Care Guidelines of the European Communities Council Directive (2010/63/E.U.) and approved by the Ethics Committee of the University of Valencia before performing the experiments.

Rats were anaesthetized with an intraperitoneal injection of 1.5 g/kg of urethane (Sigma-Aldrich/Merk, Barcelona, Spain) with supplemental doses to maintain the anesthetic level, complemented by local anesthesia with lidocaine sc (1 mL, 5%), blocking the zygomatic and ophthalmic nerves, and fibers. After the loss of corneal reflex and paw withdrawal, animals were placed inside a stereotaxic frame. Trephine holes were drilled in the skull and 100 μm-diameter cylindric, custom-made Teflon-coated stainless steel recording electrodes (AM Systems, Sequim, WA, USA) were placed, according to the stereotactic coordinates from Bregma [99]; these were always placed ipsilaterally in the left hemisphere at the dHPC (AP −3.4 mm; L 2.5 mm; DV 2.4 mm), intermediate hippocampus (iHPC) (AP −5.8 mm; L 5.8 mm; DV 5 mm), and vHPC (AP −4.7 mm; L 5 mm; DV 8.7 mm and basolateral amygdala (BLA) (AP −2.3 mm; L 5 mm; DV 8.5 mm). A stainless-steel screw (Plastics One, Roanoke, VA, USA) was implanted in the occipital bone as a reference, and was fixed with dental acrylic. For DBS, we used in-house custom-made bipolar twisted electrodes made of 100 μm-diameter Teflon-coated stainless steel wire, with 1 mm between both tips. Stimulating electrodes were bilaterally implanted into the IL region of the mPFC (AP +3.2 mm; L 0.5 mm; DV 5.4 mm). A correction factor was applied to the coordinates to increase accuracy, based on the ratio between the experimental and the theoretical distance from bregma to interaural references (experimental distance/9 mm). Additionally, different penetration angles were used to reach the desired coordinates (details in Supplementary Table S1). Recorded and stimulated regions are illustrated in Figure 1A,B. Body temperature was maintained throughout the operation with an isothermal pad at 37 °C.

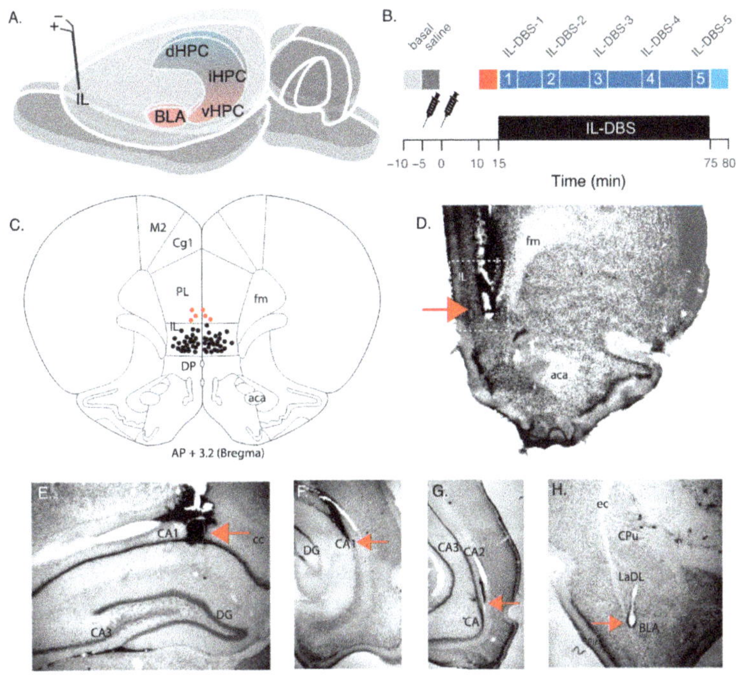

Figure 1. (**A**) Experimental setup. Top: recording and stimulating regions. Bottom: recording protocol with periods selected for statistical analysis. (**B**) Schematic diagram showing DBS electrode tip positions. Red dots indicate the electrode tips in the excluded exemplars. All stimuli were delivered bilaterally. (**C**) Histological sample showing the electrode track and tip in IL. (**D**) Electrode track and tip (red arrow) in dHPC. (**E**) Electrode track and tip (red arrow) in iHPC. (**F**) Electrode track and tip (red arrow) in vHPC. (**G**) Electrode track and tip (red arrow) in BLA. (**H**) Electrode track and tip (red arrow) in IL. aca: anterior commissure; BLA: basolateral amygdala; CA1, CA2, CA3: Cornu Ammonis fields; cc: corpus callosum; CPu: caudate putamen nucleus; DG: dentate gyrus; dHPC: dorsal hippocampus; fm: forceps minor; iHPC: intermediate hippocampus; IL: infralimbic cortex; LaDL: lateral amygdaloid nucleus, dorsolateral part; vHPC: ventral hippocampus.

2.2. Drug Administration

As a control, before the administration of the anxiogenic drug, the animals were injected with 2 mL/kg saline solution ip FG-7142 (Sigma-Aldrich, St. Louis, MO, USA), which was administered ip at a single dose of 7.5 mg/kg diluted in 12.5 mL of β-cyclodextrin and 1 M chlorohydric acid (HCl), pH 5.0, to a final volume of 2 mL/kg [74].

Under urethane, FG-7142 induces the release of acetylcholine in the vHPC [100], an effect that was recently found under chronic restraint stress, which is a model of anxiety [101].

2.3. Recording and Stimulation Procedure

One hour after surgery, recording began. The experimental procedure (Figure 1B) involved a continuous recording under anesthesia in the following conditions: (1) 300 s as baseline (henceforth, "basal" epoch); (2) 300 s following the administration of saline solution ("saline" epoch); (3) administration of the anxiogenic drug and, subsequently, recording for 15 min ("FG-7142" epoch); (4) 1 h of IL-DBS (bipolar stimulation at 130 Hz, 100 μA, and 80 μs) ("DBS" epoch); (5) 300 s in IL-DBS-off mode ("post-DBS" epoch). An additional group (6 animals with implanted electrodes) only received saline and FG-7142 but were in DBS-off mode during all the recording to visualize the evolution of the response to the drug and the intervention alone (Figure 2).

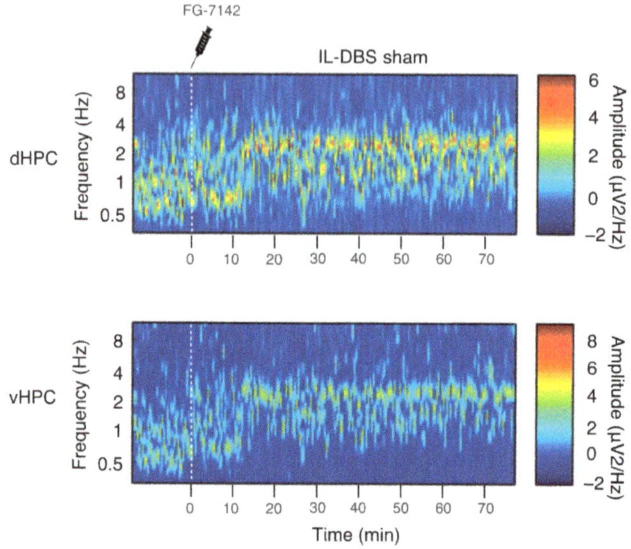

Figure 2. Profile of FG-7142 persistent effects in an IL-DBS sham-operated rat with electrodes inserted but in DBS-off mode during all of the experiments. Observe that spontaneous reversal was not apparent during the recorded time course.

LFPs were preamplified (model p511 AC Grass Preamplifier) and amplified (MPLI 4G21; Cibertec, Madrid, Spain), band-pass filtered (0.3–300 Hz), acquired, and digitized at 1 kHz (CED Micro; Cambridge Electronics Design, Cambridge, UK). Further details are reported elsewhere [67].

2.4. Histological Analysis

After the experiments, animals were deeply anesthetized with an overdose of sodium pentobarbital (100 mg/kg, 20%; Dolethal, Vetoquinol, Madrid, Spain) and transcardially perfused with 500 mL of 0.1% heparinized saline (0.9%, pH 7), followed by 500 mL of 4% paraformaldehyde (Sigma-Aldrich, St. Louis, MO, USA). Brains were removed and maintained in 30% sucrose for cryopreservation. Coronal sections of 40 μm were obtained by a freezing microtome (Leica, Madrid, Spain), collected in the same solution, and stored for processing. Sections were then stained by the Giemsa technique to subsequently verify the placement of electrodes and the injection site (Figure 1C–G). Following verification, three animals with misplaced electrodes were excluded from the study.

2.5. Data Analysis

All the analyses were performed offline with MATLAB software (The MathWorks, Natick, MA, USA; RRID:SCR_001622), using self-developed and built-in routines. First, LFPs were downsampled to 500 Hz, digitally notch-filtered with a Butterworth bandstop filter of around 50 Hz and harmonics until 200 Hz, and z-score normalized.

2.5.1. Spectral Analysis

The recordings were analyzed based on the Fast Fourier Transform. Power spectral density was calculated by the Welch method, with a 5 s pwelch window with 50% overlap and nfft 1024, implemented with the Signal Processing MATLAB Toolbox. The analyzed bands were slow oscillations (SW < 1.5 Hz), delta (1.5–2.5 Hz), low theta (2.5–5 Hz), high theta (5–12 Hz), beta (16–30 Hz), low gamma (30–60 Hz), mid gamma (60–90 Hz), and high gamma (90–120 Hz). Spectral power and relative power were calculated for each band in consecutive 60 s windows to visualize the temporal evolution of each band. Relative power was calculated as band power/power in the 0–250 Hz.

2.5.2. Wavelet Analysis

We used a continuous wavelet transform to improve the analysis on the time-frequency domain [102]. In addition, spectrograms and wavelet-based filters allowed us to better visualize the temporal evolution of the oscillations.

Given that theta oscillations play a relevant role in hippocampal processing and within limbic structures, we analyzed this oscillation in further detail by detecting epochs with predominant low theta activity ("theta segments"). We defined theta segments as 2.5–5 Hz continuous oscillations constituting at least 30% of the total oscillatory activity for each time point and calculated in consecutive 60 s windows. The analysis of theta segments allowed the quantification of the temporal ratio (proportion of time with predominant theta segments/s), the mean duration, and the number of segments for each window.

We also used the wavelet coefficient matrix to obtain coherograms for visualizing the coupling between channels. Phase-locking values (PLV) were defined as a measure of the stationarity of the phase differences in 10 s temporal windows and, therefore, of the phase-depending synchrony. The index used here was the weighted phase lag index (WPLI), in which the contribution of the observed phase leads and lags is weighted by the magnitude of the imaginary component of the cross-spectrum. This index increases the specificity by reducing the contribution of noise sources or volume conduction and the statistical power to detect changes in phase synchronization [103].

2.5.3. Cross-Frequency Coupling

Amplitude–amplitude coupling was computed in RStudio (RRID:SCR_000432) as the Pearson linear correlation between the spectral power in two bands for the same channel.

Phase–amplitude coupling (PAC) was measured in MATLAB through the modulation index (MI), as defined by Tort and colleagues [104] and described before [67]. The MI assumed normalized values between 0 and 1 and was considered statistically significant when its value was >2 SD of the substitute mean MI, constructed by 200 random permutations of the amplitude distribution.

2.6. Statistical Analysis

The statistical analyses and data visualization were performed with RStudio. Recording periods (see Figure 1A) were grouped into the following: "basal" (first 300 s of the recording), "saline" (300 s before FG-7142 administration), "FG-7142" (300 s before the IL-DBS), five different periods during DBS treatment (DBS1, DBS2, DBS3, DBS4, DBS5), and "post-DBS" (300 s following the end of the IL-DBS). In each period, we analyzed a total time of 300 s composed of 5 consecutive 60 s windows.

Given that the sample size was less than 30 and normal distribution could not be assumed, nonparametric tests were used. First, the variables were compared by Friedman's chi-squared test with post hoc comparisons, with the Conover test for the pair-wise comparisons with the Bonferroni adjust method. A significance level of p-value < 0.05 was considered to determine the existence of statistically significant differences. For the Pearson linear correlation, significance levels were also obtained by the Ggally_cor and Ggpairs packages.

3. Results

3.1. Spectral Analysis and Peak Frequency

Urethane anesthesia was predominantly characterized by low-voltage oscillations below 2 Hz in the SW, and delta range, together with spontaneous short-lasting scattered faster waves. FG-7142 induced a long-lasting characteristic state, with a general switch to faster frequencies easily recognizable in all the recorded regions, and that lasted up to 2 h in sham-operate IL-DBS (Figure 2). The plateau period was typically observed between 10 and 15 min following administration. Details of a representative case with FG-7142 administration followed by IL-DBS are shown in Figure 3A.

FG-7142 induced a marked and significant reduction in SW below 1.5 Hz in all regions, changing their oscillatory pattern to a regular oscillation with a robust peak frequency shifting to 3–3.5 Hz in the low theta range. IL-DBS progressively reversed the effect, reducing the peak frequency and returning to basal values approximately 45 min later. The effects of IL-DBS on peak frequency lasted in the post-stimulation period (Figure 3B,C). Statistical results are summarized in Table 1.

Table 1. Peak frequency computed by spectral decomposition.

Period	dHPC	iHPC	vHPC	BLA
Basal	1.063 ± 0.039	1.084 ± 0.042	0.979 ± 0.051	1.105 ± 0.045
Saline	1.042 ± 0.046	1.041 ± 0.063	1.048 ± 0.069	1.084 ± 0.042
FG-7142	**3.355 ± 0.128** ***	**3.574 ± 0.100** ***	**3.629 ± 0.244** ***	**3.202 ± 0.083** ***
DBS1	**3.047 ± 0.087** ***	**3.356 ± 0.056** ***	**3.330 ± 0.087** ***	**3.526 ± 0.061** ***
DBS2	**2.380 ± 0.098** ***	**2.292 ± 0.081** ***	**1.705 ± 0.085** ***	**1.653 ± 0.109** ***
DBS3	**1.251 ± 0.051** ***	**1.421 ± 0.101** ***	**1.426 ± 0.061** ***	**1.359 ± 0.101** **
DBS4	1.147 ± 0.058	1.230 ± 0.051	**1.253 ± 0.098** **	**1.398 ± 0.046** ***
DBS5	1.083 ± 0.060	1.147 ± 0.049	1.048 ± 0.070	1.147 ± 0.058
POST-DBS	1.063 ± 0.049	1.020 ± 0.060	1.048 ± 0.069	1.063 ± 0.049

Note: mean ± se (bold: statistical significance in pairwise comparisons to basal period; *** $p < 0.001$, ** $p < 0.01$).

3.2. Relative Power of Slow Waves, Delta and Theta Band

Figure 4 and Supplementary Table S2 summarize the statistical results of a Fourier analysis of the relative power for SW, delta, and theta bands. As mentioned previously, SW drastically diminished following the administration of FG-7142 in all regions. Interestingly, both sustained activity in the 1.5–2.5 Hz range (delta), and 16–30 Hz (beta) appeared in the BLA, vHPC, and iHPC, without any changes in the dHPC. The 2.5–5 Hz band (low theta) significantly increased in the dHPC, iHPC, and BLA, with a trend in vHPC. Again, 5–12 Hz (fast theta oscillations) only appeared in the dHPC after FG-7142.

It is relevant to note that the increase observed in the relative power in most bands during the anxiety-like period was mainly due to the disappearance of the SW Delta oscillations, which also reduced their amplitude in this state; theta only increased its amplitude in the vHPC and iHPC, although its relative power was increased by the lack of SW.

Essentially, in all cases, IL-DBS reversed the effect of FG-7142 administration over these oscillations in a time-dependent manner, returning to basal values during the stimulation and lasting in the post-stimulation period.

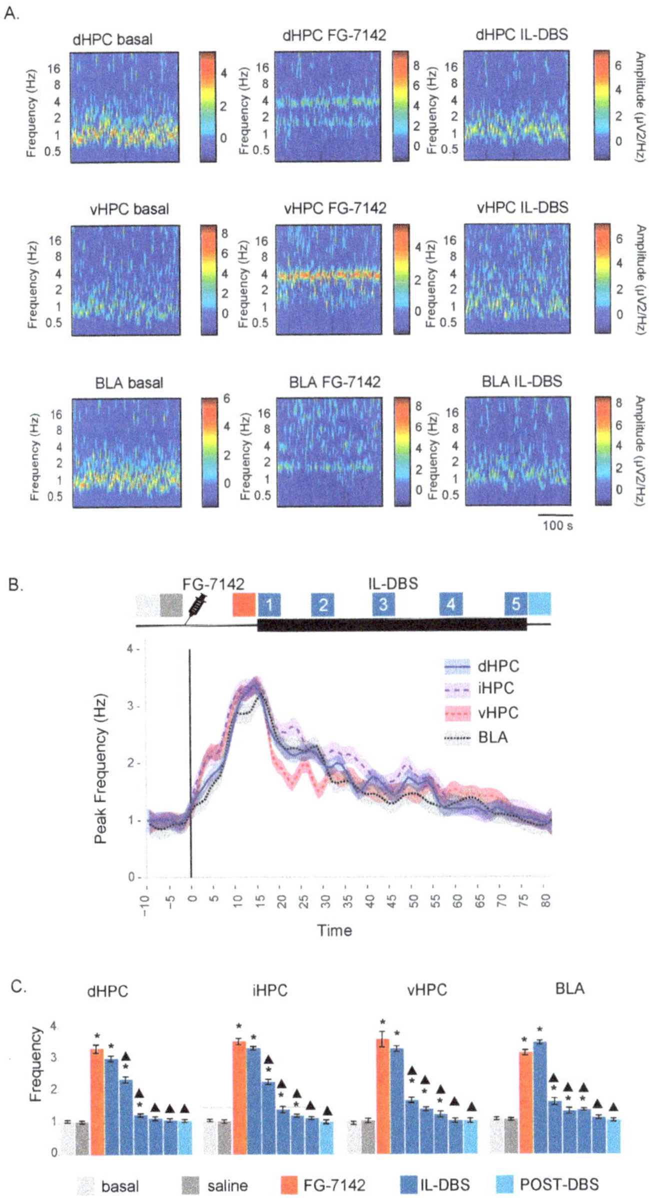

Figure 3. (**A**) Representative wavelet spectrograms in the dHPC, vHPC and BLA in basal conditions and after FG-7142 and IL_DBS interventions. Observe the increase in frequency induced by FG-7142 and the reversal of the oscillatory profile to slow waves by IL-DBS. (**B**) Time-course evolution of the peak frequency calculated by spectral decomposition. FG-7142 increases peak frequency to a similar value at 3–4 Hz in the low theta range, which is slightly lower in BLA. IL-DBS induces a progressive return to around 1 Hz, which is similar to basal values. (**C**) Statistical results of peak frequency in the 300 s periods indicated by color code in (**B**). * Statistical significance in pairwise comparisons with the basal period. Triangle: statistical significance in pairwise comparisons between IL-DBS and post-DBS with the FG-7142 period (degree of significance not indicated in order to better visualize results; please see Table 1). dHPC: dorsal hippocampus; iHPC: intermediate hippocampus; vHPC: ventral hippocampus; BLA: basolateral amygdala; IL: infralimbic cortex.

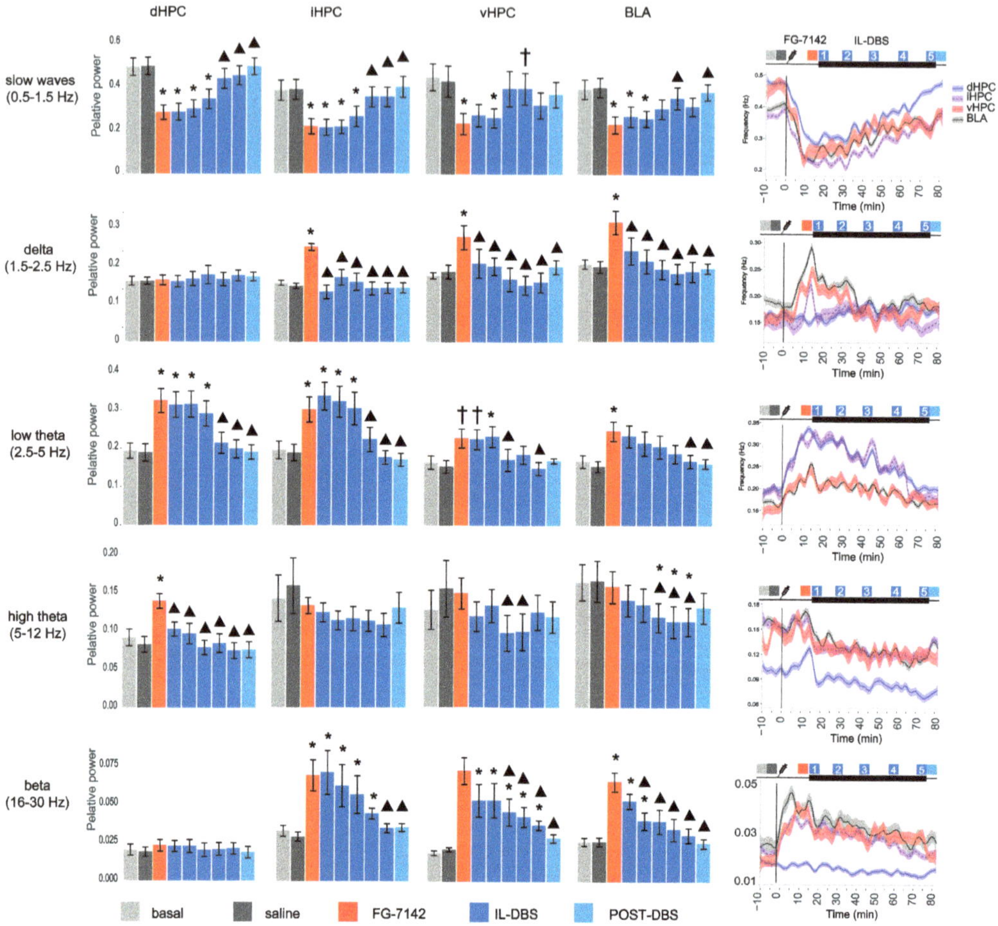

Figure 4. Statistical results of relative power of slow waves, delta, theta, and beta, calculated by spectral decomposition. * Statistical significance in pairwise comparisons with the basal period. Triangle: statistical significance in pairwise comparisons between IL-DBS and post-DBS with the FG-7142 period. Cross: statistical trend. Degree of significance not indicated to better visualize results; please see Supplementary Table S2. dHPC: dorsal hippocampus; iHPC: intermediate hippocampus; vHPC: ventral hippocampus; BLA: basolateral amygdala; IL: infralimbic cortex.

3.3. Theta Segments

Theta activity is key for information processing within the hippocampus and other limbic structures [67], and it has even been proposed as a possible anxiety biomarker [105,106]. Thus, to better characterize the effects on the theta band, we further analyzed wavelet theta segments (Figure 5 and Supplementary Table S3). FG-7142 not only showed an increase in theta oscillation amplitudes but also their persistence over time (Figure 5A,B). The theta temporal ratio experienced a net increase in all hippocampal regions but to a lesser extent in BLA, where shorter segments were found (Figure 5B,C). IL-DBS decreased both the theta temporal ratio and mean duration (Figure 5B,C). As the IL-DBS advanced, a more fractionated theta could be appreciated (more segments of shorter duration), suggesting the discontinuation of theta activity. Finally, IL-DBS reduced both the number of segments and their duration, resulting in a progressive return to basal values of the temporal ratio.

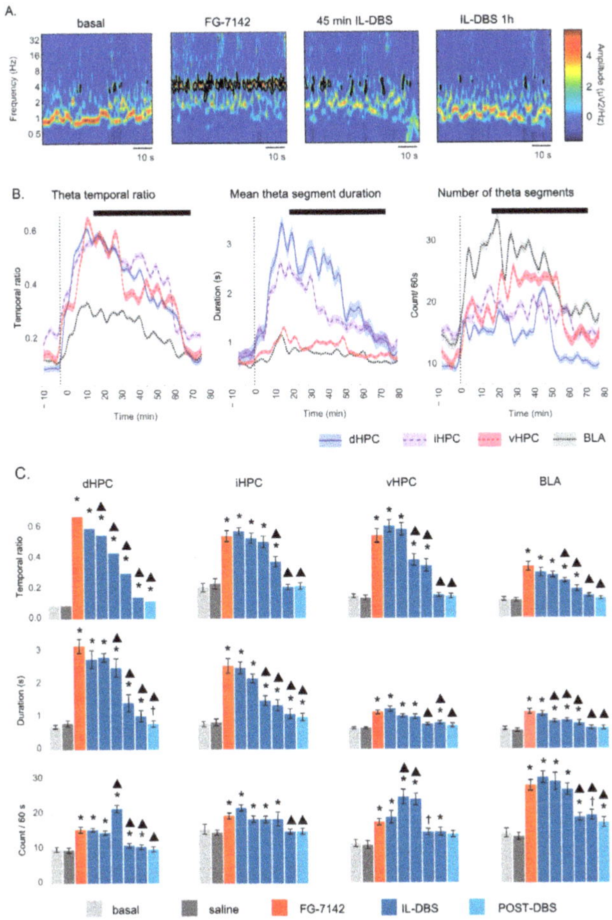

Figure 5. Theta segments: (**A**) vHPC: wavelet spectrograms. FG-7142 induces highly stable and long-lasting theta. IL-DBS disrupts theta segments, returning to basal values at 1 h. (**B**) Time course evolution of theta segments. Black line indicates the IL-DBS. (**C**) Statistical results of wavelet analysis. A more continuous theta is observed in the dHPC and iHPC, evidenced by a lower number of longer segments, while vHPC and BLA presented a more fractioned oscillation, indicated by more but shorter segments. IL-DBS first induced a disruption of the oscillations, represented by an increase in their number, together with shorter duration. Finally, theta segments diminished both in number and duration, eventually disappearing. Together, IL-DBS induced the progressive reduction in theta presence, as represented by a progressively lower temporal ratio. * Statistical significance in pairwise comparisons with the basal period. Triangle: statistical significance in pairwise comparisons with the FG-7142 period. Cross: statistical trend. Degree of significance not indicated to better visualize results; please see Supplementary Table S3. dHPC: dorsal hippocampus; iHPC: intermediate hippocampus; vHPC: ventral hippocampus; BLA: basolateral amygdala; IL: infralimbic cortex.

3.4. Effects of FG-7142 and IL-DBS on Local Gamma Power

FG-7142 administration induced an increase in mid gamma (60–90 Hz) power in the vHPC. High gamma (90–120 Hz) was also raised in the BLA and vHPC after treatment. Neither the iHPC nor the dHPC exhibited changes in gamma power in response to the anxiogenic drug.

In contrast, the IL-DBS induced an increase in gamma power in the network, which also lasted during the post-DBS period. In brief, low and high gamma power increased in the vHPC, iHPC, dHPC, and BLA, compared to both the basal and the anxiety-like states.

Mid gamma presented a similar pattern in the vHPC, dHPC, and BLA, but without any changes in the iHPC (Figure 6A,B and Supplementary Table S4).

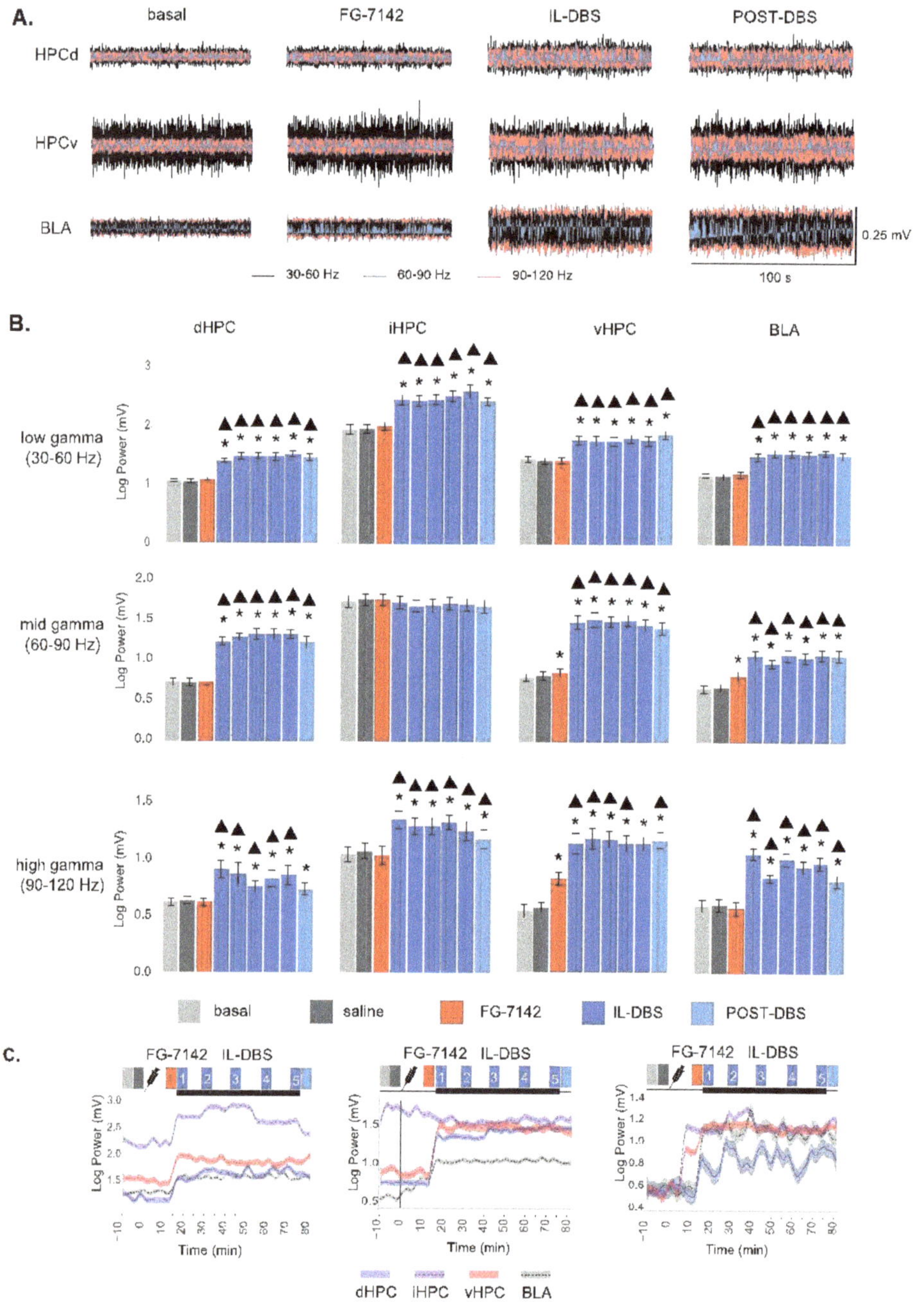

Figure 6. Effects of F-7142 and IL-DBS on gamma power: (**A**) wavelet-filtered oscillations showing the increase in all three gamma bands induced by IL-DBS. (**B**) Statistical results of gamma power computed by spectral decomposition. FG-7142

induces only statistical increases in vHPC and BLA, while a general increase in gamma power is observed during IL-DBS and post-DBS. * Statistical significance in pairwise comparisons with the basal period. Triangle: statistical significance in pairwise comparisons between IL-DBS and post-DBS with the FG-7142 period. Degree of significance not indicated to better visualize results; please see Supplementary Table S4. (**C**) Longitudinal evolution of gamma power. dHPC: dorsal hippocampus; iHPC: intermediate hippocampus; vHPC: ventral hippocampus; BLA: basolateral amygdala; IL: infralimbic cortex.

3.5. Phase Synchronization

Phase-locking allowed us to assess the synchronization between structures at certain bands, measured as WPLI, to increase accuracy. Figure 7, Supplementary Figure S1, and Supplementary Table S5 show the results. In basal conditions (anesthesia), there was a high phase-locking in SW (mean PLV > 0.8; Figure 7A,C). However, FG-7142 increased the PLV at low theta frequencies between all the hippocampal subregions (dHPC–iHPC, iHPC–vHPC, dHPC–vHPC), as well as between the dHPC–BLA and vHPC–BLA (Figure 7B,C). The most ventral subregions (vHPC–BLA, iHPC–BLA, vHPC–iHPC) increased the PLV at both delta and beta frequencies. When the IL-DBS was applied (Figure 7B,C), the PLV at SW frequency progressively increased in all regions, reaching basal values during the stimulation or in the post-DBS period; this was sooner in the vHPC–BLA and vHPC–iHPC. The anxiety-evoked PLV at low theta frequencies returned to basal values with the IL-DBS, with shorter timings in the dHPC–BLA and iHPC–BLA pairs and longer timing in the vHPC–BLA. Both the anxiety-induced delta and beta PLV between the iHPC–vHPC, iHPC–BLA, and vHPC–BLA decreased with IL-DBS. In contrast, with the IL-DBS, delta increased in the dHPC–iHPC and beta increased in the dHPC–BLA. Therefore, anxiety increased communication at specific frequencies (theta, delta and beta) in different subnetworks, which IL-DBS reversed.

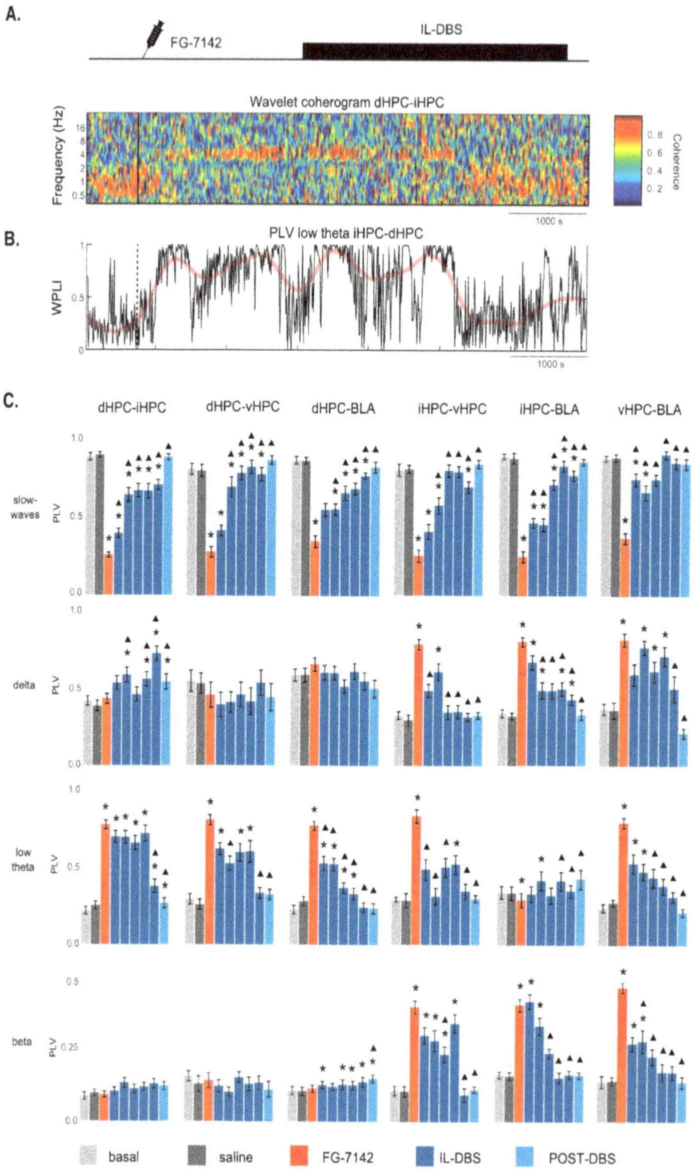

Figure 7. Effects on network synchronization induced by FG-7142 injection and IL-DBS: (**A**) A representative wavelet coherogram of dHPC-iHPC. At basal conditions, high coherence is observed at slow frequencies, which is typical of anesthesia. A clear increase in theta synchronization, together with a reduction in slow waves frequencies, can be observed in response to FG-7142. A return to basal values is induced by IL-DBS. (**B**) Time-course evolution of phase-locking value (PLV) measured as weighted phase lag index (WPLI) at low theta frequencies. WPLI values close to 1 indicate high phase synchronization at the selected frequency band (low theta in this case). Phase-locking under FG-7142 raises values close to 1. (**C**) Statistical results of WPLI. * Statistical significance in pairwise comparisons with the basal period. Triangle: statistical significance in pairwise comparisons with the FG-7142 period. Degree of significance not indicated to better visualize results; please see Supplementary Table S4. dHPC: dorsal hippocampus; iHPC: intermediate hippocampus; vHPC: ventral hippocampus; BLA: basolateral amygdala; IL: infralimbic cortex.

3.6. Cross-Frequency Coupling

Within each structure, changes in cross-frequency coupling were induced by FG-7142 and IL-DBS, both in amplitude–amplitude coupling and phase–amplitude coupling.

3.6.1. Amplitude–Amplitude Correlation

Both FG-7142 and IL-DBS produced changes in the amplitude–amplitude coupling between low-frequency oscillations in the 2.5–5 Hz range, beta activity (16–30 Hz), and gamma. Interestingly, a different pattern between regions was found (Figure 8).

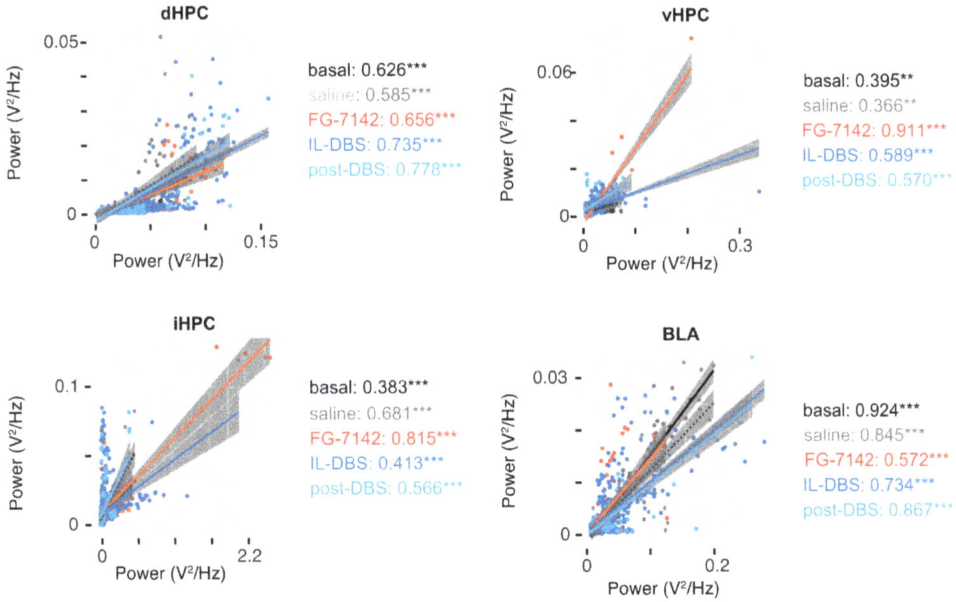

Figure 8. Amplitude–amplitude correlation between 2.5–5 Hz band and beta (16–30 Hz). Correlation at vHPC, and to a lesser extent iHPC, discriminates the effect of FG-7142 and IL-DBS well, with a high correlation following FG-7142 administration that was lower under the stimulation. r values are indicated in the right side; ** $p < 0.01$; *** $p < 0.001$. Other amplitude–amplitude correlations are represented in Supplementary Figure S2.

A topographic organization appeared, since the most evident results appeared in the vHPC and, to a lesser extent, the iHPC. In these regions, clearly different effects of the FG-7142 and DBS could be appreciated. FG-1742 generated a high correlation between the 2.5–5 Hz and faster oscillations. These effects were reversed by the IL-DBS (diminished slope), meaning similar 2.5–5 Hz amplitude values correlated with lower beta power. This pattern was less evident in the correlations calculated for dHPC and BLA areas.

Remarkably, in response to FG-7142, the correlation between the 2.5–5 Hz band and beta activity (16–30 Hz) increased in the vHPC (r = 0.911; $p < 0.001$) and in the iHPC (r = 0.815; $p < 0.001$). After IL-DBS, and during post-DBS, this value decreased (vHPC r = 0.589, iHPC r = 0.413, $p < 0.001$; vHPC r = 0.570, iHPC r = 0.566, $p < 0.001$). In contrast, few changes were observed in the dHPC. Finally, the inverse pattern appeared in BLA, with the lowest correlation occurring during FG-7142 administration.

In the dHPC, the correlation between beta and low gamma diminished in the FG-7142, DBS, and post-DBS periods, while the correlation between low, mid, and high gamma increased. The correlation between mid and high gamma was always high (r > 0.99, $p < 0.001$).

The iHPC and the vHPC exhibited the strongest correlations between the 2.5–5 Hz band and gamma during FG-7142 administration, though this diminished during IL-DBS. In this period, the iHPC showed the highest correlation between beta and mid gamma bands ($r > 0.925$, $p < 0.001$). The correlation between low and mid gamma bands was also high during the anxiogenic period in the vHPC ($r > 0.917$, $p < 0.001$). As in the dHPC in basal conditions, the correlation between mid and high gamma bands was high ($r > 0.972$, $p < 0.001$). However, in the vHPC, this correlation was reduced during IL-DBS ($r > 0.686$, $p < 0.001$).

In the BLA, the strongest correlations between the 2.5–5 Hz and faster oscillations, as well as beta gamma correlations, appeared during the post-DBS period. Similar to the dHPC, the correlation between mid and high gamma bands was always extreme ($r < 0.9$). For more details, see Supplementary Figure S2.

3.6.2. Phase-Amplitude Coupling

We obtained the MI between different bands in each structure to assess the PAC (Supplementary Table S6). Figure 9A displays a representative case in vHPC (Figure 9A, left) and BLA (Figure 9A, right). Statistical results, shown in Figure 9B, proved that FG-7142 increased delta–beta PAC in iHPC, vHPC, and BLA, as well as low theta–gamma coupling in the iHPC. However, delta–beta PAC remained similar to basal levels in the dHPC.

IL-DBS reversed the changes observed in the delta–beta coupling, returning to basal values or even lower levels in BLA. In contrast, SW–low gamma and low theta–low gamma coupling were highest during the IL-DBS, as we have previously observed [67].

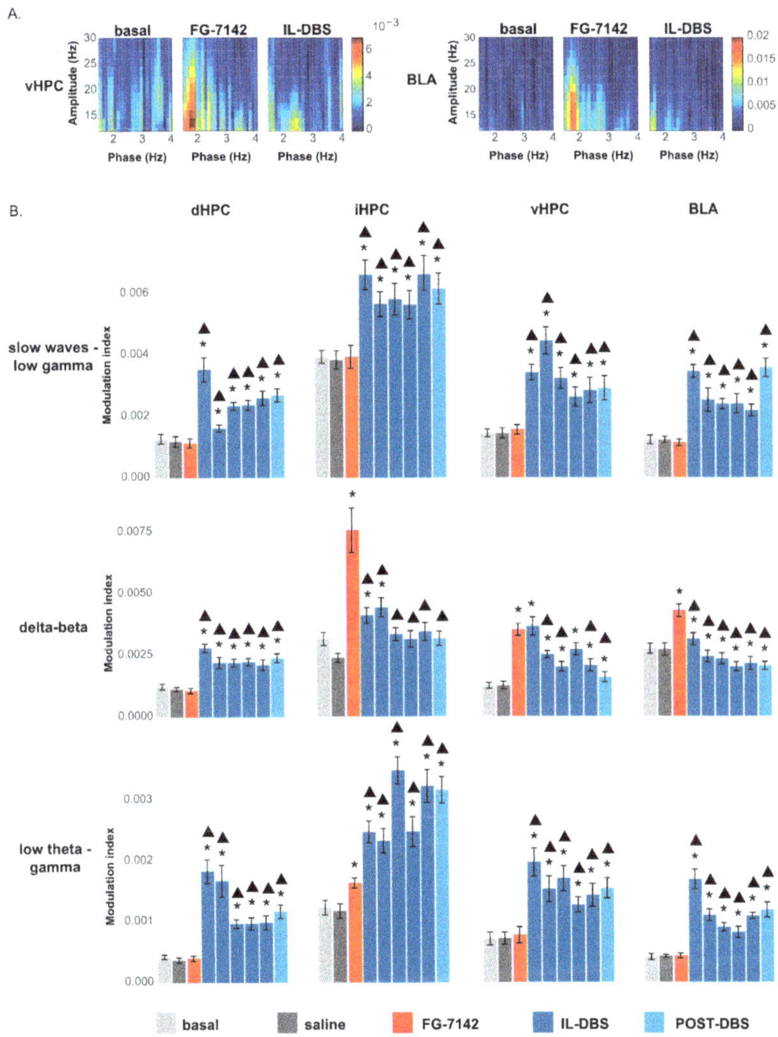

Figure 9. Effects of FG-7142 and IL-DBS over phase–amplitude coupling: (**A**) Comodulograms between 1–4 Hz and 10–30 Hz in vHPC and BLA showing an increase in coupling following administration of FG-7142 and a return to basal values with IL-DBS. (**B**) Statistical results of phase–amplitude coupling measured as the modulation index. * Statistical significance in pairwise comparisons with the basal period (degree of significance not indicated to better visualize results; please see Table S6). Triangle: statistical significance in pairwise comparisons between IL-DBS and post-DBS with the FG-7142 period. dHPC: dorsal hippocampus; iHPC: intermediate hippocampus; vHPC: ventral hippocampus; BLA: basolateral amygdala; IL: infralimbic cortex.

4. Discussion

Our study aimed to characterize oscillatory activity throughout the amygdala–hippocampal network under the effect of an anxiogenic drug, the inverse benzodiazepine FG-7142. Further, based on the high comorbidity between anxiety and depression, we analyzed the role of the IL-DBS, which exerts an antidepressant action in rats [39,40], as well as its equivalent in humans, the scACC DBS [15,27,107]. With this study, our purpose was to contribute to understandings around the neural circuits altered by anxiety, which is highly comorbid with other mental disorders, especially depression. Additionally, we aimed to shed light on how the DBS modulates these circuits.

4.1. Study Limitations

We are aware that the main limitation of the present study resides in its use of urethane anesthesia, which makes it necessary to be cautious in the frequency range of the oscillations observed. However, studying neural oscillations under urethane anesthesia is easier than doing so under freely moving conditions, since the former allows stable recordings without behavioral-induced confounding effects (i.e., hippocampal theta activity is activated during locomotion, grooming, and many other behaviors). Additionally, urethane allows a more realistic approach to neural activity than other anesthetics, and has therefore been widely used for acute electrophysiological experiments to study brain oscillations and neuronal discharges. Under urethane anesthesia, spontaneous neural oscillations alternate in a cyclic sleep-like manner [108]. Nevertheless, since its anesthetic power is lower, it needs to be supplemented with local anesthesia. However, urethane typically induces large amplitude and slow frequency oscillations that are widely distributed in the neocortex and which are similar to the oscillatory patterns characteristic of non-REM sleep [109]. In the hippocampus, these oscillations induce an alternation between slow waves (in the slow oscillations and delta frequency ranges) and short spontaneous theta periods, as our group, as well as the work of others, has previously observed [67,110–112]. SW are widely present during anesthesia and thus cannot be assumed to be a basal physiological value. However, SW also appear in unanesthetized animals and are related to the antidepressant response induced by laughing gas (N_2O), another NMDA receptor blocker [113]. Indeed, we point to this specific brain state, which is characterized by slow oscillations, as being responsive to the molecular changes related to fast-antidepressant responses.

Additionally, our lack of behavioral tests could be suggested as a weakness. However, as described before, a large body of evidence supports the anxiogenic effects of FG-7142 in rodents, cats, primates, and even humans [84,90,114–120]. Similar doses of FG-7142 injected ip in rats induce anxious behaviors at timings that are compatible with the changes described in this article.

In rodents, FG-7142 induces an increase in nonambulatory motor activity [78] but reduces exploratory behavior [80,81]. In the elevated plus-maze, FG-7142 reduces the exploration time spent in the open arms and increases the time spent in the closed arms [71]. Additionally, FG-7142 enhances behavioral suppression in response to safety signal withdrawal [82], exerts a proconflicting action, enhances shock-induced drinking suppression [79], and impairs fear extinction [83] and social interaction [84,85]. Its behavioral effects also include learned helplessness in a similar way to inescapable stress [84]. This fact is particularly relevant for our study about the IL-DBS mechanisms underlying its antidepressant actions, since learned helplessness constitutes a stress-based model of depression-like coping deficit in aversive but avoidable situations [121].

Regarding its neurobiological effects in rodents, FG-7142 also induces anxiety-related changes, including increases in corticosterone in plasma levels [86,87] and the activation of brain structures involved in stress, including the amygdala, the vHPC, the bed nucleus of the stria terminalis, and the cingulate, prelimbic, and IL cortices, as well as the brainstem nuclei of the reticular ascending arousal system, including the locus coeruleus, the periaqueductal grey, the nucleus incertus, and the dorsal raphe nucleus [78,79,96,97]. Moreover, Hackler and colleagues observed an increase in BOLD signal in the amygdala, dHPC, and hypothalamus for at least 40 min following FG-7142 administration (the authors did not report longer times) [85]. This effect is in accordance with what we observed in the sham-operated animals, without spontaneous reversal during the recording and 80 min after administration.

Additionally, the antidepressant- and anxiolytic-like action of IL-DBS in rats has been previously observed in freely behaving animals [39,40]. DBS applied at the ventromedial prefrontal cortex, and mainly restricted to the IL, reduces immobility time in the forced swimming test, which is used to evaluate learned helplessness, and increases climbing and swimming behaviors, which are usually considered as antidepressant-like actions. Additionally, DBS induces anxiolytic-like effects in the novelty-suppressed feeding test.

Therefore, in this study, our purpose was not to validate previous results but to complement them in a pharmacological model of anxiety, with the description of the neural activity in the amygdala–hippocampal network using an anxiety-inducing validated tool [77]. Additionally, chose to minimize unnecessary animal suffering.

However, further experiments in freely moving animals and studies in humans are necessary to confirm the usefulness of the studied parameters as anxiety biomarkers.

4.2. Effects of FG-7142 and IL-DBS on the Spectral Composition

Specifically, in our study, FG-7142 administration drastically reduced SW power in all recorded areas. The treatment also increased the relative power of delta and beta oscillations in the iHPC, vHPC, and BLA, and low theta ratio in the dHPC, iHPC, and BLA, with a trend in the vHPC. Low theta power increased only in vHPC and iHPC. High theta relative power was only raised in the dHPC. Rises in mid or high gamma power were also found in both the BLA and the vHPC.

Moreover, one hour of IL-DBS progressively reversed FG-7142 effects on SW, delta, theta, and beta, and was maintained in the DBS-off period. In contrast, gamma power was increased even more by the IL-DBS. In a previous study, we demonstrated that IL-DBS raises SW and gamma power in the dHPC and BLA [67] in anaesthetized animals. Additionally, in anaesthetized rats, Étievant and colleagues reported a similar effect in IL over slow oscillations after DBS, although they analyzed the full 0.25–4 Hz band [122]. We extend these previous results to a model of anxiety, showing the reversal of the pathological oscillatory profile.

SW are travelling waves mainly generated in the mPFC [123,124]. Their high amplitude is related to widespread network synchronization [125–127] and might be critical to adapting to environmental pressures [128]. Furthermore, animal models [129,130] and clinical studies of depression [131–133] presented reduced SW activity. Accordingly, Duncan and colleagues proposed reduced sleep SW activity as biomarkers of depression [134] and increased in effective antidepressant therapies [135–138]. In this sense, our results supported that IL-DBS can be an efficient treatment to restore SW oscillations associated with anxiety.

On the other hand, theta oscillations are associated with active hippocampal states, allowing memory processing [139,140], with dissociable components for spatial and emotional cues [141]. Type 1 theta (fast theta) is related to locomotion and spatial processing, and is mainly detected in the dHPC [142,143]. In rodents, low theta or type 2 theta is expressed with immobility, arousal, and emotional behaviors [144], including stress [145–148], anxiety [148,149], and fear [150–153].

These different components of hippocampal theta are organized across the dorsoventral axis [154]. For example, in humans implanted with intracranially implanted electrodes, the posterior hippocampus (equivalent to dHPC) displays high theta oscillations (~8 Hz) related to spatial processing. In comparison, the anterior hippocampus (equivalent to vHPC) exhibits low theta activity (~3 Hz) during non-spatial cognitive processing [155]. Additionally, optogenetic studies in rats have shown that the vHPC drives type 2 theta [156].

The reduction in hippocampal activity is related to anxiolytic responses. An early but extensive review by Gray and McNaughton referred to an improvement in active avoidance in conflict-generating tasks [157]. In general, hippocampal lesions result in reduced anxiety and behavioral disinhibition. More precisely, the vHPC is involved in the control of behavior under anxiogenic situations [53]. A decrease in vHPC and BLA theta has been known to occur with familiarization to a novel environment in control rats, but not in stressed rats [147], while theta power increases in the vHPC, BLA and to a lesser extent in the dHPC in stressed rats compared to control rats during the exploration of open arms in the elevated plus-maze [148]. Thus, the lowering of theta in these areas is related to a decreased anxiety level. Our results are in line with this fundamental role.

In specific behaviors involving decisions related to conflict, hippocampal theta oscillations have been proposed as anxiety biomarkers by McNaughton and colleagues [106,158,159]. In addition, drugs with anxiolytic effects reduce reticular elicited hippocampal rhythms [158,160].

Accordingly, in our study, FG-7142 induced a sustained low theta, whereas the IL-DBS first discontinued this oscillation and finally suppressed it. We hypothesize that, under anxiety, the amygdala hijacks the hippocampus in a continuous search for stress resolution, which would be reflected as a sustained theta and could compromise standard cognitive processing. IL-DBS can shortcut this sustained and pathological theta, as supported by our wavelet analyses, leaving the hippocampus available for cognitive processing.

We also found a reliable increase in gamma activity under IL-DBS, with only a moderate increase in mid and high gamma during FG-7142 administration. Fast-frequency oscillations reflect local neuronal assemblies [161–163]. Alterations in gamma have been described in mood disorders [164–166] and proposed as putative biomarkers of depression [167]. Our study agrees with animal and clinical studies that have reported similar increases in gamma power following acute ketamine administration at therapeutic levels [168–173]. Similarly to DBS, subanesthetic doses of ketamine, a noncompetitive *N*-methyl-D-aspartate (NMDA) receptor antagonist, also provides a fast antidepressant action [174], being particularly effective in anxious depression [175] and it is also helpful in relieving social anxiety disorder [176]. Cornwell and colleagues found that this rise in gamma power following ketamine administration, measured in cortical magnetoencephalographic recordings, is correlated to antidepressant responses and increased in responders vs. non-responders [177]. The increase in gamma power is more remarkable in depressive patients than in healthy controls. Even those exhibiting lower baseline gamma had better antidepressant action correlated to a higher increase in gamma power [178]. Gilbert and colleagues recently interpreted this influence in cortical networks as a therapeutic effect of modulating activation/inhibition levels while maintaining them at homeostatic levels [168]. However, most of these studies focused on cortical gamma and not hippocampal or amygdala activity. Other than gamma power, ketamine also induces antidepressant- and anxiolytic-like effects and reduces the reticular-elicited hippocampal theta in animal models [179]. Thus, IL-DBS and ketamine seem to share some electrophysiological features as fast antidepressant therapies.

4.3. Communication in the Amygdala–Hippocampal Network

Coherent oscillatory activity in distributed networks is involved in information processing [180,181]. Our study also found a decreased synchronization of SW in all regions under the anxiety-like period. We have also shown an increase in the PLV at delta and beta frequencies between the iHPC–vHPC, iHPC–BLA, and vHPC–BLA. There was a low theta band within all the hippocampal areas studied, and between dHPC–BLA, and it increased in vHPC–BLA but decreased in iHPC–BLA.

Taken together, the results suggest that, under the effects of FG-7142, the ventral subnetwork communicates via delta, low theta, and beta frequencies, while the intra-hippocampal communication affecting the dHPC operates only in the low theta range.

An increased WPLI at theta frequencies in the resting state of individuals suffering generalized social anxiety disorder has recently been described [182]. Additionally, according to an hyperanxiety animal model of chronic unpredictable stress, theta coherence between vHPC–BLA was higher when avoiding open arms than in approach actions in the elevated plus-maze [148].

The enhancement observed in 2.5–5 Hz and beta amplitude–amplitude correlation, specifically in the vHPC, complements these results, supporting the proposal of the delta–beta correlation as a putative anxiety biomarker [183–185] and extending the possibility of evaluating the PAC within these frequencies. However, it is important to be cautious in these findings' translation to human studies, since the frequency ranges differ slightly from those measured in anaesthetized rodents, in which slow rhythmical activity correspondent to theta rhythm occurs at lower frequencies [186]. Therefore, we have deliberately avoided delta or theta terms in the correlation results to reduce misinterpretations.

Finally, in the analysis of phase–amplitude coupling, we found an increase between SW–gamma, delta–beta, and low theta–gamma coupling following IL-DBS. We already described this increase in cross-frequency coupling between SW and faster frequencies in the dHPC and BLA in anaesthetized rats following IL-DBS, without any anxiety model [67].

PAC reflects the coordination of local (fast) and widespread (slow) oscillations, allowing better integration of information in a neuronal network [187]. Indeed, Salimpour and colleagues recommended PAC-oriented neuromodulation as being useful in neurological disorders [188]. In the hippocampus, theta–gamma coupling has been widely involved in memory processing [189–191]. In this case, hippocampal and BLA local activity could be better integrated following IL-DBS, contributing to the therapeutic effect.

5. Conclusions

In conclusion, our study characterizes the oscillations that emerge as a fingerprint in response to the anxiogenic drug FG-7142 in urethane-anesthetized rats. Additionally, our results provide evidence that IL-DBS reverses abnormal oscillatory processing in communication in the amygdala–hippocampal network. Further studies in freely moving animals and humans are encouraged in order to describe the oscillatory biomarkers of anxiety and to further analyze the effects of IL-DBS.

Supplementary Materials: The following are available online at https://www.mdpi.com/article/10.3390/biomedicines9070783/s1, Figure S1: Longitudinal analysis of Phase-locking value (WPLI), Figure S2: Cross-frequency amplitude-amplitude coupling, Table S1: Penetration coordinates in the recording areas, Table S2: Relative power, Table S3: Theta segments, Table S4: Gamma power, Table S5: Phase-locking value (WPLI), Table S6: Phase-amplitude coupling.

Author Contributions: Conceptualization, P.C. and A.C.-F.; data curation, H.V.-M., A.G.-M. and A.C.-F.; formal analysis, H.V.-M.; funding acquisition, P.C.; investigation, H.V.-M., A.G.-M., R.C.-J. and A.C.-F.; methodology, A.B.-S. and A.C.-F.; project administration, P.C. and A.C.-F.; resources, J.M.-R., A.L., P.C. and A.C.-F.; software, H.V.-M., A.G.-M., V.T.-M. and A.C.-F.; supervision, A.C.-F.; visualization, H.V.-M. and A.C.-F.; writing—original draft, A.C.-F.; writing—review and editing, H.V.-M., A.G.-M., R.C.-J., J.M.-R., V.T.-M., A.B.-S., A.L. and P.C. All authors have read and agreed to the published version of the manuscript.

Funding: This work was funded by the Fondo de Investigaciones Sanitarias FIS—Instituto de Salud Carlos Tercero and FEDER funds of the EU (Reference FIS-ISCIII PI16/00287). Hanna Vila-Merkle's PhD studies are funded by the Valencian Ministry of Education (Generalitat Valenciana; grant reference ACIF/2017/394).

Institutional Review Board Statement: The study was conducted according to the Animal Care Guidelines of the European Communities Council Directive (2010/63/E.U.). Additionally, the Ethics Committee of the University of Valencia (date 06.11.18; reference A1537174325669) and the Valencian Government (Generalitat Valenciana, Dirección General de Agricultura y Pesca; date 05.12.2018; reference 2018/VSC/PEA/0230) approved all procedures before the performance of the experiments.

Informed Consent Statement: Not applicable.

Data Availability Statement: Data available on request.

Acknowledgments: We thank all the LCN group for their valuable support in this work.

Conflicts of Interest: The authors declare no conflict of interest. Additionally, the funders had no role in the study's design, collection, analyses, interpretation of data, writing of the manuscript, or in the decision to publish the results.

References

1. Cryan, J.F.; Holmes, A. The ascent of mouse: Advances in modelling human depression and anxiety. *Nat. Rev. Drug Discov.* **2005**, *4*, 775–790. [CrossRef]
2. W.H.O. *Depression and Other Common Mental Disorders: Global Health Estimates*; WHO: Geneva, Switzerland, 2017.
3. Nock, M.K.; Hwang, I.; Sampson, N.A.; Kessler, R.C. Mental disorders, comorbidity and suicidal behavior: Results from the National Comorbidity Survey Replication. *Mol. Psychiatry* **2010**, *15*, 868–876. [CrossRef]
4. Nock, M.K.; Green, J.G.; Hwang, I.; McLaughlin, K.A.; Sampson, N.A.; Zaslavsky, A.M.; Kessler, R.C. Prevalence, correlates, and treatment of lifetime suicidal behavior among adolescents. *JAMA Psychiatry* **2013**, *70*, 300. [CrossRef]
5. *Diagnostic and Statistical Manual of Mental Disorders (DSM–5)*, 5th ed.; American Psychiatric Association: Washington, DC, USA, 2013.
6. Zhou, Y.; Cao, Z.; Yang, M.; Xi, X.; Guo, Y.; Fang, M.; Cheng, L.; Du, Y. Comorbid generalized anxiety disorder and its association with quality of life in patients with major depressive disorder. *Sci. Rep.* **2017**, *7*, 40511. [CrossRef] [PubMed]
7. Lamers, F.; van Oppen, P.; Comijs, H.C.; Smit, J.H.; Spinhoven, P.; van Balkom, A.J.L.M.; Nolen, W.A.; Zitman, F.G.; Beekman, A.T.F.; Penninx, B.W.J.H. Comorbidity patterns of anxiety and depressive disorders in a large cohort study. *J. Clin. Psychiatry* **2011**, *72*, 341–348. [CrossRef] [PubMed]
8. Wong, M.L.; Licinio, J. Research and treatment approaches to depression. *Nat. Rev. Neurosci.* **2001**, *2*, 243–351. [CrossRef] [PubMed]
9. Artigas, F.; Bortolozzi, A.; Celada, P. Can we increase speed and efficacy of antidepressant treatments? Part I: General aspects and monoamine-based strategies. *Eur. Neuropsychopharmacol.* **2018**, *28*, 445–456. [CrossRef]
10. Holtzheimer, P.E.; Mayberg, H.S. Stuck in a rut: Rethinking depression and its treatment. *Trends Neurosci.* **2011**, *34*, 1–9. [CrossRef] [PubMed]
11. Lozano, A.M.; Lipsman, N.; Bergman, H.; Brown, P.; Chabardes, S.; Chang, J.W.; Matthews, K.; McIntyre, C.C.; Schlaepfer, T.E.; Schulder, M.; et al. Deep brain stimulation: Current challenges and future directions. *Nat. Rev. Neurol.* **2019**, *15*, 148–160. [CrossRef]
12. Lozano, A.M.; Lipsman, N. Probing and regulating dysfunctional circuits using deep brain stimulation. *Neuron* **2013**, *77*, 406–424. [CrossRef]
13. Mayberg, H.S.; Lozano, A.M.; Voon, V.; McNeely, H.E.; Seminowicz, D.; Hamani, C.; Schwalb, J.M.; Kennedy, S.H. Deep brain stimulation for treatment-resistant depression. *Neuron* **2005**, *45*, 651–660. [CrossRef]
14. Lozano, A.M.; Mayberg, H.H.S.; Giacobbe, P.; Hamani, C.; Craddock, R.C.; Kennedy, S.S.H. Subcallosal cingulate gyrus deep brain stimulation for treatment-resistant depression. *Biol. Psychiatry* **2008**, *64*, 461–467. [CrossRef]
15. Crowell, A.L.; Riva-Posse, P.; Holtzheimer, P.E.; Garlow, S.J.; Kelley, M.E.; Gross, R.E.; Denison, L.; Quinn, S.; Mayberg, H.S. Long-term outcomes of subcallosal cingulate deep brain stimulation for treatment-resistant depression. *Am. J. Psychiatry* **2019**, *176*, 949–956. [CrossRef] [PubMed]
16. Kennedy, S.H.; Giacobbe, P.; Rizvi, S.J.; Placenza, F.M.; Nishikawa, Y.; Mayberg, H.S.; Lozano, A.M. Deep brain stimulation for treatment-resistant depression: Follow-up after 3 to 6 years. *Am. J. Psychiatry* **2011**, *168*, 502–510. [CrossRef] [PubMed]
17. Herrington, T.M.; Cheng, J.J.; Eskandar, E.N. Mechanisms of deep brain stimulation. *J. Neurophysiol.* **2016**, *115*, 19–38. [CrossRef] [PubMed]
18. Ashkan, K.; Rogers, P.; Bergman, H.; Ughratdar, I. Insights into the mechanisms of deep brain stimulation. *Nat. Rev. Neurol.* **2017**, *13*, 548–554. [CrossRef] [PubMed]
19. Malone, D.A.; Dougherty, D.D.; Rezai, A.R.; Carpenter, L.L.; Friehs, G.M.; Eskandar, E.N.; Rauch, S.L.; Rasmussen, S.A.; Machado, A.G.; Kubu, C.S.; et al. Deep brain stimulation of the ventral capsule/ventral striatum for treatment-resistant depression. *Biol. Psychiatry* **2009**, *65*, 267–275. [CrossRef]
20. Bewernick, B.H.; Hurlemann, R.; Matusch, A.; Kayser, S.; Grubert, C.; Hadrysiewicz, B.; Axmacher, N.; Lemke, M.; Cooper-Mahkorn, D.; Cohen, M.X.; et al. Nucleus accumbens deep brain stimulation decreases ratings of depression and anxiety in treatment-resistant depression. *Biol. Psychiatry* **2010**, *67*, 110–116. [CrossRef] [PubMed]
21. Schlaepfer, T.E.; Cohen, M.X.; Frick, C.; Kosel, M.; Brodesser, D.; Axmacher, N.; Joe, A.Y.; Kreft, M.; Lenartz, D.; Sturm, V. Deep brain stimulation to reward circuitry alleviates anhedonia in refractory major depression. *Neuropsychopharmacology* **2008**, *33*, 368–377. [CrossRef]
22. Krüger, S.; Seminowicz, D.; Goldapple, K.; Kennedy, S.H.; Mayberg, H.S. State and trait influences on mood regulation in bipolar disorder: Blood flow differences with an acute mood challenge. *Biol. Psychiatry* **2003**, *54*, 1274–1283. [CrossRef]
23. Simpson, J.R.; Drevets, W.C.; Snyder, A.Z.; Gusnard, D.A.; Raichle, M.E. Emotion-induced changes in human medial prefrontal cortex: II. During anticipatory anxiety. *Proc. Natl. Acad. Sci. USA* **2001**, *98*, 688–693. [CrossRef] [PubMed]
24. Zald, D.H.; Mattson, D.L.; Pardo, J.V. Brain activity in ventromedial prefrontal cortex correlates with individual differences in negative affect. *Proc. Natl. Acad. Sci. USA* **2002**, *99*, 2450–2454. [CrossRef] [PubMed]
25. Puigdemont, D.; Pérez-Egea, R.; Portella, M.J.; Molet, J.; De Diego-Adeliño, J.; Gironell, A.; Radua, J.; Gómez-Anson, B.; Rodríguez, R.; Serra, M.; et al. Deep brain stimulation of the subcallosal cingulate gyrus: Further evidence in treatment-resistant major depression. *Int. J. Neuropsychopharmacol.* **2012**, *15*, 121–133. [CrossRef] [PubMed]

26. Zhou, C.; Zhang, H.; Qin, Y.; Tian, T.; Xu, B.; Chen, J.; Zhou, X.; Zeng, L.; Fang, L.; Qi, X.; et al. A systematic review and meta-analysis of deep brain stimulation in treatment-resistant depression. *Prog. Neuro Psychopharmacol. Biol. Psychiatry* **2018**, *82*, 224–232. [CrossRef]
27. Khairuddin, S.; Ngo, F.Y.; Lim, W.L.; Aquili, L.; Khan, N.A.; Fung, M.-L.; Chan, Y.-S.; Temel, Y.; Lim, L.W. A decade of progress in deep brain stimulation of the subcallosal cingulate for the treatment of depression. *J. Clin. Med.* **2020**, *9*, 3260. [CrossRef]
28. Holtzheimer, P.E.; Husain, M.M.; Lisanby, S.H.; Taylor, S.F.; Whitworth, L.A.; McClintock, S.; Slavin, K.V.; Berman, J.; McKhann, G.M.; Patil, P.G.; et al. Subcallosal cingulate deep brain stimulation for treatment-resistant depression: A multisite, randomised, sham-controlled trial. *Lancet Psychiatry* **2017**, *4*, 839–849. [CrossRef]
29. Zhang, H.; Wang, N.; Yu, L.; Zhao, M. Efficacy and feasibility of deep brain stimulation for patients with depression. *Medicine* **2021**, *100*, e26044. [CrossRef] [PubMed]
30. Leonard, C.M. Finding prefrontal cortex in the rat. *Brain Res.* **2016**, *1645*, 1–3. [CrossRef] [PubMed]
31. Uylings, H.B.M.; Groenewegen, H.J.; Kolb, B. Do rats have a prefrontal cortex? *Behav. Brain Res.* **2003**, *146*, 3–17. [CrossRef] [PubMed]
32. Preuss, T.M. Do Rats Have Prefrontal Cortex? The Rose-Woolsey-Akert Program Reconsidered. *J. Cogn. Neurosci.* **1995**, *7*, 1–24. [CrossRef]
33. Heidbreder, C.A.; Groenewegen, H.J. The medial prefrontal cortex in the rat: Evidence for a dorso-ventral distinction based upon functional and anatomical characteristics. *Neurosci. Biobehav. Rev.* **2003**, *27*, 555–579. [CrossRef]
34. Schaeffer, D.J.; Hori, Y.; Gilbert, K.M.; Gati, J.S.; Menon, R.S.; Everling, S. Divergence of rodent and primate medial frontal cortex functional connectivity. *Proc. Natl. Acad. Sci. USA* **2020**, *117*, 21681–21689. [CrossRef]
35. Vertes, R.P. Differential Projections of the Infralimbic and Prelimbic Cortex in the Rat. *Synapse* **2004**, *51*, 32–58. [CrossRef]
36. Johansen-Berg, H.; Gutman, D.A.; Behrens, T.E.J.; Matthews, P.M.; Rushworth, M.F.S.; Katz, E.; Lozano, A.M.; Mayberg, H.S. Anatomical connectivity of the subgenual cingulate region targeted with deep brain stimulation for treatment-resistant depression. *Cereb. Cortex* **2008**, *18*, 1374–1383. [CrossRef] [PubMed]
37. Strange, B.A.; Witter, M.P.; Lein, E.S.; Moser, E.I. Functional organization of the hippocampal longitudinal axis. *Nat. Rev. Neurosci.* **2014**, *15*, 655–669. [CrossRef] [PubMed]
38. Sullivan, R.M.; Gratton, A. Lateralized effects of medial prefrontal cortex lesions on neuroendocrine and autonomic stress responses in rats. *J. Neurosci.* **2018**, *19*, 2834–2840. [CrossRef]
39. Hamani, C.; Diwan, M.; Macedo, C.E.; Brandão, M.L.; Shumake, J.; Gonzalez-Lima, F.; Raymond, R.; Lozano, A.M.; Fletcher, P.J.; Nobrega, J.N. Antidepressant-like effects of medial prefrontal cortex deep brain stimulation in rats. *Biol. Psychiatry* **2010**, *67*, 117–124. [CrossRef]
40. Jiménez-Sánchez, L.; Linge, R.; Campa, L.; Valdizán, E.M.; Pazos, Á.; Díaz, Á.; Adell, A. Behavioral, neurochemical and molecular changes after acute deep brain stimulation of the infralimbic prefrontal cortex. *Neuropharmacology* **2016**, *108*, 91–102. [CrossRef]
41. Torres-Sanchez, S.; Perez-Caballero, L.; Mico, J.A.; Celada, P.; Berrocoso, E. Effect of Deep Brain Stimulation of the ventromedial prefrontal cortex on the noradrenergic system in rats. *Brain Stimul.* **2018**, *11*, 222–230. [CrossRef]
42. Hastings, R.S.; Parsey, R.V.; Oquendo, M.A.; Arango, V.; Mann, J.J. Volumetric analysis of the prefrontal cortex, amygdala, and hippocampus in major depression. *Neuropsychopharmacology* **2004**, *29*, 952–959. [CrossRef]
43. Shin, L.M.; Rauch, S.L.; Pitman, R.K. Amygdala, medial prefrontal cortex, and hippocampal function in PTSD. *Ann. N. Y. Acad. Sci.* **2006**, *1071*, 67–79. [CrossRef]
44. Videbech, P.; Ravnkilde, B. Hippocampal volume and depression: A meta-analysis of MRI studies. *Am. J. Psychiatry* **2004**, *161*, 1957–1966. [CrossRef] [PubMed]
45. Campbell, S.; Macqueen, G. The role of the hippocampus in the pathophysiology of major depression. *J. Psychiatry Neurosci.* **2004**, *29*, 417–426.
46. Cha, J.; Greenberg, T.; Song, I.; Blair Simpson, H.; Posner, J.; Mujica-Parodi, L.R. Abnormal hippocampal structure and function in clinical anxiety and comorbid depression. *Hippocampus* **2016**, *26*, 545–553. [CrossRef] [PubMed]
47. Grillon, C. Associative learning deficits increase symptoms of anxiety in humans. *Biol. Psychiatry* **2002**, *51*, 851–858. [CrossRef]
48. Kalisch, R.; Schubert, M.; Jacob, W.; Keßler, M.S.; Hemauer, R.; Wigger, A.; Landgraf, R.; Auer, D.P. Anxiety and hippocampus volume in the rat. *Neuropsychopharmacology* **2006**, *31*, 925–932. [CrossRef] [PubMed]
49. Sapolsky, R.M. The possibility of neurotoxicity in the hippocampus in major depression: A primer on neuron death. *Biol. Psychiatry* **2000**, *48*, 755–765. [CrossRef]
50. Nestler, E.J.; Barrot, M.; DiLeone, R.J.; Eisch, A.J.; Gold, S.J.; Monteggia, L.M. *Neurobiology of Depression*; Elsevier: Amsterdam, The Netherlands, 2002; Volume 34, pp. 13–25.
51. Amaral, D.G.; Witter, M.P. The three-dimensional organization of the hippocampal formation: A review of anatomical data. *Neuroscience* **1989**, *31*, 571–591. [CrossRef]
52. Moser, M.-B.; Moser, E.I. Functional differentiation in the hippocampus. *Hippocampus* **1998**, *8*, 608–619. [CrossRef]
53. Bannerman, D.; Rawlins, J.N.; McHugh, S.; Deacon, R.M.; Yee, B.; Bast, T.; Zhang, W.-N.; Pothuizen, H.H.; Feldon, J. Regional dissociations within the hippocampus—memory and anxiety. *Neurosci. Biobehav. Rev.* **2004**, *28*, 273–283. [CrossRef]
54. Lothmann, K.; Deitersen, J.; Zilles, K.; Amunts, K.; Herold, C. New boundaries and dissociation of the mouse hippocampus along the dorsal-ventral axis based on glutamatergic, GABAergic and catecholaminergic receptor densities. *Hippocampus* **2020**, *31*, 56–78. [CrossRef]

55. Phelps, E.A.; LeDoux, J.E. Contributions of the amygdala to emotion processing: From animal models to human behavior. *Neuron* **2005**, *48*, 175–187. [CrossRef]
56. LeDoux, J. The emotional brain, fear, and the amygdala. *Cell. Mol. Neurobiol.* **2003**, *23*, 727–738. [CrossRef]
57. Rosenkranz, J.A.; Venheim, E.R.; Padival, M. Chronic stress causes amygdala hyperexcitability in rodents. *Biol. Psychiatry* **2010**, *67*, 1128–1136. [CrossRef]
58. Roozendaal, B.; McEwen, B.S.; Chattarji, S. Stress, memory and the amygdala. *Nat. Rev. Neurosci.* **2009**, *10*, 423–433. [CrossRef]
59. Vyas, A.; Jadhav, S.; Chattarji, S. Prolonged behavioral stress enhances synaptic connectivity in the basolateral amygdala. *Neuroscience* **2006**, *143*, 387–393. [CrossRef] [PubMed]
60. Stein, M.B.; Simmons, A.N.; Feinstein, J.S.; Paulus, M.P. Increased amygdala and insula activation during emotion processing in anxiety-prone subjects. *Am. J. Psychiatry* **2007**, *164*, 318–327. [CrossRef]
61. Hamilton, J.P.; Siemer, M.; Gotlib, I.H. Amygdala volume in major depressive disorder: A meta-analysis of magnetic resonance imaging studies. *Mol. Psychiatry* **2008**, *13*, 993–1000. [CrossRef]
62. Sibille, E.; Wang, Y.; Joeyen-Waldorf, J.; Gaiteri, C.; Surget, A.; Oh, S.; Belzung, C.; Tseng, G.C.; Lewis, D.A. A molecular signature of depression in the amygdala. *Am. J. Psychiatry* **2009**, *166*, 100–1024. [CrossRef] [PubMed]
63. Delaveau, P.; Jabourian, M.; Lemogne, C.; Guionnet, S.; Bergouignan, L.; Fossati, P. Brain effects of antidepressants in major depression: A meta-analysis of emotional processing studies. *J. Affect. Disord.* **2011**, *130*, 66–74. [CrossRef] [PubMed]
64. Bellani, M.; Dusi, N.; Yeh, P.H.; Soares, J.C.; Brambilla, P. The effects of antidepressants on human brain as detected by imaging studies. Focus on major depression. *Prog. Neuro Psychopharmacol. Biol. Psychiatry* **2011**, *35*, 1544–1552. [CrossRef]
65. Castro, J.E.; Varea, E.; Márquez, C.; Cordero, M.I.; Poirier, G.; Sandi, C. Role of the amygdala in antidepressant effects on hippocampal cell proliferation and survival and on depression-like behavior in the rat. *PLoS ONE* **2010**, *5*, e8618. [CrossRef]
66. Arnsten, A.F.T. Stress signalling pathways that impair prefrontal cortex structure and function. *Nat. Rev. Neurosci.* **2009**, *10*, 410–422. [CrossRef]
67. Cervera-Ferri, A.; Teruel-Martí, V.; Barceló-Molina, M.; Martínez-Ricós, J.; Luque-García, A.; Martínez-Bellver, S.; Adell, A. Characterization of oscillatory changes in hippocampus and amygdala after deep brain stimulation of the infralimbic prefrontal cortex. *Physiol. Rep.* **2016**, *4*, e12854. [CrossRef]
68. Harro, J. Animals, anxiety, and anxiety disorders: How to measure anxiety in rodents and why. *Behav. Brain Res.* **2018**, *352*, 81–93. [CrossRef] [PubMed]
69. Mohammad, F.; Ho, J.; Woo, J.H.; Lim, C.L.; Poon, D.J.J.; Lamba, B.; Claridge-Chang, A. Concordance and incongruence in preclinical anxiety models: Systematic review and meta-analyses. *Neurosci. Biobehav. Rev.* **2016**, *68*, 504–529. [CrossRef] [PubMed]
70. Braestrup, C.; Nielsen, M.; Olsen, C.E. Urinary and brain β-carboline-3-carboxylates as potent inhibitors of brain benzodiazepine receptors. *Proc. Natl. Acad. Sci. USA* **1980**, *77*, 2288–2292. [CrossRef] [PubMed]
71. Evans, A.K.; Lowry, C.A. Pharmacology of the β-Carboline FG-7142, a Partial Inverse Agonist at the Benzodiazepine Allosteric Site of the GABAA Receptor: Neurochemical, Neurophysiological, and Behavioral Effects. *CNS Drug Rev.* **2007**, *13*, 475–501. [CrossRef]
72. Pellow, S.; File, S.E. Anxiolytic and anxiogenic drug effects on exploratory activity in an elevated plus-maze: A novel test of anxiety in the rat. *Pharmacol. Biochem. Behav.* **1986**, *24*, 252–529. [CrossRef]
73. Rodgers, R.J.; Cole, J.C.; Aboualfa, K.; Stephenson, L.H. Ethopharmacological analysis of the effects of putative "anxiogenic" agents in the mouse elevated plus-maze. *Pharmacol. Biochem. Behav.* **1995**, *52*, 805–813. [CrossRef]
74. Lawther, A.J.; Clissold, M.L.; Ma, S.; Kent, S.; Lowry, C.A.; Gundlach, A.L.; Hale, M.W. Anxiogenic drug administration and elevated plus-maze exposure in rats activate populations of relaxin-3 neurons in the nucleus incertus and serotonergic neurons in the dorsal raphe nucleus. *Neuroscience* **2015**, *303*, 270–284. [CrossRef]
75. Singewald, N.; Salchner, P.; Sharp, T. Induction of c-Fos expression in specific areas of the fear circuitry in rat forebrain by anxiogenic drugs. *Biol. Psychiatry* **2003**, *53*, 275–283. [CrossRef]
76. Dorow, R. FG 7142 and its anxiety-inducing effects in humans. *Br. J. Clin. Pharmacol.* **1987**, *23*, 781–782.
77. Horowski, R. FG 7142: Is this validated tool to study anxiety now forgotten? *J. Neural Transm.* **2020**, *127*, 287–289. [CrossRef] [PubMed]
78. Abrams, J.K.; Johnson, P.L.; Hay-Schmidt, A.; Mikkelsen, J.D.; Shekhar, A.; Lowry, C.A. Serotonergic systems associated with arousal and vigilance behaviors following administration of anxiogenic drugs. *Neuroscience* **2005**, *133*, 983–997. [CrossRef]
79. Corda, M.G.; Blaker, W.D.; Mendelson, W.B.; Guidotti, A.; Costa, E. β-Carbolines enhance shock-induced suppression of drinking in rats. *Proc. Natl. Acad. Sci. USA* **1983**, *80*, 2072–2076. [CrossRef] [PubMed]
80. Stephens, D.N.; Kehr, W.; Schneider, H.H.; Schmiechen, R. β-Carbolines with agonistic and inverse agonistic properties at benzodiazepine receptors of the rat. *Neurosci. Lett.* **1984**, *47*, 333–338. [CrossRef]
81. Stephens, D.N.; Kehr, W. β-Carbolines can enhance or antagonize the effects of punishment in mice. *Psychopharmacology* **1985**, *85*, 143–147. [CrossRef]
82. Thiébot, M.H.; Dangoumau, L.; Richard, G.; Puech, A.J. Safety signal withdrawal: A behavioural paradigm sensitive to both "anxiolytic" and "anxiogenic" drugs under identical experimental conditions. *Psychopharmacology* **1991**, *103*, 415–424. [CrossRef] [PubMed]
83. Kim, J.H.; Richardson, R. A developmental dissociation in reinstatement of an extinguished fear response in rats. *Neurobiol. Learn. Mem.* **2007**, *88*, 48–57. [CrossRef]

84. Short, K.R.; Maier, S.F. Stressor controllability, social interaction, and benzodiazepine systems. *Pharmacol. Biochem. Behav.* **1993**, *45*, 827–835. [CrossRef]
85. Hackler, E.A.; Turner, G.H.; Gresch, P.J.; Sengupta, S.; Deutch, A.Y.; Avison, M.J.; Gore, J.C.; Sanders-Bush, E. 5-Hydroxytryptamine2C receptor contribution to m-chlorophenylpiperazine and N-methyl-β-carboline-3-carboxamide-induced anxiety-like behavior and limbic brain activation. *J. Pharmacol. Exp. Ther.* **2007**, *320*, 1023–1029. [CrossRef]
86. Stephens, D.N.; Schneider, H.H.; Kehr, W.; Jensen, L.H.; Petersen, E.; Honore, T. Modulation of anxiety by β-carbolines and other benzodiazepine receptor ligands: Relationship of pharmacological to biochemical measures of efficacy. *Brain Res. Bull.* **1987**, *19*, 309–318. [CrossRef]
87. Pellow, S.; File, S.E. The effects of putative anxiogenic compounds (FG 7142, CGS 8216 and Ro 15-1788) on the rat corticosterone response. *Physiol. Behav.* **1985**, *35*, 587–590. [CrossRef]
88. Thiébot, M.H.; Soubrié, P.; Sanger, D. Anxiogenic properties of beta-CCE and FG 7142: A review of promises and pitfalls. *Psychopharmacology* **1988**, *94*, 452–463. [CrossRef]
89. Takamatsu, H.; Noda, A.; Kurumaji, A.; Murakami, Y.; Tatsumi, M.; Ichise, R.; Nishimura, S. A PET study following treatment with a pharmacological stressor, FG7142, in conscious rhesus monkeys. *Brain Res.* **2003**, *980*, 275–280. [CrossRef]
90. Ongini, E.; Barzaghi, C.; Marzanatti, M. Intrinsic and antagonistic effects of β-carboline FG 7142 on behavioral and EEG actions of benzodiazepines and pentobarbital in cats. *Eur. J. Pharmacol.* **1983**, *95*, 125–129. [CrossRef]
91. Singewald, N.; Sharp, T. Neuroanatomical targets of anxiogenic drugs in the hindbrain as revealed by Fos immunocytochemistry. *Neuroscience* **2000**, *98*, 759–770. [CrossRef]
92. Lyss, P.J.; Andersen, S.L.; Leblanc, C.J.; Teicher, M.H. Degree of neuronal activation following FG-7142 changes across regions during development. *Dev. Brain Res.* **1999**, *116*, 201–203. [CrossRef]
93. Funk, D.; Li, Z.; Coen, K.; Lê, A.D. Effects of pharmacological stressors on c-fos and CRF mRNA in mouse brain: Relationship to alcohol seeking. *Neurosci. Lett.* **2008**, *444*, 254–258. [CrossRef] [PubMed]
94. Buzsáki, G.; Watson, B.O. Brain rhythms and neural syntax: Implications for efficient coding of cognitive content and neuropsychiatric disease. *Dialogues Clin. Neurosci.* **2012**, *14*, 345–367.
95. Buzsáki, G.; Draguhn, A. Neuronal olscillations in cortical networks. *Science* **2004**, *304*, 1926–1929. [CrossRef] [PubMed]
96. Singer, W. Temporal Coherence: A Versatile Code for the Definition of Relations. In *The Senses: A Comprehensive Reference*; Elsevier: Amsterdam, The Netherlands, 2008; Volume 2, pp. 1–9, ISBN 9780123708809.
97. Watson, B.O.; Buzsáki, G. Neural syntax in mental disorders. *Biol. Psychiatry* **2015**, *77*, 998–1000. [CrossRef] [PubMed]
98. Yener, G.G.; Başar, E. Brain oscillations as biomarkers in neuropsychiatric disorders. *Suppl. Clin. Neurophysiol.* **2013**, *15*, 343–363.
99. Paxinos, G.; Watson, C. *The Rat Brain in Stereotaxic Coordinates*, 6th ed.; Elsevier: Amsterdam, The Netherlands, 2006.
100. Claustre, Y.; Rouquier, L.; Desvignes, C.; Leonetti, M.; Montégut, J.; Aubin, N.; Allouard, N.; Bougault, I.; Oury-Donat, F.; Steinberg, R. Effects of the vasopressin (V1B) receptor antagonist, SSR149415, and the corticotropin-releasing factor 1 receptor antagonist, SSR125543, on FG 7142-induced increase in acetylcholine and norepinephrine release in the rat. *Neuroscience* **2006**, *141*, 1481–1488. [CrossRef] [PubMed]
101. Mei, L.; Zhou, Y.; Sun, Y.; Liu, H.; Zhang, D.; Liu, P.; Shu, H. Acetylcholine muscarinic receptors in ventral hippocampus modulate stress-induced anxiety-like behaviors in mice. *Front. Mol. Neurosci.* **2020**, *13*, 235. [CrossRef] [PubMed]
102. Torrence, C.; Compo, G.P. A practical guide to wavelet analysis. *Bull. Am. Meteorol. Soc.* **1997**, *79*, 61–78. [CrossRef]
103. Vinck, M.; Oostenveld, R.; van Wingerden, M.; Battaglia, F.; Pennartz, C.M.A. An improved index of phase-synchronization for electrophysiological data in the presence of volume-conduction, noise and sample-size bias. *Neuroimage* **2011**, *55*, 1548–1565. [CrossRef]
104. Tort, A.B.L.; Komorowski, R.; Eichenbaum, H.; Kopell, N. Measuring phase-amplitude coupling between neuronal oscillations of different frequencies. *J. Neurophysiol.* **2010**, *104*, 1195–1210. [CrossRef] [PubMed]
105. Bland, B.H.; Oddie, S.D. Theta band oscillation and synchrony in the hippocampal formation and associated structures: The case for its role in sensorimotor integration. *Behav. Brain Res.* **2001**, *127*, 119–136. [CrossRef]
106. McNaughton, N.; Swart, C.; Neo, P.; Bates, V.; Glue, P. Anti-anxiety drugs reduce conflict-specific "theta"—A possible human anxiety-specific biomarker. *J. Affect. Disord.* **2013**, *148*, 104–111. [CrossRef]
107. Holtzheimer, P.E. Subcallosal Cingulate deep brain stimulation for treatment-resistant unipolar and bipolar depression. *Arch. Gen. Psychiatry* **2012**, *69*, 150. [CrossRef]
108. Clement, E.A.; Richard, A.; Thwaites, M.; Ailon, J.; Peters, S.; Dickson, C.T. Cyclic and sleep-like spontaneous alternations of brain state under urethane anaesthesia. *PLoS ONE* **2008**, *3*, e2004. [CrossRef]
109. Steriade, M.; Nunez, A.; Amzica, F. A novel slow (<1 Hz) oscillation of neocortical neurons in vivo: Depolarizing and hyperpolarizing components. *J. Neurosci.* **1993**, *13*, 3252–3265. [CrossRef]
110. Nuñez, A.; Cervera-Ferri, A.; Olucha-Bordonau, F.; Ruiz-Torner, A.; Teruel, V. Nucleus incertus contribution to hippocampal theta rhythm generation. *Eur. J. Neurosci.* **2006**, *23*, 2731–2738. [CrossRef] [PubMed]
111. Cervera-Ferri, A.; Guerrero-Martínez, J.; Bataller-Mompeán, M.; Taberner-Cortes, A.; Martínez-Ricós, J.; Ruiz-Torner, A.; Teruel-Martí, V. Theta synchronization between the hippocampus and the nucleus incertus in urethane-anesthetized rats. *Exp. Brain Res.* **2011**, *211*, 177–192. [CrossRef] [PubMed]

112. Martínez-Bellver, S.; Cervera-Ferri, A.; Martínez-Ricós, J.; Ruiz-Torner, A.; Luque-García, A.; Blasco-Serra, A.; Guerrero-Martínez, J.; Bataller-Mompeán, M.; Teruel-Martí, V. Regular theta-firing neurons in the nucleus incertus during sustained hippocampal activation. *Eur. J. Neurosci.* **2015**, *41*, 1049–1067. [CrossRef] [PubMed]
113. Kohtala, S.; Theilmann, W.; Rosenholm, M.; Penna, L.; Karabulut, G.; Uusitalo, S.; Järventausta, K.; Yli-Hankala, A.; Yalcin, I.; Matsui, N.; et al. Cortical excitability and activation of trkb signaling during rebound slow oscillations are critical for rapid antidepressant responses. *Mol. Neurobiol.* **2019**, *56*, 4163–4174. [CrossRef]
114. Drugan, R.C.; Maier, S.F.; Skolnick, P.; Paul, S.M.; Crawley, J.N. An anxiogenic benzodiazepine receptor ligand induces learned helplessness. *Eur. J. Pharmacol.* **1985**, *113*, 453–457. [CrossRef]
115. Lukkes, J.L.; Engelman, G.H.; Zelin, N.S.; Hale, M.W.; Lowry, C.A. Post-weaning social isolation of female rats, anxiety-related behavior, and serotonergic systems. *Brain Res.* **2012**, *1443*, 1–17. [CrossRef]
116. Johnson, P.L.; Samuels, B.C.; Fitz, S.D.; Federici, L.M.; Hammes, N.; Early, M.C.; Truitt, W.; Lowry, C.A.; Shekhar, A. Orexin 1 receptors are a novel target to modulate panic responses and the panic brain network. *Physiol. Behav.* **2012**, *107*, 733–742. [CrossRef] [PubMed]
117. McGregor, I.S.; Lee, A.M.; Westbrook, R.F. Stress-induced changes in respiratory quotient, energy expenditure and locomotor activity in rats: Effects of midazolam. *Psychopharmacology* **1994**, *116*, 475–482. [CrossRef] [PubMed]
118. Kato, Y.; Gokan, H.; Oh-Nishi, A.; Suhara, T.; Watanabe, S.; Minamimoto, T. Vocalizations associated with anxiety and fear in the common marmoset (Callithrix jacchus). *Behav. Brain Res.* **2014**, *275*, 43–52. [CrossRef] [PubMed]
119. Marín, R.H.; Martijena, I.D.; Arce, A. Effect of diazepam and a β-carboline on open-field and T-maze behaviors in 2-day-old chicks. *Pharmacol. Biochem. Behav.* **1997**, *58*, 915–921. [CrossRef]
120. Steenbergen, P.J.; Richardson, M.K.; Champagne, D.L. Patterns of avoidance behaviours in the light/dark preference test in young juvenile zebrafish: A pharmacological study. *Behav. Brain Res.* **2011**, *222*, 15–25. [CrossRef]
121. Vollmayr, B.; Gass, P. Learned helplessness: Unique features and translational value of a cognitive depression model. *Cell Tissue Res.* **2013**, *354*, 171–178. [CrossRef]
122. Etiévant, A.; Oosterhof, C.; Bétry, C.; Abrial, E.; Novo-Perez, M.; Rovera, R.; Scarna, H.; Devader, C.; Mazella, J.; Wegener, G.; et al. Astroglial control of the antidepressant-like effects of prefrontal cortex deep brain stimulation. *EBioMedicine* **2015**, *2*, 898–908. [CrossRef]
123. Massimini, M. The sleep slow oscillation as a traveling wave. *J. Neurosci.* **2004**, *24*, 6862–6870. [CrossRef]
124. Murphy, M.; Riedner, B.A.; Huber, R.; Massimini, M.; Ferrarelli, F.; Tononi, G. Source modeling sleep slow waves. *Proc. Natl. Acad. Sci. USA* **2009**, *106*, 1608–1613. [CrossRef] [PubMed]
125. Esser, S.K.; Hill, S.L.; Tononi, G. Sleep homeostasis and cortical synchronization: I. Modeling the effects of synaptic strength on sleep slow waves. *Sleep* **2007**, *30*, 1617–1630. [CrossRef]
126. Riedner, B.A.; Vyazovskiy, V.V.; Huber, R.; Massimini, M.; Esser, S.; Murphy, M.; Tononi, G. Sleep homeostasis and cortical synchronization: III. A high-density EEG study of sleep slow waves in humans. *Sleep* **2007**, *30*, 1643–1657. [CrossRef]
127. Vyazovskiy, V.V.; Riedner, B.A.; Cirelli, C.; Tononi, G. Sleep homeostasis and cortical synchronization: II. A local field potential study of sleep slow waves in the rat. *Sleep* **2007**, *30*, 1631–1642. [CrossRef]
128. Maquet, P.; Degueldre, C.; Delfiore, G.; Aerts, J.; Péters, J.M.; Luxen, A.; Franck, G. Functional neuroanatomy of human slow wave sleep. *J. Neurosci.* **1997**, *17*, 2801–2812. [CrossRef]
129. Voget, M.; Rummel, J.; Avchalumov, Y.; Sohr, R.; Haumesser, J.K.; Rea, E.; Mathé, A.A.; Hadar, R.; van Riesen, C.; Winter, C. Altered local field potential activity and serotonergic neurotransmission are further characteristics of the Flinders sensitive line rat model of depression. *Behav. Brain Res.* **2015**, *291*, 299–305. [CrossRef]
130. Zheng, C.; Zhang, T. Synaptic plasticity-related neural oscillations on hippocampus-prefrontal cortex pathway in depression. *Neuroscience* **2015**, *292*, 170–180. [CrossRef]
131. Armitage, R. Microarchitectural findings in sleep EEG in depression: Diagnostic implications. *Biol. Psychiatry* **1995**, *37*, 72–84. [CrossRef]
132. Benca, R.M.; Obermeyer, W.H.; Thisted, R.A.; Gillin, J.C. Sleep and Psychiatric disorders: A meta-analysis. *Arch. Gen. Psychiatry* **1992**, *49*, 651–668. [CrossRef] [PubMed]
133. Dijk, D.J. Slow-wave sleep deficiency and enhancement: Implications for insomnia and its management. *World J. Biol. Psychiatry* **2010**, *11*, 22–28. [CrossRef] [PubMed]
134. Duncan, W.C.; Zarate, C.A. Ketamine, sleep, and depression: Current status and new questions. *Curr. Psychiatry Rep.* **2013**, *15*, 394. [CrossRef] [PubMed]
135. Ehlers, C.L.; Havstad, J.W.; Kupfer, D.J. Estimation of the time course of slow-wave sleep over the night in depressed patients: Effects of clomipramine and clinical response. *Biol. Psychiatry* **1996**, *39*, 171–181. [CrossRef]
136. Argyropoulos, S.V.; Hicks, J.A.; Nash, J.R.; Bell, C.J.; Rich, A.S.; Nutt, D.J.; Wilson, S. Redistribution of slow wave activity of sleep during pharmacological treatment of depression with paroxetine but not with nefazodone. *J. Sleep Res.* **2009**, *18*, 342–348. [CrossRef]
137. Landsness, E.C.; Goldstein, M.R.; Peterson, M.J.; Tononi, G.; Benca, R.M. Antidepressant effects of selective slow wave sleep deprivation in major depression: A high-density EEG investigation. *J. Psychiatr. Res.* **2011**, *45*, 1019–1026. [CrossRef] [PubMed]

138. Duncan, W.C.; Sarasso, S.; Ferrarelli, F.; Selter, J.; Riedner, B.A.; Hejazi, N.S.; Yuan, P.; Brutsche, N.; Manji, H.K.; Tononi, G.; et al. Concomitant BDNF and sleep slow wave changes indicate ketamine-induced plasticity in major depressive disorder. *Int. J. Neuropsychopharmacol.* **2013**, *16*, 301–311. [CrossRef] [PubMed]
139. Buzsáki, G. Theta oscillations in the hippocampus. *Neuron* **2002**, *33*, 325–340. [CrossRef]
140. Hasselmo, M.E. What is the function of hippocampal theta rhythm? Linking bahavioral data to phasic properties of field potential and unit recording data. *Hippocampus* **2005**, *15*, 936–949. [CrossRef]
141. Wells, C.E.; Amos, D.P.; Jeewajee, A.; Douchamps, V.; Rodgers, J.; O'Keefe, J.; Burgess, N.; Lever, C. Novelty and anxiolytic drugs dissociate two components of hippocampal theta in behaving rats. *J. Neurosci.* **2013**, *33*, 8650–8667. [CrossRef]
142. O'Keefe, J.; Nadel, L. *The Hippocampus as a Cognitive Map*; Oxford University Press: Oxford, UK, 1978; ISBN 9780198572060.
143. Buzsáki, G.; Moser, E.I. Memory, navigation and theta rhythm in the hippocampal-entorhinal system. *Nat. Neurosci.* **2013**, *16*, 130–138. [CrossRef]
144. Sainsbury, R.S.; Heynen, A.; Montoya, C.P. Behavioral correlates of hippocampal type 2 theta in the rat. *Physiol. Behav.* **1987**, *39*, 513–519. [CrossRef]
145. Hegde, P.; Singh, K.; Chaplot, S.; Shankaranarayana Rao, B.S.; Chattarji, S.; Kutty, B.M.; Laxmi, T.R. Stress-induced changes in sleep and associated neuronal activity in rat hippocampus and amygdala. *Neuroscience* **2008**, *153*, 20–30. [CrossRef]
146. Hegde, P.; Jayakrishnan, H.R.; Chattarji, S.; Kutty, B.M.; Laxmi, T.R. Chronic stress-induced changes in REM sleep on theta oscillations in the rat hippocampus and amygdala. *Brain Res.* **2011**, *1382*, 155–164. [CrossRef]
147. Jacinto, L.R.; Reis, J.S.; Dias, N.S.; Cerqueira, J.J.; Correia, J.H.; Sousa, N. Stress affects theta activity in limbic networks and impairs novelty-induced exploration and familiarization. *Front. Behav. Neurosci.* **2013**, *7*, 127. [CrossRef]
148. Jacinto, L.R.; Cerqueira, J.J.; Sousa, N. Patterns of theta activity in limbic anxiety circuit preceding exploratory behavior in approach-avoidance conflict. *Front. Behav. Neurosci.* **2016**, *10*, 171. [CrossRef] [PubMed]
149. Adhikari, A.; Topiwala, M.A.; Gordon, J.A. Synchronized activity between the ventral hippocampus and the medial prefrontal cortex during anxiety. *Neuron* **2010**, *65*, 257–269. [CrossRef] [PubMed]
150. Narayanan, R.T.; Seidenbecher, T.; Kluge, C.; Bergado, J.; Stork, O.; Pape, H.C. Dissociated theta phase synchronization in amygdalo-hippocampal circuits during various stages of fear memory. *Eur. J. Neurosci.* **2007**, *25*, 1823–1831. [CrossRef] [PubMed]
151. Seidenbecher, T.; Lesting, J. Amygdala-hippocampal theta synchrony in learning, memory and disease. In *Insights into the Amygdala: Structure, Functions and Implications for Disorders*; Nova Science Publishers Inc.: Hauppauge, NY, USA, 2012; ISBN 9781622570119.
152. Lesting, J.; Narayanan, R.T.; Kluge, C.; Sangha, S.; Seidenbecher, T.; Pape, H.C. Patterns of coupled theta activity in amygdala-hippocampal-prefrontal cortical circuits during fear extinction. *PLoS ONE* **2011**, *6*, e21714. [CrossRef]
153. Popa, D.; Duvarci, S.; Popescu, A.T.; Lena, C.; Pare, D. Coherent amygdalocortical theta promotes fear memory consolidation during paradoxical sleep. *Proc. Natl. Acad. Sci. USA* **2010**, *107*, 6516–6519. [CrossRef]
154. Yartsev, M.M. Distinct or gradually changing spatial and nonspatial representations along the dorsoventral axis of the hippocampus. *J. Neurosci.* **2010**, *30*, 7758–7760. [CrossRef] [PubMed]
155. Goyal, A.; Miller, J.; Qasim, S.E.; Watrous, A.J.; Zhang, H.; Stein, J.M.; Inman, C.S.; Gross, R.E.; Willie, J.T.; Lega, B.; et al. Functionally distinct high and low theta oscillations in the human hippocampus. *Nat. Commun.* **2020**, *11*, 1–10. [CrossRef]
156. Mikulovic, S.; Restrepo, C.E.; Siwani, S.; Bauer, P.; Pupe, S.; Tort, A.B.L.; Kullander, K.; Leão, R.N. Ventral hippocampal OLM cells control type 2 theta oscillations and response to predator odor. *Nat. Commun.* **2018**, *9*, 3638. [CrossRef]
157. Gray, J.A.; McNaughton, N. Comparison between the behavioural effects of septal and hippocampal lesions: A review. *Neurosci. Biobehav. Rev.* **1983**, *7*, 119–188. [CrossRef]
158. McNaughton, N.; Kocsis, B.; Hajós, M. Elicited hippocampal theta rhythm: A screen for anxiolytic and procognitive drugs through changes in hippocampal function? *Behav. Pharmacol.* **2007**, *18*, 329–346. [CrossRef] [PubMed]
159. McNaughton, N. Development of a theoretically-derived human anxiety syndrome biomarker. *Transl. Neurosci.* **2014**, *5*, 137–146. [CrossRef]
160. Yeung, M.; Dickson, C.T.; Treit, D. Intrahippocampal infusion of the I h blocker ZD7288 slows evoked theta rhythm and produces anxiolytic-like effects in the elevated plus maze. *Hippocampus* **2013**, *23*, 278–286. [CrossRef] [PubMed]
161. Ray, S.; Crone, N.E.; Niebur, E.; Franaszczuk, P.J.; Hsiao, S.S. Neural correlates of high-gamma oscillations (60–200 Hz) in macaque local field potentials and their potential implications in electrocorticography. *J. Neurosci.* **2008**, *28*, 11526–11536. [CrossRef]
162. Buzsáki, G.; Wang, X.-J. Mechanisms of Gamma Oscillations. *Annu. Rev. Neurosci.* **2012**, *35*, 203–225. [CrossRef]
163. Sirota, A.; Montgomery, S.; Fujisawa, S.; Isomura, Y.; Zugaro, M.; Buzsáki, G. Entrainment of neocortical neurons and gamma oscillations by the hippocampal theta rhythm. *Neuron* **2008**, *60*, 683–697. [CrossRef]
164. Bi, K.; Chattun, M.R.; Liu, X.; Wang, Q.; Tian, S.; Zhang, S.; Lu, Q.; Yao, Z. Abnormal early dynamic individual patterns of functional networks in low gamma band for depression recognition. *J. Affect. Disord.* **2018**, *238*, 366–374. [CrossRef]
165. Lee, P.-S.; Chen, Y.-S.; Hsieh, J.-C.; Su, T.-P.; Chen, L.-F. Distinct neuronal oscillatory responses between patients with bipolar and unipolar disorders: A magnetoencephalographic study. *J. Affect. Disord.* **2010**, *123*, 270–275. [CrossRef]
166. Liu, T.Y.; Chen, Y.S.; Su, T.P.; Hsieh, J.C.; Chen, L.F. Abnormal early gamma responses to emotional faces differentiate unipolar from bipolar disorder patients. *Biomed Res. Int.* **2014**, *2014*. [CrossRef]
167. Fitzgerald, P.J.; Watson, B.O. Gamma oscillations as a biomarker for major depression: An emerging topic. *Transl. Psychiatry* **2018**, *8*, 177. [CrossRef] [PubMed]

168. Gilbert, J.R.; Zarate, C.A. Electrophysiological biomarkers of antidepressant response to ketamine in treatment-resistant depression: Gamma power and long-term potentiation. *Pharmacol. Biochem. Behav.* **2020**, *189*, 172856. [CrossRef] [PubMed]
169. Hong, L.E.; Summerfelt, A.; Buchanan, R.W.; O'Donnell, P.; Thaker, G.K.; Weiler, M.A.; Lahti, A.C. Gamma and delta neural oscillations and association with clinical symptoms under subanesthetic ketamine. *Neuropsychopharmacology* **2010**, *35*, 632–640. [CrossRef] [PubMed]
170. Maksimow, A.; Särkelä, M.; Långsjö, J.W.; Salmi, E.; Kaisti, K.K.; Yli-Hankala, A.; Hinkka-Yli-Salomäki, S.; Scheinin, H.; Jääskeläinen, S.K. Increase in high frequency EEG activity explains the poor performance of EEG spectral entropy monitor during S-ketamine anesthesia. *Clin. Neurophysiol.* **2006**, *117*, 1660–1668. [CrossRef] [PubMed]
171. Muthukumaraswamy, S.D.; Shaw, A.D.; Jackson, L.E.; Hall, J.; Moran, R.; Saxena, N. Evidence that subanesthetic doses of ketamine cause sustained disruptions of NMDA and AMPA-mediated frontoparietal connectivity in humans. *J. Neurosci.* **2015**, *35*, 11694–11706. [CrossRef]
172. Shaw, A.D.; Muthukumaraswamy, S.D.; Saxena, N.; Sumner, R.L.; Adams, N.E.; Moran, R.J.; Singh, K.D. Generative modelling of the thalamo-cortical circuit mechanisms underlying the neurophysiological effects of ketamine. *Neuroimage* **2020**, *221*, 117189. [CrossRef]
173. Zacharias, N.; Musso, F.; Müller, F.; Lammers, F.; Saleh, A.; London, M.; de Boer, P.; Winterer, G. Ketamine effects on default mode network activity and vigilance: A randomized, placebo-controlled crossover simultaneous fMRI/EEG study. *Hum. Brain Mapp.* **2020**, *41*, 107–119. [CrossRef] [PubMed]
174. Matveychuk, D.; Thomas, R.K.; Swainson, J.; Khullar, A.; MacKay, M.-A.; Baker, G.B.; Dursun, S.M. Ketamine as an antidepressant: Overview of its mechanisms of action and potential predictive biomarkers. *Ther. Adv. Psychopharmacol.* **2020**, *10*, 204512532091665. [CrossRef] [PubMed]
175. Ionescu, D.F.; Luckenbaugh, D.A.; Niciu, M.J.; Richards, E.M.; Slonena, E.E.; Vande Voort, J.L.; Brutsche, N.E.; Zarate, C.A. Effect of baseline anxious depression on initial and sustained antidepressant response to Ketamine. *J. Clin. Psychiatry* **2014**, *75*, e932–e938. [CrossRef]
176. Taylor, J.H.; Landeros-Weisenberger, A.; Coughlin, C.; Mulqueen, J.; Johnson, J.A.; Gabriel, D.; Reed, M.O.; Jakubovski, E.; Bloch, M.H. Ketamine for social anxiety disorder: A randomized, placebo-controlled crossover trial. *Neuropsychopharmacology* **2018**, *43*, 325–333. [CrossRef]
177. Cornwell, B.R.; Salvadore, G.; Furey, M.; Marquardt, C.A.; Brutsche, N.E.; Grillon, C.; Zarate, C.A. Synaptic potentiation is critical for rapid antidepressant response to ketamine in treatment-resistant major depression. *Biol. Psychiatry* **2012**, *72*, 555–561. [CrossRef] [PubMed]
178. Nugent, A.C.; Ballard, E.D.; Gould, T.D.; Park, L.T.; Moaddel, R.; Brutsche, N.E.; Zarate, C.A. Ketamine has distinct electrophysiological and behavioral effects in depressed and healthy subjects. *Mol. Psychiatry* **2019**, *24*, 1040–1052. [CrossRef]
179. Engin, E.; Treit, D.; Dickson, C.T. Anxiolytic- and antidepressant-like properties of ketamine in behavioral and neurophysiological animal models. *Neuroscience* **2009**, *161*, 359–369. [CrossRef] [PubMed]
180. Engel, A.K.; Senkowski, D.; Schneider, T.R. Multisensory integration through neural coherence. In *The Neural Bases of Multisensory Processes*; CRC Press: Boca Raton, FL, USA, 2011; ISBN 9781439812198.
181. Sauseng, P.; Klimesch, W. What does phase information of oscillatory brain activity tell us about cognitive processes? *Neurosci. Biobehav. Rev.* **2008**, *32*, 1001–1013. [CrossRef] [PubMed]
182. Xing, M.; Tadayonnejad, R.; MacNamara, A.; Ajilore, O.; DiGangi, J.; Phan, K.L.; Leow, A.; Klumpp, H. Resting-state theta band connectivity and graph analysis in generalized social anxiety disorder. *NeuroImage Clin.* **2017**, *13*, 24–32. [CrossRef]
183. Schutter, D.J.L.G.; Van Honk, J. Salivary cortisol levels and the coupling of midfrontal delta-beta oscillations. *Int. J. Psychophysiol.* **2005**, *55*, 127–129. [CrossRef]
184. Knyazev, G.G. Cross-frequency coupling of brain oscillations: An impact of state anxiety. *Int. J. Psychophysiol.* **2011**, *80*, 236–245. [CrossRef] [PubMed]
185. Van Peer, J.M.; Roelofs, K.; Spinhoven, P. Cortisol administration enhances the coupling of midfrontal delta and beta oscillations. *Int. J. Psychophysiol.* **2008**, *677*, 144–150. [CrossRef] [PubMed]
186. Leung, L.W.S. Spectral analysis of hippocampal EEG in the freely moving rat: Effects of centrally active drugs and relations to evoked potentials. *Electroencephalogr. Clin. Neurophysiol.* **1985**, *60*, 65–77. [CrossRef]
187. Canolty, R.T.; Knight, R.T. The functional role of cross-frequency coupling. *Trends Cogn. Sci.* **2010**, *14*, 506–515. [CrossRef]
188. Salimpour, Y.; Anderson, W.S. Cross-frequency coupling based neuromodulation for treating neurological disorders. *Front. Neurosci.* **2019**, *13*, 125. [CrossRef]
189. Lisman, J. The theta/gamma discrete phase code occuring during the hippocampal phase precession may be a more general brain coding scheme. *Hippocampus* **2005**, *15*, 913–922. [CrossRef] [PubMed]
190. Lisman, J.; Buzsáki, G. A neural coding scheme formed by the combined function of gamma and theta oscillations. *Schizophr. Bull.* **2008**, *34*, 974–980. [CrossRef] [PubMed]
191. Axmacher, N.; Henseler, M.M.; Jensen, O.; Weinreich, I.; Elger, C.E.; Fell, J. Cross-frequency coupling supports multi-item working memory in the human hippocampus. *Proc. Natl. Acad. Sci. USA* **2010**, *107*, 3228–3233. [CrossRef] [PubMed]

biomedicines

MDPI

Article

Fine-Tuning the PI3K/Akt Signaling Pathway Intensity by Sex and Genotype-Load: Sex-Dependent Homozygotic Threshold for Somatic Growth but Feminization of Anxious Phenotype in Middle-Aged PDK1 K465E Knock-In and Heterozygous Mice

Mikel Santana-Santana [1,2], José-Ramón Bayascas [1,3,*] and Lydia Giménez-Llort [1,2,*]

[1] Institut de Neurociències, Universitat Autònoma de Barcelona, 08016 Barcelona, Spain; mikel.santana@e-campus.uab.cat

[2] Department of Psychiatry and Forensic Medicine, School of Medicine, Universitat Autònoma de Barcelona, 08016 Barcelona, Spain

[3] Department of Biochemistry and Molecular Biology, School of Medicine, Universitat Autònoma de Barcelona, 08016 Barcelona, Spain

* Correspondence: lidia.gimenez@uab.cat (J.-R.B.); joseramon.bayascas@uab.cat (L.G.-L.)

Abstract: According to the Research Domain Criteria (RDoC), phenotypic differences among disorders may be explained by variations in the nature and degree of neural circuitry disruptions and/or dysfunctions modulated by several biological and environmental factors. We recently demonstrated the in vivo behavioral translation of tweaking the PI3K/Akt signaling, an essential pathway for regulating cellular processes and physiology, and its modulation through aging. Here we describe, for the first time, the in vivo behavioral impact of the sex and genetic-load tweaking this pathway. The anxiety-like phenotypes of 61 mature (11–14-month-old) male and female PDK1 K465E knock-in, heterozygous, and WT mice were studied. Forced (open-field) anxiogenic environmental conditions were sensitive to detect sex and genetic-load differences at middle age. Despite similar neophobia and horizontal activity among the six groups, females exhibited faster ethograms than males, with increased thigmotaxis, increased wall and bizarre rearing. Genotype-load unveiled increased anxiety in males, resembling female performances. The performance of mutants in naturalistic conditions (marble test) was normal. Homozygotic-load was needed for reduced somatic growth only in males. Factor interactions indicated the complex interplay in the elicitation of different negative valence system's items and the fine-tuning of PI3K/Akt signaling pathway intensity by genotype-load and sex.

Keywords: RDoC; PI3K/Akt; signaling pathway; sex; genetic load; fine tuning; anxiety; aging

Citation: Santana-Santana, M.; Bayascas, J.-R.; Giménez-Llort, L. Fine-Tuning the PI3K/Akt Signaling Pathway Intensity by Sex and Genotype-Load: Sex-Dependent Homozygotic Threshold for Somatic Growth but Feminization of Anxious Phenotype in Middle-Aged PDK1 K465E Knock-In and Heterozygous Mice. *Biomedicines* **2021**, *9*, 747. https://doi.org/10.3390/biomedicines9070747

Academic Editor: Masaru Tanaka

Received: 11 May 2021
Accepted: 22 June 2021
Published: 28 June 2021

1. Introduction

The expression of psychiatric symptoms such as anxiety across lifespan still needs important research efforts to dissect and understand their modulation's biological and environmental basis [1]. Here, the new understanding of psychopathology in terms of dysregulation and dysfunction in essential behavioral features through neurobiology and behavioral neuroscience can provide a promising research scenario [2,3]. In this new conceptualization, fear, aggression, and distress are three draft constructs within the negative valence system (NVS), one of the five domains in the NIMH's Research Domain Criteria (RDoC) matrix [2,4]. This RDoC matrix comprises the interplay between behavioral dimensions or functional constructs inspected by seven different 'units of analysis', namely, genetic and molecular basis, cells and neuronal circuits, physiology of the phenotypes, behavior, and self-report [3]. The molecular genetic basis of NVS phenotypes is considered to be in its infancy, yet with few candidate genes nominated for anxiety disorders [5]. In this context, basic research on signal transduction provides an advanced close examination of the impact of cell membrane receptors and second messengers on cellular biochemistry and physiology. However, the downstream actions unveiling how these genetic aspects translate into anxiety-related NVS constructs are challenging to characterize, mainly when related to biological factors as sex or the genetic load in aging scenarios, since female mice are underrepresented in research [6] and aging animals are scarcely studied [7].

Different PDK1/Akt mutant mice have consistently manifested a higher depressive and/or anxiety-like behavior [8–11]. The 3-phosphoinositide-dependent protein kinase-1 (PDK1) [12], an enzyme that activates Akt among other AGC kinases [13,14], is a key transmitter of extracellular signals of the phosphatidylinositol 3-kinase (PI3K) signaling, a pathway extensively involved in controlling neuronal development and function [15]. Its functional role in cellular biochemistry and physiology, as well as cancer and metabolism, has been largely explored [16], although in recent years, further evidence has been generated about its role in bipolar disorder, depression, anxiety, and schizophrenia [17–23]. In addition, antidepressants, antipsychotics, and mood stabilizers modify Aktactivity [17,24–26]. Moreover, the PDK1/Akt pathway has been also linked with suicide, alcohol drinking, and post-traumatic stress disorder [27–29]. Recently, a non-pharmacological intervention attenuated the cognitive deficit and depressive/anxiety-like behaviors induced by a stressor through the recovery of hippocampal Akt activity [30]. In addition, after postnatal maternal separation, mice treated with an early life non-pharmacological intervention showed ameliorated depressive and anxiety-like behavior through enhanced phosphorylated Akt in the hippocampus [31].

Here, mutant mice for this signaling pathway provide an experimental tool to depict the nuances of its downstream modulation. Mutation of PDK1 Lys465, a residue forms key interactions with the D3 and D4 phosphates of the PtdIns(3,4,5)P3 second messenger, to a Glu residue abolished binding of PDK1 to phosphoinositides and localization at the plasma membrane [32]. This signaling lesion selectively affected the phosphorylation and activation of PKB/Akt isoforms, but left intact the activation of other AGC kinase-family members [33]. These mice present smaller body size and insulin resistance [33]. At the brain level, they also exhibit pronounced Akt signaling deficits in both the cortex and the hippocampus during young adulthood (3–4 months of age) but tend to be attenuated by middle age (11–14 months of age) [34,35]. We recently showed that the double mutation of the PDK1 PH-domain (PDK1−/−) resulted in an enhancement of NVS shown as an increase of responses of fear and anxiety-like behaviors in anxiogenic situations [36]. Interestingly, this seemed to be specific to young adulthood and was found regulated at middle age. In contrast, as measured in a spatial working memory task, cognitive deficits were found in both young and mature mutants and independently of the level of their anxious-like profiles. These distinct age- and function-dependent impacts would agree with the distinct cortical and limbic deficits in the Akt signaling in their brains [34]. The elicitation of age- and regional-dependent specific patterns suggests that fine-tuning the PKB/Akt signal intensity that enables diverse physiological responses also has in vivo translation into the NVS, and age is a key regulatory factor.

Although women are significantly more likely than men to develop an anxiety disorder throughout the lifespan [37], fewer than 45% of animal studies into mood disorders used females [38,39]. The contribution of sex and genetic load in the anxious-like behavioral phenotype in this particular animal model is still unknown. Our previous report suggested that sex differences should be further explored [36]. Regarding genetic load, we hypothesize that heterozygous mice (PDK1+/−) may differ behaviorally from wild-type mice and/or homozygous mice due to differences in the intensity of the Akt signal under physiological conditions. On the other hand, recently, Akt deficiency in Akt isoform mutant mice altered anxiety-like behavior in an isoform- and sex-specific manner [40]. However, those sex-specific behavioral differences could not be explained by Akt expression or activation differences between the sexes.

Therefore, the present study aimed to explore further the contribution of sex and genetic load in the expression of the somatic and anxious-like behavioral phenotype of the PDK1-K465E PH-domain knock-in mice.

2. Materials and Methods

2.1. Generation of $PDK1^{K465E/K465E}$ Mice and Genotyping Analysis

The generation and genotyping of the PDK1 K465E/K465E knock-in mice expressing the single-amino-acid substitution of lysine 465 to glutamic acid in the PDK1 PH domain were described previously [17]. The mice were subjected to PCR genotyping of genomic DNA isolated from ear biopsy using primers K465E F (5′-GGG TGA AGC ATG GAA TCT GTG TCT T) and K465E R (5′-GCC AGG ATA CCT AAG AGT ACC TAG AA). PCR amplification resulted in a 196-bp product from the wild-type allele and a 236-bp product from the targeted allele.

2.2. Animals

A total of 61 mature age (MA, 11–14-month-old) mice, $PDK1^{-/-}$ (14 males, 16 females), $PDK1^{+/-}$ (8 males, 10 females) and $PDK1^{+/+}$ (also referred to as WT, 6 males, 7 females) were used.

Mice were maintained at the Animal House Facility of the Universitat de Lleida under standard husbandry conditions (housed three to four per cage in Macrolon cages, 35 × 35 × 25 cm, with food and water ad libitum, 22 ± 2 °C, a 12 h light: dark cycle and relative humidity 50–60%). Behavioral assessments and data analysis were performed blind to the experiment, in a counterbalanced manner, in the light cycle, from 9:00 to 13:00 h. All procedures were in accordance with Spanish legislation on 'Protection of Animals Used for Experimental and Other Scientific Purposes' and the EU Directive (2010/63/UE) on this subject. The study complies with the ARRIVE guidelines developed by the NC3Rs and aims to reduce the number of animals used [41].

2.3. Behavioral Assessments

Animals were behaviorally assessed for NVS in the open field [42] and the marble-burying tests [43], two unconditioned tests differing in their anxiogenic conditions. A graphical abstract, also including the conclusions, illustrates the methodological setting and procedures (Figure 1).

As measured by body weight, somatic growth was recorded on Day 0 prior to the behavioral battery of tests to monitor possible confounding factors. Lack of sensorimotor problems was already described in these animals in the precedent work [36].

Day 0. Somatic Growth/Bodyweight. Bodyweight was used to measure the somatic growth and physical condition/health status of animals.

Day 1. Open field test (OF). Animals were individually placed in the center of an illuminated (20 lux) open field (homemade woodwork, white box, 55 cm × 55 cm × 25 cm) and observed for 5 min. First, the ethogram of action programs (sequence of behavioral events) was analyzed. Thus, the duration of freezing behavior (latM, latency of movement) and the latency of the behavioral events that follow it were recorded: leaving the central square (latC), reaching the periphery (thigmotaxis) (latP) and performing first wall rearing (latR). Second, the time course and total levels of exploratory activity were measured as horizontal (C, number of crossings) and vertical (Rw, rearing with wall support) locomotor activity. Finally, as previously described [44] we evaluated the presence of bizarre behaviors assessed through the number of stereotyped rearings without wall support (Rc).

Day 2. Marble-Burying Test (MB). The procedure used was as previously described [45]. The mice were placed individually facing the wall in a standard home cage with six glass marbles (1 cm × 1 cm × 1 cm) on a 5-cm-thick layer of clean wood cuttings. The marbles were spaced in three rows of two marbles per row in one half of the cage. The mice were left in the cage with marbles for a 30-min period. The test was terminated by removing the mice. The number of marbles that were buried, changed position (partially buried or turned), and were left intact (I) were measured.

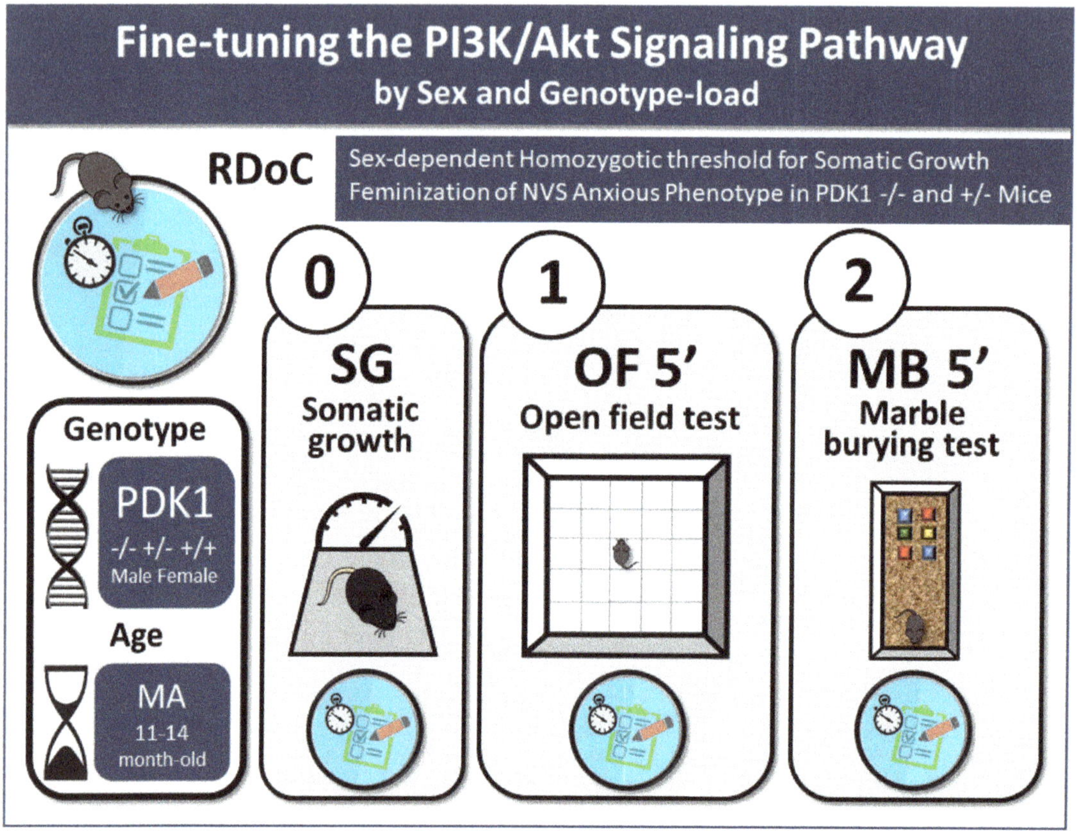

Figure 1. Graphical abstract. Fine-tuning the PI3K/Akt signaling pathway by sex and genotype-load. Experimental design: 3-days battery to assess somatic growth and the Research Domain Criteria (RDoC) negative valence system (NVS) in male and female PDK1−/−, PDK1+/− and PDK1+/+ mice at mature age (MA) are illustrated. Main findings are also indicated.

2.4. Statistics

Statistical analyses were performed using SPSS 15.0 software. All data are presented as mean ± SEM, and are illustrated as bars that illustrate the mean values in each group segregated by genotype and/or sex, as indicated in the legends. To evaluate the effects of the genotype (G) and sex (S) group, a 3 × 2 factorial analysis design was applied. Differences were studied through Multivariate General Lineal model analysis, followed by post hoc Sidak test comparisons when it was possible. For categorical variables, the Fisher's exact test was used. Graphics were made with GraphPad Prims 6, and p-value < 0.05 was considered statistically significant.

3. Results

3.1. Somatic Growth/Bodyweight

The bodyweight of animals showed sex, genotype, and interaction effects. A part of sexual dimorphism (Figure 2A, S, $F_{(1,55)} = 22.035$, $p = 0.000$), significantly lower body weight of PDK1$^{-/-}$ mice than WT and heterozygous mice was observed (Figure 2B, G, $F_{(1,55)} = 15.353$; $p = 0.000$; PDK1$^{+/+}$, ***, $p = 0.000$; PDK1$^{+/-}$, ***, $p = 0.001$). When analyzed per sex and genotype (Figure 2C, G × S, $F_{(1,55)} = 22.035$, $p = 0.000$), post hoc comparisons showed that the higher body weight in males is preserved in all the genotypes (Figure 2C, PDK1$^{+/+}$, s, $p = 0.024$; PDK1$^{+/-}$, sss, $p = 0.001$; PDK1$^{-/-}$, s, $p = 0.030$). Moreover, in females, somatic growth followed a progressive decrease with genotype load (Figure 2C, PDK1$^{+/+}$, g, $p = 0.018$), but heterozygous males had normal weight (Figure 2C, PDK1$^{+/+}$, ggg, $p = 0.000$; PDK1$^{+/-}$, ggg, $p = 0.000$).

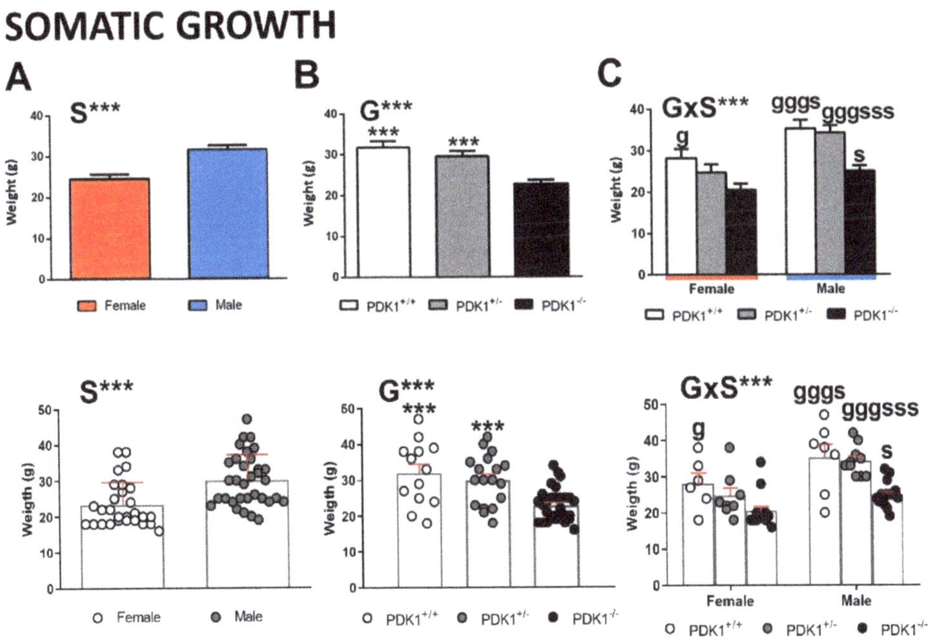

Figure 2. Somatic growth/ body weight in female and male mature PDK1$^{-/-}$, heterozygous PDK1$^{+/-}$ and homozygous WT (PDK1$^{+/+}$) mice. Top panel: Data are expressed as mean ± SEM. Bottom panel: Individual data are depicted. Bars illustrate the genotype or sex groups. Factorial analysis: (**A**) S, sex effect; (**B**) G, genotype effect; (**C**) G × S, genotype × sex interaction effects; *** $p < 0.001$. *Post-hoc* test: genotype: ^{g} $p < 0.05$, ^{ggg} $p < 0.01$ vs. the corresponding KO (PDK1$^{-/-}$, black bar) group; s (sex), ^{s} $p < 0.05$, ^{sss} $p < 0.001$ vs. the corresponding male of the same genotype.

3.2. Open Field Test

Figures 3 and 4 depict the main behavioral domains, events, and units of analysis in the open-field test, showing the distinct sex-dependent performances of homozygous and heterozygous PDK1 mutants compared to WT groups.

Fear and Thigmotaxis—Immediate response to exposure to the open-field was similar among groups, with no differences in the latency of first movement (not shown). Sex differences were found in the latency to leave the center (Figure 3A, S, $F_{(1,55)} = 5.538$; $p = 0.022$) and to reach the periphery (Figure 3B, S, $F_{(1,55)} = 11.057$; $p = 0.002$) with females being faster than males. Post hoc multicomparison analysis showed that this difference was due to sex dimorphism in the behavior of WT mice (Figure 3A, lat center, ss, $p = 0.006$), since PDK+/− and PDK1−/− males also left the center faster than WT males, albeit this difference only reached the statistical significance in the heterozygous group (Figure 3A, lat center, g, $p = 0.018$). This genotype × sex interaction reached statistical significance in the latency to reach the periphery (Figure 3B, G × S, $F_{(2,55)} = 4.028$; $p = 0.023$). Post hoc multicomparison analysis showed that WT females arrived faster than males (Figure 3B, lat periphery, sss, $p = 0.000$) and that both PDK1+/− and PDK1−/− males also reached the periphery sooner than WT (Figure 3B, gg, $p = 0.003$ and gg, $p = 0.008$, respectively).

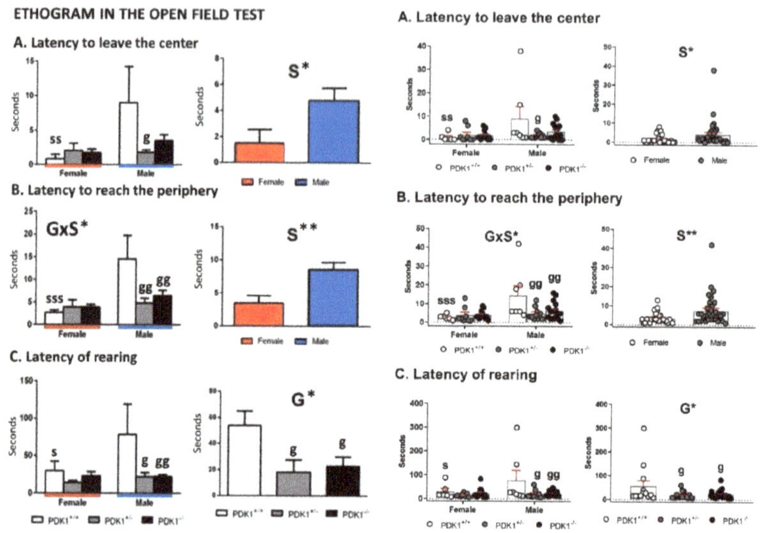

Figure 3. Ethogram in the open-field test in female and male mature PDK1$^{-/-}$, heterozygous PDK1$^{+/-}$ and homozygous WT (PDK1$^{+/+}$) mice. ((**A–C**) **Left panel**): Data are expressed as mean ± SEM or incidence. Bars illustrate the genotype groups. ((**A–C**) **Right panel**): Individual data are depicted. Factorial analysis: G, genotype effect; S, sex effect, * $p < 0.05$, ** $p < 0.01$. *Post-hoc* test: genotype: ^{g} $p < 0.05$, ^{gg} $p < 0.01$ vs. the corresponding WT (PDK1$^{+/+}$) group; s (sex), ^{s} $p < 0.05$, ^{ss} $p < 0.01$, ^{sss} $p < 0.001$ vs. the corresponding male of the same genotype.

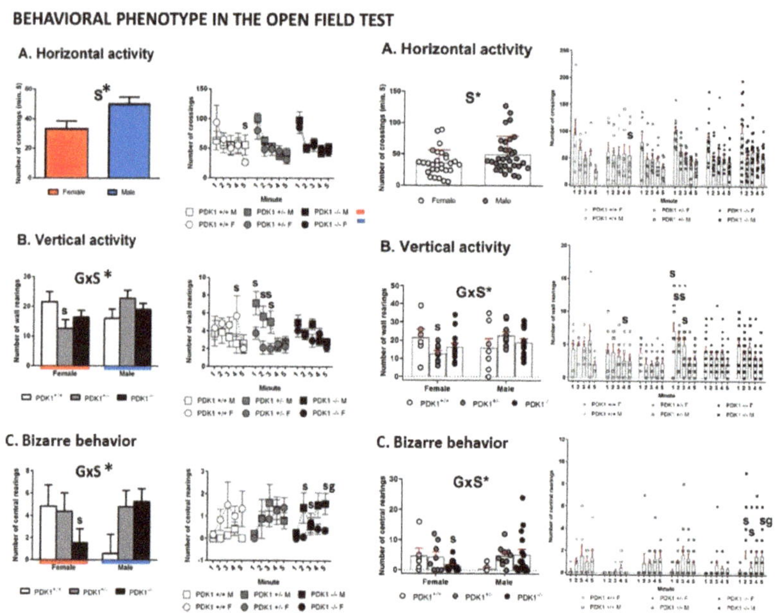

Figure 4. Exploratory and bizarre behaviors in the open-field test in female and male mature PDK1$^{-/-}$, heterozygous PDK1$^{+/-}$ and homozygous WT (PDK1$^{+/+}$) mice. ((**A–C**) **Left panel**): Data are expressed as mean ± SEM or incidence. ((**A–C**) **Right panel**): Individual data are depicted. Bars illustrate the genotype groups, as indicated in the Y-axis. Symbols illustrate the different groups (left panel) or individual values (right panel), as depicted in the legends or abscissae. Factorial analysis: G, genotype effect; S, sex effect, * $p < 0.05$. Post hoc test: g (genotype), ^{g} $p < 0.05$ vs. the corresponding WT (PDK1$^{+/+}$) group; s (sex), ^{s} $p < 0.05$, ^{ss} $p < 0.01$ vs. the corresponding male of the same genotype.

Vertical behavior—Latency of rearing showed a genotype main effect (Figure 3C, G, $F_{(1,55)} = 3.675$; $p = 0.032$), where both PDK1+/− and PDK1 −/− genotypes performed rearing earlier than WT (Figure 3C, *, $p = 0.035$ and *, $p = 0.040$, respectively). Post hoc multicomparison analysis also showed that latency of rearing was shorter in female WT as compared to males (Figure 3C, s, $p = 0.031$) and that both PDK1+/− and PDK1−/− males performed rearing earlier than WT males (Figure 3C, g, $p = 0.016$ and gg, $p = 0.008$, respectively). As shown in Figure 4, the min-by-min analysis of the temporal course of horizontal locomotor activity indicated similar habituation curves in the three genotypes. In the last minute of the test, the female sex performed less activity than males (Figure 4A, S, $F_{(1,55)} = 5.763$; $p = 0.020$). Post hoc multiple comparison analysis indicated that this sex effect was mostly due to the sexual dimorphism of WT mice in minute 5 (Figure 4A, s, $p = 0.043$).

Vertical activity (Wall Rearing): No main but interaction effects were found (Figure 4B, G × S, $F_{(2,55)} = 3.340$; $p = 0.043$). Post hoc multiple comparison analysis showed differences in the heterozygotes where males outperformed more than heterozygote females in minutes 1 (s, $p = 0.036$), 2 (ss, $p = 0.006$), and 3 (s, $p = 0.025$), resulting in a total higher total vertical activity (Figure 4B, s, $F_{(1,55)} = 6.631$, $p = 0.013$). WT females showed a higher rearing behavior in minute 4 (s, $p = 0.047$).

Bizarre behavior (Rearings in the center): No main but interaction effects were also found in the rearings performed in the center of the apparatus (Figure 4C, G × S, $F_{(2,55)} = 3.360$; $p = 0.043$). Post hoc multiple comparison analysis showed homozygote mutant females performed less than homozygote mutant males in minutes 2 (s, $p = 0.034$), 3 (s, $p = 0.048$), 5 (s, $p = 0.018$), resulting in a total lower vertical rearing activity in the center (Figure 4C, s, $F_{(1,55)} = 4.700$, $p = 0.035$). Moreover, in minute 5, homozygote mutant males exhibited more than wild-type mice (Figure 4C, g, $p = 0.039$).

3.3. Marble Burying Test

The qualitative (three levels of interaction) and quantitative (number) analysis of the marble-burying test did not show any statistically significant effect and/or differences between groups (see Figure 5). However, in contrast to the standard quantitative evaluation protocol, the consideration of several levels of interaction with small objects enabled us to uncover the predominant behaviors. That is, in the three strains, the most common behavioral interaction did not result in the complete burying of the marbles but their change of position (turned or partially buried).

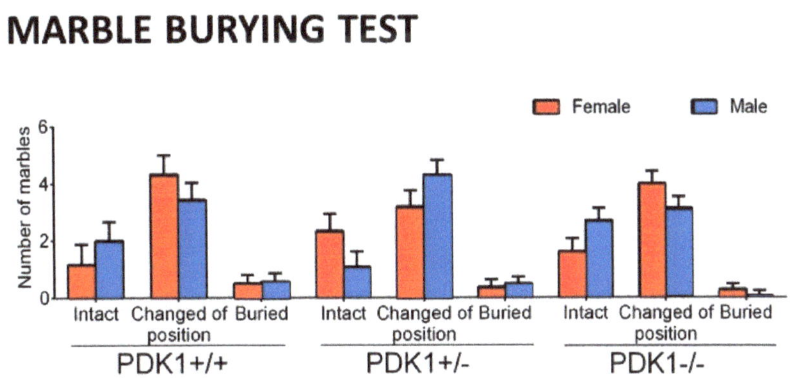

Figure 5. Marble burying test in female and male mature PDK1$^{-/-}$, heterozygous PDK1$^{+/-}$ and homozygous WT (PDK1$^{+/+}$) mice. Top panel: Data are expressed as mean ± SEM or incidence. Bottom panel: Individual data are depicted. Bars illustrate the genotype groups, as indicated in the Y-axis. Symbols illustrate the different groups or individual values, as depicted in the legends or abscissae. Factorial analysis: G, genotype effect; S, sex effect; all $p > 0.05$, *n.s.*

4. Discussion

In the present work, we describe for the first time the in vivo effects of the PDK1 mutation in the PH domain depending on age and genetic load. Mature (11–14 months of age) male and female PDK1$^{-/-}$ and PDK1$^{+/-}$ PH-domain knock-in mice were studied and compared to age- and sex-matched WT mice with normal aging. The results unveil the fine-tuning of the signaling pathways by sex and genetic load, with a feminization of the behavioral profiles.

4.1. Homozygous-Load of the Mutant Gene Is Needed for the Reduced Somatic Growth Effects Only in Mutant Males

As previously described [33,35,36], somatic growth, measured through bodyweight, was found reduced in both male and female PDK1$^{-/-}$ mice. It is known that homozygous male and female PDK1$^{-/-}$ are −35% smaller from birth than WT littermates [33]. In that precedent work, magnetic resonance imaging-obtained images or physical sections of fixed organs using the Cavalieri method described reduced brain volume (−20%) but also of metabolic (liver), immune (spleen, −20%), male gonadal (testis, −50%) organs and a slight reduction in kidney size (albeit did not reach statistical significance) in PDK1$^{-/-}$ mice compared to littermates [33]. Disector principle, a quantitative and unbiased stereological approach to estimate cell volume, also indicated that a reduction in organ volume translated into a reduction of cell size. Thus, in the case of adrenal glands of PDK1$^{-/-}$ animals, a −40% reduction in the relative cell size of zona fasciculata cells was found compared to littermates. Interestingly, the present report shows that heterozygosis was enough to sustain normal weight. However, further analysis segregated by sex unveiled that the half genetic load of wild type PDK1 could guarantee normal somatic growth only in males since heterozygous females were already sensitive to this somatic effect of PDK1/Akt signaling pathway. We hypothesize that this sex-dependent modulation of size translates into the previously reported organ sizes, glucose resistance, hyperinsulinemia, and insulin resistance [33], and future experiments are needed to study it further.

4.2. Similar Neophobia and Locomotion, but Increased Anxiety-Like Phenotype in Mutant Females and Feminized Anxious-Like Phenotype of Mutant Males

In the PDK1$^{-/-}$ mice, the cortical and hippocampal deficits in the PDK1/Akt signaling [34] and the anxious-like phenotype [36] are found attenuated at 11–14 months of age as compared to young adulthood. In the present work, we provide further evidence of a fine-tuning modulation of this signaling pathway by sex and genetic load. Neophobia, an amygdala-dependent immediate fear response to novelty, was similar among the six groups of animals. However, after that, mutant females exhibited a coping with stress strategy characterized by shorter latencies to develop the ethogram, thigmotaxis, increased wall rearing, and presence of bizarre rearings. As previously described, according to their temporal (repetitive/stereotyped or not) and spacial (horizontal/vertical) features, behaviors apparently without a purpose but considered coping-with-stress strategies can be classified as stereotyped stretching, stereotyped rearing, backward movement, and jumping [44]. These disrupted behaviors are scarcely observed in young animals and still difficult to record at middle age, as shown here by the low number in male WT. However, in C57bL/6 mice, we described bizarre behavior that could be conspicuous at 6 months of age when confronting the anxiogenic environments such as the open-field test, mainly in females due to their increased anxious-like profiles as compared to males, or when these responses are found exacerbated by neuropathological conditions [10,44,46]. Here, the bizarre emergent behavior was vertical rearing, which resembles escape behavior in the behavioral despair test. More importantly, in the present work, this female pattern was emulated by homozygous PDK1$^{-/-}$ and heterozygous PDK1$^{+/-}$ male mice, to the extent that the male WT profile was dissonant with the one exhibited by all the other groups. We have shown that bizarre behaviors delay the exploratory activity in adults [44] and aged mice [46], and can be modulated by early-life interventions [44]. Therefore, the selective effects of sex and PDK/Akt signaling genotype-load on the vertical but not the horizontal activity, as shown by normal habituation curves, is noticeable and suggests that underlying mechanisms are mediated by anxiety but not by hyperactivity [47,48].

4.3. *Performance of Mutants Can Resemble Normal under Naturalistic Anxiogenic Conditions*

In the precedent work [36], we demonstrated that in the PDK1 homozygous mice, anxiety but not working memory was modulated by age with a reduction in its expression at 11–13 months of age. This would also explain that here, similarly to previous work [44], the anxiogenic environment of the open and illuminated field test was found to be the best to observe the elicitation of bizarre behaviors, as well the fine-tuning of genotype and sex modulation, but when the behavior of animals was assessed in the marble burying test, behaviors did not differ. Thus, in the current work, similar signatures were shown by the different groups and the 'moved or semi-buried marbles' was found the dominant behavioral readout at the end of the 30 min test. Compared to an anxiogenic open-field test, marble burying is a neuroethological paradigm eliciting spontaneous responses of vigorous and deep digging of beddings to bury the pieces (food pellets or small objects) the animal finds in its environment [49,50]. The interpretation of this test is in constant debate, since it is sensitive to anxiolytic but also antipsychotic drugs [45,51], and it is proposed for modeling compulsive-like characteristics of OCD or autism spectrum disorders [51,52]. Here, as in other research, its use was aimed to in vivo identification of biological impacts in mice [53,54], in our case of genetic load and sex. Furthermore, digging can also be understood as a measure of general activity rather than a measure of repetitive or anxiety-related behavior [51,55–57] and conversely, the animal's general activity can be a confounding factor. Due to this controversy, the open-field or other anxiety tests that also monitor the general activity are a must for interpretations and discard confounding factors. In all cases, in the present work, the impact of sex and genetic load on specific vertical but not on locomotor activity may also agree with the similar signatures observed in this paradigm. This would also agree with reports on drug-induced dose-dependent reduction in marble-burying independently of its locomotor effects [58] or our most recent report in a model for neuropathological aging [47].

5. Conclusions

Of the two unconditioned tests used, the forced (open-field) but not naturalistic (marble arena) anxiogenic environmental conditions were sensitive to detect sex and genetic-load differences at middle age in the PDK1 mutant mice. Thus, despite similar initial fear response (freezing indicating increased neophobia) and horizontal locomotion among the six groups of animals, females exhibited faster ethograms than males, with increased thigmotaxis with shorter latencies to reach the periphery and perform wall rearings, and increased wall and bizarre rearing. Genotype-load unveiled increased anxiety in males in elicitation of male ethograms and profiles resembling the performances characteristic of the female phenotype. While a heterozygous genotype-load was enough to elicit reduced somatic growth (bodyweight) in females, an homozygotic load of PDK1 was needed to exert this somatic effect in males. In summary, factor interactions indicated the complex interplay in the involvement of PI3K/Akt signaling pathway in the elicitation of different NVS's construct items and somatic growth and the relevance of genotype-load and sex in the fine-tuning of its intensity.

Author Contributions: Conceptualization, L.G.-L.; animal model, J.-R.B.; behavioral performance, L.G.-L.; behavioral analysis, statistics and illustrations, M.S.-S.; writing—original draft preparation, M.S.-S. and L.G.-L.; writing—review and editing, M.S.-S., L.G.-L. and J.-R.B.; funding acquisition, J.-R.B. All authors have read and agreed to the published version of the manuscript.

Funding: This research was funded by Ministerio de Economía y Competitividad (MINECO), Programa Estatal de Investigación, Desarrollo e Innovación Orientada a los Retos de la Sociedad (SAF2014-52813-R) to J.-R.B.

Institutional Review Board Statement: The study was conducted according to the guidelines of the Declaration of Helsinki, and approved by the Ethics Committee of Departament de Medi Ambient i Habitatge, Generalitat de Catalunya (CEEAH 2291/DMAH 7493) the 17 March 2014.

Informed Consent Statement: Not applicable.

Data Availability Statement: Not applicable.

Acknowledgments: We thank Jessica Pairada and Núria Moix, Estabulari de Rosegadors of the Universitat de Lleida, for animal care.

Conflicts of Interest: The authors declare no conflict of interest. The funders had no role in the design of the study; in the collection, analyses, or interpretation of data; in the writing of the manuscript, or in the decision to publish the results.

References

1. Lenze, E.J.; Wetherell, J.L. A lifespan view of anxiety disorders. *Dialogues Clin. Neurosci.* **2011**, *13*, 381–399. [CrossRef]
2. National Institute of Mental Health. Research Domain Criteria. (Internet) NIHM. Available online: https://www.nimh.nih.gov/research/research-funded-by-nimh/rdoc/index.shtml (accessed on 29 February 2020).
3. Asher, J. Genes and Circuitry, Not Just Clinical Observation, to Guide Classification for Research (Internet). NIMH; 2010. Available online: https://www.nimh.nih.gov/news/science-news/2010/genes-and-circuitry-not-just-clinical-observation-to-guide-classification-for-research.shtml (accessed on 29 February 2020).
4. Cuthbert, B.N.; Insel, T.R. Toward the future of psychiatric diagnosis: The seven pillars of RDoC. *BMC Med.* **2013**, *11*, 126. [CrossRef]
5. Savage, J.E.; Sawyers, C.; Roberson-Nay, R.; Hettema, J.M. The genetics of anxiety-related negative valence system traits. *Am. J. Med. Genet. Part B Neuropsychiatr. Genet.* **2017**, *174*, 156–177. [CrossRef]
6. Prendergast, B.J.; Onishi, K.G.; Zucker, I. Female mice liberated for inclusion in neuroscience and biomedical research. *Neurosci. Biobehav. Rev.* **2014**, *40*, 1–5. [CrossRef] [PubMed]
7. Mitchell, S.J.; Scheibye-Knudsen, M.; Longo, D.L.; de Cabo, R. Animal Models of Aging Research: Implications for Human Aging and Age-Related Diseases. *Annu. Rev. Anim. Biosci.* **2015**, *3*, 283–303. [CrossRef]
8. Ackermann, T.F.; Hörtnagl, H.; Wolfer, D.P.; Colacicco, G.; Sohr, R.; Lang, F.; Hellweg, R.; Lang, U.E. Phosphatidylinositide Dependent Kinase Deficiency Increases Anxiety and Decreases GABA and Serotonin Abundance in the Amygdala. *Cell. Physiol. Biochem.* **2008**, *22*, 735–744. [CrossRef] [PubMed]
9. Leibrock, C.; Ackermann, T.F.; Hierlmeier, M.; Lang, F.; Borgwardt, S.; Lang, U.E. Akt2 Deficiency is Associated with Anxiety and Depressive Behavior in Mice. *Cell. Physiol. Biochem.* **2013**, *32*, 766–777. [CrossRef] [PubMed]
10. Cordón-Barris, L.; Pascual-Guiral, S.; Yang, S.; Giménez-Llort, L.; Lope-Piedrafita, S.; Niemeyer, C.; Claro, E.; Lizcano, J.M.; Bayascas, J.R. Mutation of the 3-Phosphoinositide-Dependent Protein Kinase 1 (PDK1) Substrate-Docking Site in the Developing Brain Causes Microcephaly with Abnormal Brain Morphogenesis Independently of Akt, Leading to Impaired Cognition and Disruptive Behaviors. *Mol. Cell. Biol.* **2016**, *36*, 2967–2982. [CrossRef]
11. Bergeron, Y.; Bureau, G.; Laurier-Laurin, M.-É.; Asselin, E.; Massicotte, G.; Cyr, M. Genetic Deletion of Akt3 Induces an Endophenotype Reminiscent of Psychiatric Manifestations in Mice. *Front. Mol. Neurosci.* **2017**, *10*, 102. [CrossRef] [PubMed]
12. Alessi, D.R.; James, S.R.; Downes, C.; Holmes, A.B.; Gaffney, P.R.; Reese, C.B.; Cohen, P. Characterization of a 3-phosphoinositide-dependent protein kinase which phosphorylates and activates protein kinase Bα. *Curr. Biol.* **1997**, *7*, 261–269. [CrossRef]
13. Mora, A.; Komander, D.; van Aalten, D.M.; Alessi, D.R. PDK1, the master regulator of AGC kinase signal transduction. *Semin. Cell Dev. Biol.* **2004**, *15*, 161–170. [CrossRef]
14. Pearce, L.R.; Komander, D.; Alessi, D. The nuts and bolts of AGC protein kinases. *Nat. Rev. Mol. Cell Biol.* **2010**, *11*, 9–22. [CrossRef] [PubMed]
15. Waite, K.; Eickholt, B.J. The Neurodevelopmental Implications of PI3K Signaling. *Curr. Top. Microbiol. Immunol.* **2010**, *346*, 245–265. [CrossRef]
16. Bayascas, J.R. PDK1: The Major Transducer of PI 3-Kinase Actions. *Curr. Top. Microbiol. Immunol.* **2010**, *346*, 9–29. [CrossRef] [PubMed]
17. Jope, R.S.; Roh, R.S. Glycogen Synthase Kinase-3 (GSK3) in Psychiatric Diseases and Therapeutic Interventions. *Curr. Drug Targets* **2006**, *7*, 1421–1434. [CrossRef]
18. Beaulieu, J.-M.; Gainetdinov, R.; Caron, M.G. Akt/GSK3 Signaling in the Action of Psychotropic Drugs. *Annu. Rev. Pharmacol. Toxicol.* **2009**, *49*, 327–347. [CrossRef]
19. Freyberg, Z.; Ferrando, S.J.; Javitch, J.A. Roles of the Akt/GSK-3 and Wnt Signaling Pathways in Schizophrenia and Antipsychotic Drug Action. *Am. J. Psychiatry* **2010**, *167*, 388–396. [CrossRef]
20. Jope, R.S. Glycogen Synthase Kinase-3 in the Etiology and Treatment of Mood Disorders. *Front. Mol. Neurosci.* **2011**, *4*, 16. [CrossRef] [PubMed]

21. Sachs, B.D.; Rodriguiz, R.M.; Siesser, W.B.; Kenan, A.; Royer, E.L.; Jacobsen, J.P.R.; Wetsel, W.C.; Caron, M.G. The effects of brain serotonin deficiency on behavioural disinhibition and anxiety-like behaviour following mild early life stress. *Int. J. Neuropsychopharmacol.* **2013**, *16*, 2081–2094. [CrossRef] [PubMed]
22. Singh, K. An emerging role for Wnt and GSK3 signaling pathways in schizophrenia. *Clin. Genet.* **2013**, *83*, 511–517. [CrossRef]
23. Beurel, E.; Grieco, S.F.; Jope, R.S. Glycogen synthase kinase-3 (GSK3): Regulation, actions, and diseases. *Pharmacol. Ther.* **2015**, *148*, 114–131. [CrossRef] [PubMed]
24. Shi, H.-S.; Zhu, W.-L.; Liu, J.; Luo, Y.-X.; Si, J.-J.; Wang, S.-J.; Xue, Y.-X.; Ding, Z.-B.; Shi, J.; Lu, L. PI3K/Akt Signaling Pathway in the Basolateral Amygdala Mediates the Rapid Antidepressant-like Effects of Trefoil Factor 3. *Neuropsychopharmacology* **2012**, *37*, 2671–2683. [CrossRef]
25. Wang, W.; Lu, Y.; Xue, Z.; Li, C.; Wang, C.; Zhao, X.; Zhang, J.; Wei, X.; Chen, X.; Cui, W.; et al. Rapid-acting antidepressant-like effects of acetyl-l-carnitine mediated by PI3K/AKT/BDNF/VGF signaling pathway in mice. *Neuroscience* **2015**, *285*, 281–291. [CrossRef] [PubMed]
26. Tao, W.; Dong, Y.; Su, Q.; Wang, H.; Chen, Y.; Xue, W.; Chen, C.; Xia, B.; Duan, J.; Chen, G. Liquiritigenin reverses depression-like behavior in unpredictable chronic mild stress-induced mice by regulating PI3K/Akt/mTOR mediated BDNF/TrkB pathway. *Behav. Brain Res.* **2016**, *308*, 177–186. [CrossRef] [PubMed]
27. Dwivedi, Y.; Rizavi, H.S.; Zhang, H.; Roberts, R.C.; Conley, R.R.; Pandey, G.N. Modulation in Activation and Expression of Phosphatase and Tensin Homolog on Chromosome Ten, Akt1, and 3-Phosphoinositide-Dependent Kinase 1: Further Evidence Demonstrating Altered Phosphoinositide 3-Kinase Signaling in Postmortem Brain of Suicide Subjects. *Biol. Psychiatry* **2010**, *67*, 1017–1025. [CrossRef]
28. Neasta, J.; Ben Hamida, S.; Yowell, Q.V.; Carnicella, S.; Ron, D. AKT Signaling Pathway in the Nucleus Accumbens Mediates Excessive Alcohol Drinking Behaviors. *Biol. Psychiatry* **2011**, *70*, 575–582. [CrossRef]
29. Dahlhoff, M.; Siegmund, A.; Golub, Y.; Wolf, E.; Holsboer, F.; Wotjak, C. AKT/GSK-3β/β-catenin signalling within hippocampus and amygdala reflects genetically determined differences in posttraumatic stress disorder like symptoms. *Neuroscience* **2010**, *169*, 1216–1226. [CrossRef] [PubMed]
30. Sun, L.; Cui, K.; Xing, F.; Liu, X. Akt dependent adult hippocampal neurogenesis regulates the behavioral improvement of treadmill running to mice model of post-traumatic stress disorder. *Behav. Brain Res.* **2020**, *379*, 112375. [CrossRef]
31. Huang, H.; Wang, Q.; Guan, X.; Zhang, X.; Zhang, Y.; Cao, J.; Li, X. Effects of enriched environment on depression and anxiety-like behavior induced by early life stress: A comparison between different periods. *Behav. Brain Res.* **2021**, *411*, 113389. [CrossRef]
32. Komander, D.; Fairservice, A.; Deak, M.; Kular, G.S.; Prescott, A.; Downes, C.P.; Safrany, S.; Alessi, D.; Van Aalten, D.M.F. Structural insights into the regulation of PDK1 by phosphoinositides and inositol phosphates. *EMBO J.* **2004**, *23*, 3918–3928. [CrossRef]
33. Bayascas, J.R.; Wullschleger, S.; Sakamoto, K.; García-Martínez, J.M.; Clacher, C.; Komander, D.; van Aalten, D.M.F.; Boini, K.M.; Lang, F.; Lipina, C.; et al. Mutation of the PDK1 PH Domain Inhibits Protein Kinase B/Akt, Leading to Small Size and Insulin Resistance. *Mol. Cell. Biol.* **2008**, *28*, 3258–3272. [CrossRef]
34. Yang, S.; Pascual-Guiral, S.; Ponce, R.; Giménez-Llort, L.; Baltrons, M.A.; Arancio, O.; Palacio, J.R.; Clos, V.M.; Yuste, V.J.; Bayascas, J.R. Reducing the Levels of Akt Activation by PDK1 Knock-in Mutation Protects Neuronal Cultures against Synthetic Amyloid-Beta Peptides. *Front. Aging Neurosci.* **2018**, *9*, 435. [CrossRef] [PubMed]
35. Zurashvili, T.; Cordón-Barris, L.; Ruiz-Babot, G.; Zhou, X.; Lizcano, J.M.; Gómez, N.; Giménez-Llort, L.; Bayascas, J.R. Interaction of PDK1 with Phosphoinositides Is Essential for Neuronal Differentiation but Dispensable for Neuronal Survival. *Mol. Cell. Biol.* **2013**, *33*, 1027–1040. [CrossRef] [PubMed]
36. Giménez-Llort, L.; Santana-Santana, M.; Bayascas, J.R. The Impact of the PI3K/Akt Signaling Pathway in Anxiety and Working Memory in Young and Middle-Aged PDK1 K465E Knock-In Mice. *Front. Behav. Neurosci.* **2020**, *14*, 61. [CrossRef] [PubMed]
37. McLean, C.P.; Asnaani, A.; Litz, B.T.; Hofmann, S.G. Gender differences in anxiety disorders: Prevalence, course of illness, comorbidity and burden of illness. *J. Psychiatr. Res.* **2011**, *45*, 1027–1035. [CrossRef]
38. Zucker, I.; Beery, A. Males still dominate animal studies. *Nat. Cell Biol.* **2010**, *465*, 690. [CrossRef]
39. Beery, A.; Zucker, I. Sex bias in neuroscience and biomedical research. *Neurosci. Biobehav. Rev.* **2011**, *35*, 565–572. [CrossRef]
40. Wong, H.; Levenga, J.; Laplante, L.; Keller, B.; Cooper-Sansone, A.; Borski, C.; Milstead, R.; Ehringer, M.; Hoeffer, C. Isoform-specific roles for AKT in affective behavior, spatial memory, and extinction related to psychiatric disorders. *eLife* **2020**, *9*, 56630. [CrossRef]
41. Kilkenny, C.; Browne, W.J.; Cuthill, I.C.; Emerson, M.; Altman, D.G. Improving Bioscience Research Reporting: The ARRIVE Guidelines for Reporting Animal Research. *PLoS Biol.* **2010**, *8*, e1000412. [CrossRef]
42. Hall, C.S.; Ballachey, E.L. A study of the rat's behavior in a field: A contribution to method in comparative psychology. *Univ. Calif. Publ. Psychol.* **1932**, *6*, 1–12.
43. Deacon, R.M.J. Digging and marble burying in mice: Simple methods for in vivo identification of biological impacts. *Nat. Protoc.* **2006**, *1*, 122–124. [CrossRef]
44. Baeta-Corral, R.; Giménez-Llort, L. Bizarre behaviors and risk assessment in 3xTg-AD mice at early stages of the disease. *Behav. Brain Res.* **2014**, *258*, 97–105. [CrossRef] [PubMed]
45. Torres-Lista, V.; López-Pousa, S.; Giménez-Llort, L. Marble-burying is enhanced in 3xTg-AD mice, can be reversed by risperidone and it is modulable by handling. *Behav. Process.* **2015**, *116*, 69–74. [CrossRef] [PubMed]

46. Castillo-Mariqueo, L.; Giménez-Llort, L. Translational Modeling of Psychomotor Function in Normal and AD-Pathological Aging With Special Concerns on the Effects of Social Isolation. *Front. Aging* **2021**, *2*, 5. [CrossRef]
47. Gimenez-Llort, L.; Alveal-Mellado, D. Digging Signatures in 13-Month-Old 3xTg-AD Mice for Alzheimer's Disease and Its Disruption by Isolation Despite Social Life Since They Were Born. *Front. Behav. Neurosci.* **2021**, *14*, 611384. [CrossRef]
48. Muntsant, A.; Giménez-Llort, L. Impact of Social Isolation on the Behavioral, Functional Profiles, and Hippocampal Atrophy Asymmetry in Dementia in Times of Coronavirus Pandemic (COVID-19): A Translational Neuroscience Approach. *Front. Psychiatry* **2020**, *11*, 572583. [CrossRef]
49. Pinel, J.P.; Treit, D. Burying as a defensive response in rats. *J. Comp. Physiol. Psychol.* **1978**, *92*, 708–712. [CrossRef]
50. Gyertyán, I. Analysis of the marble burying response: Marbles serve to measure digging rather than evoke burying. *Behav. Pharmacol.* **1995**, *6*, 24–31.
51. De Brouwer, G.; Fick, A.; Harvey, B.H.; Wolmarans, D.W. A critical inquiry into marble-burying as a preclinical screening paradigm of relevance for anxiety and obsessive–compulsive disorder: Mapping the way forward. *Cogn. Affect. Behav. Neurosci.* **2019**, *19*, 1–39. [CrossRef]
52. Mahmood, H.M.; Aldhalaan, H.M.; Alshammari, T.K.; Alqasem, M.A.; Alshammari, M.A.; Albekairi, N.A.; AlSharari, S.D. The Role of Nicotinic Receptors in the Attenuation of Autism-Related Behaviors in a Murine BTBR T + tf/J Autistic Model. *Autism Res.* **2020**, *13*, 1311–1334. [CrossRef]
53. Broekkamp, C.L.; Rijk, H.W.; Joly-Gelouin, D.; Lloyd, K.L. Major tranquillizers can be distinguished from minor tranquillizers on the basis of effects on marble burying and swim-induced grooming in mice. *Eur. J. Pharmacol.* **1986**, *126*, 223–229. [CrossRef]
54. Deacon, R.M.; Bannerman, D.; Kirby, B.; Croucher, A.; Rawlins, J.P. Effects of cytotoxic hippocampal lesions in mice on a cognitive test battery. *Behav. Brain Res.* **2002**, *133*, 57–68. [CrossRef]
55. Greene-Schloesser, D.M.; Van Der Zee, E.A.; Sheppard, D.K.; Castillo, M.R.; Gregg, K.A.; Burrow, T.; Foltz, H.; Slater, M.; Bult-Ito, A. Predictive validity of a non-induced mouse model of compulsive-like behavior. *Behav. Brain Res.* **2011**, *221*, 55–62. [CrossRef] [PubMed]
56. Mitra, S.; Bastos, C.; Chesworth, S.; Frye, C.; Bult-Ito, A. Strain and sex based characterization of behavioral expressions in non-induced compulsive-like mice. *Physiol. Behav.* **2017**, *168*, 103–111. [CrossRef] [PubMed]
57. Dixit, P.V.; Sahu, R.; Mishra, D.K. Marble-burying behavior test as a murine model of compulsive-like behavior. *J. Pharmacol. Toxicol. Methods* **2020**, *102*, 106676. [CrossRef] [PubMed]
58. Jimenez-Gomez, C.; Osentoski, A.; Woods, J.H. Pharmacological evaluation of the adequacy of marble burying as an animal model of compulsion and/or anxiety. *Behav. Pharmacol.* **2011**, *22*, 711–713. [CrossRef] [PubMed]

biomedicines

Review

Immune Influencers in Action: Metabolites and Enzymes of the Tryptophan-Kynurenine Metabolic Pathway

Masaru Tanaka [1,2], Fanni Tóth [1], Helga Polyák [2], Ágnes Szabó [2], Yvette Mándi [3] and László Vécsei [1,2,*]

1 MTA-SZTE—Neuroscience Research Group, H-6725 Szeged, Hungary; tanaka.masaru.1@med.u-szeged.hu (M.T.); toth.fanni@med.u-szeged.hu (F.T.)
2 Interdisciplinary Excellence Centre, Department of Neurology, Faculty of Medicine, University of Szeged, H-6725 Szeged, Hungary; polyak.helga@med.u-szeged.hu (H.P.); szabo.agnes.4@med.u-szeged.hu (Á.S.)
3 Department of Medical Microbiology and Immunology, Faculty of Medicine, University of Szeged, H-6720 Szeged, Hungary; mandi.yvette@med.u-szeged.hu
* Correspondence: vecsei.laszlo@med.u-szeged.hu; Tel.: +36-62-545-351

Abstract: The tryptophan (TRP)-kynurenine (KYN) metabolic pathway is a main player of TRP metabolism through which more than 95% of TRP is catabolized. The pathway is activated by acute and chronic immune responses leading to a wide range of illnesses including cancer, immune diseases, neurodegenerative diseases and psychiatric disorders. The presence of positive feedback loops facilitates amplifying the immune responses vice versa. The TRP-KYN pathway synthesizes multifarious metabolites including oxidants, antioxidants, neurotoxins, neuroprotectants and immunomodulators. The immunomodulators are known to facilitate the immune system towards a tolerogenic state, resulting in chronic low-grade inflammation (LGI) that is commonly present in obesity, poor nutrition, exposer to chemicals or allergens, prodromal stage of various illnesses and chronic diseases. KYN, kynurenic acid, xanthurenic acid and cinnabarinic acid are aryl hydrocarbon receptor ligands that serve as immunomodulators. Furthermore, TRP-KYN pathway enzymes are known to be activated by the stress hormone cortisol and inflammatory cytokines, and genotypic variants were observed to contribute to inflammation and thus various diseases. The tryptophan 2,3-dioxygenase, the indoleamine 2,3-dioxygenases and the kynurenine-3-monooxygenase are main enzymes in the pathway. This review article discusses the TRP-KYN pathway with special emphasis on its interaction with the immune system and the tolerogenic shift towards chronic LGI and overviews the major symptoms, pro- and anti-inflammatory cytokines and toxic and protective KYNs to explore the linkage between chronic LGI, KYNs, and major psychiatric disorders, including depressive disorder, bipolar disorder, substance use disorder, post-traumatic stress disorder, schizophrenia and autism spectrum disorder.

Keywords: chronic inflammation; low-grade inflammation; immune tolerance; inflammatory factor; kynurenine; kynurenic acid; depression; bipolar disorder; substance use disorder; post-traumatic stress disorder; schizophrenia; autism spectrum disorder

Citation: Tanaka, M.; Tóth, F.; Polyák, H.; Szabó, Á.; Mándi, Y.; Vécsei, L. Immune Influencers in Action: Metabolites and Enzymes of the Tryptophan-Kynurenine Metabolic Pathway. *Biomedicines* **2021**, 9, 734. https://doi.org/10.3390/biomedicines9070734

Academic Editor: Rosanna Di Paola

Received: 10 June 2021
Accepted: 23 June 2021
Published: 25 June 2021

1. Introduction

Chronic low-grade inflammation (LGI) has been linked to the prodromal stage of a broad range of chronic illnesses such as cardiovascular-, metabolic-, immunologic-, neurodegenerative- and psychiatric diseases [1]. Chronic LGI is characterized by the long-term of unresolved inflammatory condition in which proinflammatory and anti-inflammatory factors are continuously released and fail to cease their actions (Figure 1a). The long-lasting release of the inflammatory factors initiates compensatory immune suppression and consequently causes immune tolerance, a condition in which the immune system is unresponsive to particular antigens that normally elicit an immune response (Figure 1b).

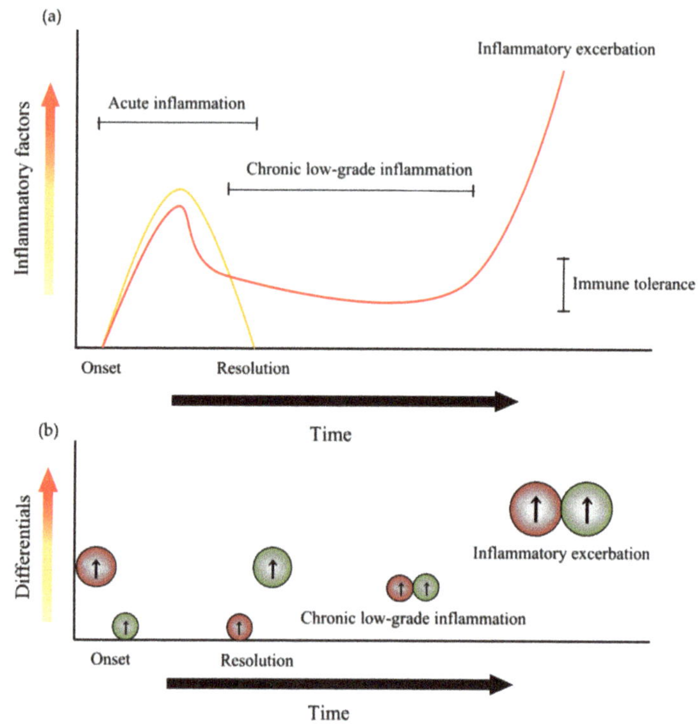

Figure 1. Acute inflammation, chronic low-grade inflammation and the status of pro-inflammatory and anti-inflammatory factors. (**a**) Acute inflammation onsets with the increase of inflammatory factors and is resolved with the decrease of inflammatory cytokines (yellow line). Chronic low-grade inflammation (LGI) is characterized by a period of relatively low-level inflammatory factors that induce immune tolerance. Eventually, inflammatory factors increase, leading to inflammatory exacerbation and contributing to the pathogenesis of various diseases (red line). (**b**) Relative levels of pro-inflammatory (in red) and anti-inflammatory (in green) factors after the onset and before the resolution of acute inflammation, during LGI and at inflammatory exacerbation.

C-reactive protein (CRP) is a well-established biomarker of inflammation and in LGI the plasma concentration of CRP is between 3 mg/L–10 mg/L. LGI was found to be negatively associated with self-rated physical health score in Health-Related Quality of Life (HRQL) in healthy individuals, but not associated with mental health score in HRQL [2]. Thus, an additional biomarker is necessary to seek the linkage between LGI and mental illnesses. Furthermore, the central nervous system (CNS) is an immune-privileged site that may become the source of inflammatory factors to maintain the immune tolerance. The privileged status of the CNS immune system depends on the integrity of the blood-brain barrier (BBB) and the subsequent influence of inflammatory factors from other parts of the body such as muscles and gut microbiota. The long-term immune tolerance proceeds to significantly higher secretion of inflammatory factors which is linked to inflammatory exacerbation and consequently, pathogenesis of a wide range of neurologic- and psychiatric diseases [3] (Figure 1b).

The tryptophan (TRP)-kynurenine (KYN) metabolic pathway is gaining growing attention as the immune regulator which plays a crucial role of the pathogenesis of a wide range of diseases from cancer to psychiatric disorders. The pathway is a major branch of L-TRP metabolism that is significantly activated during inflammation reaction. Over 95% of L-TRP transforms into a palette of small bioactive molecules with oxidant, antioxidant, neurotoxic, neuroprotective and/or immunomodulatory property. Particularly, KYN, kynurenic acid (KYNA), xanthurenic acid (XA) and cinnabarinic acid (CA) are ligands of the aryl hydrocarbon receptor (AhR) which plays a crucial role in the modulation of inflammation and the subsequent resolution, and the induction of immune tolerance [4].

AhR is a transcription factor that regulates gene expression, but it modulates inflammation through genomic and non-genomic pathways [5]. KYNs are proposed to be emerging players in immunoregulatory networks through AhRs and can be targets for immunotherapy [6]. Strong skeletal muscle mass plays an important role in maintaining effective immune functions. Physical exercise influences the muscle TRP-KYN metabolism and thus energy homeostasis. Intervention through physical exercise program is under thorough study for obesity and chronic illnesses including diseases affecting the CNS [7–9].

The activation of the TRP-KYN pathway reversed the progression of the experimental autoimmune encephalomyelitis mouse disease, an animal model of multiple sclerosis (MS) [10]. Monitoring the status of reduction-oxidation as well as KYNs was proposed for useful biomarkers in MS [11]. Cognitive performance, the activation of immune system, and the TRP-KYN pathway were linked in the elderly as well as neurodegenerative diseases [12,13]. KYNA was reported to possess antidepressant-like effects and KYNA analogues were described as potential anti-dementia drugs [14,15]. The TRP-KYN pathway is involved in migraine headache and is one of the potential targets as anti-migraine drugs [16]. Modulation of the pathway was found to reduce or prevent substance abuse [17]. Furthermore, AhR also participates in the gut-brain axis. A novel link between gut microbiota and schizophrenia (SCZ) has been explored in the KYN system [18]. The commensal microflora and microbial AhR agonists are under extensive research in search of the gut microflora-produced biomolecules in influence on CNS and thus novel opportunities for AhR-targeted medications [19]. This review article discusses the metabolites and enzymes of the TRP-KYN metabolic pathway with a special emphasis on its interaction with the immune system, and the major symptoms, pro- and anti-inflammatory cytokines and toxic and protective KYNs of major psychiatric disorders.

2. The Kynurenine System

The essential amino acid TRP is metabolized into several different bioactive molecules such as nicotinamide adenine dinucleotide (NAD^+), serotonin (5-hydroxytryptamine, 5-HT), and melatonin (MT). Only 1–5% of TRP is utilized through the methoxyindole pathway, synthesizing 5-HT and MT; however, 90–95% of TRP is utilized in the TRP-KYN metabolic pathway which is leading to the synthesis of NAD^+ and other bioactive molecules. Many cell types and organs have important roles in the pathway, such as the brain, liver, intestine and immune cells. NAD^+ is a main cofactor of the electron transport in the mitochondrial respiratory chain, which is essential for the synthesis of adenosine triphosphate (ATP), ATP also plays an important role in the brain's glycogen storage and in several enzyme reactions. In addition to NAD^+, several bioactive molecules are synthesized in the pathway [20].

Firstly, L-TRP is converted to N-formyl-kynurenine by tryptophan 2,3-dioxygenase (TDO) or indoleamine 2,3-dioxygenase (IDO) 1 or 2. N-formyl-kynurenine is degraded to L-KYN by formamidase. L-KYN is metabolized by three ways: to KYNA by kynurenine aminotransferase (KATs), to 3-hydroxy-kynurenine (3-HK) by kynurenine 3-monooxygenase (KMO) and to anthranilic acid (AA) by kynureninase. KAT enzymes also transform 3-HA to XA. 3-HK and AA are transformed to 3-hydroxyanthranilic acid (3-HAA) by kynureninase or in a non-specific hydroxylation, respectively. In this case, 3-HAA is converted to picolinic acid (PIC) by 2-amino-3-carboxymuconate-semialdehyde decarboxylase, and to quinolinic acid (QUIN) by 3-hydroxyanthranilate dioxygenase. XA is converted to CA by autoxidation. CA is also produced from 3-HK or QUIN. Eventually, QUIN is transformed into nicotinic acid ribonucleotide, then to nicotinic acid, leading to the formation of NAD^+ [20] (Figure 2).

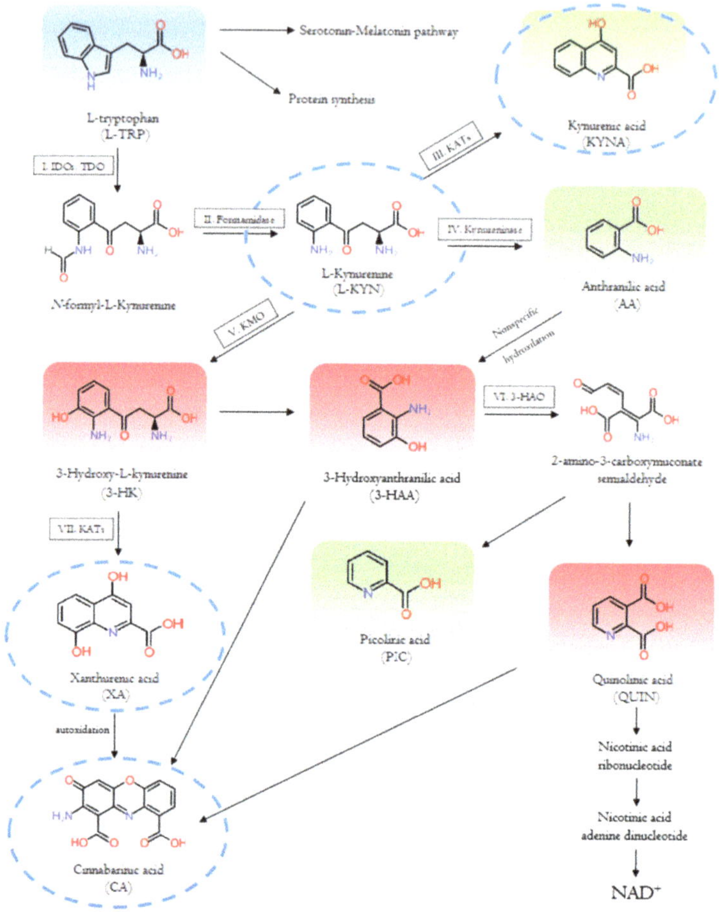

Figure 2. The tryptophan-kynurenine metabolic pathway and bioactive kynurenine metabolites. The pathway depends on the type of cells. In some cells some enzyme is missing, and thus, some metabolite is not produced. The kynurenine metabolites are multifarious molecules with various properties. The aryl hydrocarbon receptor (AhR) ligands are circled with a blue dotted line; toxic kynurenines (KYNs) are in red shade, and protective KYNs are in green shade [20].

2.1. *Enzymes and Metabolites of the Tryptophan-Kynurenine Pathway*

Many studies have reported association between the TRP-KYN metabolic pathway, its metabolites and enzymes and the immune systems. TRP degradation via the pathway is activated by an acute immune response in a wide range of diseases, including immune disorders, neurodegenerative and psychiatric diseases, as well as cancer [21–25]. The enzymes involved in the pathway play a major role in various immunological and inflammatory processes. Furthermore, the metabolites of the pathway are also involved in numerous pathological and physiological processes [13,25]. These metabolites can be neuroprotective, neurotoxic, oxidant, antioxidant and/or immune modifiers [26]. In addition, KYN metabolites have proinflammatory, anti-inflammatory and immunosuppressive properties [27]. They regulate the proliferation and function of several immune cells [28]. The pathway is important in mediating the equilibrium between activation and inhibition of the immune system. It is a controller of innate and adaptive immune responses [29].

2.1.1. The Interaction with the Immune System

The interaction of the TRP-KYN metabolic pathway with the immune system were demonstrated in viral or bacterial inflammatory processes [30], including in autoimmune diseases such as systemic lupus erythematosus (SLE) and Sjögren's syndrome (SjS). Analysis of peripheral blood of SjS patients found higher expression of IDO-1 in the patients' dendritic cells, compared to the dendritic cells of healthy controls [31] (Table 1). In SjS patients, high levels of IDO were reported in T cells and in antigen-presenting cells (APC), compared to healthy controls [31,32]. In SLE patients' plasma and cerebrospinal fluid (CSF), lower TRP levels and elevated QUIN levels were observed compared to healthy controls [33]. There was a significant positive correlation between the KYN/TRP ratio and tumor necrosis factor (TNF)-α levels, indicating a link between the pro-inflammatory pathway and KYNs [33] (Table 1).

Table 1. The enzymes of the tryptophan-kynurenine pathway and related diseases.

Enzymes	Substrates	Products	Diseases
TDO	Tryptophan	L-kynurenine	Human brain tumors [34] Other tumor types [35,36]
IDO	Tryptophan	L-kynurenine	Tumors [36,37] Neurological and neurodegenerative diseases [25] Depression [38] Systemic lupus erythematosus [33] Sjörgen's syndrome [31,32]
KAT	L-kynurenine 3-hydroxy-L-kynurenine	Kynurenic acid Xanthurenic acid	Multiple sclerosis [39] Parkinson's disease [40] Alzheimer's disease [41] Huntington's disease [42–44] Epilepsy [25] Amyotrophic lateral sclerosis [45] Schizophrenia [46–48]
KMO	L-kynurenine	3-hydroxy-L-kynurenine	Bipolar disorder [49] Autoimmunity related diseases [50]

KYNs are key factors in T cell mediated immune responses. KYN can inhibit antigen-specific T cell proliferation and cause apoptosis [29]. KYNs lead to cell death in the T helper type 1 (Th1) cells, at the same time they upregulate T helper type 2 (Th2) cells. This switches the balance between the Th1–Th2 ratio to Th2 [29,51]. Elevation of the TNF-stimulated gene 6 (TSG-6) expression by KYNA and novel KYNA analogues may be one of the mechanisms responsible for their suppressive effect on TNF-α production [52]. Targeting the metabolic pathway with the purpose of repairing the imbalances of KYN metabolites can be a potential approach to improve symptoms.

2.1.2. Tryptophan 2,3-Dioxygenase

The TDO enzyme is mainly expressed in liver tissue and is responsible for the breakdown of TRP [36,53]. The TDO enzyme also occurs in the brain. Two variants were identified and expressed at different levels in the brain of mouse, and it was proposed that its role is crucial in postnatal development [54,55]. Furthermore, the TDO-AhR pathway is activated and related to the malignant progression and low survival in brain tumors. The TDO-induced KYN represses the body's anti-tumor immune response, thereby promoting tumor cells motility and survival through the AhR system [34]. During inflammation of the microenvironment and tumor progression, KYN is pronounced in adequate amounts to activate AhR in humans [34] (Table 1). In addition, an increased TDO expression was described in many tumor types, for example, breast cancer, melanoma or lung cancer [35,36] (Table 1). The main determinant of TRP availability is the TDO enzyme, the expression of

TDO can be stimulated by estrogens, corticosteroids, heme, as well as TRP itself [35,56,57]. NADH and NADPH inhibit TDO expression through a negative feedback loop [54] (Table 1, Figure 3).

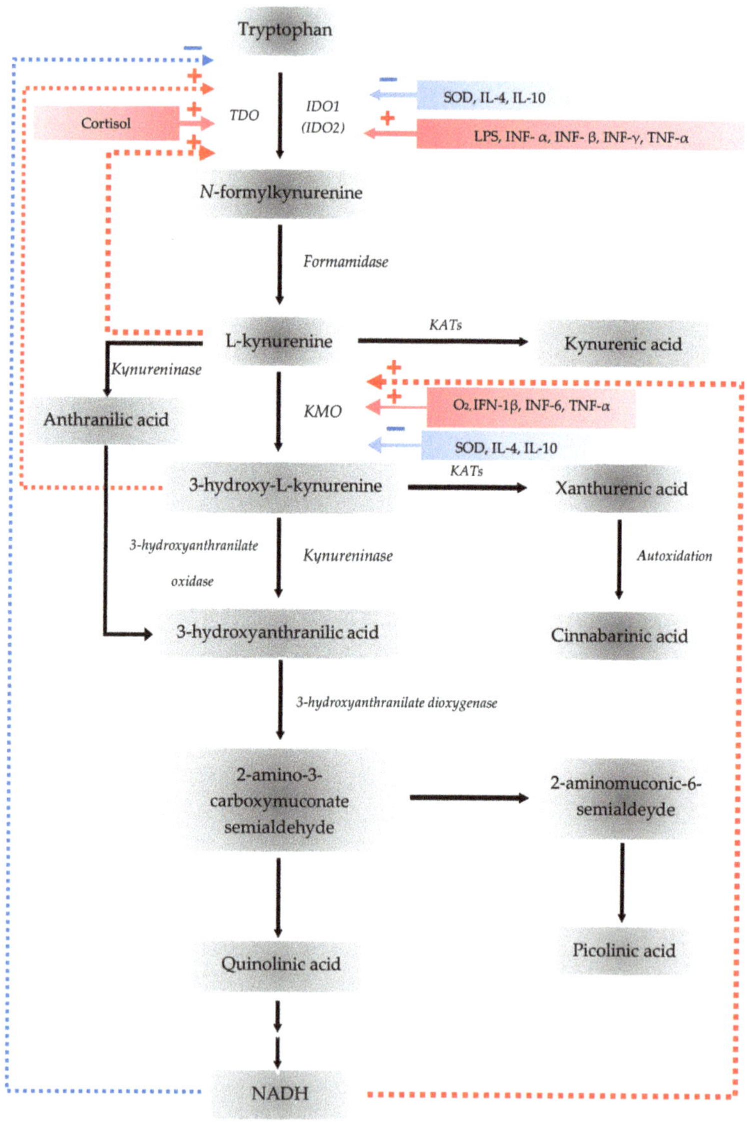

Figure 3. Stimulators (red) and inhibitors (blue) of the tryptophan-kynurenine metabolic pathway. The tryptophan 2,3-dioxygenase (TDO) is stimulated by cortisol and 3-hydroxyanthranilic acid (3-HA) but inhibited by nicotinamide adenine dinucleotide (NADH) forming a negative feedback loop. The indoleamine 2,3-dioxygenases (IDOs) are stimulated by interferon (IFN)-β, IFN-γ, tumor necrosis factor (TNF)-α and lipopolysaccharide (LPS) but inhibited by IL-4, IL-10 and superoxide dismutase (SOD). Kynurenine 3-monooxygenase (KMO) is stimulated by IFN-1 β, IFN-6, TNF-α, oxygen molecule (O_2) but inhibited by IL-4, IL-10 and SOD. KMO is also inhibited by NADH forming another negative feedback loop.

2.1.3. Indoleamine 2,3-Dioxygenase

IDOs are responsible for the first step in extrahepatic TRP metabolism. IDOs are expressed by APCs, vascular endothelium, epithelial - and tumor cells [58]. This is a widely inducible enzyme, which occurs in most tissues in human [36,59]. IFN-γ-susceptible elements regulate the IDO gene that bind to activate signal transducer and activator of transcription 1, nuclear factor-κB and IFN regulatory factor-1 [60]. However, IDO can be most strongly induced by IFN-γ, as well as many different inflammatory cytokines and mediators, while nitric oxide or the predominance of TRP inhibits these enzymes [54,61]. The IDO induction is inhibited by certain anti-inflammatory cytokines and is potentiated by pro-inflammatory cytokines, such as TNF-α [54]. Consequently, it is hypothesized that the state of the IDO enzymes, is affected by the balance between pro- and anti-inflammatory cytokines [54]. Guillemin et al. have described that several brain cells, including astrocytes, microglial cells, endothelial cells or the human neurons expressed the IDO enzymes [62]. The effect of IDOs on the immune system was first described in the prevention of T-cell-mediated fetal rejection, when it was demonstrated that IDO enzymes synthesized in placental cells protect the fetus from maternal T cell-mediated attack [63]. Furthermore, studies described that IDO is expressed in several tissue types, such as the human lung, small intestine, over and above the placenta already mentioned, and it is upregulated during inflammatory processes, since the IDO enzymes have a physiologically key role in regulating the immune response to antigenic challenges on the surface of the gastrointestinal mucosa [58,64]. The majority of tumor cells overexpress IDOs, either in tumor cells themselves or in tumor-associated cells such as macrophages, dendritic cells or endothelial cells [37]. Due to the inducible nature of the IDO enzymes, it is expressed in the tumor after a certain degree of inflammation which, in turn, activate the tumor. Expression of IDOs is induced by T-cell activation or inflammation which is subsequently suppressed [37]. This is beneficial if the IDO controls harmful inflammation or creates APC tolerance to apoptotic cells, but it is extremely harmful if it suppresses the immune response against the tumor [37] (Table 1, Figure 3). The elevated expression of IDOs is an unfavorable prognostic factor in ovarian cancer, melanoma, breast cancer, brain tumors, glioma and colon cancer, among others [35,37]. The upregulation of IDOs is associated with increased T cell infiltration and inflammation, which indicates anti-tumor immune response and favorable prognosis [37]. In addition, a number of studies presented altered IDO expression in various neurological diseases. An elevated IDO enzyme activity has been described in cerebral ischemia, Parkinson's disease (PD), Huntington's disease (HD) and other neurodegenerative diseases, among others [25] (Table 1). The activation of IDO results in a complex immunomodulatory effect which is considered to be essential for the development of both physiological and pathological immune tolerance. Furthermore, the parallel occurrence of autoimmune and immunological process can be a self-defense response of the body [25].

Natural killer (NK) cells take part in innate immunity, destroying pathogens and transformed cells. IDO metabolites can suppress NK cell proliferation and function [65]. KYN has a pro-apoptotic effect on NK cells, which is mediated by ROS [66]. IDO can regulate invariant natural killer (iNKT) cell response and KYN, 3-HK and 3-HAA switch the cytokine balance to Th2, decreasing interferon (IFN)-γ [67]. IDO inhibition shifts the cytokine response to Th1 with a decrease in interleukin (IL)-4.

2.1.4. Kynurenine Aminotransferases

KATs catalyze the conversion L-KYN to KYNA. In the human brain there are four isoforms of KATs, including KAT I, glutamine transaminase K/cysteine conjugate beta-lyase (CCBL) 1, KAT II, aminoadipate aminotransferase, KAT III, glutamine transaminase L/cysteine conjugate beta-lyase CCBL 2 and KAT IV, glutamic-oxaloacetic transaminase 2/mitochondrial aspartate aminotransferase [68]. The isoform liable for KYNA synthesis is the KAT II in human brain [68,69]. These enzymes have a broad substrate specificity and function, being biologically active as homodimer with pyridoxal 5′-phosphate-dependent enzyme family [68,70,71]. In addition to the irreversible transamination of L-KYN to KYNA, KATs can catalyze the conversion of 3-HK to XA [70]. The permeability of KYNA through the BBB is low [72]. KATs activity occurs in astrocyte cells [69,73]. KYNA targets on a number of sites in the CNS and participates in several neurodegenerative diseases involving cognitive impairment [71,74–76]. KYNA alters cytokine release from human iNKT cells via G-protein coupled receptor 35 (GPR35) [77]. The increased levels of plasma KYNs was observed in disorders with iNKT cell involvement such as autoimmune diseases and multiple sclerosis [78,79]. The KYNA-centric hypothesis holds that KYNA is well capable of modulating neuropathological conditions [80]. Therefore, isoenzymes involved in the formation of KYNA are considered to be potential targets in the regulation of cerebral KYNA [68,81–84].

Changes in KYNA concentrations have been described in several different neurological disorders, including MS, PD, Alzheimer's disease, HD, epilepsy, amyotrophic lateral sclerosis, as well as SCZ [25,39–46] (Table 1). The inhibition of TNF-α can be a potential treatment for various inflammatory diseases [85]. KYNA suppresses the production of TNF-α in mononuclear cells and in $CD14^+$ peripheral blood monocytes. KYNA inhibits TNF-α at a transcriptional level [86]. An elevated brain TNF-α level plays a pivotal role in the pathogenesis of neurodegenerative disorders [87]. KYNA inhibition of TNF-α production may consequently be a significant factor in neuroprotection.

Compared to healthy controls SCZ patients have higher KYNA levels in the CSF and in CNS regions [48] (Table 1). In SCZ the Th1 response is in part inhibited, whilst the Th2 response is over-activated leading to a Th1/Th2 imbalance, which is linked to astrocyte activation [88]. Astrocytes can generate vast amounts of KYN and KYNA [62]. The functional abundance of astrocytes can result in additional KYNA accumulation. Since astrocytes lack KYN hydroxylase, this leads to KYNA accumulation in the CNS. Consequently, immune-mediated disturbance of glutamatergic-dopaminergic neurotransmission can bring about the clinical symptoms of SCZ [47] (Table 1).

There is a link between TRP, KYN and KYNA peripheral blood levels and depressive symptoms during IFN-α treatment [89]. Van Gool et al. also found a connection between IFN-α immunotherapy and psychiatric side effect [90]. IFN-α induces IDO, which converts TRP to KYN leading to a shortage of 5-HT, which may result in depression [38,91] (Table 1). IDO induction, a switch toward the TRP-KYN metabolic pathway and the disruption of the equilibrium between neurotoxic and neuroprotective actions all confirm the significance of KYN system activation in depression [92]. Psychological stress elevates brain KYN levels and switches TRP metabolism to the TRP-KYN metabolic pathway [14,93].

2.1.5. Kynurenine 3-Monooxygenase

KMO is responsible for the conversion of L-KYN to 3-HK. It is a mitochondrial flavoprotein, using nicotinamide adenosine dinucleotide phosphate (NADPH) and O_2 for the catalyzed reaction [94]. In various neurodegenerative diseases an elevated 3-HK level has been observed, as an endogenous oxidative stress generator [39,95]. An elevated KYNA level has been observed in the CSF of patients with SCZ, as KMO is responsible for the conversion of L-KYN to 3-HK, based on the fact that the amount of L-KYN available for KYNA synthesis decreases; thus, the increase in KYNA in SCZ is due to increased KYN and overexpression of KAT, irrespective of changes in KMO [96]. L-KYN has been reported to support the regulatory T-cells and tumor formation through the AhR as well as the activation of the adenylate- and guanylate-cyclase pathways [27,97,98]. Presumably, an increase in kynurenine metabolism via over-expression of KMO may provide a protection against tumorigenesis [27]. Nevertheless, upregulation of KMO can cause the formation of other neuroactive molecules, such as QUIN, HAA and 3-HK which have a ROS-generating effect [27]. Inhibition of KMO, in turn, enhances the formation of neuroprotective KYNA, which plays an important role in immunomodulation [27,99–101]. The KMO expression is regulated in lipopolysaccharide-induced systemic inflammation along with a significant increase in pro-inflammatory cytokines in the CNS of rats [102]. Furthermore, KMO activity has been studied in bipolar disorder (BD), a reduced KMO gene expression has been described in the prefrontal cortex of patients with BD with psychotic feature compared with BP patients without psychotic traits [49] (Table 1).

KMO expression and activity have been studied in autoimmune diseases. The link to the immune system appears to exist via AhRs which play a key role in regulating the differentiation of pro-inflammatory Th17 cells [50]. Increasing KYN metabolism through KMO can be protective against tumor formation. Nevertheless, KMO upregulation also produces the following metabolites 3-HK and QUIN with reactive oxygen species (ROS) generating properties and neurotoxic effects [103]. T helper type 17 (Th17) cells express the enzyme KMO. Addition of exogenous KYN or inhibition of KMO activity caused an amelioration in Th17 lineage differentiation in a mouse model of autoimmune gastritis [50]. KMO facilitates KYN metabolism, decreasing KYN levels and subsequently reducing Th17 cell formation and IL-17 production. Thus, KMO inhibition intensified inflammation through the formation of Th17 cells [50].

The inhibition of KMO elevates KYNA production. KYNA has immunomodulatory effects via GPR35 receptors and AHRs [101]. GPR35 is highly expressed in human $CD14^+$ monocytes, T cells, neutrophils and dendritic cells, while it is expressed in lower levels in B cells, eosinophils, basophils and iNKT cells [77,104]. KYNA attenuates inflammation by restricting TNF production in macrophages via GPR35 receptors [104]. In $KMO^{-/-}$ mice serum, lower cytokine and chemokine levels, whilst higher KYN and KYNA levels were found compared to the wild type [105]. Elevated levels of KYN and KYNA are the vital components in the decreased inflammatory responses found in $KMO^{-/-}$ animals.

3. Symptoms, Inflammatory Status and Kynurenines in Psychiatric Disorders

This section overviews and discusses the major symptoms, inflammatory status and the kynurenine system of psychiatric disorders in clinical human studies. The reference priority is given to the following order: meta-analysis, systematic review, case-control study and expert review. Depression, anxiety and cognitive impairment are the most common symptoms of psychiatric disorders that may concur and/or sway during progression and comorbidity frequently occurs in mental illnesses, which renders the exact diagnosis even more difficult. Scrupulous studies are underway to untangle the thread of pathophysiology of mental disorders and their comorbidities not only in clinical medicine, but also in animal studies [106–109]. Psychological stress, especially depression has been found to be a risk factor for dementia, a prognostic biomarker for stokes and a therapeutic target for meaning-centered psychotherapy in depression, and animal-assisted and pet-robot interventions in dementia [110–113]. Four main representative psychiatric symptoms including positive, negative and cognitive symptoms, and anxiety are reviewed. Psychiatric disorders present inflammatory signs in serum, CSF and/or the brain tissue samples in which pro-inflammatory and anti-inflammatory cytokine levels can be detected and measured. The simultaneous alternations of KYN metabolism take place under inflammation, disturbing a balance of toxic and protective KYN metabolites.

3.1. Major Depressive Disorder

MDD is a mental disorder with at least two weeks of low mood, often accompanied by low self-esteem, loss of interest, low energy and pain without a cause. Less than one-fifth of MDD patients experiences positive psychotic symptoms such as either delusions, hallucinations or both [114]. The mean score of the Hamilton Rating Scale for Depression, Scale for the Assessment of Negative Symptoms (SANS) and negative symptom scale of Positive and Negative Symptom Scale of the patients with MDD were significantly higher than those of control subjects, validating the clinical significance of negative symptoms and depressive symptoms in MDD patients [115]. Cognitive impairment in patients with MDD is often overlooked and may precede after symptoms of MDD, such as sleep, appetite and affective symptoms [116]. Generalized anxiety disorder (GAD) often co-occur in MDD.

Many symptoms overlap with MDD and GAD, such as irritability, restlessness, sleep problems and concentration difficulty [117] (Table 2).

Table 2. The enzymes of the tryptophan-kynurenine pathways and related disease.

		Major Depressive Disorder	Bipolar Disorder	Generalized Anxiety Disorder	Substance Use Disorder	Post-Traumatic Stress Disorder	Schizophrenia	Autism Spectrum Disorder
Symptoms	Positive	+	++	++	++	++	++	+
	Negative	++	++	++	+	++	++	+
	Cognitive	+	+	++	++	++	-	+
	Anxiety	++	++	++	++	++	++	++
Inflammatory factors	Proinflammatory	↑	↑	↑	↑	↑	↑	↑
	Anti-inflammatory	↑	↑	↓	↓	↓,?	↑	↑
Kynurenines	Toxic	↑	?	↑	?	?	↑	↑
	Protective	↓	? (serum), ↑ (CSF)	?	?	?	↑,?	↓

+: noticeable; ++: prominent; -: not typical;↑: increase; ↓: decrease; ?: questionable or unknown.

Regarding inflammatory cytokines, meta-analyses reported strong evidence of significantly increased levels of CRP, IL-1, IL-6, TNF-α and sIL-2R in serum of MDD patients [118–123]. Decreased levels of CRP and IL-6 were observed after antidepressant treatment [124]. Higher concentration of CCL2/MCP-1 was also reported in MDD patients. CSF levels of IL-6 and IL-8 were significantly increased in patients with MDD [125] (Table 2).

Regarding the KYN system, meta-analyses reported the decreased levels of plasma TRP, KYN and KYNA in patients with MDD, and the increased level of QUIN was observed in antidepressant-free patients. The increased QUIN immunoreactivity was detected in the prefrontal cortex and hippocampus of the postmortem brain tissues from patients with MDD [126,127]. Magnetic resonance spectroscopy showed a higher turnover of cells with KYN and the 3-HAA/KYN ratio in adolescent depression. The findings are in accordance with the activation of the TRP-KYN pathway by pro-inflammatory cytokines activating IDO, and KMO enzymes toward 3-HK and QUIN branches, leading to higher levels of toxic 3-HK and QUIN [128] (Table 2).

3.2. Bipolar Disorder

BD is a mental disorder that causes alternating periods of depression and mania. Positive symptoms regularly occur to BD with prevalence rates ranging from 20 to 50% in acute bipolar mania [129]. Cognitive impairment is present in the minority of BD patients. SANS, Brief Psychiatric Rating Scale and Social and Occupational Functioning Assessment Scale showed that negative symptoms were present in more than a quarter of the patients. The patients had more sever affective flattening, alogia, anhedonia-asociality and avolition-apathy [130]. Cognitive deficits of verbal and visual memory, and executive tasks have been demonstrated during depressive episodes, while executive dysfunction and attention deficits have been reported during manic episodes [131,132]. Many patients with BD experience at least one anxiety attack [133] (Table 2).

Regarding inflammatory cytokines, four meta-analyses of serum or plasma samples from BD patients invariably reported significantly increased levels of TNF-α and sIL-2R; IL-4, IL-6, IL-1RA, sIL-6R and TNFR1 levels were significantly increased in two meta-analyses; IL-10 levels were significantly increased in one meta-analysis [123,134–136]. A meta-analysis of CSF samples from BD patients reported increased IL-1β levels [125] (Table 2).

Regarding the KYN system a case-control study showed that KYNA levels were reduced and the 3-HK/KYN and 3-HK/KYNA ratio was increased in BD compared to healthy control [137]. However, a meta-analysis reported no significant difference of TRP and KYN levels, KYN/TRP and KYNA/QUIN ratios in serum from BD patients [138] KYNA was significantly increased in CSF of BD patients [124] (Table 2).

3.3. Generalized Anxiety Disorder

GAD is a mental disorder characterized by excessive, uncontrollable and irrational anxiety. GAD is associated with the severity of positive symptoms such as delusions and hallucinations [139]. More than quarter of GAD patients showed negative symptoms [140]. Patients with GAD have an impaired cognitive function, particularly in attention and working memory [141] (Table 2).

On the status of inflammatory cytokines, CRP of blood, serum or plasma samples was significantly raised in GAD by meta-analysis, and IFN-γ and TNF-α levels were significantly increased in GAD in at least two or more studies [142]. Lower levels of IL-10 and higher ratios of TNF-α/IL10, TNF-α/IL4, IFN-γ/IL10 and IFN-γ/IL4 were observed in the serum of GAD patients, showing significantly increased pro- to anti-inflammatory cytokine ratios, which suggests a distinct cytokine imbalance [143] (Table 2).

On the KYN system, the plasma KYN levels were decreased in endogenous anxiety and normalized after treatment [144]. Metabolomic studies reported decreased KYN levels in patients diagnosed with Type D personality that is characterized by negative affectivity and social inhibition [145]. Stress and inflammation appear to activate the TRP-KYN pathway, depleting 5-HT and melatonin and thus making more susceptible to anxiety (Table 2).

3.4. Substance Use Disorder

Substance use disorder (SUD) affects a person's brain and behavior leading to an inability to control the use of a drug or medication. In addition to an impaired control, patients show social impairment, risky use and pharmacological indicators including tolerance and withdrawal. Common substances are alcohol, sedatives, caffeine, hallucinogens, inhalants, stimulants and tabaco, among others [146]. SUD is frequently comorbid with other mental illnesses. Positive symptoms are more prominent among substance abusing SCZ patients [147]. The onset of positive symptoms occurs in nearly three-fourths of cannabis users after cannabis abuse [148]. Serious hallucinations and delusions are frequent in alcohol addicted SCZ patients [149]. Negative symptoms are less common in patients with substance use disorder probably because patients with social withdrawal have more difficulties to obtain abused substance [150]. Increased rates of criminal activity and violent behavior are more common in SCZ patients with SUD [151]. Cognitive impairments are prevalent among patients with SUD. Alcohol affects total and memory domain scores more than cannabis, while opioids affect visuospatial domain more than cannabis or stimulants [152]. SUD occurs at an increasing rate in patients with GAD. Substance use and anxiety are considered to occur in a vicious cycle [153] (Table 2).

Few studies regarding inflammatory cytokines were reported. Cocaine increased the mRNA expression of IL-1ß receptor in the ventral tegmental area, reducing cocaine seeking. It may suggest that chronic cocaine use induces proinflammatory signaling contributing to cocaine seeking [154]. A single nucleotide polymorphism in the IL-10 gene is associated with decrease expression of IL-10 and is linked to alcoholism. It was suggested that increased proinflammatory and reduced anti-inflammatory signals are predisposing factors for alcoholism [155] (Table 2).

No clinical study was found regarding the serum or CSF level of KYNs in patients with SUD. The TRP-KYN metabolic pathway is considered to play an important role in SUD and was discussed as a potential target for SUD therapy [17]. Patients with cocaine use disorder (CUD) frequently develop MDD. The plasma 5-hydroxytryptamine (5-HT) concentration was significantly higher and the KYN/5-HT ratio was significantly lower in patients with CUD-induced MDD than those with MDD, while there were no differences between CUD-primary MDD and MDD. It suggests that the TRP-KYN pathway participates less in CUD-induced MDD and the presence of other mechanisms of the development of depression [156] (Table 2).

3.5. Post-Traumatic Stress Disorder

Post-traumatic stress disorder (PTSD) develops after a terrifying experience in individuals who suffer from flashbacks, nightmares, severe anxiety and uncontrollable thoughts regarding the event. Substantial evidence supports that PTSD is caused by insufficient integration of a trauma memory into the hippocampal-cortical memory networks, forming fragmented, incomplete and disorganized intrusive memories [157]. Most patients with PTSD complained of chronic sleep disturbances characterized by significantly reduced slow wave sleep (SWS), light sleep stages, awakenings, arousals and increased rapid eye movement (EEG). SWS drives memory consolidation by repeated reactivation of newly encoded memory. Thus, lowered sleep quality facilitates the formation of intrusive memories [158]. PTSD is frequently comorbid with SCZ. More than a half of patients with PTSD experienced psychotic positive symptoms, but emerging evidence suggests that PTSD with secondary psychosis might be different from PTSD without psychosis [159]. Patients with PTSD activate the fight-flight-freeze response and reduce overall brain functioning, leading to several negative symptoms [160]. PTSD causes long-term cognitive dysfunction such as memory, attention, planning and problem solving [161]. PTSD frequently cooccur with GAD and their symptoms overlap [162] (Table 2).

Inflammation has been linked to PTSD. Increased proinflammatory cytokines IL-1β, IL-6, IFN-γ and TNF-α were found elevated in the serum of patients with PTSD and partly correlated with the severity of PTSD [163]. Decreased levels of anti-inflammatory cytokine IL-4 were reported in patients with PTSD. The alteration of the serum anti-inflammatory cytokines IL-4 and IL-10 remains inconclusive in PTSD [164]. Higher levels of serum anti-inflammatory cytokine TGF-β were found to be predicative indicators for the development of PTSD one month after accidents [165] (Table 2).

No clinical study was reported regarding the peripheral or CSF samples of KYNs in patients with PTSD. KYN metabolites are monitored in clinical settings as evidence of inflammatory responses contributing to sleep deprivation and the formation of intrusive memories [164].

3.6. Schizophrenia

SCZ is a mental disorder in which patients abnormally interpret reality and suffer from hallucinations, delusions and extremely disordered thinking and behavior. Patients with SCZ usually experience positive symptoms such as hallucinations, delusions, flight of ideas, negative symptoms such as apathy, emotionless, lack of social functioning and cognitive symptoms including difficulty in concentration and attention, and memory impairments. However, cognitive symptoms are subtle and are often detected only when neuropsychological tests are performed [166]. The prevalence of GAD was significantly higher in patients with SCZ and the prevalence of panic disorder, social anxiety disorder and obsessive-compulsive disorder was significantly higher in SCZ patients [167] (Table 2).

The peripheral activation of the immune system was observed in SCZ. Three meta-analyses on serum cytokines of SCZ patients were reported accordingly. (1) IL-1β, IL-6 and TGF-β were increased in acutely relapsed and first-episode psychosis and the cytokine levels were normalized with antipsychotic treatment. Soluble IL-2 receptor (sIL-2R) stayed high in acute psychosis and after antipsychotic treatment [168]. (2) IL-6, TNF-α, sIL-2R and IL-1 receptor antagonist were significantly increased in acutely exacerbating and IL-6 levels significantly decreased following treatment. IL-1β and sIL-2R were significantly increased in chronic SCZ [123]. (3) MCP-1 (CCL2), MIP-1β (CCL4), eotaxin-1 (CCL11) and IL-8 were elevated in pooled analysis of all SCZ patients, while MCP-1 was elevated in first-episode psychosis (FEP) and IL-8, eotaxin-1 and MIP-1β were elevated in multiple-episode psychosis [169] (Table 2).

The activation of the central immune system was also observed. Three meta-analysis on CSF cytokines of SCZ were reported accordingly. (1) IL-1β was decreased significantly decreased in SCZ, but there was no significant difference in CSF levels of IL-1α, IL-2 or IL-6 between SCZ and healthy controls [168]. (2) IL-1β, IL-6 and IL-8 were significantly increased IL-2R were significantly decreased in SCZ [125]. (3) IL-6 and IL-8 were significantly elevated in SCZ and IL-6 levels were higher in early-stage SCZ than chronic SCZ [170] (Table 2). CRP, IL-6 and TNF-α are overlapping biomarkers in SCZ and cardiovascular diseases and anti-inflammatory drugs were proposed for the treatment of SCZ [171].

Regarding the KYN system, the serum KYN and KYN/TRP ratio was higher in SCZ [172]. A meta-analysis of CSF samples showed increased KYN and KYNA levels and another meta-analysis of plasma, CSF, brain tissue or saliva showed increased levels of KYNA in SCZ [125,173] (Table 2). Thus, the KYN system is activated in SCZ and elevated KYNA levels are considered to contribute to the cognitive impairments of SCZ. Recently, another meta-analysis reported that KYNA levels and the KYNA/3-HK ratio were not altered and the KYNA/KYN ratio was decreased in SCZ, suggesting the presence of differential pattern between SCZ and mood disorders [174]. The combination of acetylcholine inhibitor galantamine and N-methyl-D-aspartate receptor memantine was proposed as antioxidant treatment SCZ and for the treatment of SCZ cognitive impairments [175,176].

3.7. Autism Spectrum Disorder

Autism Spectrum Disorder (ASD), defined by the Diagnostic and Treatment Manual for Mental Disorders, Fifth Edition (DSM-5), is characterized by persistent deficits in social communication interaction and restricted-repetitive patterns of behavior, interests or activities. A specific subtype of ASD is linked to comorbid psychosis, showing positive symptoms of delusion, hallucination, thought disorder, mania and depression and negative symptoms of psychosis appear to share many features with ASD [177]. Cognitive deficits including mental deterioration, are associated with social and communication difficulties that involve components of cognition, communication and social understanding [178]. Meta-analyses reported that ASD children had higher anxiety levels than normally developing ones, that high-functioning ASD adolescents are at high risk of developing anxiety disorders, and that autism population showed higher prevalence of anxiety disorders, the highest being attention-deficit hyperactivity disorders, in decreasing orders, sleep-wake disorders, disruptive, impulse-control and conduct disorders depressive disorders, obsessive-compulsive disorder BD and SCZ spectrum disorders [179,180] (Table 2).

Regarding inflammatory cytokines, two Meta-analyses showed increases of IL-1β, IL-6, IL-8, IFN-γ, TNF-α, eotaxin and monocyte chemotactic protein-1, while TGF-β1 were significantly lower in ASD [181,182]. However, a case-control study reported that significantly higher levels of IL-4, IL-5 and IL-13, with Th-2 predominance in plasma and peripheral blood mononuclear cells of ASD children [183] (Table 2).

The alteration of the KYN system was also observed. The mean serum level of KYNA was significantly lower, while the KYN/KYNA ratio was significantly higher in children with ASD. The same relative values were found when comparing the childhood autism subgroup with the controls [184]. Significantly higher KYN/TRP ratio and KYN and QUIN levels were observed in blood samples of ASD patients, while no significant difference of KYNA and significantly lower picolinic acid level were detected in ASD [185] (Table 2).

All psychiatric disorders presented an evidence of the innate inflammatory activation by increased pro-inflammatory cytokines. MDD, BD, SCZ and ASD witnessed the activation of the secondary adaptive immune response by increased anti-inflammatory cytokines, while GAD, and SUD showed reduced levels of anti-inflammatory cytokines. PTSD showed no changes or mixed results depending on the cause of stress. Regardless of the activation of the secondary adaptive immune response, the inflammatory profiles of all psychiatric disorders described in this review, have shifted away from healthy state (Table 2).

Either causative or resultant of acute and chronic inflammation, the altered balance of toxic and protective KYN metabolites was observed. Toxic KYN metabolites are increased in MDD, GAD, SCZ, ASD and the CSF samples of BD. Modulatory KYN metabolites were increased in SCZ; decreased in MDD and ASD; unchanged in the serum of BP; unknown in GAD and SUD.

4. Conclusions and Future Perspective

LGI defined by the serum concentration of CRP has well established the relationship with physical health score in healthy individual, but not mental health score. Thus, the CRP measurement is not adequate for the assessment of mental health. LGI is also characterized by a long period of slightly elevated serum concentrations of proinflammatory and anti-inflammatory factors and accompanying immune tolerance. Elevated levels of proinflammatory cytokines are consistent findings in major psychiatric disorders, but the levels of anti-inflammatory cytokines are mixed, and their roles in the pathogenesis remain obscure. Some inflammatory cytokines and factors cannot be simply categorized into pro- or anti-inflammatory; thus, comprehensive analysis according to their specific functions in immune reaction may further complement this study.

The involvement of toxic KYNs in mental disorders has gained credit and this study reinforced current understanding of their interactions with the immune system in LGI. However, the roles of toxic KYNs in BP, SUD and PTSD are to be explored. The roles of protective KYNs such as KYNA, AA, PA and CA are even more obscure or unknown. The decreased levels of KYNA are considered to contribute to the pathogenesis of MDD and ASD, while the increased level of KYNA is considered to be at least one of the culprits in the exacerbation of SCZ.

Generally, the measurement of TRP/KYN ratio is used for assessment of the activation of the TRP-KYN pathway and 3-HK/KYNA and QUIN/KYNA ratios are used for relative toxicity of the KYN system. However, emerging evidence has suggested KYN metabolites cannot be simply categorized into toxic or protective. For example, KYNA is excitatory in low dose at α-amino-3-hydroxy-5-methyl-4-isoxazolepropionic acid (AMPA) receptor, while inhibitory in high dose at AMPA receptor. Our preliminary data indicated that KYNA elicits cognitive enhancement in a low dose, but not in higher doses. 3-HK is generally considered to be oxidative and thus toxic, but it may serve as antioxidant in particular environment. Metabolomic analysis of KYN metabolites and their related molecules may help identify a certain profile contributing to LGI and its exacerbation. Furthermore, the influence of nutritional, metabolic and sleep status on the structure and the function of the brain is of particular interest [186–188].

The immune privileged site of CNS encapsulated by the BBB may complicate the assessment of inflammatory status in the brain. The BBB is semipermeable; thus, the entry of circulating molecules into the CNS depends on the state of the BBB. The integrity measurements of the BBB may ensure the assessment of LGI in the CNS and functional imaging studies may reveal a relationship with psychiatric symptoms in mental illnesses [189]. Together, they are expected to warrant as additional indicators for a battery of biomarkers which may serve as risk, diagnostic, prognostic, predicative and/or therapeutic biomarker in psychiatric diagnosis.

Finally, the classification of psychiatric disorders mainly depends on the manifestation of signs and symptoms, which inevitably includes a broad range of heterogenous population into study samples, leading to inconclusive results. Frequent comorbidities of mental illnesses even more complicate the procedures of grouping subjects. Application of research domain criteria and artificial intelligence diagnostic system which integrate many levels of information may become a useful assist in focusing on homogenous populations with the reduction of statistical deviations [190].

Understanding the roles of chronic LGI in the development of mental illnesses, the TRP-KYN metabolic pathway in chronic LGI including mechanism of the immune switch, dynamic structural changes of the BBB and the participation of components of the body in neuroinflammation will certainly help explore possible preventive, interventional and therapeutic measures through the TRP-KYN pathway.

Author Contributions: Conceptualization, M.T., Y.M. and L.V.; methodology, not applicable.; software, not applicable; validation, not applicable; formal analysis, not applicable; investigation, not applicable.; resources, not applicable; data curation, not applicable.; writing—original draft preparation, M.T., F.T., H.P. and Á.S.; writing—review and editing, M.T., F.T., H.P. Á.S., Y.M. and L.V.; visualization, M.T. and Á.S.; supervision, L.V.; project administration, L.V.; funding acquisition, L.V. All authors have read and agreed to the published version of the manuscript.

Funding: This research was funded by GINOP 2.3.2-15-2016-00034, GINOP 2.3.2-15-2016-00048, TUDFO/47138-1/2019-ITM and TKP2020 Thematic Excellence Programme 2020. Helga Polyák was supported by the ÚNKP-20-3—New National Excellence Program of the Ministry for Innovation and Technology from the source of the National Research, Development and Innovation Fund; and EFOP 3.6.3-VEKOP-16-2017-00009. The APC was funded by University of Szeged Open Access Fund (4942).

Institutional Review Board Statement: Not applicable.

Informed Consent Statement: Not applicable.

Data Availability Statement: Not applicable.

Conflicts of Interest: The authors declare no conflict of interest.

Abbreviations

AA	anthranilic acid
AhR	aryl hydrocarbon receptor
AMPA	α-amino-3-hydroxy-5-methyl-4-isoxazolepropionic acid
APC	antigen-presenting cell
ASD	autism spectrum disorder
ATP	adenosine triphosphate
BBB	blood-brain barrier
BD	bipolar disorder
CA	cinnabarinic acid
CCBL	cysteine conjugate beta-lyase
CNS	central nervous system
CRP	C-reactive protein
CSF	cerebrospinal fluid
CUD	cocaine use disorder
DSM-5	Diagnostic and Treatment Manual for Mental Disorders, Fifth Edition
EEG	electroencephalography
FEP	first-episode psychosis
GAD	generalized anxiety disorder
GPR35	G-protein coupled receptor 35
3-HAA	3-hydroxyanthranilic acid
3-HK	3-hydroxy-kynurenine
HD	Huntington's disease
HRQL	Health-Related Quality of Life
5-HT	serotonin, 5-hydroxytryptamine
IDO	indoleamine 2,3-dioxygenase
IFN	interferon
IL	interleukin
iNKT	invariant natural killer cell
KATs	kynurenine aminostransferase
KMO	kynurenine 3-monooxygenase
KP	kynurenine pathway

KYN	kynurenine
KYNA	kynurenic acid
LGI	low-grade inflammation
MCP	monocyte chemoattractant protein
MDD	major depressive disorder
MS	multiple sclerosis
MT	melatonin
NAD^+	nicotinamide adenine dinucleotide
NADPH	nicotinamide adenosine dinucleotide phosphate
NK	natural killer cell
PD	Parkinson's disease
PIC	picolinic acid
PTSD	post-traumatic stress disorder
QUIN	quinolinic acid
ROS	reactive oxygen species
SANS	Scale for the Assessment of Negative Symptoms
SCZ	schizophrenia
sIL-2R	soluble IL-2 receptor
SjS	Sjögren's syndrome
SLE	systemic lupus erythematosus
SUD	substance use disorder
SWS	slow wave sleep
TDO	tryptophan 2,3-dioxygenase
Th1	T helper type 1
Th17	T helper type 17
Th2	T helper type 2
TNF	tumor necrosis factor
TRP	tryptophan
XA	xanthurenic acid

References

1. Margină, D.; Ungurianu, A.; Purdel, C.; Tsoukalas, D.; Sarandi, E.; Thanasoula, M.; Tekos, F.; Mesnage, R.; Kouretas, D.; Tsatsakis, A. Chronic Inflammation in the Context of Everyday Life: Dietary Changes as Mitigating Factors. *Int. J. Environ. Res. Public Health* **2020**, *17*, 4135. [CrossRef] [PubMed]
2. Dinh, K.M.; Kaspersen, K.A.; Mikkelsen, S.; Pedersen, O.B.; Petersen, M.S.; Thørner, L.W.; Hjalgrim, H.; Rostgaard, K.; Ullum, H.; Erikstrup, C. Low-grade inflammation is negatively associated with physi;cal Health-Related Quality of Life in healthy individuals: Results from The Danish Blood Donor Study (DBDS). *PLoS ONE* **2019**, *14*, e0214468. [CrossRef] [PubMed]
3. Rogovskii, V. Immune Tolerance as the Physiologic Counterpart of Chronic Inflammation. *Front. Immunol.* **2020**, *11*, 2061. [CrossRef] [PubMed]
4. Tanaka, M.; Bohár, Z.; Vécsei, L. Are Kynurenines Accomplices or Principal Villains in Dementia? Maintenance of Kynurenine Metabolism. *Molecules* **2020**, *25*, 564. [CrossRef] [PubMed]
5. Bock, K.W. Aryl hydrocarbon receptor (AHR)-mediated inflammation and resolution: Non-genomic and genomic signaling. *Biochem. Pharmacol.* **2020**, *182*, 114220. [CrossRef] [PubMed]
6. Proietti, E.; Rossini, S.; Grohmann, U.; Mondanelli, G. Polyamines and Kynurenines at the Intersection of Immune Modulation. *Trends Immunol.* **2020**, *41*, 1037–1050. [CrossRef] [PubMed]
7. Dadvar, S.; Ferreira, D.; Cervenka, I.; Ruas, J.L. The weight of nutrients: Kynurenine metabolites in obesity and exercise. *J. Intern. Med.* **2018**, *284*, 519–533. [CrossRef] [PubMed]
8. Martin, K.S.; Azzolini, M.; Lira Ruas, J. The kynurenine connection: How exercise shifts muscle tryptophan metabolism and affects energy homeostasis, the immune system, and the brain. *Am. J. Physiol. Cell Physiol.* **2020**, *318*, C818–C830. [CrossRef]
9. Joisten, N.; Walzik, D.; Metcalfe, A.J.; Bloch, W.; Zimmer, P. Physical Exercise as Kynurenine Pathway Modulator in Chronic Diseases: Implications for Immune and Energy Homeostasis. *Int. J. Tryptophan Res.* **2020**, *8*, 13. [CrossRef]
10. Sundaram, G.; Lim, C.K.; Brew, B.J.; Guillemin, G.J. Kynurenine pathway modulation reverses the experimental autoimmune encephalomyelitis mouse disease progression. *J. Neuroinflammation* **2020**, *17*, 176. [CrossRef]
11. Tanaka, M.; Vécsei, L. Monitoring the Redox Status in Multiple Sclerosis. *Biomedicines* **2020**, *8*, 406. [CrossRef]
12. Solvang, S.H.; Nordrehaug, J.E.; Tell, G.S.; Nygård, O.; McCann, A.; Ueland, P.M.; Midttun, Ø.; Meyer, K.; Vedeler, C.A.; Aarsland, D.; et al. The kynurenine pathway and cognitive performance in community-dwelling older adults. The Hordaland Health Study. *Brain Behav. Immun.* **2019**, *75*, 155–162. [CrossRef]
13. Tanaka, M.; Toldi, J.; Vécsei, L. Exploring the Etiological Links behind Neurodegenerative Diseases: Inflammatory Cytokines and Bioactive Kynurenines. *Int. J. Mol. Sci.* **2020**, *21*, 2431. [CrossRef]

14. Tanaka, M.; Bohár, Z.; Martos, D.; Telegdy, G.; Vécsei, L. Antidepressant-like effects of kynurenic acid in a modified forced swim test. *Pharmacol. Rep.* **2020**, *72*, 449–455. [CrossRef]
15. Tanaka, M.; Török, N.; Vécsei, L. Novel Pharmaceutical Approaches in Dementia. In *NeuroPsychopharmacotherapy*; Riederer, P., Laux, G., Nagatsu, T., Le, W., Riederer, C., Eds.; Springer: Cham, Switzerland, 2021. [CrossRef]
16. Tanaka, M.; Török, N.; Vécsei, L. Editorial: Are 5-HT1 receptor agonists effective anti-migraine drugs? *Expert Opin. Pharmacother.* **2021**, *12*, 1–5. [CrossRef]
17. Morales-Puerto, N.; Giménez-Gómez, P.; Pérez-Hernández, M.; Abuin-Martínez, C.; Gil de Biedma-Elduayen, L.; Vidal, R.; Gutiérrez-López, M.D.; O'Shea, E.; Colado, M.I. Addiction and the kynurenine pathway: A new dancing couple? *Pharmacol. Ther.* **2021**, *223*, 107807. [CrossRef]
18. Wang, Y.; Yuan, X.; Kang, Y.; Song, X. Tryptophan-kynurenine pathway as a novel link between gut microbiota and schizophrenia: A review. *Trop. J. Pharm. Res.* **2019**, *18*, 897–905. [CrossRef]
19. Barroso, A.; Mahler, J.V.; Fonseca-Castro, P.H.; Quintana, F.J. The aryl hydrocarbon receptor and the gut-brain axis. *Cell Mol. Immunol.* **2021**, *18*, 259–268. [CrossRef]
20. Encyclopedia. Available online: https://encyclopedia.pub/8633 (accessed on 21 June 2021).
21. Dehhaghi, M.; Kazemi Shariat Panahi, H.; Heng, B.; Guillemin, G.J. The Gut Microbiota, Kynurenine Pathway, and Immune System Interaction in the Development of Brain Cancer. *Front. Cell Dev. Biol.* **2020**, *8*. [CrossRef]
22. Polyák, H.; Cseh, E.K.; Bohár, Z.; Rajda, C.; Zádori, D.; Klivényi, P.; Toldi, J.; Vécsei, L. Cuprizone markedly decreases kynurenic acid levels in the rodent brain tissue and plasma. *Heliyon* **2021**, *7*, e06124. [CrossRef]
23. Németh, H.; Toldi, J.; Vécsei, L.; Kynurenines. Parkinson's disease and other neurodegenerative disorders: Preclinical and clinical studies. *J. Neural. Transm.* **2006**, *70*, 285–304. [CrossRef]
24. Muneer, A. Kynurenine Pathway of Tryptophan Metabolism in Neuropsychiatric Disorders: Pathophysiologic and Therapeutic Considerations. *Clin. Psychopharmacol. Neurosci.* **2020**, *18*, 507–526. [CrossRef] [PubMed]
25. Vécsei, L.; Szalárdy, L.; Fülöp, F.; Toldi, J. Kynurenines in the CNS: Recent advances and new questions. *Nat. Rev. Drug Discov.* **2013**, *12*, 64–82. [CrossRef] [PubMed]
26. Török, N.; Tanaka, M.; Vécsei, L. Searching for Peripheral Biomarkers in Neurodegenerative Diseases: The Tryptophan-Kynurenine Metabolic Pathway. *Int. J. Mol. Sci.* **2020**, *21*, 9338. [CrossRef]
27. Boros, F.A.; Vécsei, L. Immunomodulatory Effects of Genetic Alterations Affecting the Kynurenine Pathway. *Front. Immunol.* **2019**, *10*, 2570. [CrossRef]
28. Biernacki, T.; Sandi, D.; Bencsik, K.; Vécsei, L. Kynurenines in the Pathogenesis of Multiple Sclerosis: Therapeutic Perspectives. *Cells* **2020**, *9*, 1564. [CrossRef]
29. Mándi, Y.; Vécsei, L. The kynurenine system and immunoregulation. *J. Neural. Transm.* **2012**, *11*, 197–209. [CrossRef]
30. Suhs, K.W.; Novoselova, N.; Kuhn, M.; Seegers, L.; Kaever, V.; Muller-Vahl, K.; Trebst, C.; Skripuletz, T.; Stangel, M.; Pessler, F. Kynurenine Is a Cerebrospinal Fluid Biomarker for Bacterial and Viral Central Nervous System Infections. *J. Infect. Dis.* **2019**, *220*, 127–138. [CrossRef]
31. Furuzawa-Carballeda, J.; Hernandez-Molina, G.; Lima, G.; Rivera-Vicencio, Y.; Ferez-Blando, K.; Llorente, L. Peripheral regulatory cells immunophenotyping in primary Sjogren's syndrome: A cross-sectional study. *Arthritis Res. Ther.* **2013**, *15*, R68. [CrossRef]
32. Legany, N.; Berta, L.; Kovacs, L.; Balog, A.; Toldi, G. The role of B7 family costimulatory molecules and indoleamine 2,3-dioxygenase in primary Sjogren's syndrome and systemic sclerosis. *Immunol. Res.* **2017**, *65*, 622–629. [CrossRef]
33. Akesson, K.; Pettersson, S.; Stahl, S.; Surowiec, I.; Hedenstrom, M.; Eketjall, S.; Trygg, J.; Jakobsson, P.J.; Gunnarsson, I.; Svenungsson, E.; et al. Kynurenine pathway is altered in patients with SLE and associated with severe fatigue. *Lupus Sci. Med.* **2018**, *5*, e000254. [CrossRef]
34. Opitz, C.A.; Litzenburger, U.M.; Sahm, F.; Ott, M.; Tritschler, I.; Trump, S.; Schumacher, T.; Jestaedt, L.; Schrenk, D.; Weller, M.; et al. An endogenous tumour-promoting ligand of the human aryl hydrocarbon receptor. *Nature* **2011**, *478*, 197–203. [CrossRef]
35. Lanser, L.; Kink, P.; Egger, E.M.; Willenbacher, W.; Fuchs, D.; Weiss, G.; Kurz, K. Inflammation-Induced Tryptophan Breakdown is Related with Anemia, Fatigue, and Depression in Cancer. *Front. Immunol.* **2020**, *11*. [CrossRef]
36. Sforzini, L.; Nettis, M.A.; Mondelli, V.; Pariante, C.M. Inflammation in cancer and depression: A starring role for the kynurenine pathway. *Psychopharmacology* **2019**, *236*, 2997–3011. [CrossRef]
37. Munn, D.H.; Mellor, A.L. IDO in the Tumor Microenvironment: Inflammation, Counter-regulation and Tolerance. *Trends Immunol.* **2016**, *37*, 193–207. [CrossRef]
38. Wichers, M.C.; Maes, M. The role of indoleamine 2,3-dioxygenase (IDO) in the pathophysiology of interferon-alpha-induced depression. *J. Psychiatry Neurosci.* **2004**, *29*, 11–17.
39. Füvesi, J.; Rajda, C.; Bencsik, K.; Toldi, J.; Vécsei, L. The role of kynurenines in the pathomechanism of amyotrophic lateral sclerosis and multiple sclerosis: Therapeutic implications. *J. Neural. Transm.* **2012**, *119*, 225–234. [CrossRef]
40. Zádori, D.; Klivényi, P.; Toldi, J.; Fülöp, F.; Vécsei, L. Kynurenines in Parkinson's disease: Therapeutic perspectives. *J. Neural Transm.* **2012**, *119*, 275–283. [CrossRef]
41. Zádori, D.; Klivényi, P.; Vámos, E.; Fülöp, F.; Toldi, J.; Vécsei, L. Kynurenines in chronic neurodegenerative disorders: Future therapeutic strategies. *J. Neural Transm.* **2009**, *116*, 1403–1409. [CrossRef]
42. Beal, M.F.; Matson, W.R.; Swartz, K.J.; Gamache, P.H.; Bird, E.D. Kynurenine Pathway Measurements in Huntington's Disease Striatum: Evidence for Reduced Formation of Kynurenic Acid. *J. Neurochem.* **1990**, *55*, 1327–1339. [CrossRef]

43. Beal, M.F.; Matson, W.R.; Storey, E.; Milbury, P.; Ryan, E.A.; Ogawa, T.; Bird, E.D. Kynurenic acid concentrations are reduced in Huntington's disease cerebral cortex. *J. Neurol. Sci.* **1992**, *108*, 80–87. [CrossRef]
44. Jauch, D.; Urbańska, E.M.; Guidetti, P.; Bird, E.D.; Vonsattel, J.-P.G.; Whetsell, W.O.; Schwarcz, R. Dysfunction of brain kynurenic acid metabolism in Huntington's disease: Focus on kynurenine aminotransferases. *J. Neurol. Sci.* **1995**, *130*, 39–47. [CrossRef]
45. Iłżecka, J.; Kocki, T.; Stelmasiak, Z.; Turski, W.A. Endogenous protectant kynurenic acid in amyotrophic lateral sclerosis. *Acta Neurol. Scand.* **2003**, *107*, 412–418. [CrossRef]
46. Erhardt, S.; Schwieler, L.; Nilsson, L.; Linderholm, K.; Engberg, G. The kynurenic acid hypothesis of schizophrenia. *Physiol. Behav.* **2007**, *92*, 203–209. [CrossRef] [PubMed]
47. Müller, N.; Myint, A.M.; Schwarz, M.J. Kynurenine pathway in schizophrenia: Pathophysiological and therapeutic aspects. *Cur. Pharm. Res.* **2011**, *17*, 130–136. [CrossRef] [PubMed]
48. Müller, N.; Schwarz, M. Schizophrenia as an inflammationmediated dysbalance of glutamatergic neurotransmission. *Neurotox. Res.* **2006**, *10*, 131–148. [CrossRef] [PubMed]
49. Lavebratt, C.; Olsson, S.; Backlund, L.; Frisén, L.; Sellgren, C.; Priebe, L.; Nikamo, P.; Träskman-Bendz, L.; Cichon, S.; Vawter, M.P.; et al. The KMO allele encoding Arg 452 is associated with psychotic features in bipolar disorder type 1, and with increased CSF KYNA level and reduced KMO expression. *Mol. Psychiatry* **2014**, *19*, 334–341. [CrossRef]
50. Stephens, G.L.; Wang, Q.; Swerdlow, B.; Bhat, G.; Kolbeck, R.; Fung, M. Kynurenine 3-monooxygenase mediates inhibition of Th17 differentiation via catabolism of endogenous aryl hydrocarbon receptor ligands. *Eur. J. Immunol.* **2013**, *43*, 1727–1734. [CrossRef]
51. Fallarino, F.; Grohmann, U.; Vacca, C.; Bianchi, R.; Orabona, C.; Spreca, A.; Fioretti, M.C.; Puccetti, P. T cell apoptosis by tryptophan catabolism. *Cell Death Differ.* **2002**, *9*, 1069–1077. [CrossRef]
52. Mándi, Y.; Endrész, V.; Mosolygó, T.; Burián, K.; Lantos, I.; Fülöp, F.; Szatmári, I.; Lőrinczi, B.; Balog, A.; Vécsei, L. The Opposite Effects of Kynurenic Acid and Different Kynurenic Acid Analogs on Tumor Necrosis Factor-α (TNF-α) Production and Tumor Necrosis Factor-Stimulated Gene-6 (TSG-6) Expression. *Front. Immunol.* **2019**, *10*, 1406. [CrossRef]
53. Savitz, J. The Kynurenine Pathway: A Finger in Every Pie. *Mol. Psychiatry* **2020**, *25*, 131–147. [CrossRef]
54. Badawy, A.A.-B. Kynurenine Pathway of Tryptophan Metabolism: Regulatory and Functional Aspects. *Int. J. Tryptophan Res.* **2017**, *10*. [CrossRef]
55. Kanai, M.; Nakamura, T.; Funakoshi, H. Identification and characterization of novel variants of the tryptophan 2,3-dioxygenase gene: Differential regulation in the mouse nervous system during development. *Neurosci. Res.* **2009**, *64*, 111–117. [CrossRef]
56. Cervenka, I.; Agudelo, L.Z.; Ruas, J.L. Kynurenines: Tryptophan's metabolites in exercise, inflammation, and mental health. *Science* **2017**, *357*. [CrossRef]
57. Ogbechi, J.; Clanchy, F.I.; Huang, Y.-S.; Topping, L.M.; Stone, T.W.; Williams, R.O. IDO activation, inflammation and musculoskeletal disease. *Exp. Gerontol.* **2020**, *131*, 110820. [CrossRef]
58. Wu, H.; Gong, J.; Liu, Y. Indoleamine 2, 3-dioxygenase regulation of immune response (Review). *Mol. Med. Rep.* **2018**, *17*, 4867–4873. [CrossRef]
59. Prendergast, G.C.; Malachowski, W.J.; Mondal, A.; Scherle, P.; Muller, A.J. Indoleamine 2,3-Dioxygenase and Its Therapeutic Inhibition in Cancer. *Int. Rev. Cell Mol. Biol.* **2018**, *336*, 175–203. [CrossRef]
60. Prendergast, G.C.; Smith, C.; Thomas, S.; Mandik-Nayak, L.; Laury-Kleintop, L.; Metz, R.; Muller, A.J. Indoleamine 2,3-dioxygenase pathways of pathgenic inflammation and immune escape in cancer. *Cancer Immunol. Immunother.* **2014**, *63*, 721–735. [CrossRef]
61. Badawy, A.A.-B.; Guillemin, G. The Plasma [Kynurenine]/[Tryptophan] Ratio and Indoleamine 2,3-Dioxygenase: Time for Appraisal. *Int. J. Tryptophan Res.* **2019**, *12*. [CrossRef]
62. Guillemin, G.J.; Smythe, G.; Takikawa, O.; Brew, B.J. Expression of indoleamine 2, 3-dioxygenase and production of quinolinic acid by human microglia, astrocytes, and neurons. *Glia* **2005**, *49*, 15–23. [CrossRef]
63. Munn, D.H.; Zhou, M.; Attwood, J.T.; Bondarev, I.; Conway, S.J.; Marshall, B.; Brown, C.; Mellor, A.L. Prevention of Allogeneic Fetal Rejection by Tryptophan Catabolism. *Science* **1998**, *281*, 1191–1193. [CrossRef]
64. Ciorba, M.A.; Bettonville, E.E.; McDonald, K.G.; Metz, R.; Prendergast, G.C.; Newberry, R.D.; Stenson, W.F. Induction of IDO-1 by Immunostimulatory DNA Limits Severity of Experimental Colitis. *J. Immunol.* **2010**, *184*, 3907–3916. [CrossRef]
65. Frumento, G.; Rotondo, R.; Tonetti, M.; Damonte, G.; Benatti, U.; Ferrara, G.B. Tryptophan-derived catabolites are responsible for inhibition of T and natural killer cell proliferation induced by indoleamine 2, 3-dioxygenase. *J. Exp. Med.* **2002**, *196*, 459–468. [CrossRef]
66. Song, H.; Park, H.; Kim, Y.S.; Kim, K.D.; Lee, H.K.; Cho, D.H.; Yang, J.W.; Hur, D.Y. L-kynurenine-induced apoptosis in human NK cells is mediated by reactive oxygen species. *Int. Immunopharmacol.* **2011**, *11*, 932. [CrossRef]
67. Molano, A.; Illarionov, P.; Besra, G.S.; Putterman, C.; Porcelli, S.A. Modulation of invariant natural killer T cell cytokine responses by indoleamine 2, 3-dioxygenase. *Immunol. Lett.* **2008**, *117*, 81–90. [CrossRef]
68. Han, Q.; Cai, T.; Tagle, D.A.; Li, J. Structure, expression, and function of kynurenine aminotransferases in human and rodent brains. *Cell Mol. Life Sci.* **2010**, *67*, 353–368. [CrossRef]
69. Guidetti, P.; Hoffman, G.E.; Melendez-Ferro, M.; Albuquerque, E.X.; Schwarcz, R. Astrocytic localization of kynurenine aminotransferase II in the rat brain visualized by immunocytochemistry. *Glia* **2007**, *55*, 78–92. [CrossRef]

70. Boros, F.; Bohár, Z.; Vécsei, L. Genetic alterations affecting the kynurenine pathway and their association with diseases. *Mut. Res.* **2018**, *776*, 32–45. [CrossRef] [PubMed]
71. Nematollahi, A.; Sun, G.; Jayawickrama, G.S.; Church, W.B. Kynurenine Aminotransferase Isozyme Inhibitors: A Review. *Int. J. Mol. Sci.* **2016**, *17*. [CrossRef] [PubMed]
72. Fukui, S.; Schwarcz, R.; Rapoport, S.I.; Takada, Y.; Smith, Q.R. Blood–Brain Barrier Transport of Kynurenines: Implications for Brain Synthesis and Metabolism. *J. Neurochem.* **1991**, *56*, 2007–2017. [CrossRef] [PubMed]
73. Guillemin, G.J.; Kerr, S.J.; Smythe, G.A.; Smith, D.G.; Kapoor, V.; Armati, P.J.; Croitoru, J.; Brew, B.J. Kynurenine pathway metabolism in human astrocytes: A paradox for neuronal protection. *J. Neurochem.* **2001**, *78*, 842–853. [CrossRef]
74. Schwarcz, R.; Bruno, J.P.; Muchowski, P.J.; Wu, H.-Q. Kynurenines in the mammalian brain: When physiology meets pathology. *Nat. Rev. Neurosci.* **2012**, *13*, 465–477. [CrossRef]
75. Sellgren, C.; Kegel, M.; Bergen, S.; Ekman, C.; Olsson, S.; Larsson, M.; Vawter, M.; Backlund, L.; Sullivan, P.; Sklar, P.; et al. A genome-wide association study of kynurenic acid in cerebrospinal fluid: Implications for psychosis and cognitive impairment in bipolar disorder. *Mol. Psychiatry* **2014**, *19*, 334–341. [CrossRef]
76. Stazka, J.; Luchowski, P.; Urbanska, E.M. Homocysteine, a risk factor for atherosclerosis, biphasically changes the endothelial production of kynurenic acid. *Eur. J. Pharmacol.* **2005**, *517*, 217–223. [CrossRef]
77. Fallarini, S.; Magliulo, L.; Paoletti, T.; de Lalla, C.; Lombardi, G. Expression of functional GPR35 in human iNKT cells. *Biochem. Biophys. Res. Commun.* **2010**, *398*, 420–425. [CrossRef]
78. Yamamura, T.; Sakuishi, K.; Illes, Z.; Miyake, S. Understanding the behavior of invariant NKT cells in autoimmune diseases. *J. Neuroimmunol.* **2007**, *191*, 8–15. [CrossRef]
79. Hartai, Z.; Klivenyi, P.; Janaky, T.; Penke, B.; Dux, L.; Vecsei, L. Kynurenine metabolism in multiple sclerosis. *Acta Neurol. Scand.* **2005**, *112*, 93–96. [CrossRef]
80. Bai, M.Y.; Lovejoy, D.B.; Guillemin, G.J.; Kozak, R.; Stone, T.W.; Koola, M.M. Galantamine-Memantine Combination and Kynurenine Pathway Enzyme Inhibitors in the Treatment of Neuropsychiatric Disorders. *Complex Psychiatry* **2021**. [CrossRef]
81. Coyle, J.T. Glial metabolites of tryptophan and excitotoxicity: Coming unglued. *Exper. Neurol.* **2006**, *197*, 4–7. [CrossRef]
82. Schwarcz, R. The kynurenine pathway of tryptophan degradation as a drug target. Cur. *Opin. Pharmacol.* **2004**, *4*, 12–17. [CrossRef]
83. Schwarcz, R.; Pellicciari, R. Manipulation of Brain Kynurenines: Glial Targets, Neuronal Effects, and Clinical Opportunities. *J. Pharmacol. Exp. Ther.* **2002**, *303*, 1–10. [CrossRef] [PubMed]
84. Vamos, E.; Pardutz, A.; Klivenyi, P.; Toldi, J.; Vecsei, L. The role of kynurenines in disorders of the central nervous system: Possibilities for neuroprotection. *J. Neurol. Sci. Vasc. Dement.* **2009**, *283*, 21–27. [CrossRef] [PubMed]
85. Mazza, J.; Rossi, A.; Weinberg, J.M. Innovatives uses of tumor necrosis factor alpha inhibitors. *Dermatol. Clin.* **2010**, *28*, 559–575. [CrossRef] [PubMed]
86. Tiszlavicz, Z.; Németh, B.; Fülöp, F.; Vécsei, L.; Tápai, K.; Ocsovszky, I.; Mándi, Y. Different inhibitory effects of kynurenic acid and a novel kynurenic acid analogue on tumour necrosis factor-a (TNF-a) production by mononuclear cells, HMGB1 production by monocytes and HNP1-3 secretion by neutrophils. *Naunyn Schmiedebergs Arch. Pharmacol.* **2011**, *383*, 447–455. [CrossRef]
87. Oztan, O.; Turksoy, V.A.; Daltaban, I.S.; Gunduzoz, M.; Tutkun, L.; Iritas, S.B.; Hakan, A.K. Pro-inflammatory cytokine and vascular adhesion molecule levels in manganese and lead-exposed workers. *Int. J Immunother. Cancer Res.* **2019**, *5*, 1–7. [CrossRef]
88. Müller, N.; Schwarz, M.J. Immune system and schizophrenia. *Cur. Immunol. Rev.* **2010**, *6*, 213–220. [CrossRef]
89. Raison, C.L.; Dantzer, R.; Kelley, K.W.; Lawson, M.A.; Woolwine, B.J.; Vogt, G.; Spivey, J.R.; Saito, K.; Miller, A.H. CSF concentrations of brain tryptophan and kynurenines during immune stimulation with IFN-alpha: Relationship to CNS immune responses and depression. *Mol. Psychiatry* **2010**, *15*, 393–403. [CrossRef]
90. Van Gool, A.R.; Verkerk, R.; Fekkes, D.; Bannink, M.; Sleijfer, S.; Kruit, W.H.J.; van der Holt, B.; Scharpe, S.; Eggermont, A.M.M.; Stoter, G.; et al. Neurotoxic and neuroprotective metabolites of kynurenine in patients with renal cell carcinoma treated with interferon-alpha: Course and relationship with psychiatric status. *Psychiatry Clin. Neurosci.* **2008**, *62*, 597–602. [CrossRef]
91. Török, N.; Maszlag-Török, R.; Molnár, K.; Szolnoki, Z.; Somogyvári, F.; Boda, K.; Tanaka, M.; Klivényi, P.; Vécsei, L. Single Nucleotide Polymorphisms of Indoleamine 2,3-Dioxygenase Influenced the Age Onset of Parkinson's Disease. *Preprints* **2020**, 2020100172. [CrossRef]
92. Miura, H.; Ozaki, N.; Sawada, M.; Isobe, K.; Ohta, T.; Nagatsu, T. A link between stress and depression: Shifts in the balance between the kynurenine and serotonin pathways of tryptophan metabolism and the etiology and pathophysiology of depression. *Stress* **2008**, *11*, 198–209. [CrossRef]
93. Mucci, F.; Marazziti, D.; Della Vecchia, A.; Baroni, S.; Morana, P.; Carpita, B.; Mangiapane, P.; Morana, F.; Morana, B.; Dell'Osso, L. State-of-the-Art: Inflammatory and Metabolic Markers in Mood Disorders. *Life* **2020**, *10*, 82. [CrossRef]
94. Okamoto, H.; Hayaishi, O. Flavin adenine dinucleotide requirement for kynurenine hydroxylase of rat liver mitochondria. *Biochem. Biophys. Res. Commun.* **1967**, *29*, 394–399. [CrossRef]
95. Okuda, S.; Nishiyama, N.; Saito, H.; Katsuki, H. 3-Hydroxykynurenine, an Endogenous Oxidative Stress Generator, Causes Neuronal Cell Death with Apoptotic Features and Region Selectivity. *J. Neurochem.* **1998**, *70*, 299–307. [CrossRef]
96. Moroni, F. Tryptophan metabolism and brain function: Focus on kynurenine and other indole metabolites. *Eur. J. Pharmacol.* **1999**, *375*, 87–100. [CrossRef]

97. Nguyen, N.T.; Nakahama, T.; Le, D.H.; Van Son, L.; Chu, H.H.; Kishimoto, T. Aryl hydrocarbon receptor and kynurenine: Recent advances in autoimmune disease research. *Front. Immunol.* **2014**, *5*, 551. [CrossRef]
98. Pilotte, L.; Larrieu, P.; Stroobant, V.; Colau, D.; Dolusic, E.; Frédérick, R.; De Plaen, E.; Uyttenhove, C.; Wouters, J.; Masereel, B.J.; et al. Reversal of tumoral immune resistance by inhibition of tryptophan 2,3-dioxygenase. *Proc. Natl. Acad. Sci. USA* **2012**, *109*, 2497–2502. [CrossRef]
99. Andiné, P.; Lehmann, A.; Ellrén, K.; Wennberg, E.; Kjellmer, I.; Nielsen, T.; Hagberg, H. The excitatory amino acid antagonist kynurenic acid administered after hypoxic-ischemia in neonatal rats offers neuroprotection. *Neurosci. Lett.* **1988**, *90*, 208–212. [CrossRef]
100. Foster, A.C.; Vezzani, A.; French, E.D.; Schwarcz, R. Kynurenic acid blocks neurotoxicity and seizures induced in rats by the related brain metabolite quinolinic acid. *Neurosci. Lett.* **1984**, *48*, 273–278. [CrossRef]
101. Wirthgen, E.; Hoeflich, A.; Rebl, A.; Günther, J. Kynurenic acid: The Janus-faced role of an immunomodulatory tryptophan metabolite and its link to pathological conditions. *Front. Immunol.* **2017**, *8*, 1957. [CrossRef]
102. Connor, T.J.; Starr, N.; O'Sullivan, J.B.; Harkin, A. Induction of indolamine 2,3-dioxygenase and kynurenine 3-monooxygenase in rat brain following a systemic inflammatory challenge: A role for IFN-γ? *Neurosci. Lett.* **2008**, *441*, 29–34. [CrossRef]
103. Jacobs, K.R.; Castellano-Gonzalez, G.; Guillemin, G.J.; Lovejoy, D.B. Major Developments in the Design of Inhibitors along the Kynurenine Pathway. *Cur. Med. Chem.* **2017**, *24*, 2471–2495. [CrossRef]
104. Wang, J.; Simonavicius, N.; Wu, X.; Swaminath, G.; Reagan, J.; Tian, H.; Ling, L. Kynurenic acid as a ligand for orphan G protein-coupled receptor GPR35. *J. Biol. Chem.* **2006**, *281*, 22021–22028. [CrossRef]
105. Kubo, H.; Hoshi, M.; Mouri, A.; Tashita, C.; Yamamoto, Y.; Nabeshima, T.; Saito, K. Absence of kynurenine 3-monooxygenase reduces mortality of acute viral myocarditis in mice. *Immunol. Lett.* **2016**, *181*, 94–100. [CrossRef]
106. Tanaka, M.; Vécsei, L. Editorial of Special Issue "Crosstalk between Depression, Anxiety, and Dementia: Comorbidity in Behavioral Neurology and Neuropsychiatry". *Biomedicines* **2021**, *9*, 517. [CrossRef]
107. Ibos, K.E.; Bodnár, É.; Bagosi, Z.; Bozsó, Z.; Tóth, G.; Szabó, G.; Csabafi, K. Kisspeptin-8 Induces Anxiety-Like Behavior and Hypolocomotion by Activating the HPA Axis and Increasing GABA Release in the Nucleus Accumbens in Rats. *Biomedicines* **2021**, *9*, 112. [CrossRef]
108. Muntsant, A.; Jiménez-Altayó, F.; Puertas-Umbert, L.; Jiménez-Xarrie, E.; Vila, E.; Giménez-Llort, L. Sex-Dependent End-of-Life Mental and Vascular Scenarios for Compensatory Mechanisms in Mice with Normal and AD-Neurodegenerative Aging. *Biomedicines* **2021**, *9*, 111. [CrossRef]
109. Giménez-Llort, L.; Marin-Pardo, D.; Marazuela, P.; Hernández-Guillamón, M. Survival Bias and Crosstalk between Chronological and Behavioral Age: Age- and Genotype-Sensitivity Tests Define Behavioral Signatures in Middle-Aged, Old, and Long-Lived Mice with Normal and AD-Associated Aging. *Biomedicines* **2021**, *9*, 636. [CrossRef]
110. Cantón-Habas, V.; Rich-Ruiz, M.; Romero-Saldaña, M.; Carrera-González, M. Depression as a Risk Factor for Dementia and Alzheimer's Disease. *Biomedicines* **2020**, *8*, 457. [CrossRef]
111. Kowalska, K.; Krzywoszański, Ł.; Droś, J.; Pasińska, P.; Wilk, A.; Klimkowicz-Mrowiec, A. Early Depression Independently of Other Neuropsychiatric Conditions, Influences Disability and Mortality after Stroke (Research Study-Part of PROPOLIS Study). *Biomedicines* **2020**, *8*, 509. [CrossRef]
112. Balogh, L.; Tanaka, M.; Török, N.; Vécsei, L.; Taguchi, S. Crosstalk between Existential Phenomenological Psychotherapy and Neurological Sciences in Mood and Anxiety Disorders. *Biomedicines* **2021**, *9*, 340. [CrossRef]
113. Park, S.; Bak, A.; Kim, S.; Nam, Y.; Kim, H.S.; Yoo, D.H.; Moon, M. Animal-Assisted and Pet-Robot Interventions for Ameliorating Behavioral and Psychological Symptoms of Dementia: A Systematic Review and Meta-Analysis. *Biomedicines* **2020**, *8*, 150. [CrossRef] [PubMed]
114. Ohayon, M.; Schatzberg, A. Prevalence of depressive episodes with psychotic features in the general population. *Am. J. Psychiatry* **2002**, *159*, 1855–1861. [CrossRef] [PubMed]
115. Galynker, I.; Cohen, L.; Cai, J. Negative symptoms in patients with major depressive disorder: A preliminary report. Neuropsychiatry. *Neuropsychol. Behav. Neurol.* **2000**, *13*, 171–176.
116. McIntyre, R.; Cha, D.; Soczynska, J. Cognitive deficits and functional outcomes in major depressive disorder: Determinants, substrates, and treatment interventions. *Depress. Anxiety* **2013**, *30*, 515–527. [CrossRef]
117. Ballenger, J. Anxiety and depression: Optimizing treatments. Prim Care Companion. *J. Clin. Psychiatry* **2000**, *2*, 71–79. [CrossRef]
118. Howren, M.B.; Lamkin, D.M.; Suls, J. Associations of depression with C-reactive protein, IL-1, and IL-6: A meta-analysis. *Psychosom. Med.* **2009**, *71*, 171–186. [CrossRef]
119. Dowlati, Y.; Herrmann, N.; Swardfager, W.; Liu, H.; Sham, L.; Reim, E.K.; Lanctôt, K.L. A meta-analysis of cytokines in major depression. *Biol. Psychiatry* **2010**, *67*, 446–457. [CrossRef]
120. Liu, Y.; Ho, R.C.; Mak, A. Interleukin (IL)-6, tumour necrosis factor alpha (TNF-α) and soluble interleukin-2 receptors (sIL-2R) are elevated in patients with major depressive disorder: A meta-analysis and meta-regression. *J. Affect. Disord.* **2012**, *139*, 230–239. [CrossRef]
121. Valkanova, V.; Ebmeier, K.P.; Allan, C.L. CRP, IL-6 and depression: A systematic review and meta-analysis of longitudinal studies. *J. Affect. Disord.* **2013**, *150*, 736–744. [CrossRef]

122. Haapakoski, R.; Mathieu, J.; Ebmeier, K.P.; Alenius, H.; Kivimäki, M. Cumulative meta-analysis of interleukins 6 and 1β, tumour necrosis factor α and C-reactive protein in patients with major depressive disorder. *Brain Behav. Immun.* **2015**, *49*, 206–215. [CrossRef]
123. Goldsmith, D.R.; Rapaport, M.H.; Miller, B.J. A meta-analysis of blood cytokine network alterations in psychiatric patients: Comparisons between schizophrenia, bipolar disorder and depression. *Mol. Psychiatry* **2016**, *21*, 1696–1709. [CrossRef]
124. Hiles, S.A.; Baker, A.L.; de Malmanche, T.; Attia, J. A meta-analysis of differences in IL-6 and IL-10 between people with and without depression: Exploring the causes of heterogeneity. *Brain Behav. Immun.* **2012**, *26*, 1180–1188. [CrossRef]
125. Wang, A.K.; Miller, B.J. Meta-analysis of Cerebrospinal Fluid Cytokine and Tryptophan Catabolite Alterations in Psychiatric Patients: Comparisons Between Schizophrenia, Bipolar Disorder, and Depression. *Schizophr. Bull.* **2018**, *44*, 75–83. [CrossRef]
126. Ogawa, S.; Fujii, T.; Koga, N.; Hori, H.; Teraishi, T.; Hattori, K.; Noda, T.; Higuchi, T.; Motohashi, N.; Kunugi, H. Plasma L-tryptophan concentration in major depressive disorder: New data and meta-analysis. *J. Clin. Psychiatry* **2014**, *75*, e906–e915. [CrossRef]
127. Ogyu, K.; Kubo, K.; Noda, Y.; Iwata, Y.; Tsugawa, S.; Omura, Y.; Wada, M.; Tarumi, R.; Plitman, E.; Moriguchi, S.; et al. Kynurenine pathway in depression: A systematic review and meta-analysis. *Neurosci, Biobehav. Rev.* **2018**, *90*, 16–25. [CrossRef]
128. Réus, G.; Jansen, K.; Titus, S.; Carvalho, A.F.; Gabbay, V.; Quevedo, J. Kynurenine pathway dysfunction in the pathophysiology and treatment of depression: Evidences from animal and human studies. *J. Psychiatr. Res.* **2015**, *68*, 316–328. [CrossRef]
129. Dunayevich, E.; Keck, P.E., Jr. Prevalence and description of psychotic features in bipolar mania. *Cur. Psychiatry Rep.* **2000**, *2*, 286–290. [CrossRef]
130. Ameen, S.; Ram, D. Negative symptoms in the remission phase of bipolar disorder. *Ger. J. Psychiatry* **2007**, *10*, 1–7.
131. Malhi, G.S.; Ivanovski, B.; Hadzi-Pavlovic, D.; Mitchell, P.B.; Vieta, E.; Sachdev, P. Neuropsychological deficits and functional impairment in bipolar depression, hypomania and euthymia. *Bipolar Disord.* **2007**, *9*, 114–125. [CrossRef]
132. Martínez-Arán, A.; Vieta, E.; Colom, F.; Torrent, C.; Sánchez-Moreno, J.; Reinares, M.; Benabarre, A.; Goikolea, J.M.; Brugué, E.; Daban, C.; et al. Cognitive impairment in euthymic bipolar patients: Implications for clinical and functional outcome. *Bipolar Disord.* **2004**, *6*, 224–232. [CrossRef]
133. Das, A. Anxiety disorders in bipolar I mania: Prevalence, effect on illness severity, and treatment implications. *Indian J. Psychol. Med.* **2013**, *35*, 53–59. [CrossRef]
134. Modabbernia, A.; Taslimi, S.; Brietzke, E.; Ashrafi, M. Cytokine alterations in bipolar disorder: A meta-analysis of 30 studies. *Biol. Psychiatry* **2013**, *74*, 15–25. [CrossRef]
135. Munkholm, K.; Braüner, J.V.; Kessing, L.V.; Vinberg, M. Cytokines in bipolar disorder vs. healthy control subjects: A systematic review and meta-analysis. *J.; Psychiatr, Res.* **2013**, *47*, 1119–1133. [CrossRef]
136. Munkholm, K.; Vinberg, M.; Vedel Kessing, L. Cytokines in bipolar disorder: A systematic review and meta-analysis. *J. Affect. Disord.* **2013**, *144*, 16–27. [CrossRef]
137. Birner, A.; Platzer, M.; Bengesser, S.A.; Dalkner, N.; Fellendorf, F.T.; Queissner, R.; Pilz, R.; Rauch, P.; Maget, A.; Hamm, C.; et al. Increased breakdown of kynurenine towards its neurotoxic branch in bipolar disorder. *PLoS ONE* **2017**, *12*, e0172699. [CrossRef]
138. Arnone, D.; Saraykar, S.; Salem, H.; Teixeira, A.L.; Dantzer, R.; Selvaraj, S. Role of Kynurenine pathway and its metabolites in mood disorders: A systematic review and meta-analysis of clinical studies. *Neurosci. Biobehav. Rev.* **2018**, *92*, 477–485. [CrossRef]
139. Hartley, S.; Barrowclough, C.; Haddock, G. Anxiety and depression in psychosis: A systematic review of associations with positive psychotic symptoms. *Acta Psychiatr. Scand.* **2013**, *128*, 327–346. [CrossRef]
140. Wigman, J.T.; van Nierop, M.; Vollebergh, W.A.; Lieb, R.; Beesdo-Baum, K.; Wittchen, H.U.; van Os, J. Evidence that psychotic symptoms are prevalent in disorders of anxiety and depression, impacting on illness onset, risk, and severity—Implications for diagnosis and ultra-high risk research. *Schizophr. Bull.* **2012**, *38*, 247–257. [CrossRef]
141. Yang, Y.; Zhang, X.; Zhu, Y.; Dai, Y.; Liu, T.; Wang, Y. Cognitive impairment in generalized anxiety disorder revealed by event-related potential N270. *Neuropsychiatr. Dis. Treat.* **2015**, *11*, 1405–1411. [CrossRef] [PubMed]
142. Costello, H.; Gould, R.L.; Abrol, E.; Howard, R. Systematic review and meta-analysis of the association between peripheral inflammatory cytokines and generalized anxiety disorder. *BMJ Open* **2019**, *9*, e027925. [CrossRef] [PubMed]
143. Hou, R.; Garner, M.; Holmes, C.; Osmond, C.; Teeling, J.; Lau, L.; Baldwin, D.S. Peripheral inflammatory cytokines and immune balance in Generalised Anxiety Disorder: Case-controlled study. *Brain Behav. Immun.* **2017**, *62*, 212–218. [CrossRef]
144. Orlikov, A.B.; Prakhye, I.B.; Ryzov, I.V. Kynurenine in blood plasma and DST in patients with endogenous anxiety and endogenous depression. *Biol. Psychiatry* **1994**, *36*, 97–102. [CrossRef]
145. Altmaier, E.; Emeny, R.T.; Krumsiek, J.; Lacruz, M.E.; Lukaschek, K.; Häfner, S.; Kastenmüller, G.; Römisch-Margl, W.; Prehn, C.; Mohney, R.P.; et al. Metabolomic profiles in individuals with negative affectivity and social inhibition: A population-based study of Type D personality. *Psychoneuroendocrinology* **2013**, *38*, 1299–1309. [CrossRef]
146. National Institute on Drug Abuse. Advancing Addiction Science. Available online: https://www.drugabuse.gov/publications/media-guide/science-drug-use-addiction-basics (accessed on 28 April 2021).
147. UpToDate. Co-Occurring Schizophrenia and Substance Use Disorder: Epidemiology, Pathogenesis, Clinical Manifestations, Course, Assessment and Diagnosis. Available online: https://www.uptodate.com/contents/co-occurring-schizophrenia-and-substance-use-disorder-epidemiology-pathogenesis-clinical-manifestations-course-assessment-and-diagnosis (accessed on 28 April 2021).

148. Connor, J.P.; Stjepanović, D.; Le Foll, B.; Hoch, E.; Budney, A.J.; Hall, W.D. Cannabis use and cannabis use disorder. *Nat. Rev. Dis. Primers* **2021**, *7*, 16. [CrossRef]
149. Addiction Center. Schizophrenia and Addiction. Available online: https://www.addictioncenter.com/addiction/schizophrenia/ (accessed on 28 April 2021).
150. Simon, N.; Belzeaux, R.; Adida, M.; Azorin, J.M. Negative symptoms in schizophrenia and substance-related disorders. *L'Encephale* **2015**, *41* Suppl. S1, 6S27–6S31. [CrossRef]
151. Whiting, D.; Lichtenstein, P.; Fazel, S. Violence and mental disorders: A structured review of associations by individual diagnoses, risk factors, and risk assessment. *Lancet Psychiatry* **2021**, *8*, 150–161. [CrossRef]
152. Bruijnen, C.; Dijkstra, B.; Walvoort, S.; Markus, W.; van der Nagel, J.; Kessels, R.; De Jong, C. Prevalence of cognitive impairment in patients with substance use disorder. *Drug Alcohol Rev.* **2019**, *38*, 435–442. [CrossRef]
153. Elmquist, J.; Shorey, R.C.; Anderson, S.E.; Stuart, G.L. The Relationship Between Generalized Anxiety Symptoms and Treatment Dropout Among Women in Residential Treatment for Substance Use Disorders. *Subst. Use Misuse* **2016**, *51*, 835–839. [CrossRef]
154. Brown, K.T.; Levis, S.C.; O'Neill, C.E.; Northcutt, A.L.; Fabisiak, T.J.; Watkins, L.R.; Bachtell, R.K. Innate immune signaling in the ventral tegmental area contributes to drug-primed reinstatement of cocaine seeking. *Brain Behav. Immune* **2018**, *67*, 130–138. [CrossRef]
155. Kohno, M.; Link, J.; Dennis, L.E.; McCready, H.; Huckans, M.; Hoffman, W.F.; Loftis, J.M. Neuroinflammation in addiction: A review of neuroimaging studies and potential immunotherapies. *Pharmacol. Biochem. Behav.* **2019**, *179*, 34–42. [CrossRef]
156. Fonseca, F.; Mestre-Pintó, J.I.; Gómez-Gómez, À.; Martinez-Sanvisens, D.; Rodríguez-Minguela, R.; Papaseit, E.; Pérez-Mañá, C.; Langohr, K.; Valverde, O.; Pozo, Ó.J.; et al. On Behalf of Neurodep Group the Tryptophan System in Cocaine-Induced Depression. *J. Clin. Med.* **2020**, *9*, 4103. [CrossRef]
157. Bedard-Gilligan, M.; Zoellner, L.A.; Feeny, N.C. Is Trauma Memory Special? Trauma Narrative Fragmentation in PTSD: Effects of Treatment and Response. *Clin. Psychol. Sci.* **2017**, *5*, 212–225. [CrossRef]
158. De Boer, M.; Nijdam, M.J.; Jongedijk, R.A.; Bangel, K.A.; Olff, M.; Hofman, W.F.; Talamini, L.M. The spectral fingerprint of sleep problems in post-traumatic stress disorder. *Sleep* **2020**, *43*, zsz269. [CrossRef]
159. Compean, E.; Hamner, M. Posttraumatic stress disorder with secondary psychotic features (PTSD-SP): Diagnostic and treatment challenges. *Prog Neuropsychopharmacol. Biol. Psychiatry* **2019**, *88*, 265–275. [CrossRef] [PubMed]
160. Maeng, L.Y.; Milad, M.R. Post-Traumatic Stress Disorder: The Relationship Between the Fear Response and Chronic Stress. *Chronic Stress* **2017**, *1*. [CrossRef] [PubMed]
161. Hayes, J.P.; Vanelzakker, M.B.; Shin, L.M. Emotion and cognition interactions in PTSD: A review of neurocognitive and neuroimaging studies. *Front. Integr. Nneurosci.* **2012**, *6*, 89. [CrossRef] [PubMed]
162. Price, M.; Legrand, A.C.; Brier, Z.; Hébert-Dufresne, L. The symptoms at the center: Examining the comorbidity of posttraumatic stress disorder, generalized anxiety disorder, and depression with network analysis. *J. Psychiatr. Res.* **2019**, *109*, 52–58. [CrossRef] [PubMed]
163. Kim, T.D.; Lee, S.; Yoon, S. Inflammation in Post-Traumatic Stress Disorder (PTSD): A Review of Potential Correlates of PTSD with a Neurological Perspective. *Antioxidants* **2020**, *9*, 107. [CrossRef]
164. Kim, Y.K.; Amidfar, M.; Won, E. A review on inflammatory cytokine-induced alterations of the brain as potential neural biomarkers in post-traumatic stress disorder. *Prog. Neuro-Psychopharmacol. Biol. Psychiatry* **2019**, *91*, 103–112. [CrossRef]
165. Cohen, M.; Meir, T.; Klein, E.; Volpin, G.; Assaf, M.; Pollack, S. Cytokine levels as potential biomarkers for predicting the development of posttraumatic stress symptoms in casualties of accidents. *Int. J. Psychiatry Med.* **2011**, *42*, 117–131. [CrossRef]
166. Berkwits, M.; Porter, R.; Jones, T.V.; Fletcher, A.J.; Beers, M.H. *The Merck Manual of Medical Information*; Merck & Co. Inc.: New York, NY, USA, 2003.
167. Kiran, C.; Chaudhury, S. Prevalence of comorbid anxiety disorders in schizophrenia. *Indian J. Psychiatry* **2016**, *25*, 35–40. [CrossRef]
168. Miller, B.J.; Buckley, P.; Seabolt, W.; Mellor, A.; Kirkpatrick, B. Meta-analysis of cytokine alterations in schizophrenia: Clinical status and antipsychotic effects. *Biol. Psychiatry* **2011**, *70*, 663–671. [CrossRef]
169. Frydecka, D.; Krzystek-Korpacka, M.; Lubeiro, A.; Stramecki, F.; Stańczykiewicz, B.; Beszłej, J.A.; Piotrowski, P.; Kotowicz, K.; Szewczuk-Bogusławska, M.; Pawlak-Adamska, E.; et al. Profiling inflammatory signatures of schizophrenia: A cross-sectional and meta-analysis study. *Brain Behav. Immunity* **2018**, *71*, 28–36. [CrossRef]
170. Gallego, J.A.; Blanco, E.A.; Husain-Krautter, S.; Madeline Fagen, E.; Moreno-Merino, P.; Del Ojo-Jiménez, J.A.; Ahmed, A.; Rothstein, T.L.; Lencz, T.; Malhotra, A.K. Cytokines in cerebrospinal fluid of patients with schizophrenia spectrum disorders: New data and an updated meta-analysis. *Schizophr. Res.* **2018**, *202*, 64–71. [CrossRef]
171. Koola, M.M.; Raines, J.K.; Hamilton, R.G.; McMahon, R.P. Can anti-inflammatory medications improve symptoms and reduce mortality in schizophrenia? *Cur. Psychiatry* **2016**, *15*, 52–57.
172. Okusaga, O.; Fuchs, D.; Reeves, G.; Giegling, I.; Hartmann, A.M.; Konte, B.; Friedl, M.; Groer, M.; Cook, T.B.; Stearns-Yoder, K.A.; et al. Kynurenine and Tryptophan Levels in Patients with Schizophrenia and Elevated Antigliadin Immunoglobulin G Antibodies. *Psychosom. Med.* **2016**, *78*, 931–939. [CrossRef]
173. Plitman, E.; Iwata, Y.; Caravaggio, F.; Nakajima, S.; Chung, J.K.; Gerretsen, P.; Kim, J.; Takeuchi, H.; Chakravarty, M.M.; Remington, G.; et al. Kynurenic acid in schizophrenia: A systematic review and meta-analysis. *Schizophr. Bull.* **2017**, *43*, 764–777. [CrossRef]

174. Marx, W.; McGuinness, A.J.; Rocks, T.; Ruusunen, A.; Cleminson, J.; Walker, A.J.; Gomes-da-Costa, S.; Lane, M.; Sanches, M.; Diaz, A.P.; et al. The kynurenine pathway in major depressive disorder, bipolar disorder, and schizophrenia: A meta-analysis of 101 studies. *Mol. Psychiatry* **2020**. [CrossRef]
175. Koola, M.M.; Praharaj, S.K.; Pillai, A. Galantamine-Memantine Combination as an Antioxidant Treatment for Schizophrenia. *Cur. Behav. Neurosci. Rep.* **2019**, *6*, 37–50. [CrossRef]
176. Koola, M.M.; Sklar, J.; Davis, W.; Nikiforuk, A.; Meissen, J.K.; Sawant-Basak, A.; Aaronson, S.T.; Kozak, R. Kynurenine pathway in schizophrenia: Galantamine-memantine combination for cognitive impairments. *Schizophr. Res.* **2018**, *193*, 459–460. [CrossRef]
177. Bell, V.; Dunne, H.; Zacharia, T.; Brooker, K.; Shergill, S. A symptom-based approach to treatment of psychosis in autism spectrum disorder [corrected]. *BJPsych. Open* **2018**, *4*, 1–4. [CrossRef]
178. Leekam, S. Social cognitive impairment and autism: What are we trying to explain? *Philos Trans. R. Soc.* **2016**, *371*, 20150082. [CrossRef]
179. Van Steensel, F.J.A.; Heeman, E.J. Anxiety Levels in Children with Autism Spectrum Disorder: A Meta-Analysis. *J. Child Fam. Stud.* **2017**, *26*, 1753–1767. [CrossRef]
180. Lai, M.C.; Kassee, C.; Besney, R.; Bonato, S.; Hull, L.; Mandy, W.; Szatmari, P.; Ameis, S.H. Prevalence of co-occurring mental health diagnoses in the autism population: A systematic review and meta-analysis. *Lancet Psychiatry* **2019**, *6*, 819–829. [CrossRef]
181. Masi, A.; Quintana, D.S.; Glozier, N.; Lloyd, A.R.; Hickie, I.B.; Guastella, A.J. Cytokine aberrations in autism spectrum disorder: A systematic review and meta-analysis. *Mol. Psychiatry* **2015**, *20*, 440–446. [CrossRef]
182. Saghazadeh, A.; Ataeinia, B.; Keynejad, K.; Abdolalizadeh, A.; Hirbod-Mobarakeh, A.; Rezaei, N. A meta-analysis of pro-inflammatory cytokines in autism spectrum disorders: Effects of age, gender, and latitude. *J. Psychiatr. Res.* **2019**, *115*, 90–102. [CrossRef]
183. Molloy, C.A.; Morrow, A.L.; Meinzen-Derr, J.; Schleifer, K.; Dienger, K.; Manning-Courtney, P.; Altaye, M.; Wills-Karp, M. Elevated cytokine levels in children with autism spectrum disorder. *J. Neuroimmunol.* **2006**, *172*, 198–205. [CrossRef]
184. Bryn, V.; Verkerk, R.; Skjeldal, O.H.; Saugstad, O.D.; Ormstad, H. Kynurenine Pathway in Autism Spectrum Disorders in Children. *Neuropsychobiology* **2017**, *76*, 82–88. [CrossRef] [PubMed]
185. Lim, C.K.; Essa, M.M.; de Paula Martins, R.; Lovejoy, D.B.; Bilgin, A.A.; Waly, M.I.; Al-Farsi, Y.M.; Al-Sharbati, M.; Al-Shaffae, M.A.; Guillemin, G.J. Altered kynurenine pathway metabolism in autism: Implication for immune-induced glutamatergic activity. *Autism Res.* **2016**, *9*, 621–631. [CrossRef]
186. Kordestani Moghadam, P.; Nouriyengejeh, S.; Seyedhoseini, B.; Pourabbasi, A. The Study of Relationship between Nutritional Behaviors and Metabolic Indices: A Systematic Review. *Adv. Biomed. Res.* **2020**, *9*, 66. [CrossRef]
187. Kordestani-Moghadam, P.; Assari, S.; Nouriyengejeh, S.; Mohammadipour, F.; Pourabbasi, A. Cognitive Impairments and Associated Structural Brain Changes in Metabolic Syndrome and Implications of Neurocognitive Intervention. *J. Obes. Metab. Syndr.* **2020**, *29*, 174–179. [CrossRef] [PubMed]
188. Kordestani Moghadam, P.; Nasehi, M.; Khodagholi, F.; Reza Zarrindast, M. Vulnerability of Left Amygdala to Total Sleep Deprivation and Reversed Circadian Rhythm in Molecular Level: Glut1 as a Metabolic Biomarker. *Galen. Med. J.* **2019**, *8*, 970. [CrossRef]
189. Kim, J.; Kim, Y.K. Crosstalk between Depression and Dementia with Resting-State fMRI Studies and Its Relationship with Cognitive Functioning. *Biomedicines* **2021**, *9*, 82. [CrossRef]
190. Komatsu, H.; Watanabe, E.; Fukuchi, M. Psychiatric Neural Networks and Precision Therapeutics by Machine Learning. *Biomedicines* **2021**, *9*, 403. [CrossRef]

biomedicines

MDPI

Article

Genotype Load Modulates Amyloid Burden and Anxiety-Like Patterns in Male 3xTg-AD Survivors despite Similar Neuro-Immunoendocrine, Synaptic and Cognitive Impairments

Aida Muntsant [1,2] and Lydia Giménez-Llort [1,2,*]

1 Institut de Neurociències, Universitat Autònoma de Barcelona, 08193 Barcelona, Spain; aida.muntsant@uab.cat

2 Department of Psychiatry and Forensic Medicine, School of Medicine, Universitat Autònoma de Barcelona, 08193 Barcelona, Spain

* Correspondence: lidia.gimenez@uab.cat; Tel.: +34-93-581-2378

Abstract: The wide heterogeneity and complexity of Alzheimer's disease (AD) patients' clinical profiles and increased mortality highlight the relevance of personalized-based interventions and the need for end-of-life/survival predictors. At the translational level, studying genetic and age interactions in a context of different levels of expression of AD-genetic-load can help to understand this heterogeneity better. In the present report, a singular cohort of long-lived (19-month-old survivors) heterozygous and homozygous male 3xTg-AD mice were studied to determine whether their AD-genotype load can modulate the brain and peripheral pathological burden, behavioral phenotypes, and neuro-immunoendocrine status, compared to age-matched non-transgenic controls. The results indicated increased amyloid precursor protein (APP) levels in a genetic-load-dependent manner but convergent synaptophysin and choline acetyltransferase brain levels. Cognitive impairment and HPA-axis hyperactivation were salient traits in both 3xTg-AD survivor groups. In contrast, genetic load elicited different anxiety-like profiles, with hypoactive homozygous, while heterozygous resembled controls in some traits and risk assessment. Complex neuro-immunoendocrine crosstalk was also observed. Bodyweight loss and splenic, renal, and hepatic histopathological injury scores provided evidence of the systemic features of AD, despite similar peripheral organs' oxidative stress. The present study provides an interesting translational scenario to study further genetic-load and age-dependent vulnerability/compensatory mechanisms in Alzheimer's disease.

Keywords: Alzheimer's disease; genetic load; survival; end-of-life; frailty; heterogeneity; BPSD; NPS; neuro-immunoendocrine crosstalk

Citation: Muntsant, A.; Giménez-Llort, L. Genotype Load Modulates Amyloid Burden and Anxiety-Like Patterns in Male 3xTg-AD Survivors Despite Similar Neuro-Immunoendocrine, Synaptic and Cognitive Impairments. *Biomedicines* **2021**, *9*, 715. https://doi.org/10.3390/biomedicines9070715

Academic Editors: Masaru Tanaka and Nóra Török

Received: 11 May 2021
Accepted: 20 June 2021
Published: 23 June 2021

1. Introduction

Alzheimer's disease (AD) is the leading cause of dementia, one of the principal causes of disability in late adulthood. It is a multi-factorial disorder caused by the interaction of biological, environmental factors, where age-related changes play a determinant role [1]. At the neuropathological level, Alzheimer's disease is mainly defined by an extracellular accumulation of amyloid-β (Aβ) plaques and reactive gliosis and cellular tau-containing neurofibrillary tangles (NFTs) accompanied by synaptic dysfunction and cholinergic-dependent progressive memory decline [2]. Whereas cognitive dysfunction defines the diagnosis of the core clinical symptoms, neuropsychiatric symptoms (NPS) [3], also called Behavioral and Psychological Symptoms of Dementia (BPSD), are observed in 90% of patients. The broad array of NPS include agitation, anxiety, verbal, or physical aggression, sundowning behavior, wandering, depression, challenging and disruptive behaviors, hallucinations, among other alterations [4]. These NPS are highly associated with the burden of disease, lower quality of life and caregiver burnout [5], and earlier institutionalization [6].

Neurodegenerative disorders such as dementia are associated with increased mortality compared to aged control populations [7–9]. Although sex-specific clinicopathological mechanism is not well understood and are largely unexplored [10], males presented deranged neuro-immuno-endocrine system despite their less harmful neuropathological status [11,12]. Moreover, the vast heterogeneity and complexity of patients' clinical profiles and temporal progression of the disease highlight the relevance of personalized-based interventions [13]. However, despite there is more than one potential therapeutic target for this disease, currently approved interventions are just a few; they target loss of cholinergic function and excitotoxicity but exert modest benefits restricted to symptomatology [14]. Disease-modifying treatments are still under intensive research and development [15]. Better understanding the implication of genetic and phenotypic factors may also provide novel mechanisms for clustering AD patients [16,17] and would be determinant also when translated to experimental models [18].

Thanks to the shorter life span of most non-human animals, translational research can provide a fleet-footed scenario for studying genetic and age interactions in the context of different levels of AD-genetic expression. Also, this short temporal frame is very appreciated for long-term monitoring and study of factors potentially involved in disease modulation from morphological, structural, functional, and behavioral levels. Among the animal models of AD, we have proposed long-term survivors of the widely used 3xTg-AD mice as a model for heterogeneity in end-of-life dementia [19]. This model, based on the familial AD mutations PS1/M146V and APPSwe, also harboring the tauP301L human transgene, progressively develops temporal- and regional-specific development of amyloid-β plaques and tau-containing neurofibrillary tangles observed in the human brain of AD patients [20,21]. It also mimics other hallmarks of the disease such as synaptic dysfunction and decreased long-term potentiation [21,22], neuroinflammation, reactive gliosis [23,24], brain oxidative stress [25,26] as well as changes in neurotransmitter systems [27] and impairment in neuro-immunoendocrine status [28]. Cognitive deficits [29,30] and a wide spectrum of neuropsychiatric (NPS)-like disturbances have also been described [18,31,32]. Whether they are sensitive to genetic-load and in which way remains to be determined.

Since the establishment of 3xTg-AD and NTg mouse colonies in our laboratory we have repeatedly observed that the animals overcoming 15 months of age show milder impairment of cognitive and NPS-like behaviors than expected for their neuropathological status. Females usually presented greater survivors' rates than males, for this reason we have previously described behavioral and functional phenotype of long-term survivors, 18-month-old female 3xTg-AD mice [19]. The present work studied a singular cohort of long-lived (19-month-old survivors) heterozygous and homozygous male 3xTg-AD with an extraordinary survival rate. In this particular scenario, we explored how the AD-genetic load interferes with the normal aging scenario and its implication in the pathological burden and neuro-immunoendocrine status involving not only the HPA axis but also peripheral organs. Finally, how the genetic load translates into these survivors' cognitive and NPS behavioral phenotype was also explored. These results highlight that amyloid precursor protein (APP) levels increased in a genetic load-dependent manner, but similar synaptophysin and choline acetyltransferase brain levels. Cognitive impairment was invariable as the distinct trait of Alzheimer's disease; however, anxiety-like behavior seemed more related to the genetic-load. Convergence of physical status and sensorimotor profiles were more related to normal aging processes. On the other hand, complex neuro-immunoendocrine crosstalk was observed with peripheral histopathology, but no correlations with frailty index nor oxidative stress parameters were found. These results suggest the existence of vulnerability/compensatory mechanisms in transgenic mice.

2. Materials and Methods

2.1. Animals

Homozygous triple-transgenic 3xTg-AD mice harboring human PS1/M146V, APPSwe, and tauP301L transgenes were genetically engineered at the University of California

Irvine, as previously described [21]. Briefly, two independent transgenes (encoding human APPSwe and human tauP301L, both under control of the mouse Thy1.2 regulatory element) were co-injected into single-cell embryos harvested from homozygous mutant PS1M146V knock-in (PS1KI) mice. The PS1 knock-in mice were originally generated after embryonic transfer into pure C57BL/6.

A cohort of seventeen mice from the Spanish colonies of 3xTg-AD (n = 9, homozygous, n = 5 heterozygous, n = 4) and C57BL/6 (n = 8) wild-type mice (from now, referred as non-transgenic mice, NTg) from litters of a breeding program established after embryonic transfer to C57BL/6 strain background were used in this study. All animals were housed and maintained (Makrolon, 35 × 35 × 25 cm^3) under standard laboratory conditions (12 h light/dark, cycle starting at 8:00 a.m., food and water ad libitum, 22 ± 2 °C, 50–60% humidity) at Universitat Autònoma de Barcelona. Behavioral tests were performed from 9:00 h to 13:00 h. Behavioral assessments, biochemical and neuropathological analyses were performed blind to the experiment in a counterbalanced manner.

All procedures followed Spanish legislation on 'Protection of Animals Used for Experimental and Other Scientific Purposes' and the EU Council directive (2010/63/EU) on this subject. The protocol CEEAH 3588/DMAH 9452 was approved the 8 March 2019 by Departament de Medi Ambient i Habitatge, Generalitat de Catalunya. The study complies with the ARRIVE guidelines developed by the NC3Rs and aims to reduce the number of animals used [33].

2.2. Experimental Design

At 18 months of age, mice's physical and mental health status started to be characterized and concluded at 19 months [18.70 ± 0.17 (17.5–19.31)]. After that, samples for physiological, biochemical, and pathological analysis were collected. Survival was continuously monitored.

2.3. Behavioral Assessment

Comprehensive screening of several physical, emotional, and cognitive functions was successively performed using a battery of tests based on three main behavioral dimensions that can be described as follows:

2.3.1. Physical Status, Reflexes, and Sensorimotor Functions

Visual reflex and posterior leg extension reflex were measured three times by holding the animal by the tail and slowly lowering it to a black surface. Motor coordination (distance covered) and equilibrium (latency to fall off) were assessed in a horizontal wood (1.3 cm wide) and a metal (1 cm diameter) rod on two consecutive 20 s trials each. Motor coordination (mean distance covered) and muscle strength (latency to fall off in the two 5 s trials) and motor strength (latency to fall off the 60 s trial) were measured in the wire hang test consisting of allowing the animal to cling from the middle of a horizontal wire (diameter: 2 mm, length: 40 cm, divided into eight 5 cm segments) with the forepaws for two trials of 5 s and a third 60 s trial. All the apparatuses were suspended 40 cm above a padded table.

2.3.2. Neuropsychiatric-Like Behaviors

Changes in emotionality increased neophobia and other signs of anxiety-like responses, all of them BPSD-like behaviors modeled in 3xTg-AD mice [18], were measured in classical unconditioned tests. The tests evaluate locomotion/exploration, anxiety-like behaviors, and emotionality under different anxiogenic conditions.

Corner Test (CT) and Open Field Test (OF)

Neophobia was assessed in the corner test for 30 s, placing the animal in the center of a clean standard home cage filled with wood save bedding. The number of corners visited, the latency of first rearing and the number of rearings were recorded. [18]. Immediately after the CT, mice were placed in the center of an open field (metalwork, white box, 42 × 38 × 15 cm) and observed for 5 min [34]. The ethogram, described by the temporal profile of the following sequence of behavioral events, was recorded: duration of freezing behavior, latency to leave the central square, and that of entering the peripheral ring and latency and total duration of self-grooming behavior. Horizontal (crossings of 10 × 10 cm squares) and vertical (rearings with wall support) locomotor activities were also measured. During the tests, defecation boli and urination were also recorded. The repeated test, 24 h later, was used to evaluate the long-term memory of these experiences [35]. Distance and time in the center/periphery were evaluated by video-tracking analysis (ANY-Maze, version 5.14, Stoelting Europe, Dublin, Ireland).

Dark–Light Box Test (DLB)

Anxiety and risk assessment were measured for 5 min after introducing the animal into the dark compartment of the DLB (Panlab S.L., Barcelona, Spain). The apparatus consisted of two compartments (black, 27 cm × 18 cm × 27 cm^3, white, 27 cm × 27 cm × 27 cm^3 illuminated by a red 20 W bulb) connected by an opening (7 cm × 7 cm^2). The experimental room was kept in darkness. Latency to enter the lit compartment, the number of entries, total time spent, distance covered, and the number of rearings and groomings in this compartment were noted. Risk assessment was measured as the latency and number of stretch attendances toward the lit area.

Marble Test (MB)

The animal was placed in a standard home cage containing nine glass marbles (1 × 1 × 1 cm^3) evenly spaced, making a square (three rows of three marbles per row only in the left area of the cage) on a 5 cm thick layer of sawdust. The mice were left in the cage with marbles for a 30 min period, after which the test was terminated by removing the mice and counting the number of marbles: intact (untouched), rotated (90 or 180°), half-buried (at least $\frac{1}{2}$ buried by sawdust), and buried (completely hidden).

2.3.3. Cognitive Function

T-Maze Test (TM)

Two different paradigms were carried out in a T-shaped maze (woodwork; two short arms of 30 × 10 cm^2; one long arm of 50 × 10 cm^2). Coping with stress strategies, risk assessment, and working memory were assessed in the spontaneous alternation task [36]. The animal was placed inside the maze's long arm with its head facing the end wall, and it was allowed to explore the maze for a maximum of 5 min. The ethogram (latencies to different goals) in this task was recorded as follows: to move and turn (freezing behavior), to reach the intersection, to cross (4 paws criteria) the intersection of the three arms, and the total time invested in exploring the three arms of the maze (test completion criteria).

On the day after, the second working memory paradigm consisted of one forced-choice followed, 60 s later, by one free choice (recall trial). Here, goals were defined as: to move and turn, to reach the intersection, the time elapsed until the animal crossed (4 paws criteria) the intersection of the three arms, and the time elapsed until the mice completed 20 s in the forced arm (time to reach the criteria). The animals that completed the forced trial in less than the cut-off time (10 min) were allowed to explore the maze in the free choice trial where both arms were accessible for 5 min. The arm chosen by the mice and the time spent to reach the correct arm during the free choice were recorded (exploration criteria).

In both paradigms, the choice of the already visited arm in the previous trial was considered an error, and the total number was calculated. Finally, defecation boli and urination were also recorded.

Morris-Water-Maze (MWM)

Three learning and memory paradigms were administered during 5 consecutive days. First, mice were trained to locate a hidden platform (7-cm diameter, 1 cm on/below the water surface) in a circular pool for mice (120 cm in diameter and 60 cm deep, 25 °C opaque water). Mice that failed to find the platform within 60 s were placed on it for 10 s, the same period was allowed for the successful animals.

Cue learning with a visible platform: On the first day, the animals were tested for the cued learning of a visual platform consisting of four trials in 1 day. In each trial, the mouse was gently released (facing the wall) from one randomly selected starting point (W-S-E-N) and allowed to swim until it escaped onto the platform, elevated 1 cm above the water level in the NE position and indicated by a visible striped flag ($5.3 \times 8.3 \times 15$ cm^3). Extra maze cues were absent in the black walls of the room.

Place learning with a hidden platform: On the following day, the place learning task consisted of four trial sessions per day for 4-days with trials spaced 30 min apart. The mouse was gently released (facing the wall) from one randomly selected starting point (N-E-W-S; E-N-S-W) and allowed to swim until it escaped onto the hidden platform, which was now located in the middle of the SW quadrant (reversal). Different geometric figures hung on each wall of the room were used as external visual clues. Variables of time (escape latency), distance covered, and swimming speed were analyzed in all the tasks' trials. The escape latency was readily measured with a stopwatch by an observer unaware of the animal's genotype and confirmed during the subsequent video-tracking analysis (ANY-Maze v. 5.14, Stoelting, Dublin, Ireland).

Two hours and 30 min after the last place task, the platform was removed, and the animal was allowed to swim for a 60 s probe trial. Quadrant preference and entries into the previous platform location were video-tracked and analyzed.

2.4. Body Weight, Mouse Clinical Frailty Index Assessment, and Survival

Bodyweight and frailty were assessed using an adaptation of the MCFI [37], including 30 clinically-like assessed non-invasive items. For 29 of these items, mice were given a score 0 if not presented, 0.5 if there was a mild deficit, and 1 for the severe deficit. Weight was scored based on the number of standard deviations from a reference mean. The clinical evaluation included the integument, the physical/musculoskeletal system, the vestibulocochlear/auditory systems, the ocular and nasal systems, the digestive system, the urogenital system, the respiratory system, signs of discomfort, and body weight. Survival was recorded continuously with a daily cadence.

2.5. HPA Axis Endocrine Status

Four days after the behavioral assessment, blood samples were collected during the euthanasia. Serum was obtained by centrifugation and stored at −80 °C. Corticosterone content (ng/mL) was analyzed using a commercial kit (Corticosterone EIA Immunodiagnostic Systems Ltd., Boldon, UK) and read at 450 nm of absorbance with Varioskan LUX ESW 1.00.38. (Thermo Fisher Scientific, Waltham, MA, USA).

2.6. Neuropathology and Synaptic Function

Brain and peripheral organs were dissected for further biochemical and/or pathological analysis. The right prefrontal cortex, entorhinal cortex, and hippocampus were dissected out, weighed, snap-frozen separately, and stored at –80 °C until processing for preparation of protein extract for biochemistry analysis. Frozen samples were lysed in cold lysis buffer containing protease and phosphatase inhibitors (Sigma-Aldrich, Saint Louis, MO, USA). Protein content was quantified with the BCA Protein Assay Kit (Thermo Fisher Scientific, Waltham, MA, USA), resolved on SDS-polyacrylamide gel electrophoresis, and detected by Western blotting using the following antibodies: 6E10 (1:500, Biolegend, San Diego, CA, USA); synaptophysin (1:2000, Dako, Glostrup, Denmark); ChAT (1:500, Thermo Fisher Scientific, Waltham, MA, USA), β-actin (1:10,000; Sigma-Aldrich, Saint Louis, MO, USA). Bands were detected with an enhanced chemiluminescent reagent in a ChemiDoc MP System (Bio-Rad Laboratories, Inc., Hercules, CA, USA) and quantified in a linear range using the ImageLab 5.2.1 software (Bio-Rad Laboratories, Inc., Hercules, CA, USA).

2.7. Peripheral Organs Pathological Status

2.7.1. Splenic, Renal and Hepatic Histopathological Evaluation

Spleen, kidneys, and liver were dissected and port-fixed by immersion 24 h in 10% formalin (Sigma-Aldrich, Saint Louis, MO, USA). The size (weight in mg) and organ indexes (relative size, % vs. bodyweight) of the spleen were also recorded as an indirect measure of the physiological status of the peripheral immune organs. All samples were washed twice with 4 °C phosphate buffered saline for about 20 min to stop fixation and rinse the fixative, immersed in ethanol 70% and kept at 4 °C until paraffin embedding. Histological processing for paraffin embedding was performed by means of an automatic processing machine (Leica TP1020, Leica Biosystems, Nussloch, Germany): EtOH 70% 30 min; EtOH 80% 20 min; EtOH 96% 2 × 20 min; EtOH 100% 2 × 30 min + 1 × 40 min; EtOH 100%-Xylene 30 min; Xylene 2 × 40 min; paraffin 2 × 1 h. The paraffin blocks were confectioned in a paraffin embedding station (Leica EG1150H, Leica Biosystems, Nussloch, Germany) and were cooled in a cold plate (Leica EG1150C, Leica Biosystems, Nussloch, Germany). Histological preparations of spleen, kidney, and liver were stained with hematoxylin-eosin, and a pathological evaluation was performed blindly by an expert pathologist following a criterion based on the intensity and the distribution of the lesion. The degree of tissue damage was calculated following an injury score grading system: 0—no damage, 1: mild, 2: moderate, 3: severe, 4: very severe. As the same basic lesion of amyloid characteristics was observed in the different organs, a systemic character of the damage was confirmed, and a total injury score with the different organs damage was used to evaluate the total systemic injury.

2.7.2. Oxidative Stress of Spleen, Kidneys, Liver, and Heart

The antioxidant capacity was studied from the evaluation of the levels of total glutathione (GSH), as well as the enzymatic activity of glutathione peroxidase (GPx) and reductase (GR) from the homogenization of different organs (liver, kidneys, spleen, and heart).

Glutathione concentrations: Total glutathione, the main non-enzymatic reducing agent of the organism, was assayed by the enzymatic recycling method previously described [38] by monitoring the change in absorbance at 412 nm adapted to 96-well plates with slight modifications [39].

Glutathione reductase activity: The activity of the enzyme glutathione was assessed following the method described by Massey and Williams [40] with slight modifications. The total activity was determined following the oxidation of NADPH spectrophotometrically at 340 nm for 300 s. The results were expressed as milliunits (mU) of enzymatic activity per mg of organ protein.

Glutathione peroxidase activity: The glutathione peroxidase activity was measured using the modified technique previously described [41,42] with slight modifications. The reaction was followed spectrophotometrically by the decrease of the absorbance at 340 nm for 300 s. The results were expressed as mU of enzymatic activity per mg of organ protein.

2.8. Statistics

Results are expressed as mean ± SEM. SPSS 15.0 (SPSS Inc., Chicago, IL, USA) and GraphPad Prism 8.0 (GraphPad Software Inc., San Diego, CA, USA) software were used. Differences between two different genotypes were evaluated with a two-tailed unpaired Student's *t*-test (U Mann Whitney, for quantitative discontinuous). One-way analysis of variance (ANOVA) for comparisons between all the groups of mice, including NTg, 3xTg-AD homozygous, and 3xTg-AD heterozygous, followed by Bonferroni's post hoc test. In the temporal courses, RMA, Repeated measures ANOVA, was used for within-subject analysis. Differences in life spans were studied through the Kaplan-Meier test. In all the tests, statistical significance was considered at $p < 0.05$.

3. Results

As summarized in the graphical abstract (Figure 1) and depicted in Figures 2–8, the main findings show that genotype-load modulated amyloid burden and anxiety-like patterns in male 3xTg-AD survivors despite similar neuro-immunoendocrine and cognitive impairments.

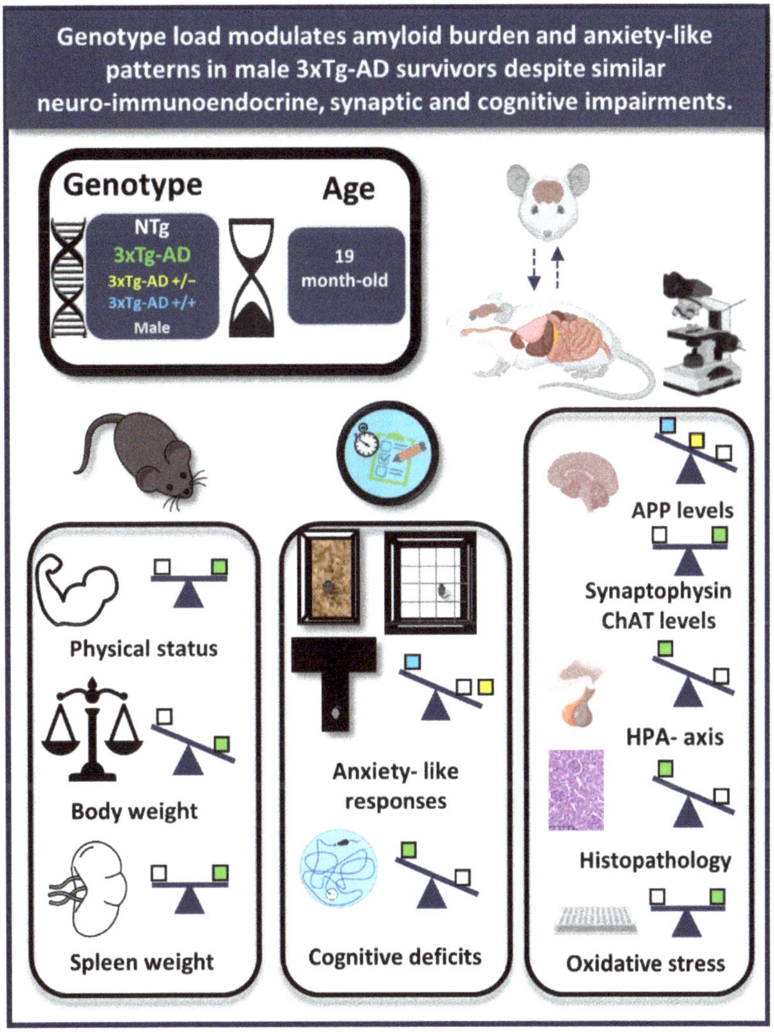

Figure 1. Graphical abstract. Genotype load modulates amyloid burden and anxiety-like patterns in male 3xTg-AD survivors despite similar neuro-immunoendocrine and cognitive impairments. Experimental design and main findings. White square: NTg mice, yellow square: heterozygous 3xTg-AD mice, blue square: homozygous 3xTg-AD mice; Green square: 3xTg-AD mice (both 3xTg-AD genotypes, since no genotype-load differences were found).

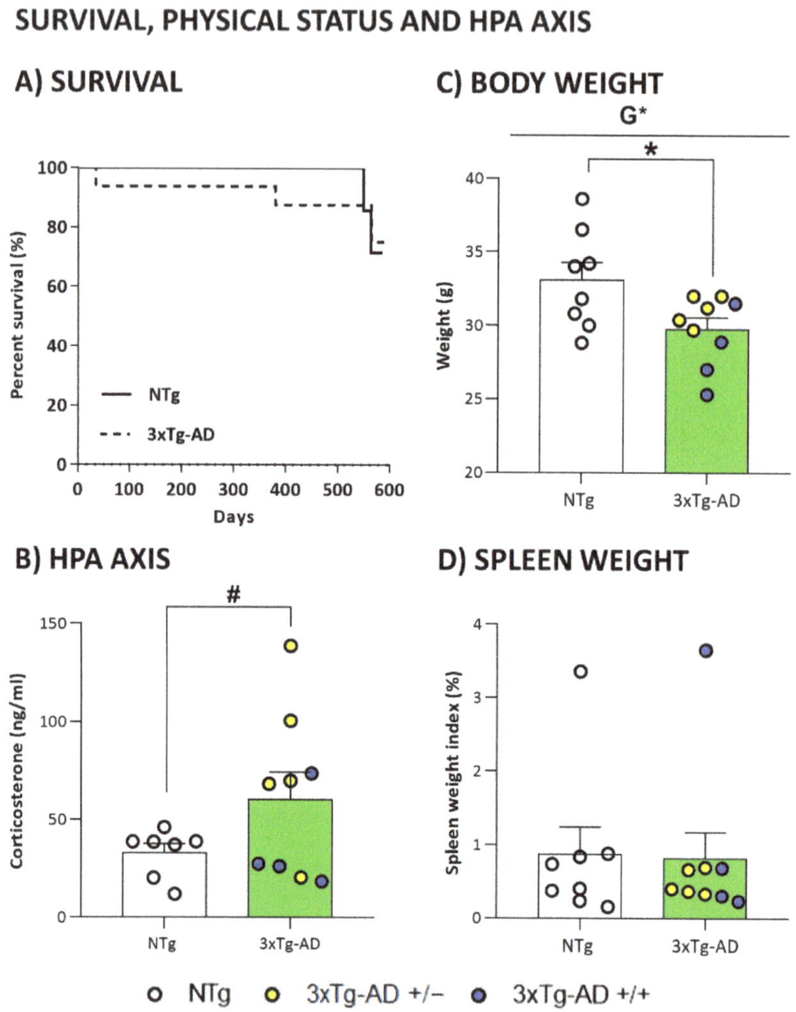

Figure 2. Survival, HPA axis endocrine status and physical health. (**A**) Survival; (**B**) Corticosterone levels; (**C**) Body weight and (**D**) spleen weight in 19-month-old mice. Results are expressed as the mean ± SEM. Male NTg, n = 8 (White circles for individual values; white bar, mean value); male 3xTg-AD n = 9 (Yellow circles, individual values of heterozygous 3xTg-AD +/− mice, n = 5; Blue circles, individual values for homozygous 3xTg-AD +/+ mice, n = 4; Green bar, mean value of both 3xTg-AD genotypes, since no genotype-load differences were found). Statistics: two-tailed unpaired Student's t-test (above the line) for Genotype differences (G): * $p < 0.05$; one-way analysis of variance (ANOVA) for comparisons between all the groups of mice followed by Bonferroni's post-hoc test. * $p < 0.05$ vs. homozygous 3xTg-AD-group; # $p < 0.05$ vs. heterozygous 3xTg-AD-group.

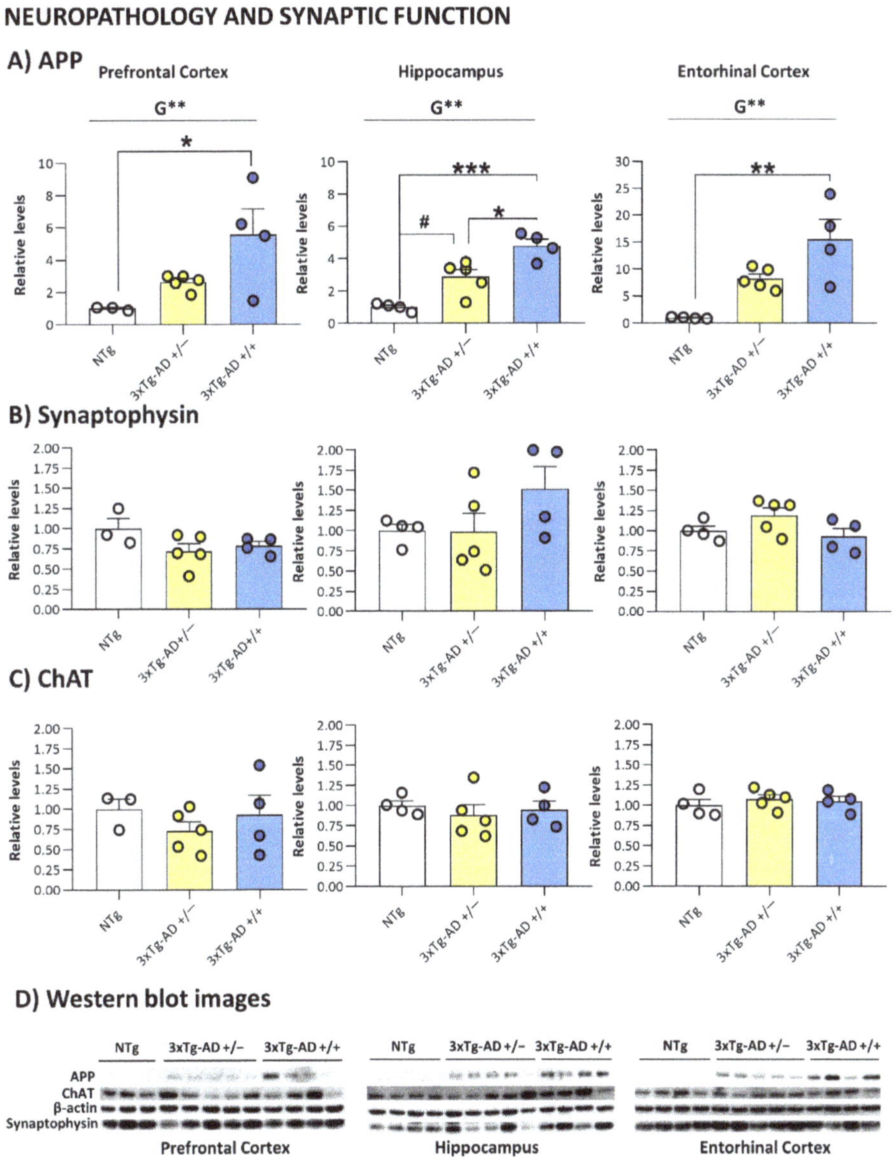

Figure 3. Neuropathology and Synaptic Function: Brain biochemical analysis of APP (**A**), synaptophysin (**B**) and ChAT (**C**) in the prefrontal cortex, hippocampus, and entorhinal cortex. (**D**) Western blot images. Results are expressed as the relative levels as fold change ± SEM. Male NTg, $n = 3$–4 (White circles for individual values; white bar, mean value); male 3xTg-AD $n = 9$ (Yellow circles, individual values of heterozygous 3xTg-AD +/− mice, $n = 5$; blue circles, individual values for homozygous 3xTg-AD +/+ mice, $n = 4$; yellow and blue bars, mean value for heterozygous and homozygous 3xTg-AD genotypes, respectively, since genotype-load differences were found). Statistics: two-tailed unpaired Student's *t*-test (above the line) for Genotype differences (G): ** $p < 0.01$; one-way analysis of variance (ANOVA) for comparisons between all the groups of mice followed by Bonferroni's post hoc test. * $p < 0.05$, ** $p < 0.01$, *** $p < 0.001$ vs. homozygous 3xTg-AD-group; # $p < 0.05$ vs. heterozygous 3xTg-AD-group.

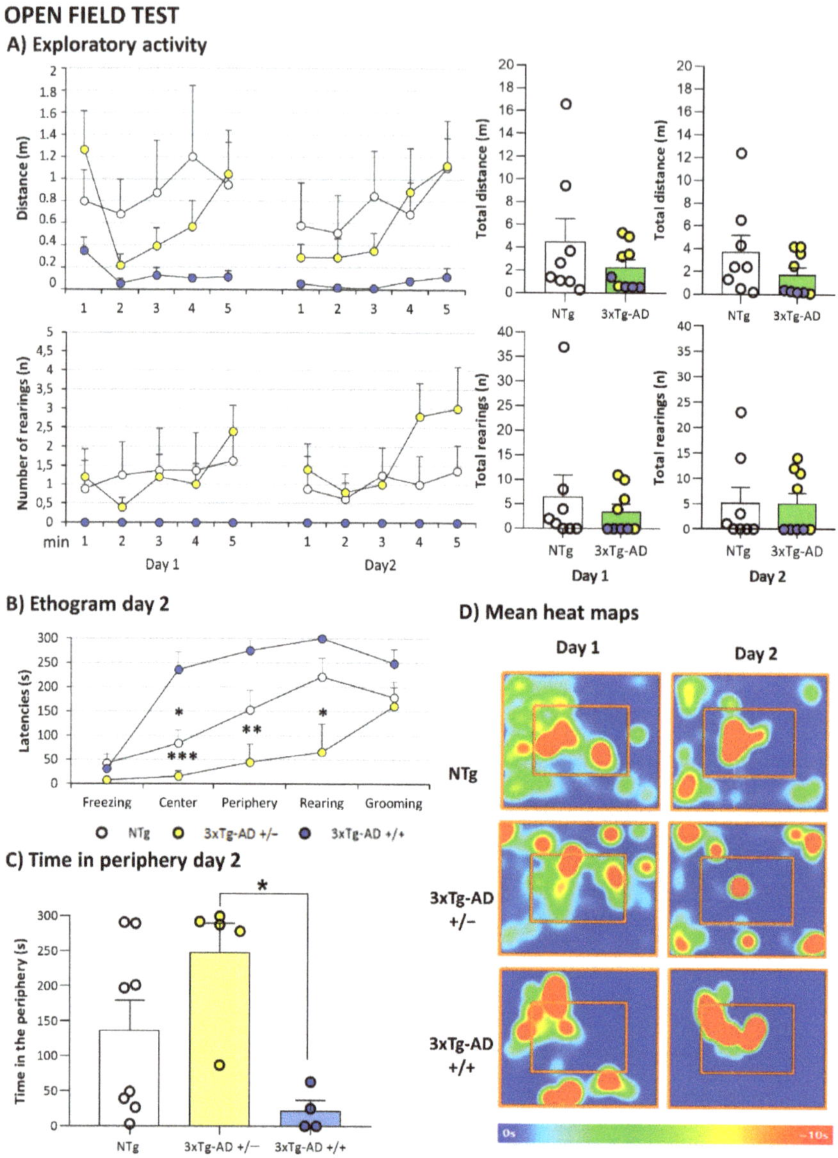

Figure 4. Mental Health: Neuropsychiatric-like phenotype in 2-day Open-field test. (**A**) Exploratory activity; (**B**) Ethogram day 2; (**C**) Time in periphery day 2 and (**D**) Heat maps representation of how much time animals spends in different parts of the apparatus during a test, with blue as the shortest time and red as the longest. Results are expressed as the mean ± SEM. Male NTg, $n = 8$ (White circles for individual values; white bar, mean value); male 3xTg-AD $n = 9$ (Yellow circles, individual values of heterozygous 3xTg-AD +/− mice, $n = 5$; blue circles, individual values for homozygous 3xTg-AD +/+ mice, $n = 4$; green bar, mean value of both 3xTg-AD genotypes, since no genotype-load differences were found; yellow and blue bars, mean value for heterozygous and homozygous 3xTg-AD genotypes, respectively, since genotype-load differences were found). Statistics: one-way analysis of variance (ANOVA) for comparisons between all the groups of mice followed by Bonferroni's post hoc test. * $p < 0.05$, ** $p < 0.01$, *** $p < 0.001$ vs. homozygous 3xTg-AD-group.

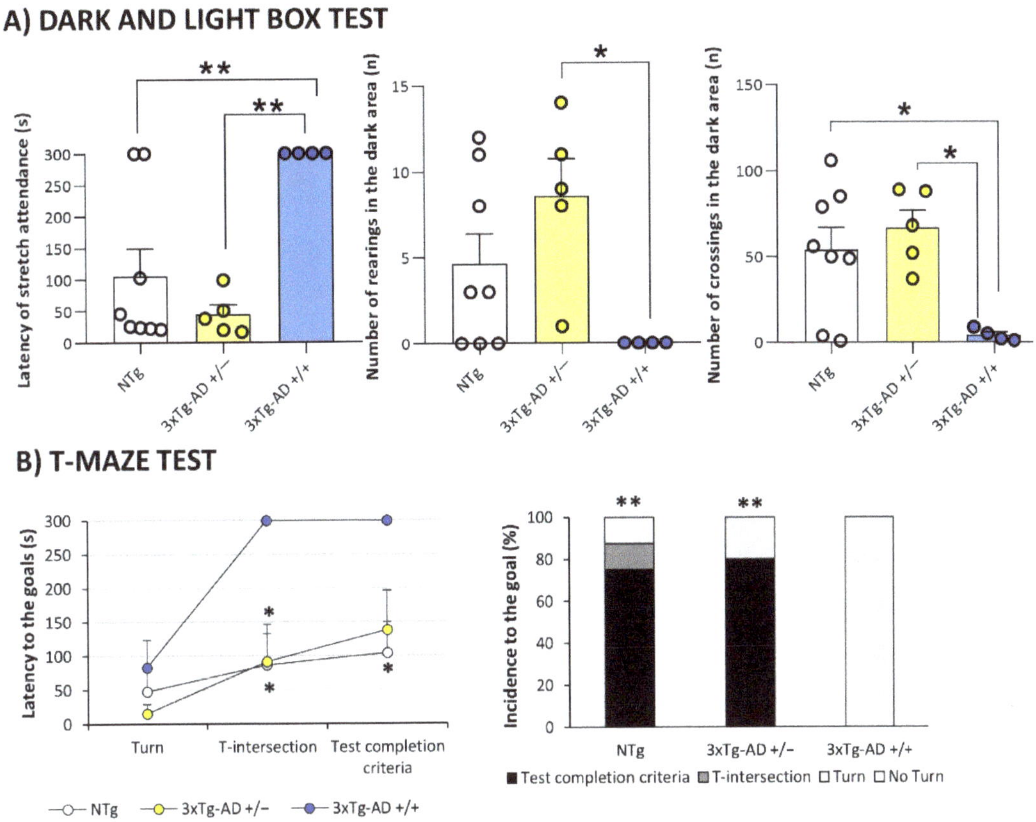

Figure 5. Mental Health: Neuropsychiatric-like phenotype and cognitive impairment in Dark and light box test (**A**) and T-Maze test (**B**). Results are expressed as the mean ± SEM. Male NTg, $n = 8$ (White circles for individual values; white bar, mean value); male 3xTg-AD $n = 9$ (Yellow circles, individual values of heterozygous 3xTg-AD +/− mice, $n = 5$; blue circles, individual values for homozygous 3xTg-AD +/+ mice, $n = 4$; yellow and blue bars, mean value for heterozygous and homozygous 3xTg-AD genotypes, respectively, since genotype-load differences were found). Statistics: one-way analysis of variance (ANOVA) for comparisons between all the groups of mice followed by Bonferroni's post hoc test. * $p < 0.05$, ** $p < 0.01$, vs. homozygous 3xTg-AD-group.

3.1. Survival

Survival curves of an initial sample of 28 male, twelve NTg, and sixteen 3xTg-AD mice are illustrated in Figure 2A. Although 3xTg-AD mice showed a younger mortality pattern than NTg mice, Log-rank analyses showed no differences when starting the experiment (71.4% in NTg vs. 87.5% in 3xTg-AD mice). During the experiment, one 3xTg-AD died. At the end of the experiment, the survival rates were 71.4% in NTg vs. 75% in 3xTg-AD mice.

3.2. HPA Axis Endocrine Status

Although no significant differences were observed between genotypes when we measured the corticosterone values (Figure 2B), heterozygous mice showed a higher level in comparison NTg mice ($p = 0.045$, post hoc test).

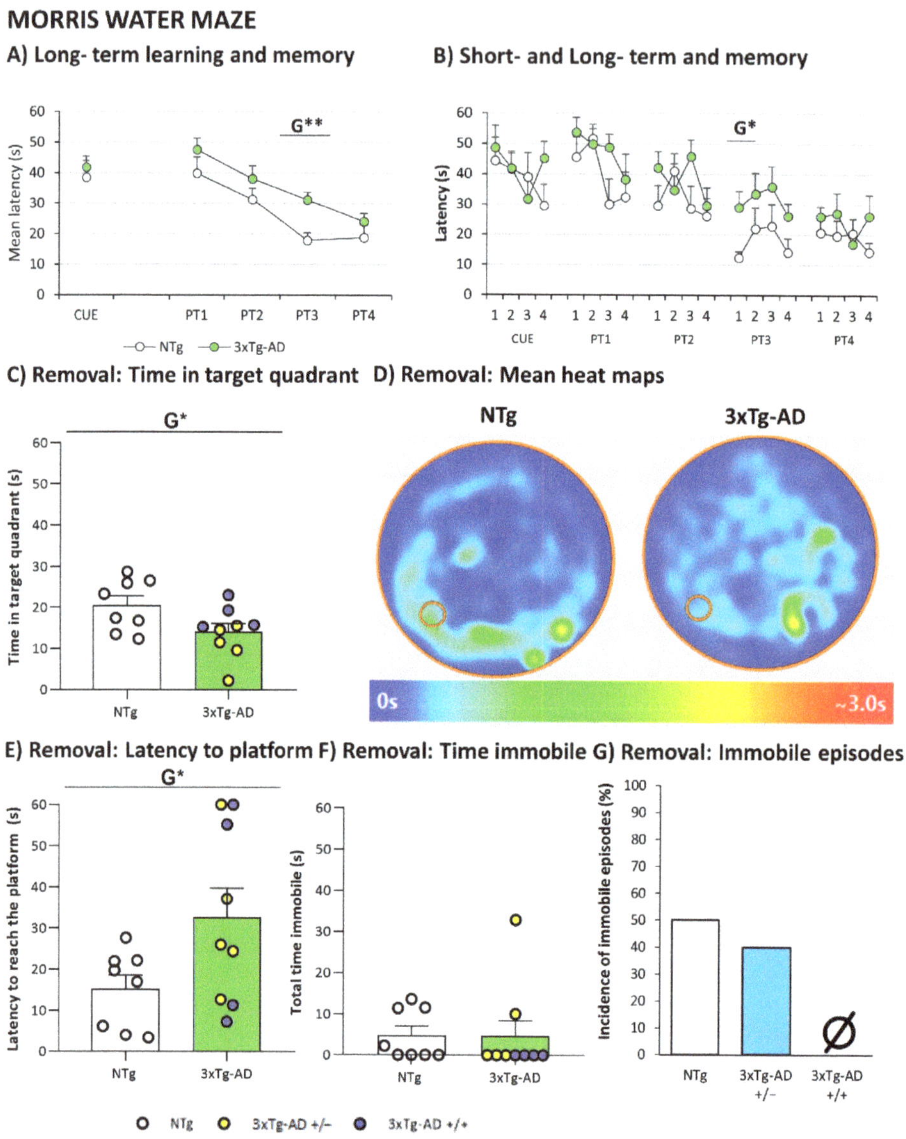

Figure 6. Mental Health: Cognitive impairment in Morris Water Maze (**A**) Long-term learning and memory; (**B**) Short- and long-term memory; (**C**) Short-term memory in Removal: Time in target quadrant; (**D**) Heat maps representation in removal. (**E**) Short-term memory in Removal: Latency to reach the platform; (**F**) Time immobile in removal; (**G**) Immobile episodes in removal. Results are expressed as the mean ± SEM. Male NTg, n = 8 (White circles for individual values; white bar, mean value); male 3xTg-AD n = 9 (Yellow circles, individual values of heterozygous 3xTg-AD +/− mice, n = 5; blue circles, individual values for homozygous 3xTg-AD +/+ mice, n = 4; green bar, mean value of both 3xTg-AD genotypes, since no genotype-load differences were found; yellow and blue bars, mean value for heterozygous and homozygous 3xTg-AD genotypes, respectively, since genotype-load differences were found). Heat maps representation of how much time animals spends in different parts of the apparatus during a test, with blue as the shortest time and red as the longest. Statistics: two-tailed unpaired Student's t-test (above line) for Genotype differences (**G**): * $p < 0.05$, ** $p < 0.01$.

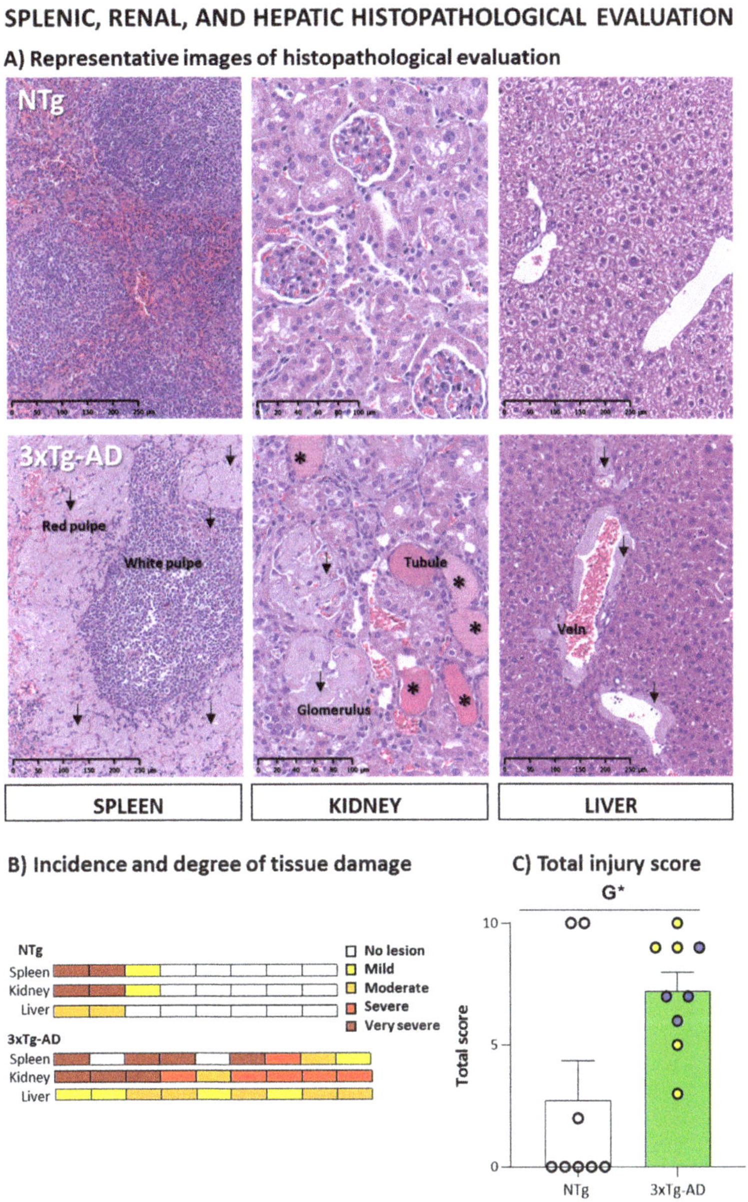

Figure 7. Pathological Status of Peripheral Organs in 19-month-old male 3xTg-AD mice and NTg counterparts: (**A**) Representative images of histopathological evaluation of peripheral organs (kidney, spleen, and liver), Black arrow: amyloidosis damage, *: proteinuria; (**B**) Incidence and degree of tissue damage; (**C**) General systemic total score. Results are expressed as the mean ± SEM. Male NTg, $n = 8$ (White circles for individual values; white bar, mean value); male 3xTg-AD $n = 9$ (Yellow circles, individual values of heterozygous 3xTg-AD +/− mice, $n = 5$; Blue circles, individual values for homozygous 3xTg-AD +/+ mice, $n = 4$; Green bar, mean value of both 3xTg-AD genotypes, since no genotype-load differences were found). Statistics: two-tailed unpaired Student's t-test (above line) for Genotype differences (G): * $p < 0.05$.

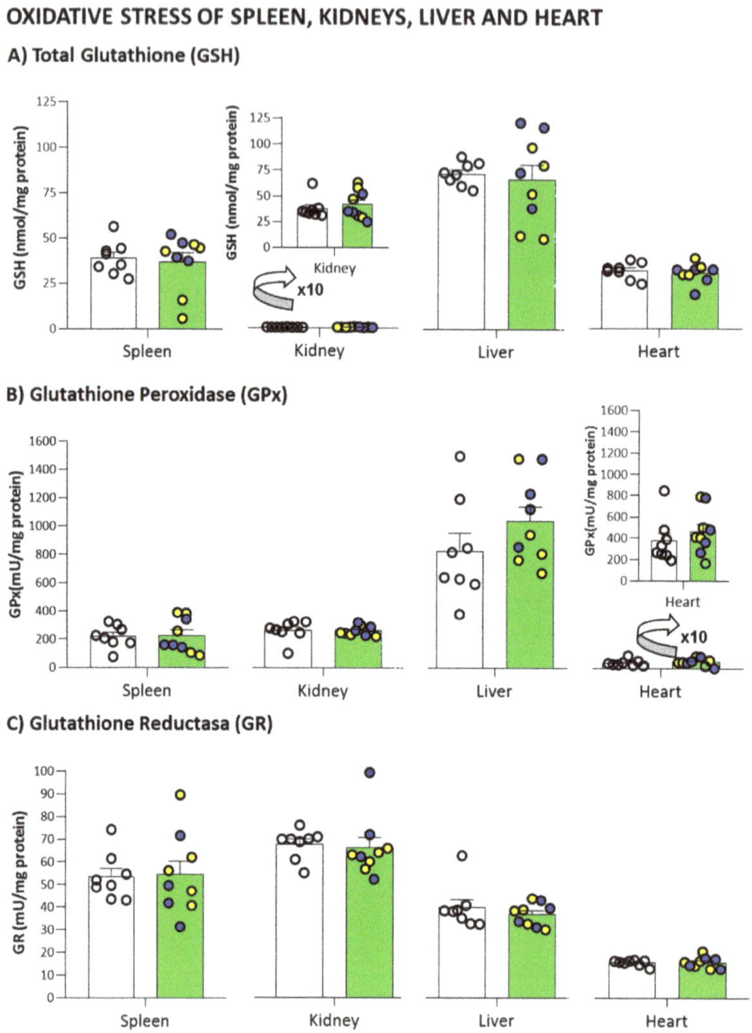

Figure 8. Pathological Status of Peripheral Organs: Oxidative stress parameters in peripheral organs: (**A**) Total Glutathione (GSH); (**B**) Glutathione Peroxidase (GPx); (**C**) Glutathione Reductase (GR) in 19-month-old male 3xTg-AD mice and NTg counterparts. Results are expressed as the mean ± SEM. Male NTg, $n = 8$ (White circles for individual values; white bar, mean value); male 3xTg-AD $n = 9$ (Yellow circles, individual values of heterozygous 3xTg-AD +/− mice, $n = 5$; Blue circles, individual values for homozygous 3xTg-AD +/+ mice, $n = 4$; Green bar, mean value of both 3xTg-AD genotypes, since no genotype-load differences were found). Statistics: n.s., no significative, $p > 0.05$.

3.3. Physical Status, Reflexes, and Sensorimotor Functions

As detailed in Table 1, frailty index, reflexes, and sensorimotor functions of 19-month-old 3xTg-AD mice did not differ from those observed in NTg mice with normal aging (genotype effects, Student *t*-test, $p > 0.05$ or even equal values). Independently of genotype, animals did not cover almost any distance, and latencies were very short. In both groups, the measures of resistance and coordination revealed high individual variability. Genotype differences were found in body weight (Figure 2C), increased in 3xTg-AD mice ($p = 0.037$, Student's *t*-test). However, this difference was only observed between homozygous and NTg mice ($p = 0.032$, post hoc test). No differences in spleen weight were observed (Figure 2D).

Table 1. Similarity of physical status and sensorimotor function in 19-month-old male 3xTg-AD mice compared to sex- and age-matched NTg mice with normal aging. Results are expressed as mean ± SEM or incidence. Student's *t*-test, n.s., no statistically significant; $p > 0.05$.

	Males, 19-Month-Old			
	NTg Mice $n = 8$	**3xTg-AD Mice** $n = 9$	**Genotype Differences**	**Genetic Load Differences**
Physical Status, Reflexes, and Sensorimotor Function				
Frailty index score	0.05 ± 0.02	0.03 ± 0.01	n.s.	n.s.
Reflexes				
Visual placing reflex (3 trials)	3/3	3/3	equal	equal
Posterior leg reflex (3 trials)	3/3	3/3	equal	equal
Wood rod test (two 20-s trials)				
Equilibrium (mean falling latency, s)	3.63 ± 1.18	1.94 ± 1.01	n.s.	n.s.
Coordination (mean distance, cm)	0.19 ± 0.09	0.06 ± 0.05	n.s.	n.s.
Wire rod test (two 20-s trials)				
Equilibrium (mean falling latency, s)	6.19 ± 2.32	7.78 ± 2.40	n.s.	n.s.
Coordination (mean distance, cm)	0.19 ± 0.19	0.28 ± 0.12	n.s.	n.s.
Wire hang test (two 5-s trials)				
Strength (mean time hold, s)	2.50 ± 0.33	3.50 ± 0.53	n.s.	n.s.
Coordination (mean distance, segments)	0 ± 0	0 ± 0	equal	equal
Wire hang test (one 60-s trial)				
Resistance (time hold, s)	29.5 ± 8.57	29.11 ± 9.33	n.s.	n.s.
Coordination (distance, segments)	1.63 ± 0.56	0.89 ± 0.39	n.s.	n.s.

3.4. Neuropathology and Synaptic Function

The analysis of immunoblotting from the prefrontal cortex, hippocampus, and entorhinal cortex protein extracts incubated with 6E10 antibody showed a genetic-load-dependent increase of APP (Figure 3A); ($p < 0.008$, Student's *t*-test). This gradient was mainly observed in the hippocampus, where significant differences were also observed between homozygous and heterozygous groups ($p < 0.016$, Bonferroni's post hoc test, homozygous vs. NTg and heterozygous mice). However, no differences ($p > 0.05$, Student's *t*-test) were found when we evaluate levels of synaptophysin (Figure 3B) a synaptogenesis and neuroplasticity marker nor choline acetyltransferase (Figure 3C), the enzyme responsible for the acetylcholine synthesis.

3.5. Neuropsychiatric Symptoms (NPS)-Like Phenotype and Cognitive Impairment under Different Anxiogenic Conditions

In the corner test, genotype differences were observed only when horizontal activity was measured in the first corner test ($p = 0.002$, Student's *t*-test) and disappeared when we repeated the test 24 h later. Although the activity between tests was decreased in all groups, statistical differences were observed in the number of corners in NTg mice ($p = 0.009$, paired *t*-test) and the number of rearings in 3xTg-AD mice ($p = 0.038$, paired *t*-test). Surprisingly, results in the open field test evidenced striking similarities between 18-month-old 3xTg-AD and NTg mice. Thus, all the analyzed behavioral variables (see Table 2 and Figure 4), including those related to the time course of elicitation of behavioral events and emotionality. Furthermore, as observed in the physical and sensorimotor aspects, both groups of mice showed high individual variability, resulting in high statistical variance. However, when we repeated the test 24 h later, significant differences in open field ethogram were observed between homozygous and heterozygous mice ($p < 0.015$, post hoc test). Lower latencies were observed in the exit of the center, entrance to the periphery, and vertical activity in heterozygous mice (Figure 4B). Moreover, heterozygous mice spent more time in the periphery than homozygous mice ($p = 0.013$, post hoc test, Figure 4C,D).

Table 2. Similarity, exploratory and BPSD-like domains, in 19-month-old male 3xTg-AD mice as compared to sex- and age-matched NTg mice with normal aging. Results are expressed as mean ± SEM. Student's *t*-test, ** $p < 0.01$, vs. NTg mice; n.s., no statistically significant, $p > 0.05$.

	Males, 19-Month-Old			
	NTg Mice *n* = 8	**3xTg-AD Mice** *n* = 9	**Genotype Differences**	**Genetic Load Differences**
BPSD-Like Behaviors and Exploratory Activity				
Corner test (one 30-s trial)				
Vertical activity (latency, s)	19.13 ± 3.78	14.89 ± 3.02	n.s.	n.s.
Vertical activity (number)	1.25 ± 0.41	2.22 ± 0.62	n.s.	n.s.
Horizontal activity (number)	6.13 ± 0.48	3.44 ± 0.50	**	n.s.
24 h Corner test (one 30-s trial)				
Vertical activity (latency, s)	25.50 ± 2.97	19.89 ± 3.65	n.s.	n.s.
Vertical activity (number)	0.75 ± 0.53	1.00 ± 0.33	n.s.	n.s.
Horizontal activity (number)	2.88 ± 0.51	3.22 ± 0.49	n.s.	n.s.
Open field test (5 min)				
Initial freezing (latency, s)	5.25 ± 1.25	5.33 ± 0.69	n.s.	n.s.
Exit of the center (latency, s)	11.13 ± 1.80	11.56 ± 2.06	n.s.	n.s.
Entrance to the periphery (latency, s)	100 ± 43.00	82.22 ± 41.49	n.s.	n.s.
Vertical activity (latency, s)	199 ± 41.88	173.56 ± 40.66	n.s.	n.s.
Self-grooming (latency, s)	190.1 ± 28.89	147.44 ± 23.45	n.s.	n.s.
Vertical activity (number)		See Figure 4A		
Horizontal activity (distance, m)		See Figure 4A		
Time immobile (s)	194.35 ± 27.91	224.89 ± 17.00	n.s.	n.s.
Time in periphery (s)	141.42 ± 38.53	151.02 ± 37.05	n.s.	n.s.
Self-grooming (number)	1.13 ± 0.35	1.11 ± 0.20	n.s.	n.s.
Defecation boli (number)	3.875 ± 0.69	2.67 ± 0.62	n.s.	n.s.
24 h Open field test (5 min)				
Initial freezing (latency, s)		See Figure 4B		
Exit of the center (latency, s)		See Figure 4B		
Entrance into the periphery (latency, s)		See Figure 4B		
Vertical activity (latency, s)		See Figure 4B		
Self-grooming (latency, s)		See Figure 4B		
Vertical activity (number)		See Figure 4A		
Horizontal activity (distance, m)		See Figure 4A		
Time immobile (s)	234.77 ± 18.76	235.66 ± 19.89	n.s.	n.s.
Time in periphery (s)		See Figure 4C		
Self-grooming (number)	1.00 ± 0.189	0.89 ± 0.261	n.s.	n.s.
Defecation boli (number)	3.88 ± 0.479	2.89 ± 0.655	n.s.	n.s.
Marble test (30 min)				
Intact marbles (number)	2.50 ± 1.23	3.67 ± 1.11	n.s.	n.s.
Rotated marbles (number)	2.88 ± 0.63	2.89 ± 0.67	n.s.	n.s.
Half-buried marbles (number)	2.13 ± 0.71	1.67 ± 0.50	n.s.	n.s.
Buried marbles (number)	1.50 ± 0.53	0.78 ± 0.50	n.s.	n.s.

In the Dark light box, no genotype differences were observed between 3xTg-AD and NTg ($p > 0.05$, Student's *t*-test). However, when we evaluated homozygous and heterozygous independently, significant differences were observed (Figure 5A). Albeit did not reach statistical significance, none of the homozygous mice entered into the lit area. Besides, during the 300 s of the test, homozygous did not perform any stretch attendance than NTg and heterozygous mice ($p < 0.009$, post hoc test). Moreover, they did not perform any rearing in the dark area during the test ($p = 0.033$, post hoc test vs. heterozygous mice). The number of crossing was also reduced ($p < 0.043$, post hoc test vs. heterozygous and NTg mice).

In the Marble test, no genotype differences were observed between 3xTg-AD and NTg in the Marble test ($p > 0.05$, Student's *t*-test), as indicated in Table 2.

In the T-maze, no genotype differences were observed between 3xTg-AD and NTg in both T-maze test. However, when we evaluated the two 3xTg-AD subgroups (Figure 5B), we observed that when we studied the coping with stress strategies in the T-maze, heterozygous and NTg showed convergence of profiles. Differences in the latency to reach the intersection of the T-maze were found in spontaneous alternation test ($p < 0.048$, Bonferroni's post hoc test, vs. heterozygous and NTg mice) and any of the homozygous mice accomplished the test completion criteria ($p = 0.037$, post hoc test vs. NTg). As detailed on the right, one NTg mice rested with their backs protected in the starting point, and one spent time but did not cross the intersection, the two others (75% of the sample) completed the test successfully. Among heterozygous, one of the animals turned but was not able to cross the intersection, the rest, 80% of the sample completed with the test completion criteria. Finally, 100% of homozygous mice, started but did not cross the intersection. In the working memory paradigm studied 24 h later all the homozygous animals failed to reach the acquisition criteria during the 5 min of the test. The test was prolonged to 10 min, but still, animals were unsuccessful (data not shown).

In the Morris water maze, cognitive deficits were the most salient distinctive trait in 3xTg-AD mouse survivors. As represented in Figure 6, cognitive deficits in spatial reference learning and memory differentiated the 19-month-old 3xTg-AD mice from age-matched NTg counterparts. In the assessment of visual perceptual learning and memory (Figure 6A), the three groups of mice showed the same mean escape latency on the first day of the cue task. On the second day, the platform was hidden and located in a reversed position; this made the new paradigm a difficult place task. Spatial reference memory assessed by means of place-learning showed differences between genotypes on the third day of the test ($p = 0.002$, Student's t-test). Swimming velocities were not different between the groups (data not shown). 2 h 30 min after the last day of place learning, an extra trial with the removal of the platform indicated the worse performance of 3xTg-AD groups compared with NTg (Figure 6C). NTg mice invested more time than the other groups in the target quadrant ($p = 0.046$, Student's t-test). Indeed, heat plots reveal that the NTg group mostly searched close to the designated platform position. Moreover, the latency of reaching the previous location was also recorded. In this case, the NTg mice reached the trained location faster than 3xTg-AD mice ($p = 0.047$, Student's t-test). However, when the time the animals stood immobile during the removal test, considered as floating time, was recorded, the NTg and heterozygous groups showed a high prevalence of floating (50% (4/8) and 40% (2/5) respectively). In contrast, 3xTgAD mice maintained movement all the time during the test (0/4).

3.6. *Peripheral Organs Pathological Status*

3.6.1. Splenic, Renal, and Hepatic Histopathological Evaluation

Figure 7 illustrates the results of the histopathological analysis of the spleen, kidney, and liver. Systemic amyloidosis damage was observed in the animals that presented lesions. Figure 7A shows representative images of microscopic analyses through Hematoxyline and Eosin staining. As detailed in Figure 7B, the incidence of amyloidosis was higher in the spleen (77%), kidney (100%), and liver (100%) 3xTg-AD mice than in NTg mice (38%, 38%, 25%, respectively).

In the spleen, amyloid deposit distribution was generalized. It was first located in the marginal zone of white pulp and progressively extended to all red pulp. This fact implies an intense hypocellularity and a functional loss of the organ. Although the presence of this damage was higher in the 3xTg-AD group, no significant statistical difference was achieved when we evaluated the injury score. As shown in Figure 2D, the spleen's size and relative size (% vs. bodyweight) were recorded as an indirect measure of its physiological status. However, no differences between groups were observed ($p > 0.05$, Student's t-test). Moreover, weight measures did not correlate with the severity of amyloidosis damage.

In the kidney, the presence of amyloid was observed mainly in the glomerulus and occasionally in the tubular interstitium. In general, the score of the lesion was from moderate to very severe. Concurrently in the more severe cases, multifocal-generalized amyloid deposition was observed in the renal interstitium. Moreover, proteinuria was also observed as distended tubs with the presence of an intense eosinophilic colloid –protein. This damage could cause an important renal dysfunction. Genotype differences were observed when we evaluated the injury score ($p = 0.046$, U Mann Whitney).

In the liver, the lesions affected centrilobular veins, portal vessels, or even higher range interstitial vascularization. Unlike what happened in the spleen and kidneys, the characteristics of the hepatic lesions were mild to moderate, with little pathological relevance. However, the results confirm the systemic nature of the disease since genotype differences were observed when we evaluated the injury score ($p = 0.027$, U Mann Whitney).

As commented, this amyloid damage did not affect all organs equally and presented some heterogeneity. The spleen and kidney presented substantial damage, whereas were mild and little relevant in the liver. However, a correlation between the three organ lesions' intensities was observed ($p < 0.001$, Spearman's correlation). Furthermore, as detailed in Figure 7C, genotype differences were observed when we evaluated the general systemic total score ($p = 0.019$, Student's t-test).

3.6.2. Oxidative Stress Parameters in Peripheral Organs

Concerning the antioxidant capacity from the homogenization of different organs (spleen, kidneys, liver, and heart) no statistical differences were observed in the levels of total glutathione (Figure 8A), as well as the enzymatic activity of glutathione peroxidase (Figure 8B) and glutathione reductase (Figure 8C).

4. Discussion

The present study was aimed to study whether the AD-genotype load can modulate the pathological burden, behavioral phenotype, and neuro-immunoendocrine status in a singular cohort of long-lived (19-month-old survivors) heterozygous and homozygous male 3xTg-AD and as compared to age-matched non-transgenic controls. Therefore, a comprehensive screening of several physical, emotional, and cognitive functions was successively performed using a battery of tests. First, we determined their physical status, including frailty and sensorimotor function, and the survival of animals being continuously monitored from birth to the end of the experiment. Second, the brain was evaluated by levels of amyloid precursor protein (APP), synaptophysin as a synaptogenesis and neuroplasticity marker, and choline acetyltransferase, the enzyme responsible for the Ach synthesis. Third, the behavioral phenotype of animals was evaluated to determine their emotional and anxiety-like profiles, and cognitive functions were assessed in spatial learning and memory tasks. Fourth, neuro-immunoendocrine crosstalk was characterized by glucocorticoid levels, an indicator of HPA axis function. Finally, the histopathological evaluation, and oxidative stress parameters of the spleen, kidney, liver, and heart were used to assess the systemic health of peripheral organs.

4.1. Convergence of Physical Status and Survival Profiles of Long-Lived Survivors

Exclusion or under-representation of older individuals is not unusual in clinical trials despite being the most significant health care resources [43]. Concretely, in clinical trials on Alzheimer's disease, the patients enrolled are not representative of their general population [44]. This problem also occurs at the preclinical level, where most experimental designs are performed in young adulthood, adults, and middle-aged animals. Heterogeneity found in the complexity of age-related scenario and the reduced survival of animals, with the concomitant increase of laboratory costs, produce scarcity research in very old mice, even more in models of neurodegenerative disease [19,45,46].

In the 3xTg-AD mice model, a frailty/survival paradoxical was described, with female exhibiting a worse neuropathological status [47] but higher mortality rates in homozygous [26,28] and heterozygous male 3xTg-AD mice [48]. However, the present cohorts present an extraordinary survival rate, higher than 70% at 19 months of age. In this singular scenario, we were interested to study the relevance of AD-genotype load and the frailty/survival paradigm in normal and neurodegenerative pathological aging.

Frailty, a common tool to measure health status, is becoming widely used in clinical decision making as disease outcomes such as Covid-19 or even mortality were better predicted by frailty index than age or comorbidity [9,49]. In mouse models, the Mouse Clinical Frailty Index [37], a translational adaptation of frailty index data in humans, is also a valuable tool in longevity and aging studies in mice. Although we have noticed and increased frailty levels in 14-month-old 3xTg-AD males compared to NTg counterparts [50], no significant differences were observed in this cohort of 19-month-old survivors. The higher scores were primarily observed in the integument and muscular-skeletal dimension, in accordance with the more common clinical presentations in aged mice, such as alopecia and dermatitis [51].

The body weight of animals was also monitored as an index of health/frailty status, and, in this case, the overweight characteristic of the 3xTg-AD Spanish colony was not found [52]. Instead of this, reduced body weight was observed predominantly in homozygous mice, similarly as described previously in isolated 3xTg-AD male mice [53].

Regarding sensorimotor function, and as observed in 18-month-old transgenic and NTg females [19], poor physical motor abilities were observed in both groups. A convergence of sensorimotor profiles was caused by lack of coordination and short latencies of falling with high individual variability.

4.2. Non-Linear HPA-Axis Activation in 3xTg-AD Males

A crosstalk between endocrine abnormalities of the hypothalamic-pituitary-adrenal (HPA) system and patients with Alzheimer's disease have been described repeatedly [54]. Elevated cortisol levels have been associated with cognitive decline dementia [55] and peripheral immunodepression [56]. These data agree with our first report in 15-month-old animals, where a significant increase in plasma corticosterone was observed in 3xTg-AD male mice, suggesting enhanced HPA axis activation accompanied with immune function alterations [28]. In the present study, we described a non-linear increase of corticosterone levels, with heterozygous mice presenting higher levels than NTg mice. This can be explained as cortisol levels seem to be associated with the progression of the disease rather than the severity. Thus, Csernansky et al. observed more significant correlations in AD-patients at the early stages of the disease [57]. It has been also described the role of microglia in the chronic-stress induced neuroinflammation and their contribution to neurodegenerative disease [58,59]. Study the impact this HPA axis hyperactivation on inflammation and further activation of glial cells would be necessary to better understand the underlying mechanism of the cognitive and anxiety-like symptoms observed in 3xTg-AD, opening new preventive and prognostic options.

4.3. Amyloid Precursor Protein (APP) Levels Increased in a Genetic-Load-Dependent Manner but Age-Dependent Convergence of Synaptophysin and Choline Acetyltransferase Brain Levels

Alzheimer's disease is defined as an accumulation of amyloid-β (Aβ) plaques and tau-containing neurofibrillary tangles (NFTs), although they can also be found in normal aging. Neuroinflammation and other metabolic and neuronal processes such as synaptic changes and changes in neurotransmitter systems also play a role in the pathogenesis of AD [2]. The 3xTg-AD model develops age-related, progressive neuropathology, including plaques and tangles mimicking human patients' temporal and neuroanatomical patterns [20,21]. In the current experimental scenario with survivors, we can study how the three different levels of AD-genetic-load (null, heterozygous, homozygous) translate into the expression of these hallmarks of AD.

The hippocampus was the most sensitive AD-target region to show the effect of genetic-load in APP levels, while in the cortical areas studied (prefrontal and entorhinal), the difference did not reach statistical significance, probably due to the variability. These results agree and complement those reported in young mutants in the original work describing the model [21].

Synaptophysin is a membrane protein of synaptic vesicles closely related to cognitive processes and synaptic plasticity [60]. Several authors have reported changes in synaptophysin expression in Alzheimer's patient's brain areas [61,62]. In 3xTg-AD mice, we have already reported that synaptophysin expression levels significantly decreased in middle-aged mice [22,63]. However, no significant genotype differences were observed in survivors studied in the present report.

Similar results were observed when we evaluated the levels of ChAT, the enzyme responsible for acetylcholine synthesis, one of the most involved neurotransmitters in the disease. Nowadays, acetylcholinesterase inhibitors still constitute the most important group of drugs for Alzheimer's disease treatment [64]. Despite the significative decreased levels observed in middle-aged mice [27,65], no significant differences were observed in these group of 19-month old survivors. Interestingly, aging-related loss of presynaptic protein synaptophysin and cholinergic inputs observed in C57BL/6J male mice [66] could explain that aging processes might be related to this convergence of synaptophysin and ChAT levels.

Therefore, amyloid levels were increased in a genetic-load-dependent manner independently of aging. However, synaptic, and cholinergic functions seem to be more dependent on aging processes/survival paradigms.

4.4. Genotype Load Modulates Anxiety-Like Patterns Despite Similar Cognitive Impairments

It has been reported that genetic load can aggravate the extent and accelerate the onset of pathological alterations in transgenic mice [67,68]. For example, it has been previously established age-dependent difference in pathology and cognitive deterioration between hemizygous and homozygous 3xTg-AD mice [21,30,69]. The present work aimed to explore the genetic-load-dependent effect on behavioral and psychological outcomes in a singular cohort of long-lived mice. Studying the impact of the genetic component at advanced stages of the disease may help to understand better the aging interactions which can be involved in the wide heterogeneity and complexity of patients' clinical profiles.

As previously observed in 18-month-old female survivors [19], no genotype differences were observed between 3xTg-AD and NTg in the corner test, open-field test, and T-maze, three classical unconditioned tests measuring neophobia, exploratory activity, and emotionality [18] neither in the dark and light box and marble test. This convergence of behavioral profiles involves considering the contribution of genetic patterns and/or aging-related decline per *se*. In this sense, our laboratory has described convergence of profiles in the context of poor aging from 12 to 18 months of age as part of the complexity of age-related scenarios and heterogeneity among all populations, including both wild-type mice and 3xTg-AD mice [19,50,53]. The survival of very old 3xTg-AD mice points to the existence of distinct brain and systemic physiological protective mechanisms for AD-pathology besides those that may exist in normal aging [50,70].

However, on the other hand, when we evaluated independently homozygous and heterozygous mice, we observed that genotype load modulated anxiety-like- profiles. When we repeated the open field test 24 h later, the ethogram exhibited higher latencies. Thus, increases were observed in the latency to exit the center, entrance to the periphery and vertical activity in homozygous, and spent more time in the center than heterozygous mice. In agreement with previous reports showing a 24 h long-term memory deficit in 3xTg-AD mice at 2, 4, 6, and 14 months of age, the behavioral response of mutants did not benefit from previous experience in contrast to NTg age-matched counterparts [35,50]. However, in this case, repeated the test increased the genetic-load differences not observed in the first day-test.

In the dark and light box test, the anxiogenic profile of homozygous 3xTg-mice was associated by a delay in the risk assessment activity and the number of crossings and rearings performed in the dark area.

The anxiogenic profile was also confirmed in the T-maze test, indicating that the profile that have been previously described in this model [18,29,31] persists in 19-month-old survivors. Noteworthy, none of the homozygous mice accomplished the test completion nor acquisition criteria. This fact indicates their aged status and/or poor motivation [19], a singular fact that we have also observed associated with severe status neurodegenerative models [71]. Moreover, the increased latencies of homozygous to achieve the crossing intersection have been related to immunosenescence and reduced survival [72].

As reported in 18-month-old female survivors [19], cognitive impairment remained the salient distinctive trait in 3xTg-AD mice as compared to NTg mice. These results are in accordance with worse performance in Morris Water Maze observed in several ages of 3xTg-AD [18,29,31,35,73]. On the other hand, the swimming performance can reflect their emotional status in an aquatic environment known to be anxiogenic for mice [74]. In this case, the floating behavior (inactivity without forward movement) characteristic of non-transgenic performance [75] was not presented in 3xTg-AD homozygous mice. However, it was observed in non-transgenic and 3xTg-AD heterozygous mice. Therefore, these results allow us to propose that the underlying mechanisms are still preserved in heterozygosis. The results in genetic load also confirmed the anxiogenic and cognitive phenotypes being modulated independently in both groups.

These results highlight the distinct contribution of genetic-load disease-related components and aging to behavioral readouts. Cognitive impairment is a distinct trait of the disease. However, anxiety-like behavior seems to be more related to genetic-load, been more affected the animals with higher genetic dosages. Despite the inherent limitations of the sample size of the present study, consistent behavioral patterns make the present results of interest for further exploration in a larger size sample. These data agree with the premorbid predisposition to anxiety and depression in familial Alzheimer's disease [76] and may explain why early-onset Alzheimer's disease patients more often present non-amnestic phenotypic variants [77].

4.5. Peripheral Organs Presented Histopathological Alterations but No Differences in Their Oxidative Stress Parameters

Neurodegenerative disorders such as dementia are associated with increased mortality compared to the general old population [7,8]. Clinical evidence suggests an interaction between the brain and systemic abnormalities that can explain this fact [78]. For instance, it has been repeatedly described that the immune system has an important role in AD pathology, both at the central nervous system and peripheral level [79,80]. Our research in the 3xTg-AD mice also supports the relevance of the neuro-immunoendocrine impairment in AD. Thus, we have described significant involvement of the peripheral immune system [28,81–85]. The impairment was also monitored through peritoneal cells in a longitudinal study from 2 to 15 months of age, mimicking premorbid, prodromal, early to advanced stages of the disease [84]. Therefore, a better understanding of neuro-immunoendocrine crosstalk could help with an early diagnosis and, as we have proposed, improve the disease monitoring of AD.

In the present study, histological analysis was performed on the spleen, kidney, and liver. Systemic amyloidosis damage was observed in the animals that presented lesions. A higher incidence was observed in 3xTg-AD mice independently of genetic-load than in NTg mice. In the spleen, amyloid deposit distribution was generalized, producing an intense hypocellularity and a functional loss of the organ. In the kidney, the presence of amyloid was observed mainly in the glomerulus, causing an important renal disfunction. Although in the liver, the lesions presented little pathological relevance, it confirmed the systemic nature of amyloidosis. Amyloid has been reported to occur spontaneously in a variety of animal species, including mice. For instance, glomerular amyloidosis is common in older mice [51]. Moreover, the grade and incidence of amyloid deposition seem to increase with age. In SAM mice, a mouse model of senescence-accelerated mouse, renal amyloidosis was more frequent in animals with complications such as abscess, skin ulcer or tumors [85]. The easy measurement of their weight and relative weight (organometrics), with clinical translation, can be used as early indicators of peripheral immunological system aging [82,83,86], as also confirmed by other laboratories [87,88]. In this case, spleen weight was recorded as an indirect measure of their physiological status. However, no differences between groups were observed. Moreover, this measure did not correlate with the severity of amyloidosis damage. Similarly, in the SAM mice, the kidney/body weight ratio did not parallel the grade of renal amyloidosis [85].

Although brain oxidative stress in AD is accepted, the contribution of the disease to peripheral oxidative redox state has been scarcely studied. We have previously shown sex-specific immuno-endocrine aging in 3xTg-AD mice. Concretely, peripheral alterations in early oxidative stress status in male and female 3xTg-AD mice, with a decrease in antioxidant defenses and an increase in xanthine oxidase activity in most peripheral tissues, among them the spleen, kidney, and liver [28,52,86,89]. However, like the present study, no genotype differences were found in reduced glutathione levels in peritoneal leukocytes at 15 months of age [84]. These studies suggest a premature immunosenescence in the prodromal stage of AD. However, a decrease in antioxidants and an increase in oxidants associated with the aging process [90] could explain this convergence of profiles in our survivors.

Taking all these data into account, the present study provides an interesting translational scenario showing complex neuro-immunoendocrine crosstalk. Furthermore, vulnerability/compensatory mechanisms in transgenic mice were observed as histopathological alterations showed organs dysfunction with no correlations in frailty index nor oxidative stress parameters.

5. Conclusions

The singular cohort of long-lived (19-month-old survivors) heterozygous and homozygous male 3xTg-AD mice studied here indicates that the AD-genotype load modulates the brain and peripheral pathological burden, behavioral phenotypes, and neuro-immunoendocrine status, compared to age-matched non-transgenic controls. The main findings pointed at the non-linear impact of genetic load in the different dimensions studied. While amyloid precursor protein (APP) levels increased in a genetic-load-dependent manner, synaptophysin and choline acetyltransferase brain levels referring to synaptic function were similar in the three groups of mice, that may agree with the decrease of synaptic function described in aged animals. Cognitive impairment and the level of activation of the HPA-axis were salient traits in both 3xTg-AD survivor groups, with no impact of genetic load. In contrast, homozygous and heterozygous exhibited different responses in classical unconditioned anxiety tests. Homozygous 3xTg-AD mice showed severe hypofunction in most tests, while heterozygous resembled controls in some anxiety variables and risk assessment, suggesting different genetic-load modulation of these states. Complex neuro-immunoendocrine crosstalk was also observed. Bodyweight loss and splenic, renal, and hepatic histopathological injury scores provided evidence of the systemic features of AD, despite similar peripheral organs' oxidative stress. The present study provides an interesting translational scenario to study further genetic-load and age-dependent vulnerability/compensatory mechanisms in Alzheimer's disease. Research with very old mice and, particularly, in long-term survivors' cohorts with specific behavioral and physiological profiles can be helpful for the better understanding of heterogenous manifestations reported in end-of-life Alzheimer's patients.

Author Contributions: Conceptualization, L.G.-L.; Methodology: A.M.; data curation: A.M.; writing-original draft preparation, L.G.-L. and A.M.; writing-review and editing, L.G.-L. and A.M.; supervision: L.G.-L.; funding acquisition, L.G.-L. All authors have read and agreed to the published version of the manuscript.

Funding: This work was funded by UAB-GE-260408 to L.G.-L. The colony of 3xTg-AD mice is sustained by ArrestAD H2020 Fet-OPEN-1-2016-2017-737390, European Union's Horizon 2020 research and innovation program under grant agreement No 737390 to L.G.-L.

Institutional Review Board Statement: The study was conducted according to the guidelines of the Declaration of Helsinki, and approved by the Ethics Committee of Departament de Medi Ambient i Habitatge, Generalitat de Catalunya (CEEAH 3588/DMAH 9452) the 8 March 2019.

Acknowledgments: We thank Frank M. LaFerla, Institute for Memory Impairments and Neurological Disorders, University of California Irvine, CA, USA for kindly providing the progenitors of the

Spanish colonies of 3xTg-AD and NTg mice. Thanks to Javier Carrasco, The INc Molecular Biology Unit for his help in corticosterone and oxidative stress determinations. And to Serveis Integrats d'Animals de Laboratori and Servei de Diagnòstic de Patologia Veterinària Universitat Autònoma de Barcelona for splenic, renal, and hepatic histopathological evaluation. Some figures of the graphical abstract were created with BioRender.com.

Conflicts of Interest: The authors declare no conflict of interest.

References

1. Lourida, I.; Hannon, E.; Littlejohns, T.J.; Langa, K.M.; Hypponen, E.; Kuzma, E.; Llewellyn, D.J. Association of Lifestyle and Genetic Risk with Incidence of Dementia. *JAMA* **2019**, *322*, 430–437. [CrossRef] [PubMed]
2. Spires-Jones, T.L.; Hyman, B.T. The Intersection of Amyloid Beta and Tau at Synapses in Alzheimer's Disease. *Neuron* **2014**, *82*, 756–771. [CrossRef] [PubMed]
3. Cummings, J.L. The Neuropsychiatric Inventory: Assessing psychopathology in dementia patients. *Neurology* **1997**, *48* (Suppl. S6), 10S–16S. [CrossRef] [PubMed]
4. Zhao, Q.-F.; Tan, L.; Wang, H.-F.; Jiang, T.; Tan, M.-S.; Tan, L.; Xu, W.; Li, J.-Q.; Wang, J.; Lai, T.-J.; et al. The prevalence of neuropsychiatric symptoms in Alzheimer's disease: Systematic review and meta-analysis. *J. Affect. Disord.* **2016**, *190*, 264–271. [CrossRef]
5. Kamiya, M.; Sakurai, T.; Ogama, N.; Maki, Y.; Toba, K. Factors associated with increased caregivers' burden in several cognitive stages of Alzheimer's disease. *Geriatr. Gerontol. Int.* **2014**, *14*, 45–55. [CrossRef]
6. De Vugt, M.E.; Stevens, F.; Aalten, P.; Lousberg, R.; Jaspers, N.; Verhey, F.R.J. A prospective study of the effects of behavioral symptoms on the institutionalization of patients with dementia. *Int. Psychogeriatr.* **2005**, *17*, 577–589. [CrossRef]
7. Van Dijk, P.T.; Dippel, D.W.; Habbema, J.D.F. Survival of Patients with Dementia. *J. Am. Geriatr. Soc.* **1991**, *39*, 603–610. [CrossRef]
8. Mitchell, S.L.; Miller, S.C.; Teno, J.M.; Kiely, D.K.; Davis, R.B.; Shaffer, M.L. Prediction of 6-Month Survival of Nursing Home Residents With Advanced Dementia Using ADEPT vs. Hospice Eligibility Guidelines. *JAMA* **2010**, *304*, 1929–1935. [CrossRef]
9. Zeng, A.; Song, X.; Dong, J.; Mitnitski, A.; Liu, J.; Guo, Z.; Rockwood, K. Mortality in Relation to Frailty in Patients Admitted to a Specialized Geriatric Intensive Care Unit. *J. Gerontol. Ser. A Boil. Sci. Med. Sci.* **2015**, *70*, 1586–1594. [CrossRef]
10. Ferretti, M.T.; Iulita, M.F.; Cavedo, E.; Chiesa, P.A.; Dimech, A.S.; Chadha, A.S.; Baracchi, F.; Girouard, H.; Misoch, S.; Giacobini, E.; et al. Sex differences in Alzheimer disease—The gateway to precision medicine. *Nat. Rev. Neurol.* **2018**, *14*, 457–469. [CrossRef]
11. Mazure, C.M.; Swendsen, J. Sex differences in Alzheimer's disease and other dementias. *Lancet Neurol.* **2016**, *15*, 451–452. [CrossRef]
12. Sinforiani, E.; Citterio, A.; Zucchella, C.; Bono, G.; Corbetta, S.; Merlo, P.; Mauri, M. Impact of Gender Differences on the Outcome of Alzheimer's Disease. *Dement. Geriatr. Cogn. Disord.* **2010**, *30*, 147–154. [CrossRef]
13. Komarova, N.L.; Thalhauser, C.J. High Degree of Heterogeneity in Alzheimer's Disease Progression Patterns. *PLoS Comput. Biol.* **2011**, *7*, e1002251. [CrossRef]
14. Cummings, J.; Lee, G.; Ritter, A.; Sabbagh, M.; Zhong, K. Alzheimer's disease drug development pipeline: 2019. *Alzheimer's Dement. Transl. Res. Clin. Interv.* **2019**, *5*, 272–293. [CrossRef]
15. Anand, R.; Gill, K.D.; Mahdi, A.A. Therapeutics of Alzheimer's disease: Past, present and future. *Neuropharmacology* **2014**, *76*, 27–50. [CrossRef]
16. Gamberger, D.; Lavrač, N.; Srivatsa, S.; Tanzi, R.E.; Doraiswamy, P.M. Identification of clusters of rapid and slow decliners among subjects at risk for Alzheimer's disease. *Sci. Rep.* **2017**, *7*, 6763. [CrossRef]
17. Escott-Price, V.; Myers, A.J.; Huentelman, M.; Hardy, J. Polygenic risk score analysis of pathologically confirmed Alzheimer disease. *Ann. Neurol.* **2017**, *82*, 311–314. [CrossRef]
18. Giménez-Llort, L.; Blázquez, G.; Cañete, T.; Johansson, B.; Oddo, S.; Tobeña, A.; LaFerla, F.; Fernández-Teruel, A. Modeling behavioral and neuronal symptoms of Alzheimer's disease in mice: A role for intraneuronal amyloid. *Neurosci. Biobehav. Rev.* **2007**, *31*, 125–147. [CrossRef]
19. Torres-Lista, V.; De La Fuente, M.; Giménez-Llort, L. Survival Curves and Behavioral Profiles of Female 3xTg-AD Mice Surviving to 18-Months of Age as Compared to Mice with Normal Aging. *J. Alzheimer's Dis. Rep.* **2017**, *1*, 47–57. [CrossRef]
20. Belfiore, R.; Rodin, A.; Ferreira, E.; Velazquez, R.; Branca, C.; Caccamo, A.; Oddo, S. Temporal and regional progression of Alzheimer's disease-like pathology in 3xTg-AD mice. *Aging Cell* **2019**, *18*, e12873. [CrossRef]
21. Oddo, S.; Caccamo, A.; Shepherd, J.D.; Murphy, M.P.; Golde, T.E.; Kayed, R.; Metherate, R.; Mattson, M.P.; Akbari, Y.; LaFerla, F.M. Triple-Transgenic Model of Alzheimer's Disease with Plaques and Tangles: Intracellular Abeta and Synaptic Dysfunction. *Neuron* **2003**, *39*, 409–421. [CrossRef]
22. Hedberg, M.M.; Clos, M.V.; Ratia, M.; Gonzalez, D.; Lithner, C.U.; Camps, P.; Muñoz-Torrero, D.; Badia, A.; Giménez-Llort, L.; Nordberg, A. Effect of Huprine X on ?-Amyloid, Synaptophysin and ?7 Neuronal Nicotinic Acetylcholine Receptors in the Brain of 3xTg-AD and APPswe Transgenic Mice. *Neurodegener. Dis.* **2010**, *7*, 379–388. [CrossRef]
23. Caruso, D.; Barron, A.; Brown, M.A.; Abbiati, F.; Carrero, P.; Pike, C.J.; Garcia-Segura, L.M.; Melcangi, R.C. Age-related changes in neuroactive steroid levels in 3xTg-AD mice. *Neurobiol. Aging* **2013**, *34*, 1080–1089. [CrossRef]

24. Kitazawa, M.; Oddo, S.; Yamasaki, T.R.; Green, K.N.; LaFerla, F.M. Lipopolysaccharide-Induced Inflammation Exacerbates Tau Pathology by a Cyclin-Dependent Kinase 5-Mediated Pathway in a Transgenic Model of Alzheimer's Disease. *J. Neurosci.* **2005**, *25*, 8843–8853. [CrossRef]
25. Ghosh, D.; LeVault, K.R.; Barnett, A.J.; Brewer, G.J. A Reversible Early Oxidized Redox State That Precedes Macromolecular ROS Damage in Aging Nontransgenic and 3xTg-AD Mouse Neurons. *J. Neurosci.* **2012**, *32*, 5821–5832. [CrossRef]
26. García-Mesa, Y.; Colie, S.; Corpas, R.; Cristòfol, R.; Comellas, F.; Nebreda, A.R.; Giménez-Llort, L.; Sanfeliu, C. Oxidative Stress Is a Central Target for Physical Exercise Neuroprotection Against Pathological Brain Aging. *J. Gerontol. Ser. A Boil. Sci. Med. Sci.* **2015**, *71*, 40–49. [CrossRef]
27. Perez, S.E.; He, B.; Muhammad, N.; Oh, K.-J.; Fahnestock, M.; Ikonomovic, M.D.; Mufson, E.J. Cholinotrophic basal forebrain system alterations in 3xTg-AD transgenic mice. *Neurobiol. Dis.* **2011**, *41*, 338–352. [CrossRef] 3xTg
28. Giménez-Llort, L.; Arranz, L.; Maté, I.; De La Fuente, M. Gender-Specific Neuroimmunoendocrine Aging in a Triple-Transgenic 3xTg-AD Mouse Model for Alzheimer's Disease and Its Relation with Longevity. *Neuroimmunomodulation* **2008**, *15*, 331–343. [CrossRef] [PubMed]
29. Sterniczuk, R.; Antle, M.C.; LaFerla, F.M.; Dyck, R. Characterization of the 3xTg-AD mouse model of Alzheimer's disease: Part 2. Behavioral and cognitive changes. *Brain Res.* **2010**, *1348*, 149–155. [CrossRef] [PubMed]
30. Billings, L.M.; Oddo, S.; Green, K.N.; McGaugh, J.L.; LaFerla, F.M. Intraneuronal Aβ Causes the Onset of Early Alzheimer's Disease-Related Cognitive Deficits in Transgenic Mice. *Neuron* **2005**, *45*, 675–688. [CrossRef] [PubMed]
31. Blázquez, G.; Cañete, T.; Tobena, A.; Giménez-Llort, L.; Fernández-Teruel, A. Cognitive and emotional profiles of aged Alzheimer's disease (3xTgAD) mice: Effects of environmental enrichment and sexual dimorphism. *Behav. Brain Res.* **2014**, *268*, 185–201. [CrossRef]
32. España, J.; Giménez-Llort, L.; Valero, J.; Miñano, A.; Rábano, A.; Rodriguez-Alvarez, J.; LaFerla, F.M.; Saura, C.A. Intraneuronal β-Amyloid Accumulation in the Amygdala Enhances Fear and Anxiety in Alzheimer's Disease Transgenic Mice. *Biol. Psychiatry* **2010**, *67*, 513–521. [CrossRef]
33. Kilkenny, C.; Browne, W.J.; Cuthill, I.C.; Emerson, M.; Altman, D.G. Improving Bioscience Research Reporting: The ARRIVE Guidelines for Reporting Animal Research. *PLoS Biol.* **2010**, *8*, e1000412. [CrossRef]
34. Hall, C.; Ballachey, E.L. *A Study of the Rat's Behavior in a Field. A Contribution to Method in Comparative Psychology*; University of California Publications in Psychology: Berkeley, CA, USA, 1932; Volume 6, pp. 1–12.
35. Torres-Lista, V.; Parrado-Fernández, C.; Alvarez-Montón, I.; Frontiñan, J.; Durán-Prado, M.; Peinado, J.R.; Johansson, B.; Alcaín, F.J.; Giménez-Llort, L. Neophobia, NQO1 and SIRT1 as premorbid and prodromal indicators of AD in 3xTg-AD mice. *Behav. Brain Res.* **2014**, *271*, 140–146. [CrossRef]
36. Douglas, R.J. Cues for spontaneous alternation. *J. Comp. Physiol. Psychol.* **1966**, *62*, 171–183. [CrossRef]
37. Whitehead, J.C.; Hildebrand, B.A.; Sun, M.; Rockwood, M.R.; Rose, R.; Rockwood, K.; Howlett, S.E. A Clinical Frailty Index in Aging Mice: Comparisons with Frailty Index Data in Humans. *J. Gerontol. Ser. A Boil. Sci. Med. Sci.* **2014**, *69*, 621–632. [CrossRef]
38. Tietze, F. Enzymic method for quantitative determination of nanogram amounts of total and oxidized glutathione: Applications to mammalian blood and other tissues. *Anal. Biochem.* **1969**, *27*, 502–522. [CrossRef]
39. Rahman, I.; Kode, A.; Biswas, S.K. Assay for quantitative determination of glutathione and glutathione disulfide levels using enzymatic recycling method. *Nat. Protoc.* **2006**, *1*, 3159–3165. [CrossRef]
40. Massey, V.; Williams, C.H. On the Reaction Mechanism of Yeast Glutathione Reductase. *J. Biol. Chem.* **1965**, *240*, 4470–4480. [CrossRef]
41. Lawrence, R.A.; Burk, R.F. Glutathione peroxidase activity in selenium-deficient rat liver. *Biochem. Biophys. Res. Commun.* **1976**, *71*, 952–958. [CrossRef]
42. Alvarado, C.; Alvarez, P.; Jimenez, L.; De La Fuente, M. Oxidative stress in leukocytes from young prematurely aging mice is reversed by supplementation with biscuits rich in antioxidants. *Dev. Comp. Immunol.* **2006**, *30*, 1168–1180. [CrossRef]
43. Zulman, D.M.; Sussman, J.B.; Chen, X.; Cigolle, C.T.; Blaum, C.S.; Hayward, R.A. Examining the Evidence: A Systematic Review of the Inclusion and Analysis of Older Adults in Randomized Controlled Trials. *J. Gen. Intern. Med.* **2011**, *26*, 783–790. [CrossRef]
44. Banzi, R.; Camaioni, P.; Tettamanti, M.; Bertele', V.; Lucca, U. Older patients are still under-represented in clinical trials of Alzheimer's disease. *Alzheimer's Res. Ther.* **2016**, *8*, 32. [CrossRef]
45. Fahlström, A.; Yu, Q.; Ulfhake, B. Behavioral changes in aging female C57BL/6 mice. *Neurobiol. Aging* **2011**, *32*, 1868–1880. [CrossRef]
46. Giménez-Llort, L.; Ramírez-Boix, P.; De La Fuente, M. Mortality of septic old and adult male mice correlates with individual differences in premorbid behavioral phenotype and acute-phase sickness behavior. *Exp. Gerontol.* **2019**, *127*, 110717. [CrossRef]
47. Hirata-Fukae, C.; Li, H.-F.; Hoe, H.-S.; Gray, A.J.; Minami, S.S.; Hamada, K.; Niikura, T.; Hua, F.; Tsukagoshi-Nagai, H.; Horikoshi-Sakuraba, Y.; et al. Females exhibit more extensive amyloid, but not tau, pathology in an Alzheimer transgenic model. *Brain Res.* **2008**, *1216*, 92–103. [CrossRef]
48. Rae, E.A.; Brown, R.E. The problem of genotype and sex differences in life expectancy in transgenic AD mice. *Neurosci. Biobehav. Rev.* **2015**, *57*, 238–251. [CrossRef]
49. Hewitt, J.; Carter, B.; Vilches-Moraga, A.; Quinn, T.J.; Braude, P.; Verduri, A.; Pearce, L.; Stechman, M.; Short, R.; Price, A.; et al. The effect of frailty on survival in patients with COVID-19 (COPE): A multicentre, European, observational cohort study. *Lancet Public Health* **2020**, *5*, e444–e451. [CrossRef]

50. Muntsant, A.; Jiménez-Altayó, F.; Puertas-Umbert, L.; Jiménez-Xarrie, E.; Vila, E.; Giménez-Llort, L. Sex-Dependent End-of-Life Mental and Vascular Scenarios for Compensatory Mechanisms in Mice with Normal and AD-Neurodegenerative Aging. *Biomedicines* **2021**, *9*, 111. [CrossRef]
51. Pettan-Brewer, C.; Treuting, P.M.M. Practical pathology of aging mice. *Pathobiol. Aging Age-Relat. Dis.* **2011**, *1*, 7202. [CrossRef]
52. Giménez-Llort, L.; García, Y.; Buccieri, K.; Revilla, S.; Suñol, C.; Cristofol, R.; Sanfeliu, C. Gender-Specific Neuroimmunoendocrine Response to Treadmill Exercise in 3xTg-AD Mice. *Int. J. Alzheimer's Dis.* **2010**, *2010*, 128354. [CrossRef] [PubMed]
53. Muntsant, A.; Giménez-Llort, L. Impact of Social Isolation on the Behavioral, Functional Profiles, and Hippocampal Atrophy Asymmetry in Dementia in Times of Coronavirus Pandemic (COVID-19): A Translational Neuroscience Approach. *Front. Psychiatry* **2020**, *11*, 572583. [CrossRef] [PubMed]
54. Ouanes, S.; Popp, J. High Cortisol and the Risk of Dementia and Alzheimer's Disease: A Review of the Literature. *Front. Aging Neurosci.* **2019**, *11*, 43. [CrossRef] [PubMed]
55. Hartmann, A.; Veldhuis, J.; Deuschle, M.; Standhardt, H.; Heuser, I. Twenty-Four Hour Cortisol Release Profiles in Patients With Alzheimer's and Parkinson's Disease Compared to Normal Controls: Ultradian Secretory Pulsatility and Diurnal Variation. *Neurobiol. Aging* **1997**, *18*, 285–289. [CrossRef]
56. Woiciechowsky, C.; Schöning, B.; Lanksch, W.R.; Volk, H.-D.; Döcke, W.-D. Mechanisms of brain-mediated systemic anti-inflammatory syndrome causing immunodepression. *J. Mol. Med.* **1999**, *77*, 769–780. [CrossRef]
57. Csernansky, J.G.; Dong, H.; Fagan, A.M.; Wang, L.; Xiong, C.; Holtzman, D.M.; Morris, J.C. Plasma Cortisol and Progression of Dementia in Subjects With Alzheimer-Type Dementia. *Am. J. Psychiatry* **2006**, *163*, 2164–2169. [CrossRef]
58. Pedrazzoli, M.; Losurdo, M.; Paolone, G.; Medelin, M.; Jaupaj, L.; Cisterna, B.; Slanzi, A.; Malatesta, M.; Coco, S.; Buffelli, M. Glucocorticoid receptors modulate dendritic spine plasticity and microglia activity in an animal model of Alzheimer's disease. *Neurobiol. Dis.* **2019**, *132*, 104568. [CrossRef]
59. Picard, K.; St-Pierre, M.-K.; Vecchiarelli, H.A.; Bordeleau, M.; Tremblay, M.È. Neuroendocrine, neuroinflammatory and pathological outcomes of chronic stress: A story of microglial remodeling. *Neurochem. Int.* **2021**, *145*, 104987. [CrossRef]
60. Nie, J.; Zhou, M.; Lü, C.; Hu, X.; Wan, B.; Yang, B.; Li, Y. Effects of triptolide on the synaptophysin expression of hippocampal neurons in the AD cellular model. *Int. Immunopharmacol.* **2012**, *13*, 175–180. [CrossRef]
61. Sze, C.-I.; Troncoso, J.C.; Kawas, C.; Moution, P.; Price, D.L.; Martin, L.J. Loss of the Presynaptic Vesicle Protein Synaptophysin in Hippocampus Correlates with Cognitive Decline in Alzheimer Disease. *J. Neuropathol. Exp. Neurol.* **1997**, *56*, 933–944. [CrossRef]
62. Proctor, D.T.; Coulson, E.; Dodd, P.R. Reduction in Post-Synaptic Scaffolding PSD-95 and SAP-102 Protein Levels in the Alzheimer Inferior Temporal Cortex is Correlated with Disease Pathology. *J. Alzheimer's Dis.* **2010**, *21*, 795–811. [CrossRef]
63. Revilla, S.; Suñol, C.; García-Mesa, Y.; Giménez-Llort, L.; Sanfeliu, C.; Cristòfol, R. Physical exercise improves synaptic dysfunction and recovers the loss of survival factors in 3xTg-AD mouse brain. *Neuropharmacology* **2014**, *81*, 55–63. [CrossRef]
64. Cummings, J.L.; Isaacson, R.S.; Schmitt, F.A.; Velting, D.M. A practical algorithm for managing Alzheimer's disease: What, when, and why? *Ann. Clin. Transl. Neurol.* **2015**, *2*, 307–323. [CrossRef]
65. Orta-Salazar, E.; Aguilar-Vázquez, A.; Martínez-Coria, H.; Anda, S.L.-D.; Rivera-Cervantes, M.; Beas-Zarate, C.; Feria-Velasco, A.; Díaz-Cintra, S. REST/NRSF-induced changes of ChAT protein expression in the neocortex and hippocampus of the 3xTg-AD mouse model for Alzheimer's disease. *Life Sci.* **2014**, *116*, 83–89. [CrossRef]
66. Xu, L.; Long, J.; Su, Z.; Xu, B.; Lin, M.; Chen, Y.; Long, D. Restored presynaptic synaptophysin and cholinergic inputs contribute to the protective effects of physical running on spatial memory in aged mice. *Neurobiol. Dis.* **2019**, *132*, 104586. [CrossRef]
67. Richard, B.C.; Kurdakova, A.; Baches, S.; Bayer, T.A.; Weggen, S.; Wirths, O. Gene Dosage Dependent Aggravation of the Neurological Phenotype in the 5XFAD Mouse Model of Alzheimer's Disease. *J. Alzheimer's Dis.* **2015**, *45*, 1223–1236. [CrossRef]
68. Willuweit, A.; Velden, J.; Godemann, R.; Manook, A.; Jetzek, F.; Tintrup, H.; Kauselmann, G.; Zevnik, B.; Henriksen, G.; Drzezga, A.; et al. Early-Onset and Robust Amyloid Pathology in a New Homozygous Mouse Model of Alzheimer's Disease. *PLoS ONE* **2009**, *4*, e7931. [CrossRef]
69. Billings, L.M.; Green, K.N.; McGaugh, J.L.; LaFerla, F.M. Learning Decreases A *56 and Tau Pathology and Ameliorates Behavioral Decline in 3xTg-AD Mice. *J. Neurosci.* **2007**, *27*, 751–761. [CrossRef]
70. Giménez-Llort, L.; Marin-Pardo, D.; Marazuela, P.; Hernández-Guillamón, M. Survival Bias and Crosstalk between Chronological and Behavioral Age: Age- and Genotype-Sensitivity Tests Define Behavioral Signatures in Middle-Aged, Old, and Long-Lived Mice with Normal and AD-Associated Aging. *Biomedicines* **2021**, *9*, 636. [CrossRef]
71. Pagès, G.; Giménez-Llort, L.; García-Lareu, B.; Ariza, L.; Navarro, M.; Casas, C.; Chillón, M.; Bosch, A. Intrathecal AAVrh10 corrects biochemical and histological hallmarks of mucopolysaccharidosis VII mice and improves behavior and survival. *Hum. Mol. Genet.* **2019**, *28*, 3610–3624. [CrossRef]
72. Guayerbas, N.; Puerto, M.; Ferrández, M.D.; De La Fuente, M. A diet supplemented with thiolic anti-oxidants improves leucocyte function in two strains of prematurely ageing mice. *Clin. Exp. Pharmacol. Physiol.* **2002**, *29*, 1009–1014. [CrossRef]
73. Gulinello, M.; Gertner, M.; Mendoza, G.; Schoenfeld, B.P.; Oddo, S.; LaFerla, F.; Choi, C.H.; McBride, S.M.; Faber, D.S. Validation of a 2-day water maze protocol in mice. *Behav. Brain Res.* **2009**, *196*, 220–227. [CrossRef]
74. D'Hooge, R.; De Deyn, P.P. Applications of the Morris water maze in the study of learning and memory. *Brain Res. Rev.* **2001**, *36*, 60–90. [CrossRef]
75. Baeta-Corral, R.; Giménez-Llort, L. Persistent hyperactivity and distinctive strategy features in the Morris water maze in 3xTg-AD mice at advanced stages of disease. *Behav. Neurosci.* **2015**, *129*, 129–137. [CrossRef] [PubMed]

76. Ringman, J.M.; Liang, L.-J.; Zhou, Y.; Vangala, S.; Teng, E.; Kremen, S.; Wharton, D.; Goate, A.; Marcus, D.S.; Farlow, M.R.; et al. Early behavioural changes in familial Alzheimer's disease in the Dominantly Inherited Alzheimer Network. *Brain* **2015**, *138*, 1036–1045. [CrossRef] [PubMed]
77. Mendez, M.F. Early-onset Alzheimer Disease and Its Variants. *Contin. Lifelong Learn. Neurol.* **2019**, *25*, 34–51. [CrossRef] [PubMed]
78. Wang, J.; Gu, B.J.; Masters, C.L.; Wang, Y.-J. A systemic view of Alzheimer disease—Insights from amyloid-β metabolism beyond the brain. *Nat. Rev. Neurol.* **2017**, *13*, 612–623. [CrossRef] [PubMed]
79. Richartz, E.; Stransky, E.; Batra, A.; Simon, P.; Lewczuk, P.; Buchkremer, G.; Bartels, M.; Schott, K. Decline of immune responsiveness: A pathogenetic factor in Alzheimer's disease? *J. Psychiatr. Res.* **2005**, *39*, 535–543. [CrossRef]
80. Heneka, M.T.; O'Banion, M.K. Inflammatory processes in Alzheimer's disease. *J. Neuroimmunol.* **2007**, *184*, 69–91. [CrossRef]
81. Arranz, L.; De Castro, N.M.; Baeza, I.; Giménez-Llort, L.; De la Fuente, M. Effect of Environmental Enrichment on the Immunoendocrine Aging of Male and Female Triple-Transgenic 3xTg-AD Mice for Alzheimer's Disease. *J. Alzheimer's Dis.* **2011**, *25*, 727–737. [CrossRef]
82. Giménez-Llort, L.; Maté, I.; Manassra, R.; Vida, C.; De La Fuente, M. Peripheral immune system and neuroimmune communication impairment in a mouse model of Alzheimer's disease. *Ann. N. Y. Acad. Sci.* **2012**, *1262*, 74–84. [CrossRef]
83. Gimenez-Llort, L.; Torres-Lista, V.; Fuente, M. Crosstalk between Behavior and Immune System During the Prodromal Stages of Alzheimer's Disease. *Curr. Pharm. Des.* **2014**, *20*, 4723–4732. [CrossRef]
84. Maté, I.; Cruces, J.; Giménez-Llort, L.; De La Fuente, M. Function and Redox State of Peritoneal Leukocytes as Preclinical and Prodromic Markers in a Longitudinal Study of Triple-Transgenic Mice for Alzheimer's Disease. *J. Alzheimer's Dis.* **2014**, *43*, 213–226. [CrossRef]
85. Ogawa, H. Senile cardiac amyloidosis in senescence accelerated mouse(SAM). *Jpn. Circ. J.* **1988**, *52*, 1377–1383. [CrossRef]
86. De La Fuente, M.; Manassra, R.; Mate, I.; Vida, C.; Hernanz, A.; Giménez-Llort, L. Early oxidation and inflammation state of the immune system in male and female triple transgenic mice for Alzheimer's Disease (3xTgAD). *Free Radic. Biol. Med.* **2012**, *53*, S165. [CrossRef]
87. Marchese, M.; Cowan, D.; Head, E.; Ma, D.; Karimi, K.; Ashthorpe, V.; Kapadia, M.; Zhao, H.; Davis, P.; Sakic, B. Autoimmune Manifestations in the 3xTg-AD Model of Alzheimer's Disease. *J. Alzheimer's Dis.* **2014**, *39*, 191–210. [CrossRef]
88. Yang, S.-H.; Kim, J.; Lee, M.J.; Kim, Y. Abnormalities of plasma cytokines and spleen in senile APP/PS1/Tau transgenic mouse model. *Sci. Rep.* **2015**, *5*, 15703. [CrossRef]
89. Hernanz, A.; Vida, C.; Manassra, R.; Giménez-Llort, L.; De La Fuente, M. P2-063: Early peripheral oxidative stress status in male and female triple-transgenic mice for alzheimer's disease. *Alzheimer's Dement.* **2014**, *10*, P492–P493. [CrossRef]
90. De Toda, I.M.; Vida, C.; Garrido, A.; De La Fuente, M. Redox Parameters as Markers of the Rate of Aging and Predictors of Life Span. *J. Gerontol. Ser. A Boil. Sci. Med. Sci.* **2019**, *75*, 613–620. [CrossRef]

biomedicines

MDPI

Article

Survival Bias and Crosstalk between Chronological and Behavioral Age: Age- and Genotype-Sensitivity Tests Define Behavioral Signatures in Middle-Aged, Old, and Long-Lived Mice with Normal and AD-Associated Aging

Lydia Giménez-Llort [1,2,*,†], Daniela Marin-Pardo [1,2,†], Paula Marazuela [3] and Mar Hernández-Guillamón [3]

1 Institut de Neurociències, Universitat Autònoma de Barcelona, E-08193 Barcelona, Spain; daniela.marin@e-campus.uab.cat

2 Department of Psychiatry and Forensic Medicine, School of Medicine, Universitat Autònoma de Barcelona, E-08193 Barcelona, Spain

3 Vall d'Hebron Research Institute (VHIR), E-08035 Barcelona, Spain; paula.marazuela@vhir.org (P.M.); mar.hernandez.guillamon@vhir.org (M.H.-G.)

* Correspondence: lidia.gimenez@uab.cat; Tel.: +34-93-581-23-78

† First co-authorship.

Citation: Giménez-Llort, L.; Marin-Pardo, D.; Marazuela, P.; Hernández-Guillamón, M. Survival Bias and Crosstalk between Chronological and Behavioral Age: Age- and Genotype-Sensitivity Tests Define Behavioral Signatures in Middle-Aged, Old, and Long-Lived Mice with Normal and AD-Associated Aging. *Biomedicines* **2021**, *9*, 636. https://doi.org/10.3390/biomedicines9060636

Academic Editors: Masaru Tanaka and Nóra Török

Received: 5 May 2021
Accepted: 24 May 2021
Published: 2 June 2021

Abstract: New evidence refers to a high degree of heterogeneity in normal but also Alzheimer's disease (AD) clinical and temporal patterns, increased mortality, and the need to find specific end-of-life prognosticators. This heterogeneity is scarcely explored in very old male AD mice models due to their reduced survival. In the present work, using 915 (432 APP23 and 483 C57BL/6 littermates) mice, we confirmed the better survival curves in male than female APP23 mice and respective wildtypes, providing the chance to characterize behavioral signatures in middle-aged, old, and long-lived male animals. The sensitivity of a battery of seven paradigms for comprehensive screening of motor (activity and gait analysis), neuropsychiatric and cognitive symptoms was analyzed using a cohort of 56 animals, composed of 12-, 18- and 24-month-old male APP23 mice and wildtype littermates. Most variables analyzed detected age-related differences. However, variables related to coping with stress, thigmotaxis, frailty, gait, and poor cognition better discriminated the behavioral phenotype of male APP23 mice through the three old ages compared with controls. Most importantly, non-linear age- and genotype-dependent behavioral signatures were found in long-lived animals, suggesting crosstalk between chronological and biological/behavioral ages useful to study underlying mechanisms and distinct compensations through physiological and AD-associated aging.

Keywords: survival; aging; Alzheimer's disease; heterogeneity; long-life; gait analysis; cognition; BPSD

1. Introduction

Success in aging and increased life expectancy are historical achievements of the last century. However, the fast rate of social aging and age-related chronic diseases urge a bio-psycho-social safety net able to hamper the global burden that it is projected to happen in the next decades [1–3]. In addition, the individual differences in the complex process of aging leads to old age being the most heterogeneous period of life, thus demanding multidisciplinary gerontology and geriatric approaches [4]. Concerning mental health, World Health Organization (WHO)'s last report warns that the prevalence of psychiatric and neurological disorders in older adults, which already account for 6.6% of the total disability-adjusted life years (DALYs), will also increase [5]. Foremost, these disorders are likely to happen in an already complex multimorbid scenario that in most cases will include frailty and age-related medical conditions, strongly affecting the quality of life of old people and their caregivers. In this worrisome forecast, prevalence and correlates of psychiatric disorders among nursing home residents without dementia are the topic of interest of the systematic review and meta-analysis [6].

In this context, the syndromic nature of Alzheimer's disease (AD), the most common neurodegenerative disease representing more than 80% of the cases of dementia worldwide in older people, exemplifies the challenges of such a complex scenario [7]. Thus, besides progressive loss of judgment, memory, and high functions as clinical hallmarks of AD, a wide array of neuropsychiatric symptoms (NPS), also referred to as 'Behavioral and Psychological Symptoms of Dementia (BPSD)' including behavioral and daily life activity impairments, exacerbate the functional impairment of patients and the burden of disease [8,9]. They are present in 90% of patients as the disease progresses, with noteworthy prevalence, such as the 20–80% for agitation; 9–63% for delusion; 11–46% for aggression, 4–41% for hallucinations [10]. BSPD are also considered the core symptoms of different dementia subtypes from early on in the case of dementia, with Lewy bodies or its behavioral variant frontotemporal dementia, and is thus becoming essential for diagnosis [11]. Principal component analysis condensed cognitive/behavioral variables into seven factors, namely: general-cognitive, constructional abilities, hyperactivity, psychosis, anxiety, mood-excitement and mood-depression/apathy, concluding that cognition and other behavioral aspects are independent dimensions [12,13]. Clinical management of BPSD is challenging, requesting the support of non-pharmacological interventions [14,15], mostly in the case of antipsychotics since they have been associated with an increased mortality risk [10,11,15,16] as was also demonstrated in animal models [17]. Due to this complexity and heterogeneity in the human manifestation of AD neuropathology, modeling the whole array of cognitive and behavioral deficits in animal models has been a challenge during the last two decades [18]. At the biological level, the neurobiological basis for the cognitive and behavioral heterogeneity in Alzheimer's disease reflects such a complexity [7]. Thus, besides synaptic dysfunction, beta-amyloid, and tau neuropathological hallmarks of Alzheimer's disease, other key pathological factors such as brain oxidative stress, neuroinflammation, neurovascular dysfunction, and neuroimmunoendocrine crosstalk have been associated with it [19,20].

Recently, new evidence refers to a high degree of heterogeneity in the patterns and temporal progression of clinical symptoms in Alzheimer's disease, indicating several subgroups of patients [21]. At the translational level, this heterogeneity has also been demonstrated in animal models for the disease [22–24]. On the other hand, new perspectives on psychological science also point at emerging data supporting the default-executive coupling hypothesis of aging, where gains on cognitive aging fill the gap that results from a framing effect and focus on losses in cognitive ability as hallmarks of aging [25,26]. In this regard, experimental gerontologists highlight the relevance of using aged animals to mimic the complexity of the physiological and multifactorial pathological aging processes in humans [27,28]. This is most important when studying the age and disease interaction effects in the expression of phenotypic characteristics of late-onset neurodegenerative processes and the screening for drug discovery [18,29]. However, the number of research works using old (+18 months of age) and very old (+21 months of age) or naturally long-lived animals have to overcome the sparsity of studies [30–32], to confront methodological difficulties due to the natural constraints of aged animals [33,34] and severe limitations due to mortality bias [35,36]. Since BPSD are highly prevalent also in old people without dementia [6], translational research using AD-models can also provide the benefit of the observation of the age-matched old wildtype specimens as a source of knowledge of the normal aging process, as is presented here.

Compared with aged control populations, dementia is associated with increased mortality [37,38], and this vulnerability can be enhanced in some AD patients when atypical antipsychotics are used for the management of their BPSD [10,14–16]. In this context, the heterogeneity in the progress of clinical symptoms in the older AD patients is considered a problem for public health planning that urgently needs prognostic indicators specific to this aged population [21,39]. Among them, comorbidity, functional disability, and demographic characteristics such as older age, male gender, and low education are identified as those increasing the risk of death [37,40,41]. Similarly, despite the females of several animal models of AD exhibiting a worse neuropathological status than males [42,43], increased mortality rates in males has been reported in many of them [35,44,45], and is related to an impaired neuroimmunoendocrine system [19,35,46,47]. At the experimental level, this reduced survival in males can result in a mortality bias in studies using old and very old animals (by standard, 18 and 24 months of age, respectively), where male subjects with worse life prognostics cannot be included because they are already dead [22,23,48].

Interestingly, in the APP23 model [49], we have observed that male mice harboring APP23 mutations can reach old and very old ages and can therefore be a useful model to elucidate unbiased age-dependent disease features in the male sex. Therefore, in the present project, we first confirmed long-lived survival curves in male APP23 compared to APP23 females and respective control wildtype (WT) mice that were grown and aged under the same living conditions. Then, three cohorts of 12, 18, and 24 months of age male APP23 mice were successively evaluated in a battery of seven behavioral tests [18] for the comprehensive screening of exploratory activity and gait analysis, cognitive and NPS-like symptoms, as compared to their WT counterparts, the gold-standard C57BL/6 mice strain, with normal aging.

2. Materials and Methods

2.1. Animals

APP23 transgenic male mice (Hemizygote B6, D2-TgN[Thy-APP23]-23-Tg mice, Novartis, Basel, Switzerland) [49] overexpress the mutant human-type APP protein with the Swedish mutation (K670M/N671L) under the control of the murine brain and neuron-specific Thy-1 promoter (thymocyte antigen-1). Hemizygous APP23 mice were backcrossed with the wildtype (WT) C57BL/6 mice (Janvier Labs, Le Genest-Saint-Isle, France), and the APP genotype was tested by Transnetyx (Cordova, TN, USA). The APP23 mice and their wild-type littermates were aged in the Rodent Platform—Lab Animal Service (LAS), the Vall d'Hebron Research Institute animal facility to obtain the final study cohort. Animals were maintained under standard laboratory conditions of food (SAFE A004, Panlab, S.L., Barcelona, Spain) and water ad libitum, 22 ± 2 °C, a 12-h dark/light cycle, 50–60% humidity.

2.2. Experimental Design

The experimental design was defined in three steps. First, survival curves were calculated based on the two colonies of 432 APP23 mice and 483 WT C57BL/6 mice. After that, behavioral assessments were performed in 58 male mice, 29 APP23 mice and their 29 WT C57BL/6 mice littermates. Three sets of animals of 12, 18, and 24 months of age, were transferred to Servei d'Estabulari UAB, Universitat Autònoma de Barcelona, which is located at a distance of 17.4 km from Vall d'Hebron Research Institute (a 15 min ride). All the animals were housed three to four per cage and maintained (Makrolon, 35 × 35 × 25 cm^3) under standard laboratory conditions (12 h light/dark, cycle starting at 8:00 h, food and water available ad libitum, 22 ± 2 °C, 50–60% humidity). One week after arrival, the animals were successively assessed using a battery of seven tests to evaluate four behavioral and functional dimensions: sensorimotor, cognitive, emotional, and daily life activities. All procedures followed Spanish legislation on 'Protection of Animals Used for Experimental and Other Scientific Purposes' and the EU Council directive (2010/63/EU) on this subject. The protocol CEEAH 3588/DMAH 9452 was approved the 8th of March 2019 by Departament de Medi Ambient i Habitatge, Generalitat de Catalunya. The study complies with the ARRIVE guidelines developed by the NC3Rs and aims to reduce the number of animals used [50].

2.3. Behavioral Assessments

Behavioral assessments [18] were performed from 9:00 h to 13:00 h, in a counterbalanced manner and blind to the experiment. Assessments were performed blind to the experiment in a counterbalanced manner. The experimental groups were the following: 12m-WT (n = 10), 12m-APP23 (n = 9), 18m-WT (n = 10), 18m-APP23 (n = 11), 24m-WT (n = 9), and 24m-APP23 (n = 9).

2.3.1. Day 1. Corner and Open-Field Tests (CT and OF)

Animals were individually placed in the center of a clean standard home cage, filled with wood shave bedding. Neophobia was evaluated in the corner test (CT) for 30 s through the number of corners visited (CTc), latency to perform the first rearing (CTlatR), and the number of rearings (CTr). Immediately after, mice were placed in the center of an open-field (OF), beige metal drawer (metalwork, 50 × 40 × 25 cm) and were observed for 5 min. The sequence of behavioral events that define the animal's ethogram was recorded as follows: duration of freezing behavior (LatM, latency to move), latency to leave the central square (LatC) and that of entering the peripheral ring (LatP), as well as latency and total duration of self-grooming behavior (LatG and tG, respectively). Horizontal (crossings of 10 × 10 squares) and vertical (rearings with wall support) locomotor activities were also measured. Bizarre behaviors observed in this test (stereotyped stretching, stereotyped rearing, backward movements, and jumps) were also measured according to previously reported criterion [51]. During the tests, defecation boli and urination were also recorded.

In the present work, we propose gait analysis of locomotion in the open field to measure the number of forward locomotion episodes (walking preceded and followed by a rest) and the number of crossings covered on each, as complementary to measures to horizontal and vertical activity time courses [18] and classical total counts.

2.3.2. Day 2. Recognition Tests (OF2 and OR)

The day after, the animals were retested in the open-field (OF2) to evaluate the behavioral response when they confronted the same anxiogenic environment again. Analysis of activity was done during the first minute of the test, the time period where we have previously described AD-genotype differences [52]. Immediately after, animals were moved to a standard home cage, where they remained for one minute before being reintroduced to the field where two objects were now allocated to administer the novel object recognition test. The animals were assessed (4 h apart) for their ability to recognize a familiar object (S, sample) from a new one (N). Each of these sessions consisted of a "sample trial" followed by a "test trial." In the sample trial, the animals were placed in the open-field (a known environment) and left to explore (nose directed to the object not less than 1 cm) two identical objects, S1 and S2 (glass bottles, 15 × 12 cm, 5 cm diameter), equally spaced in the floor of the apparatus until they reached the criteria of exploration of both for 20 s. The time required to reach the criteria was named "time 1." One minute later, animals were reintroduced in the apparatus for 5 min (test trial) where two different non-explored objects were located: an identical copy of the sample object (S3) and a completely new object (N, rectangular aluminum can, 15 × 10 cm, 4 cm high). Preference for the new object was measured through the index TN−TS/TN+TS where TS and TN are the time spent exploring "S3" and "N," respectively.

2.3.3. Day 3. Spontaneous Alternation in the T-Maze (TM-SA)

On the third day, the black T-shaped maze (woodwork) consisted of two short arms of 25 × 8 cm and a long arm of 30 × 8 cm. The animals were placed inside the long arm of the maze with its head facing the end wall. The latencies of the first movement, start walking, arriving at the intersection of the arms, and completing the exploration of the maze were recorded. Finally, defecation boli and urination were also recorded.

2.3.4. Day 4 to 9. Morris Water Maze Test (MWM)

Mice were trained, four trials per day, spaced 30 min apart, to locate a platform (14 cm diameter) in a circular pool for mice (120 cm diameter, 80 cm height, 25 °C opaque water), and were covered with a completely black curtain. Mice were gently released (facing the wall) from one randomly selected starting cardinal point and allowed to swim until they escaped onto the platform. On the first day, a cue task (CUE, DAY 1) assessed the visual perceptual learning and memory of a visible platform, elevated 1 cm above the water level in the N position and indicated by a visible striped flag (5.3 × 8.3 × 15 cm). Extra maze cues were absent in the black curtain. During the next four consecutive days (PT1-PT4, DAY2-DAY5), the mice searched for a hidden platform that was located in the middle of the S quadrant. White geometric figures hung on each wall of the room were used as external visual clues. In all trials, mice failing to find the platform were placed on it for 10 s, the same period as the successful animals. On the last day, 2 h after the last trial of the place-learning task, a probe trial without the platform was administered during 60 s to assess spatial memory for the previously trained platform location.

In all the learning tasks, the variables of time (escape latency), distance, and speed were also recorded by a computerized tracking system (ANY-Maze v. 5.14, Stoelting, Dublin, Ireland). The number of crossings over the removed platform position (annulus crossings), the time spent, the distance traveled in each quadrant, and the swimming speed were also analyzed.

2.4. Statistics

Statistical analyses were performed using GraphPad Prism 6 and SPSS Statistics 20.0 software. All data are presented as mean ± SEM or percentage. To evaluate the effects of (S) sex, (G) genotype and (A) age factorial analysis design was applied. Differences were studied through multivariate General Lineal Model analysis (mGLM), followed by post-hoc Duncan's test comparisons. Differences between (G) genotype and (A) age × (T) time interval interactions in the different MWM tasks were analyzed by Repeated Measures ANOVA (RMA). Cox regression was used for multivariate analysis of survival. In all cases, statistical significance was considered at $p < 0.05$.

3. Results

3.1. Genotype and Sex-Dependent Increased Mortality Rates

Survival curve (see Figure 1) based on 916 cases and 220 events or natural deaths showed genotype-dependent increased mortality in APP23 mice (G, *** $p < 0.001$), with a severe initial drop of survival, mainly during the first two months of age. Although sex did not influence the risk of mortality in WT littermates, the effect of APP23 genotype in the overall survival was significantly different depending on the sex (S, *** $p < 0.001$). Mortality risk in female APP23 mice was 12.3 times higher than female WT littermates and 2.1 times higher than male littermates with their same AD-genotype. In the case of males, the ratio was 3.6 times higher mortality in the APP23 genotype than male WT littermates.

3.2. Strong Contribution of Age and Specificity of Genotype Factor on Key Variables for AD-Related Phenotype

As summarized in Table 1, the effect of age was shown in most behavioral variables (A, *** $p < 0.001$) while genotype differences mainly were related to horizontal and vertical activities, thigmotaxis, and coping with stress strategies. Overall, T-maze resulted in being the most sensitive test to genotype effects.

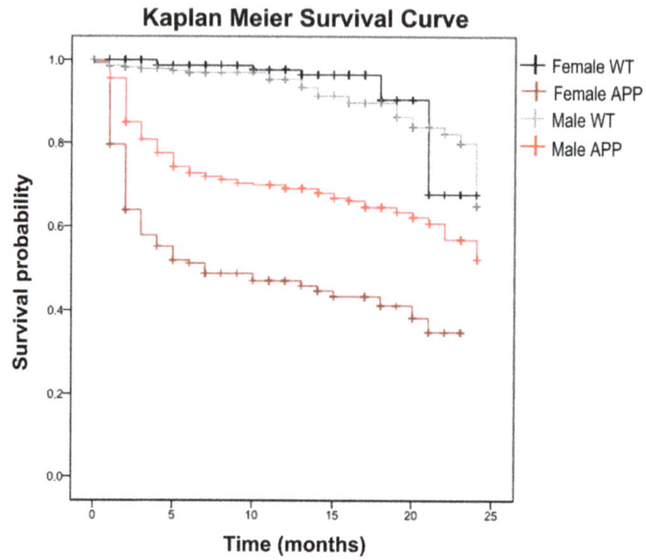

	Male WT	Male APP23	Female WT	Female APP23
N (survival)	294	275	189	157
Mean lifespan, months (95% CI)	22.3 (21.6–22.9)	17.1 (15.9–18.2)	22.4 (21.5–23.2)	11.6 (9.9 –3.1)
Number (%) of mice, dead	29 (9.9%)	95 (34.5%)	10 (5.3%)	86 (54.8%)
Number (%) of mice, censored	265 (90.1%)	180 (65.5%)	179 (94.7%)	71 (45.2%)

Figure 1. Survival—Effect of age and AD-genotype on survival. Data are expressed by mean and 95% CI, or percentage.

Table 1. Genotype and age factors and interaction effects on behavioral tests and variables from middle-age to long-life.

Behavioral Tests and Variables	Statistics	Genotype	Age	G × A	Significance
Corner test					
Total visited corners	F (2,52) = 7.392	-	A ***	-	$p = 0.001$
	F (2,52) = 4.126	G *	-	-	$p = 0.047$
Total numbers of rearings	F (2,52) = 13.374	-	A ***	-	$p = 0.000$
Latency of rearing (s)	F (2,52) = 10.210	-	A ***	-	$p = 0.000$
Open field test					
Freezing—Latency of first movement (s)	F (2,52) = 13.362	-	A ***	-	$p = 0.000$
	F (2,52) = 3.664	-	-	G × A *	$p = 0.032$
Latency to exit the center (s)	F (2,52) = 6.640	-	A **	-	$p = 0.003$
	F (2,52) = 11.169	G **	-	-	$p = 0.002$
Latency of rearing (s)	F (2,52) = 2.905	-	-	G × A (*)	$p = 0.064$
	F (2,52) = 2.649	-	A (*)	-	$p = 0.080$
Latency of self-grooming (s)	F (2,52) = 5.917	G *	-	-	$p = 0.018$
Total horizontal activity (*n* crossings)	F (2,52) = 12.909	-	A ***	-	$p = 0.000$
	F (2,52) = 6.043	G*	-	-	$p = 0.017$
"in the center (*n* crossings)	F (2,52) = 3.044	-	-	G × A (*)	$p = 0.056$
"in the periphery (*n* crossings)	F (2,52) = 11.655	-	A ***	-	$p = 0.000$
	F (2,52) = 9.404	G **	-	-	$p = 0.003$
Total vertical activity (*n* of rearings)	F (2,52) = 18.966	-	A ***	-	$p = 0.000$

Table 1. *Cont.*

Behavioral Tests and Variables	Statistics	Genotype	Age	G × A	Significance
Context and object recognition tests					
Latency to enter into the periphery	F(2,52) = 13.448	-	A ***	-	p = 0.000
Total horizontal activity					
"in the center (n of crossings)	F(2,52) = 3.325	-	A *	-	p = 0.044
"in the periphery (n of crossings)	F(2,52) = 3.339	-	A *	-	p = 0.043
Time exploring new object (s)	F(2,52) = 3.746	-	A *	-	p = 0.030
T-maze					
Latency to cross the intersection (s)	F(2,51) = 27.978	G ***	-	-	p = 0.000
Total time exploring both arms (s)	F(2,51) = 6.005	-	A **	-	p = 0.005
	F(2,51) = 4.107	G *	-	-	p = 0.048
Total time to complete the test (s)	F(2,51) = 19.484	G ***	-	-	p = 0.000
Total number of errors (n)	F(2,51) = 3.139	-	A (*)	-	p = 0.052
Total vertical activity (n of rearings)	F(2,51) = 9.700	G **	-	-	p = 0.003
	F(2,51) = 3.631	-	-	G × A *	p = 0.034

Statistical analysis: Factorial analysis, G, genotype, A, age, * $p < 0.05$, ** $p < 0.01$, *** $p < 0.001$; (*) one-tailed.

In the corner test, the horizontal locomotor activity, as measured by the number of visited corners (Figure 2A), was higher in APP23 mice as compared to WT animals (G*, $p < 0.05$). However, an age effect pointed at 12 and 24 month animals being more active in comparison with those of 18 months of age ($p < 0.05$, in both cases). In the case of vertical activity, the latency to perform the first rearing (Figure 2C) progressively increased with age (A***, $p < 0.001$). Conversely, the total number of rearings (Figure 2B) recorded decreased as well (A***, $p < 0.001$). Both variables indicated that vertical activity dramatically decreased in the 24-month-old APP23 mice compared to the WT littermates (* $p < 0.05$), unveiling a genotype difference at this age.

The ethogram describing the temporal sequence of behavioral events of animals in the open-field test (Figure 2D) showed that the actions exhibited had a strong effect on age, together with genotype or genotype x age interaction effects. That is, the latency of the first movement (OFlatm) and to leave the central area (OFlatc) were strongly dependent on age (A***, $p < 0.001$ and A**, $p < 0.01$, respectively) but also modulated by genotype (OFlatm, A × G*, $p < 0.05$; OFlatc, $p < 0.01$). The performance of the first vertical exploration in the periphery was modulated by age (A*, $p < 0.05$) and age x genotype interaction (A × G*, $p < 0.05$) with shorter latencies in the APP23 mice as compared to WT littermates due to the presence of stereotyped vertical rearing (without wall support). Self-grooming was affected by genotype with shorter latency.

The total activity exhibited in the open field test on Day 1 (Figure 2E–H) indicated that the main effects were attributed to age factor (A***, $p < 0.001$) in both the total horizontal (Figure 2E) and vertical (Figure 2F) activities, with a progressive reduction of both variables with aging. Genotype differences were also found in the horizontal activity exhibited on the first day (Figure 2E, G*, $p < 0.05$), with a higher total number of crossing shown by APP23 mice than WT littermate mice. Statistically significant differences were mainly shown at 12 and 24 months of age, and they were due to the activity performed in the periphery (Figure 2G, G**, $p < 0.05$). At 12 months of age, the genotype-dependent increase of activity was observed in both the periphery and the central area, while at the older ages, the APP23 mice showed lower activity in the center as compared to WT, albeit that these differences did not reach the statistical significance until the second day of the test (see Figure 3B; G*, $p < 0.05$; A*, $p < 0.05$).

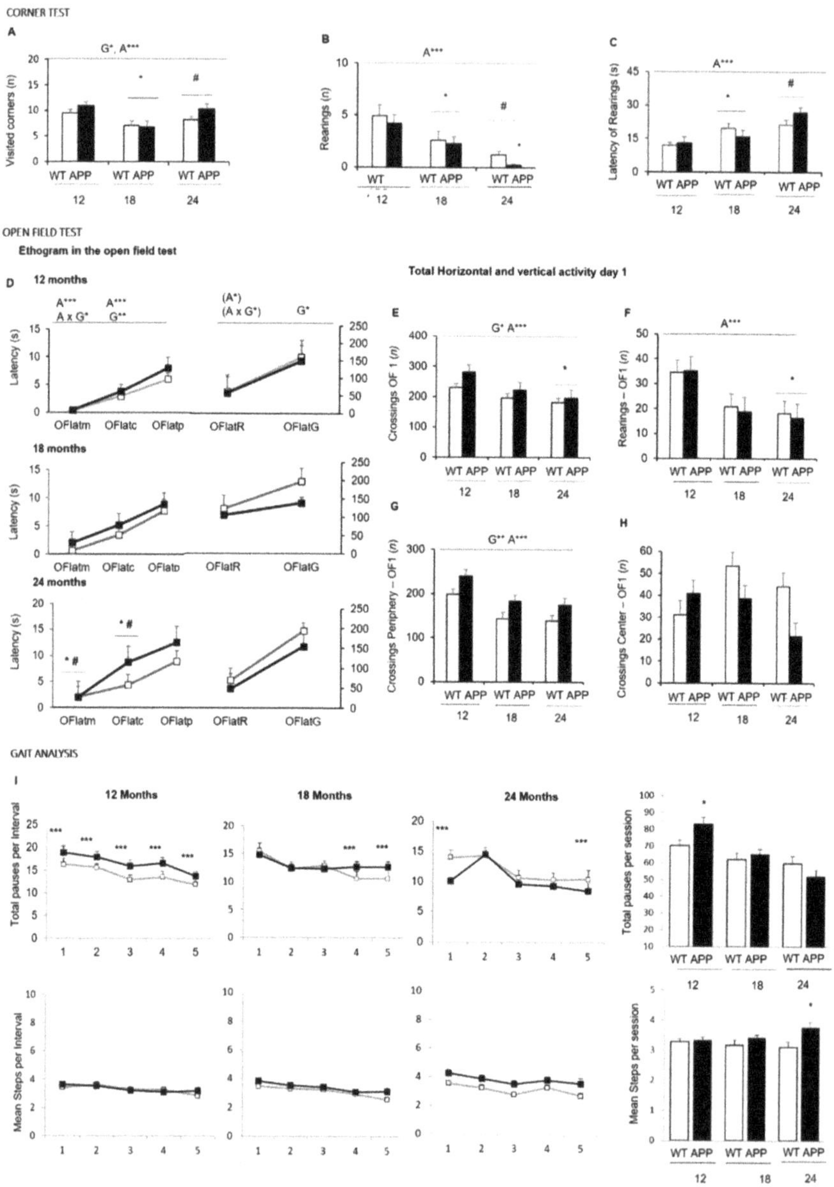

Figure 2. NPS-like behaviors and gait analysis in the corner and open-field test—Effect of age and AD-genotype on the neophobia and exploratory activity elicited in a new home cage (corner test, (**A**–**C**)) and the open-field test (**D**–**I**) at 12, 18, and 24 months of age. Data are expressed by Mean ± SEM. WT: wildtype mice; APP: APP23 mice. Corner test: Visited corners (**A**), number (**B**), and latency of rearings (**C**). Open field test: Ethogram, the temporal sequence of behavioral events in the open field test, Variables: OFlatm, latency of the first movement; OFlatc, latency to leave the central area; OFlatp, latency to enter into the periphery; OFlatR, latency of the first rearing; OFlatG, latencies of the first grooming (**D**). Total horizontal (**E**) and vertical (**F**) activity in the open-field test. Total horizontal activity in the periphery (**G**) and the central area (**H**). Gait analysis: Total number of pauses (**I**) and mean number of crossings in each time interval and in the total time of the open field test. Analysis of variance 2 × 3: Effects of genotype (G), Age (A) * $p < 0.05$, ** $p < 0.01$, *** $p < 0.001$. Post-hoc analysis: * $p < 0.05$ vs. 12 months of age, # $p < 0.05$, vs. 18 months of age; * $p < 0.05$ vs. the corresponding WT control group.

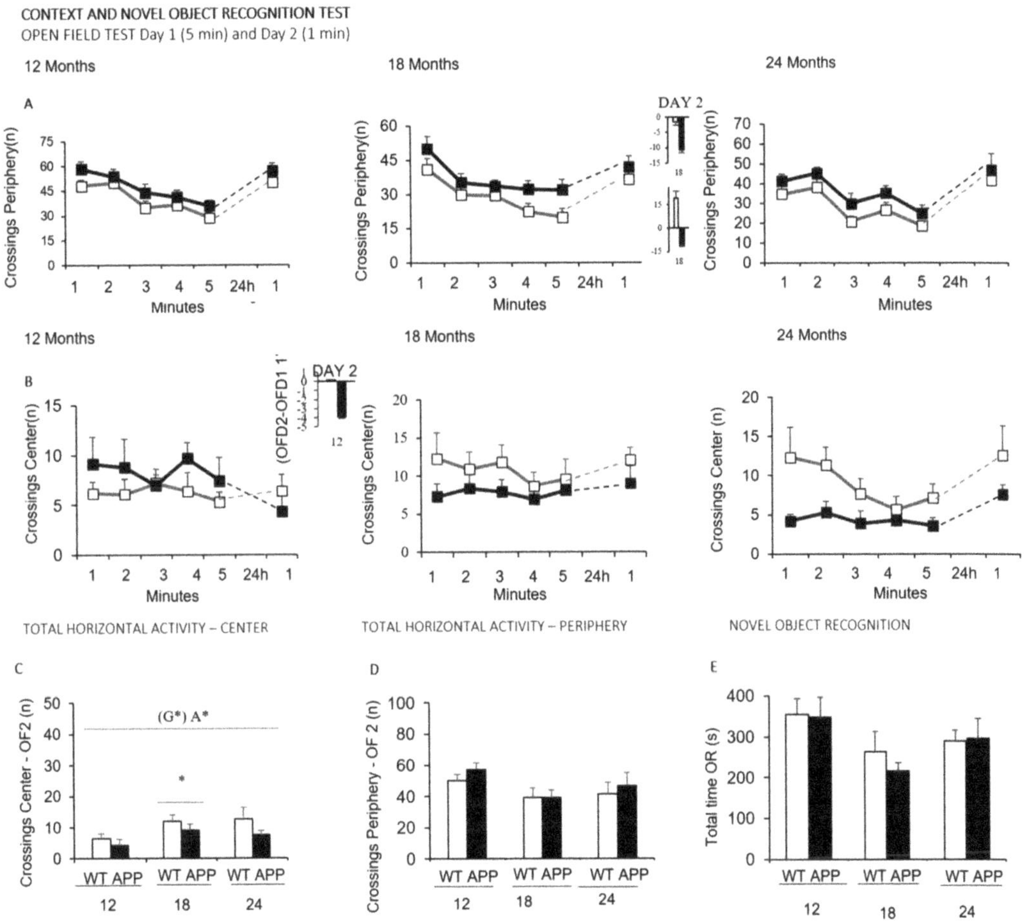

Figure 3. Context and novel object recognition tasks. Data are expressed by mean ± SEM. Time course of the horizontal activity (number of crossings) exhibited in the periphery (**A**) and the center (**B**) of the open-field test on Day 1 and 2, in 12-, 18- and 24-month-old WT (white squares) and APP23 (black squares). (**C**) Total horizontal activity (number of crossings) in the periphery on Day 2, in 12-, 18- and 24-month-old WT (white bars) and APP23 mice (black bars), (**D**) Total horizontal activity (number of crossings) in the center on Day 2, in 12-, 18- and 24-month-old WT (white bars) and APP23 mice (black bars). (**E**) Total time of exploration of the novel object (seconds) in the object recognition test in 12-, 18- and 24-month-old WT (white bars) and APP23 mice (black bars). Analysis of variance 2 × 3: Effects of genotype (G), Age (A), * $p < 0.05$. Post-hoc analysis: * $p < 0.05$ vs. 12 months of age.

The increased horizontal activity of APP23 mice compared to WT was further examined through a gait analysis as illustrated in Figure 2I. The performance also showed genotype effects. Thus, at 12 months of age, the increased total activity of APP23 mice did not result from a walking performance covering a greater number of crossings per unit of movement per se, but due to a higher number of walking episodes per interval of time. The total number of episodes was significantly higher as well (G*, $p < 0.05$). With aging, the number of episodes was reduced. At 24 months of age, the variable that evidenced the genotype effects was the number of crossings covered, which was higher in APP23 than their WT littermate group (* $p < 0.05$).

The two recognition tasks performed during the novel object recognition test administered on Day 2 are illustrated in Figure 3. That is, the horizontal activity exhibited when the animals were re-exposed to the open field test (Figure 3A–D) and the discrimination of a novel object in the novel object recognition test (Figure 3E). As shown, when the animals were introduced in the corner of the periphery, both genotypes performed a similar locomotor activity. However, the comparison with their performances on their first experience in the open field test (18 months of age, OFD2-OFD1, minute 1) as well as the before–after activity levels unveiled genotype differences at 12 (Figure 3A) and 18 (Figure 3B) months of age. In the next part, the novel object recognition test showed a low sensitivity to the genotype, only noticed at the oldest age by a lower difference in the latency to explore the novel and familiar objects than WT littermates.

In the T-maze (Figure 4), at all the ages studied and as compared to WT littermates, the APP23 mice took a longer time to reach the intersection of the vertical arm (not shown) and once there to cross it (Figure 4A, G***, $p < 0.001$). In addition, they also spent more time in both arms (Figure 4B, G*, $p < 0.05$) and required more time to complete the test (Figure 4C, G***, $p < 0.001$). The factor age was also a determinant for the time spent in the arms (Figure 4B, A**, G*, $p < 0.01$). The analysis of errors revisiting the arms that had been already explored indicated a significant age effect (A*, $p < 0.05$) with a decrease at 18 and 24 months of age as compared to 12 months ($p < 0.05$). Furthermore, a decrease in the number of rearings in the APP23 mice, with a genotype x age interaction (G × A*, $p < 0.05$), was found.

To further clarify the results and explain the interrelationships among the various tasks, correlation analyses were performed using data from all the animals in this study (not shown). In the animals' sensorimotor activity measurements, the most prominent correlation was between the open field activity, more specifically on the crossings in the periphery, and the exploration activity obtained in the test corners ($p < 0.005$). Additionally, there was a correlation between the crosses in the periphery of the open field and the exploration time of the arms of the T-maze ($p < 0.005$). On the other hand, a correlation was obtained between the number of corners visited and the amount of exploratory activity performed on the first day of the open field ($p < 0.05$).

Figure 5 illustrates the performance of animals in three paradigms of the Morris water maze, namely, the cue, place task, and probe trial. No differences between groups were found in the first CUE task for visual perceptual learning in any of the variables studied. However, a trial-by-trial analysis of their first performance in the maze showed distinct behaviors depending on the age. Thus, both groups performed equally at 12 months of age and tended to differentiate at 18 months and finally did it at a very old age. After that, genotype x day interactions were found in the mean escape latencies in the place task for spatial reference memory, at the three ages studied (Figure 5A–C: G × D*, all F's [3,45] = 3.30, $p < 0.05$). Thus, the acquisition curves of both genotypes differed through the four days of the test, with a worse performance of APP23 mice as compared to the WT littermates shown as a longer delay to find the platform on the third (PT3, * $p < 0.05$) and fourth (PT4, * $p < 0.05$) day of the test. Genotype differences in swimming speed were shown at 12 months of age (Figure 5G, G**, F [1,15] = 10.79, $p < 0.01$), with a slower pattern in APP23 mice. Therefore, distances covered to reach the platform were also calculated (Figure 5D) but showed a smother distinction in the temporal course between genotypes. At older ages, both groups of mice slowed their navigation speeds, and genotype differences were lost (Figure 5H,I). Statistically significant differences observed in escape latency translated into the variable of distance only at 24 months of age (Figure 5F, PT4, * $p < 0.05$). In the probe trial (Figure 5J–L), independent of genotype, preference for the target vs. opposed quadrant was only shown at 12 and 24 months of age, while in the 18-month-old groups, the time of permanence was biased to the adjacent left quadrant. Surprisingly, the preference of 24-month-old APP23 mice for the target quadrant was significantly higher than their WT littermate counterparts (Figure 5L, * $p < 0.05$).

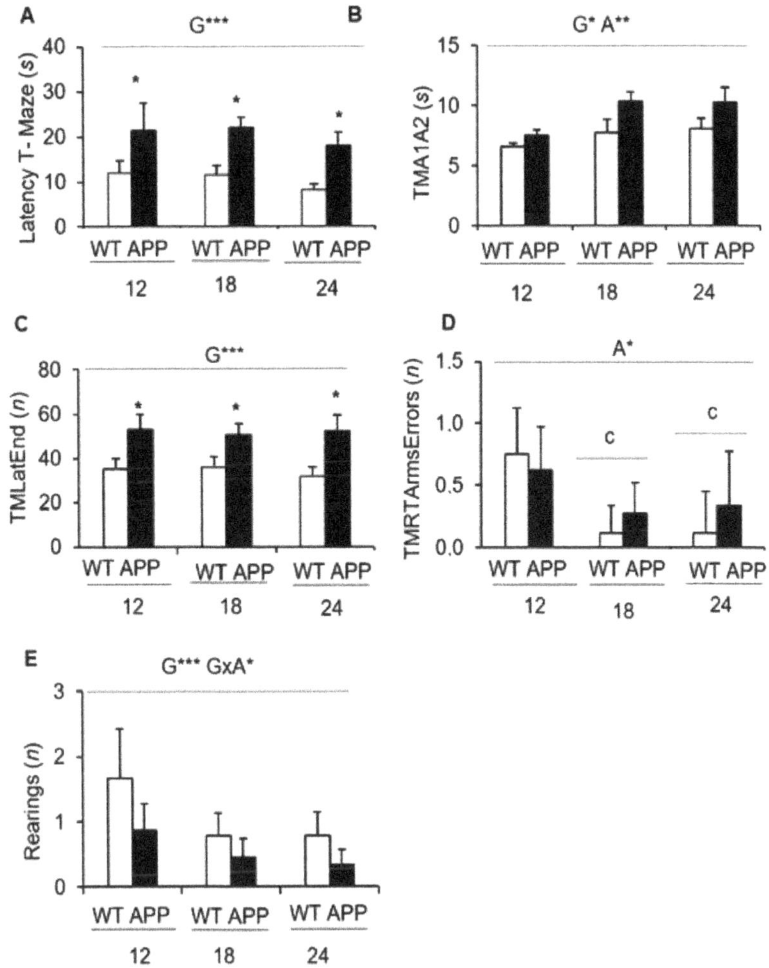

Figure 4. Coping with stress strategies, risk assessment, and spontaneous alternation in the T-Maze. (**A**) Latency to cross the intersection; (**B**) Total time invested in the exploration of the left and right arms; (**C**), Time to complete the exploration of the maze; (**D**), Total number of errors performed during the exploration of the maze; (**E**) Vertical exploratory activity. Data are expressed by means ± SEM. WT: wildtype mice; APP: APP23 mice. Analysis of variance 2 × 2: Effects of genotype (G), age (A), genotype × age (G × A), * $p < 0.05$, ** $p < 0.01$, *** $p < 0.001$. Post-hoc analysis: ^{c} $p < 0.05$ vs. 12 months of age; * $p < 0.05$ vs. the corresponding WT control group.

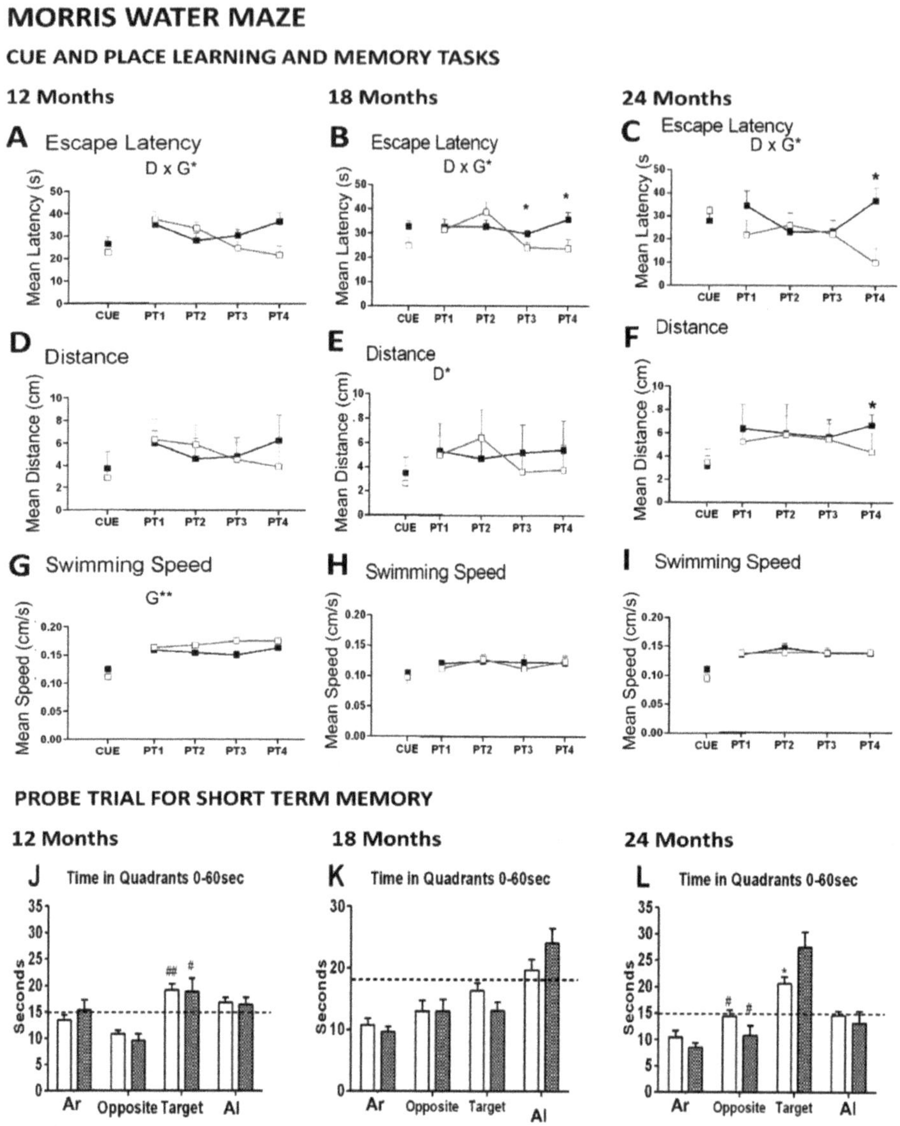

Figure 5. Quantitative analysis of the performance of wildtype (WT) and APP23 mice at 12, 18, and 24 months of age in three paradigms of the MWM. Data are expressed by means ± SEM. Day-by-day quantitative analysis of the CUE and PT place leaning task by means of (**A–C**) mean escape latency, (**D–F**) distance and (**G–I**) swimming speed. Open squares or bars: WT mice; Solid squares or bars: APP23 mice. ANOVA, D, day factor; G, genotype factor, Post-hoc Student *t*-test; * $p < 0.05$, ** $p < 0.01$ vs. the corresponding control group. (**J–L**) Probe trial for short term memory assessed by means of the time in each quadrant; adjacent right (Ar), Opposite, Target and adjacent left (Al) quadrants. Statistics: Student *t*-test; * $p < 0.05$ vs. the corresponding control group. Target vs. opposite vs. # $p < 0.05$, ## $p < 0.01$.

4. Discussion

In the present work, we determined the age and AD-genotype sensitivity of a battery of behavioral tests in APP23 mice of male sex at middle (12 months), old (18 months), and very old (24 months) ages, and compared them to age-matched C57BL/6 mice with normal aging. First, we confirmed that survival curves of APP23 mice were those suitable to assess long-lived animals, since the scarcity of the literature comparing male animals from middle to very old ages is due to increased mortality risk in this sex, increased heterogeneity in the aging process, and also in AD at end-of-life dementia stages.

Genetically engineered AD models, primarily based on the overexpression of presinilin1 or APP mutant human genes causing early-onset Familial AD (FAD), are used to study hallmark behavioral and neuropathological mechanisms of SAD, the sporadic and most common form of Alzheimer's disease despite some gaps [53,54]. For instance, the APP23 mice, overexpressing the mutant human-type APP protein with the Swedish mutation (K670M/N671L), is a widely used animal model of AD since it genetically develops amyloidosis and presents cognitive and behavioral symptoms similar to those found in patients [55]. However, both SAD and FAD models are limited by the difficulty to fully recapitulate the complexity and progression of this neurodegenerative disease in humans [18,30,54]. Most importantly, this consideration also refers to the challenge to unveil the factors that may underlie the heterogeneity described at end-of-life dementia and the individuals' survival. The neuro-immuno-endocrine hypothesis could explain the morbidity–mortality paradox among sexes that also accounts for AD [56–58], and we have already described it in mice [19,35,46]. However, more recently, distinct genotype and sex differences in life expectancy among different mouse models of AD and inbred strains have been reported in comprehensive reviews [44,45].

Survival—The survival analysis was based on a total of 916 cases from our APP23 and wildtype cohorts with the same gold-standard C57BL/6 genetic background. It showed genotype and sex-dependent increased mortality rates in the mutant mice, with a severe initial drop of survival during the first two months of age, which was more dramatic in APP23 females. Interestingly, APP/PS1 males also exhibit longer lifespans than females [59]. Survival curves demonstrated that APP23 males were able to reach a long life span, rending this animal model suitable for studying the impact of the disease in a male aging scenario. That is, 12- 18- and 24-month-old subjects would serve to study the disease at the middle, old, and very old ages, respectively, and as compared to age-matched C57BL/6 wildtype mice. There is a chance that it is strongly restricted in other genetically engineered AD models where mortality rates of males are a limiting point to address advanced aging in AD [17,22]. As mentioned before, the study of the age-matched wildtype mice also contributed to provide data to the scarcely reported normal aging process in the gold-standard C57BL/6 mice strain, from middle, old, and very-old ages.

Factorial effects and battery of tests—In this research, the behavioral profiles of APP23 and WT mice with normal aging were evaluated through a battery of seven tests. Namely, the corner test, open field test, the novel object recognition test, the T-maze, and three paradigms in the Morris water maze determine the effects of genotype and aging process on their motor, emotional, and cognitive functions. On a general basis, aging was shown as the most determinant factor for most behavioral variables studied, achieving the strongest statistically significant values, whereas genotype factor was specific of those variables related to dysfunctional impairment in AD. This is in agreement with previous results reported by our laboratory using another animal model of AD. There, the age factor from adulthood to maturity (7 to 11 months of age) was also a determinant for variables related to sensory and motor function, while genotype differences specifically pointed at cognitive and BPSD-hallmarks of disease [51]. After the mean life span, the factor of age was shadowing the genetic differences, and a mortality bias was also noted [17,22]. In the present work, the great majority of the variables that were found to be age-sensitive belong to the corner test and the open field, in agreement with the worsening of fear and anxiety-like symptoms with the progress of the disease. Here, genotype differences selectively pointed at hyperactive horizontal activity patterns, in decrement of vertical exploration, resembling those described in 3xTg-AD mice [18].

Corner and open-field tests—Fear and anxiety-like behaviors are the most common neuropsychiatric-like alterations associated with dementia that can be studied in mice models of AD [18] since they appear in their early stages, worsen with the progress of the disease, and most standard behavioral tests can record their presence [60]. Therefore, the battery of tests started with the corner and open-field tests to record the quantitative and qualitative features of these behaviors elicited in these two anxiogenic enclosures. When the APP23 mice were introduced in a new home cage of transference to the open field, the mild neophobia recorded was increased compared to that exhibited by WT littermates and worsened with age. Thus, the mutant mice performed a greater number of visited corners, and the reduction of vertical activity at 24 months of age was more severe, unveiling genotype differences in this variable.

This response was in agreement with the subsequent behavioral sequence of events observed in the open-field, illustrated as an ethogram likeminded with the sequence of 'action programs' described by Lát in 1973 [61]. The APP23 animals showed increased latencies to develop the ethogram immediately after direct exposure to the open and illuminated arena. They differed in the momentary freezing, with a longer fear response when confronting the new environment. Furthermore, they differed in the flight-to-fight copying with a stress strategy developed that elicited the early presence of bizarre vertical behaviors (stereotyped rearing without walk support, as described in [51] and anticipatory self-grooming indicative of increased anxiety [18]). With aging, the overall activity and the thigmotaxis behavior showed a reduction in all the groups. This effect was more notorious in the mutant mice. Thus, while 12-month-old APP23 mice were more active than their WT littermates in all (the central and peripheral) areas of the field, the activity of 18- and 24-month-old APP23 mice was strongly reduced in the center, indicating a worsening of anxiety in the elder ages/stages of the disease. In contrast, the increased allocentric exploration close to the protected areas of the mutants was persistent from middle-age until the oldest age. Age and genotype differences were lost the next day, as assessed in the open-field retest. When confronting the open field for the first time, the hyperactive pattern shown is consistent with previous studies describing hyperactivity in APP23 mice when assessed in this test and a Y-labyrinth [62]. However, other laboratories have reported a hypoactive pattern in this animal model [63]. The discrepancies may correspond to the specific anxiogenic conditions elicited by the tests, similarly to hyperactivity of 3xTg-AD mice when assessed under soft light conditions in activity cages. In contrast, they exhibited a clear anxiogenic hypoactive pattern in the open and illuminated open field, the dark lightbox, and the elevated T-maze [17,18].

Gait analysis of locomotor activity—The quantitative and qualitative assessment of locomotion, with distinction of inactivity, and slow and fast movements, allows discriminating patterns of hyperactivity [64]. Here, based on that, the analysis of locomotion measured the walking speed (crossings per interval of time) and its time course through the 5 min of the test [18] and contrasted is to the classical total counts. For the first time, in the present work, we propose measuring two more features of ambulation: the pace (mean distance covered in each walk) and the number of walking episodes. These variables allowed distinguishing the locomotor performance of APP23 mice from the normal gait phenotype of their WT littermate counterparts. Thus, the mean walking distance of a pace during the different minutes of the open-field test was about three–four crossings. This agrees with the number of crossings the animal needs to cover to move from one corner to the closest one, or to cross the arena without reaching the center. Here, all through the test, 24-months-old APP23 performed longer walking distances than their age-matched counterparts and the other groups, probably due to their lower activity in the center. It is important to note that the increased total activity of APP23 mice at 12 and 18 months of age did not result from a walking performance covering a greater number of crossings per pace, but due to a higher number of paces, walking episodes per interval of time.

On the other hand, in the three mutant groups, the total paces per interval of time were also increased at several time points of their temporal courses, and the value trend decreased with age. This variable related to kinetics was more sensitive to discriminate mutants at 12 months of age from their age-matched counterparts. The homologous, the swimming speed in the Morris water maze, also allowed unveiling genotype differences at 12 months of age, though in that case, APP23 mice were swimming slower than controls. Interestingly, longitudinal population-based studies have shown a decline in spontaneous or so-called preferred walking speed (PWS) in older people associated with brain structural changes in gray and white matter volumes [65]. At the clinical level, a slower fast-walking speed (FWS) is used as a marker of frailty and mortality [66–69]. Besides, the slowest PWS and FWS, and a smaller walking speed reserve (the difference between both) have been associated with poorer cognitive stage [70]. Furthermore, recently, an international cross-sectional gait and Alzheimer interaction tracking study has consistently described an abnormal gait phenotype since the earliest stages of dementia [71]. The Spatio-temporal gait parameters are worse in woman patients and at advanced/severe stages of dementia, although they seem more relevant to non-amnestic forms of cognitive impairment and non-AD dementias [70].

Cognitive function: Habituation and Recognition tests—In the present work, the hyperactivity pattern of APP23 was consistently apparent from middle to very old ages. Hyperactivity can reflect an altered ability to habituate [72], as shown in the psychostimulant effects of caffeine [73] and A_1R knockout mutant mice [74]. In fact, habituation is considered as a form of rudimentary learning and memory process for recent events [61], and where an animal learns to ignore stimulus with no predictive value [74]. Several other aspects of the cognitive profile were analyzed during the following days through different paradigms.

First, we wanted to assess the cognitive function involved in other recognition tasks. As we have previously shown, the performance of young and adult 3xTg-AD animals in the first minute of a repeated open-field test is sensitive to AD-genotype [52]. In fact, the re-exposure to a fearful environment is the basis of many conditioned memory tests (i.e., [75]). Therefore, on the second day of tests, we assessed the recognition of the open and illuminated field and, after that, the preference for a novel object from one previously inspected was recognized as familiar. The performance on the first minute of the open field repeated test closely resembled the neophobia response previously shown by the same animals in the corner test. Animals maintained their locomotor activity in the periphery and slightly increased the one performed in the center. Overall, that resulted in the loss of genotype differences previously found on the first exposure to the open field. Concerning the novel object recognition test per se, no significant differences were detected between any of the groups as well. The most found was a genotype difference in 24-months-old APP23 mice, with worse latency to explore the novel object than the familiar, but this was due to a better performance in the WT mice. The lack of AD sensitivity of these recognition tasks regarding their use to assess learning and memory could be related to the animal's anxiety-like phenotype and/or a reduced interest for exploration, the two main potential confounds that can bias the animal's cognitive performance. This would agree with the genotype and age-dependent reduction of vertical exploratory activity already shown on the first experience in the open field test and the hyperactive horizontal locomotor pattern.

T-maze—Whereas the open field allowed us to observe significant differences associated with age, and to a lesser degree with the genotype, the assessment of animals in the T-maze provided the most AD-sensitive variables. This T-shaped labyrinth is a scenario mainly used to evaluate spatial working memory [76] with the involvement of the hippocampus, septum, prefrontal cortex, and the basal forebrain [77–79]. In addition, the latency to reach the intersection of the maze differs according to coping-with-stress strategies expressed by the animal. This is to the extent that this variable was used for psychological selection of prematurely accelerated aging mice (PAM) and non-PAM mice after demonstrating that it correlates with a worse neuro-immunoendocrine function, indicators of accelerated aging, and premature death [80]. We have also extensively shown that the spontaneous alternation in the black corridors resembling burrows is able to unveil the nuances of cognitive function and anxious-like profiles in both male and female mice, from young to old age under healthy and diverse neuropathological conditions [81–83]. More recently, some authors have dissected other cognitive aspects [84].

Since the beginning of the test, the ethogram or sequence of behavioral events exhibited by APP23 mice in this maze was strongly affected by genotype. Thus, from a 'facing the wall' starting position, the latencies to turn, reach the T-intersection, and cross it with the four paws were significantly delayed in the mutants. The mean time to explore the two arms was increased with age and the AD-genotype. However, this delay was not due to time invested in the vertical exploratory activity, as it was poor and worse with the AD-genotype already since middle age. As a result, APP23 mice took a longer to complete the test as compared to their age-matched wildtype mice, a variable that exhibited a clear and robust genotype effect too. The contribution of errors re-entering an already visited arm was also scarce, with 18- and 24-months-old groups performing slightly better than middle-aged groups. At these ages, there was a trend of worse performance in APP23 mice. In other AD models, such as the 3xTg-AD mice, no differences in the number of execution errors were also found at middle age, but the efficiency to complete the different phases of the test is diminished in 3xTg-AD mice and slightly is affected by long-term treatment with the antipsychotic risperidone [17].

The present results define an altered ethogram in the T-maze and point at the delay to cross the intersection as the most AD-sensitive variable. This variable suggests a worse decision-making process, mainly depending on the prefrontal cortex, which could result from this model's extensive cortical neuropathology. Compared, the delays in the performance of the 3xTg-AD mice are also found to turn and reach the intersection of the T-maze, but once there, the delay in crossing is not so enhanced, as shown here for the APP23 mice. However, a similar delay suggesting chances in risk assessment is seen in this model when the spontaneous choice of entering an anxiogenic white and lit enclosure is assessed in the dark–light box [18,48,60]. Interestingly, that variable was improved by early postnatal handling, an early life intervention based on a tactile sensorial stimulation experience known to modulate cognitive and anxiety-like behaviors in rodents [51]. The APP/PS1 [85] and Tg2576 [86] mice, as well as selective dopaminergic receptors, cause a blockade in the pre-limbic region of the prefrontal cortex [86] or STOP-null mice modeling schizophrenia [87], also show a reduction of spontaneous alternation, suggesting its relation to frontal hypofunctionality. In the present work, the correlation analysis of the variables of T-maze with other tests indicated that the performance in the maze was strongly related to the variables of the other tests referring to increased emotivity/anxiety (self-grooming, navigation speeds) and apathy (latency of vertical and object exploration).

Cognitive function: Morris water maze—Finally, in the Morris Water maze, short- and long-term spatial reference learning and memory were assessed [88]. The performances of animals in two learning and memory tasks administered during five consecutive days were evaluated through the classical mean escape latency and the distance covered to reach the platform since a genotype effect was found in the swimming speed at 12 months of age. All animals performed equally in the cued learning, an easy task that assesses visual perceptual learning. Still, it is interesting to note that the performance in their first experience in the maze differed with aging, as very old APP23 confronted the stressful situation of being immersed in a water tank with faster latencies and shorter distances than their WT littermate counterparts. As mentioned before, the navigation was slower in APP23 at middle age but not after that. Here, the impact of aging could explain that the swimming speed be reduced in old and very old animals as compared to the younger groups. If so, the slow swimming speeds of middle-aged APP23 mice compared to their WT littermate group but similar to the speed shown at 18 and 24 months of age, would suggest that they were performing as older than expected for their chronological age. Although the anxious profile of 3xTg-AD mice explains their faster swimming speeds from early stages of the disease [89], we have previously shown a similar situation regarding AD-behavioral performances being similar to those corresponding to WT at older ages, both at the biological [90] and behavioral level [19]. In contrast, the genotype differences become strikingly smoother in long-term AD mice survivors due to a mortality bias (death of the worse animals) on one hand and age-dependent impoverished performances in the WT groups on the other [22]. Here, the performances of 24-month-old animals were not as bad as could be expected in a progression from 18 months of age, whereas cognitive impairment was a salient behavior and followed the expected deterioration.

After the removal of the platform, the performance of animals did not indicate differences in short-term memory per se. This lack of genotype differences in the probe trial two hours after the last trial of the place task was surprising as expected from the worse performance of mutants in the last or two last days of this task that involves the contribution of long-term but also short-term learning and memory. However, it is noteworthy to mention that the lack of sensitivity of probe trial to the genotype in APP23 mice is in agreement with previous results reported by other laboratory experts in this animal model [55,91]. On the other hand, we have recently demonstrated a mortality bias, with animals that died during the behavioral assessments or those with worse life prognostics who had been excluded from the final analysis, explaining the lack of expected results in 16-month-old 3xTg-AD males [17]. However, cognitive deficits in the Morris water maze were the salient behavior in 18-month-old survivor females despite a flat phenotype, not distinguishable from their control strain [22]. Here, the distinct preferences for the adjacent areas indicate, for instance, less-focused goal-directed swimming strategies at 18 months of age [91]. This suggests that a swimming strategy analysis would further understand the compensatory behavioral mechanism that resulted in such a paradox probe trial report [91].

Limitations—The main limitation of the present study is intrinsic to the heterogeneity of the aging process and the extreme difficulties to obtain the desired sample size of old and very old animals, not only of mutants with such high mortality rates, but also of their wildtype littermates with normal aging. In order to counteract the age-related heterogeneity, important efforts were needed to obtain concurrent middle-aged (12-month-old), aged (18-month-old) and very old (24-month-old) animals with the APP23 and WT genotypes, so they shared the same living conditions; moreover, to adapt research agendas so that the cohorts could be assessed within a narrow frame of time in the calendar. On the other hand, as discussed, the use of a battery of tests must assume that carry-over effects cannot be discarded, despite the benefits that assessing the same construct (i.e., anxiety) in tests differing in the level of anxiogenic conditions has to ensure convergent validity of results. These efforts resulted in a low intra- and inter-group variability, and we have reproduced the findings in subsequent experimental research in a consistent manner. However, interlaboratory reliability would be needed to confirm that the results obtained in our colonies can be reproduced in the colonies of other research institutions. An important limitation would refer to gender medicine demands for the concurrent comparative study of males and females, so future efforts should be devoted to achieve this goal despite the difficulty that it may represent when handling very old ages and survivors.

5. Conclusions and Future Directions

In the present work, the behavioral profiles at 12, 18, and 24 months of age of male APP23 mice and non-transgenic (WT C57BL/6) littermate counterparts with normal aging were assessed using three independent cohorts but in a narrow temporal frame in the calendar. Animals were successively evaluated in a battery of seven behavioral tests to screen motor, non-cognitive and cognitive-like symptoms comprehensively. Presence of 'Behavioral and Psychological Symptoms of Dementia' (BPSD)–like behaviors in APP23 mice was confirmed in three classical unconditioned tests evaluating locomotion, exploration, anxiety-like behaviors, and emotionality under three different anxiogenic conditions.

The main findings can be summarized in five points as follows:

(1). Survival curves of 920 mice of APP23 and WT C57BL/6 littermates confirmed genotype and sex-dependent increased mortality rates, and long-living males.
(2). Compared to WT littermates, the APP23 mice showed an increased number of visited corners but decreased vertical exploratory activity, evidencing increased neophobia in the corner test. Similarly, APP23 groups showed increased latencies to develop the ethogram of behaviors immediately after the direct exposure to an open and illuminated field (not shown) and increased locomotion, with increased thigmotaxis (or search for the protected peripheral area), primarily noticeable at 12 months of age.
(3). In the T-maze, a black T-shaped corridor resembling burrows, the latency to reach the intersection was consistently shown to be increased at all ages and the longer time required for APP23 mice to complete the exploration of all the arms of the maze. As part of the differences in the status of their cognitive functions exhibited during the exploration of new environments, we assessed APP23 mice for putative cognitive deficits in discriminative tasks (novelty/familiarity) for context (remembering the anxiogenic open field scenario) and object recognition.
(4). The novel object recognition test showed low sensitivity to the genotype, only noticed at the oldest age through the lowest difference in the delay in exploring the novel and familiar objects compared to WT littermates.
(5). Cognitive deficits in Spatial reference learning and memory were assessed in the Morris water maze through a 4-day place learning task using a hidden platform followed by a probe trial for long-term memory where the platform had been removed. Worse performance of 12-month-old APP23 mice was shown as compared to WT littermates during the progress of acquisition (learning and memory) in the place task, while differences were scarce in the older groups. In the probe trial, the worse spatial memory discrimination of the trained quadrant compared to the opposed quadrant was shown at 18 months of age but independently of the genotype. As we have reported in other mice models for AD, a conspicuous BPSD-like profile and age as a biological factor may result in confounding factors in an aquatic maze, considered an anxiogenic environment for mice.

In summary, most of the variables analyzed were able to show age-related differences, and those presented here are among those that, under our experimental conditions and in our hands, better discriminate the behavioral phenotype of female APP23 mice through their aging process, from middle-age (12 months of age) and old (18 months of age) to very old (24 months of age), as compared to their respective WT littermates. Most importantly, non-linear age- and genotype-dependent behavioral signatures were found in 24-month-old mice, suggesting the existence of a crosstalk between chronological and biological/behavioral ages in long-lived animals useful to study underlying mechanisms and distinct compensations through natural physiological aging and, maybe also, long-term AD-associated aging male survivors.

Author Contributions: Conceptualization, L.G.-L.; colony and survival curves, P.M.; behavioral performance and data, L.G.-L.; behavioral and statistical analysis, D.M.-P.; writing—original draft: L.G.-L.; scientific discussion and review of the manuscript: all the authors. Project and funding acquisition, M.H.-G. All authors have read and agreed to the published version of the manuscript.

Funding: This work was funded by the BrightFocus Foundation, US (A2017243S). The Neurovascular Research Laboratory is part of the INVICTUS+network, Instituto de Salud Carlos III (ISCIII), Spain [RD16/0019/0021], co-financed by the European Regional Development Fund FEDER. P.M. held a predoctoral fellowship from the Vall d'Hebron Research Institute.

Institutional Review Board Statement: The study was conducted according to the guidelines of the Declaration of Helsinki, and approved by the Ethics Committee of Departament de Medi Ambient i Habitatge, Generalitat de Catalunya (CEEAH 3588/DMAH 9452) the 8 March 2019.

Informed Consent Statement: Not applicable.

Data Availability Statement: The data presented in this study are available on request from the corresponding author.

Acknowledgments: Acknowledgement is made to the donors of Alzheimer's Disease Research, a program of BrightFocus Foundation, for support of this research.

Conflicts of Interest: The authors declare no conflict of interest. The funders had no role in the design of the study; in the collection, analyses, or interpretation of data; in the writing of the manuscript, or in the decision to publish the results.

References

1. Brookmeyer, R.; Johnson, E.; Ziegler-Graham, K.; Arrighi, H.M. Forecasting the global burden of Alzheimer's disease. *Alzheimer's Dement.* **2007**, *3*, 186–191. [CrossRef] [PubMed]
2. Jin, K.; Simpkins, J.W.; Ji, X.; Leis, M.; Stambler, I. The Critical Need to Promote Research of Aging and Aging-related Diseases to Improve Health and Longevity of the Elderly Population. *Aging Dis.* **2015**, *6*, 1–5. [CrossRef] [PubMed]
3. World Health Organization (WHO); United Nations (UN). *Population Prospects: The 2017 Revision, Key Findings and Advance Tables;* Working Paper No. ESA/P/WP/248; United Nations Department of Economic and Social Affairs/Population Division: Nairobi, Kenya, 2017.
4. Arai, H.; Ouchi, Y.; Yokode, M.; Ito, H.; Uematsu, H.; Eto, F.; Oshima, S.; Ota, K.; Saito, Y.; Sasaki, H.; et al. Toward the realization of a better aged society: Messages from gerontology and geriatrics. *Geriatr. Gerontol. Int.* **2011**, *12*, 16–22. [CrossRef] [PubMed]
5. WHO. Mental Health of Older Adults 2016. Available online: https://www.who.int/news-room/fact-sheets/detail/mental-health-of-older-adults (accessed on 27 December 2020).
6. Fornaro, M.; Solmi, M.; Stubbs, B.; Veronese, N.; Monaco, F.; Novello, S.; Fusco, A.; Anastasia, A.; De Berardis, D.; Carvalho, A.F.; et al. Prevalence and correlates of major depressive disorder, bipolar disorder and schizophrenia among nursing home residents without dementia: Systematic review and meta-analysis. *Br. J. Psychiatry* **2019**, *216*, 6–15. [CrossRef] [PubMed]
7. Cummings, J.L. Cognitive and behavioral heterogeneity in Alzheimer's disease: Seeking the neurobiological basis. *Neurobiol. Aging* **2000**, *21*, 845–861. [CrossRef]
8. Reisberg, B.; Ferris, S.H.; Franssen, E.H.; Shulman, E.; Monteiro, I.; Sclan, S.G.; Steinberg, G.; Kluger, A.; Torossian, C.; De Leon, M.J.; et al. Mortality and Temporal Course of Probable Alzheimer's Disease: A 5-Year Prospective Study. *Int. Psychogeriatr.* **1996**, *8*, 291–311. [CrossRef] [PubMed]
9. Kumar, A.; Singh, A. Ekavali A review on Alzheimer's disease pathophysiology and its management: An update. *Pharmacol. Rep.* **2015**, *67*, 195–203. [CrossRef]
10. Jeste, D.V.; Blazer, D.; Casey, D.; Meeks, T.; Salzman, C.; Schneider, L.; Tariot, P.; Yaffe, K. ACNP White Paper: Update on Use of Antipsychotic Drugs in Elderly Persons with Dementia. *Neuropsychopharmacology* **2007**, *33*, 957–970. [CrossRef]
11. Magierski, R.; Sobow, T.; Schwertner, E.; Religa, D. Pharmacotherapy of Behavioral and Psychological Symptoms of Dementia: State of the Art and Future Progress. *Front. Pharmacol.* **2020**, *11*, 1168. [CrossRef]
12. Mirakhur, A.; Craig, D.; Hart, D.J.; Mcllroy, S.P.; Passmore, A.P. Behavioural and psychological syndromes in Alzheimer's disease. *Int. J. Geriatr. Psychiatry* **2004**, *19*, 1035–1039. [CrossRef]
13. Spalletta, G.; Baldinetti, F.; Buccione, I.; Fadda, L.; Perri, R.; Scalmana, S.; Serra, L.; Caltagirone, C. Cognition and behaviour are independent and heterogeneous dimensions in Alzheimer?s disease. *J. Neurol.* **2004**, *251*, 688–695. [CrossRef] [PubMed]
14. Giménez-Llort, L.; Johansson, B. Editorial: Pharmacology of BPSD (Behavioral and Psychological Symptoms of Dementia). *Front. Pharmacol. Neuropharmacol.* **2021**. [CrossRef]
15. Yunusa, I.; El Helou, M.L. The Use of Risperidone in Behavioral and Psychological Symptoms of Dementia: A Review of Pharmacology, Clinical Evidence, Regulatory Approvals, and Off-Label Use. *Front. Pharmacol.* **2020**, *11*, 596. [CrossRef] [PubMed]
16. Piersanti, M.; Capannolo, M.; Turchetti, M.; Serroni, N.; De Berardis, D.; Evangelista, P.; Costantini, P.; Orsini, A.; Rossi, A.; Maggio, R. Increase in mortality rate in patients with dementia treated with atypical antipsychotics: A cohort study in outpatients in Central Italy. *Riv Psichiatr.* **2014**, *49*, 34–40. [PubMed]
17. Torres-Lista, V.; López-Pousa, S.; Giménez-Llort, L. Impact of Chronic Risperidone Use on Behavior and Survival of 3xTg-AD Mice Model of Alzheimer's Disease and Mice With Normal Aging. *Front. Pharmacol.* **2019**, *10*, 1061. [CrossRef] [PubMed]
18. Giménez-Llort, L.; Blázquez, G.; Cañete, T.; Johansson, B.; Oddo, S.; Tobeña, A.; LaFerla, F.; Fernandez-Teruel, A. Modeling behavioral and neuronal symptoms of Alzheimer's disease in mice: A role for intraneuronal amyloid. *Neurosci. Biobehav. Rev.* **2007**, *31*, 125–147. [CrossRef]
19. Gimenez-Llort, L.; Torres-Lista, V.; Fuente, M. Crosstalk between Behavior and Immune System during the Prodromal Stages of Alzheimer's Disease. *Curr. Pharm. Des.* **2014**, *20*, 4723–4732. [CrossRef] [PubMed]
20. Jimenez-Altayo, F.; Sànchez-Ventura, J.; Vila, E.; Giménez-Llort, L. Crosstalk between Peripheral Small Vessel Properties and Anxious-like Profiles: Sex, Genotype, and Interaction Effects in Mice with Normal Aging and 3×Tg-AD mice at Advanced Stages of Disease. *J. Alzheimer's Dis.* **2018**, *62*, 1531–1538. [CrossRef]
21. Komarova, N.L.; Thalhauser, C.J. High Degree of Heterogeneity in Alzheimer's Disease Progression Patterns. *PLoS Comput. Biol.* **2011**, *7*, e1002251. [CrossRef]

22. Torres-Lista, V.; De La Fuente, M.; Giménez-Llort, L. Survival Curves and Behavioral Profiles of Female 3xTg-AD Mice Surviving to 18-Months of Age as Compared to Mice with Normal Aging. *J. Alzheimer's Dis. Rep.* **2017**, *1*, 47–57. [CrossRef]
23. Ramírez-Boix, P.; Giménez-Llort, L. Comorbid sensorimotor and emotional profiles in the forced swim test immobility and predictive value of a single assay in very old female mice. *Exp. Gerontol.* **2019**, *120*, 107–112. [CrossRef] [PubMed]
24. Muntsant, A.; Giménez-Llort, L. Impact of Social Isolation on the Behavioral, Functional Profiles, and Hippocampal Atrophy Asymmetry in Dementia in Times of Coronavirus Pandemic (COVID-19): A Translational Neuroscience Approach. *Front. Psychiatry* **2020**, *11*, 572583. [CrossRef]
25. Spreng, R.N.; Turner, G.R. The Shifting Architecture of Cognition and Brain Function in Older Adulthood. *Perspect. Psychol. Sci.* **2019**, *14*, 523–542. [CrossRef] [PubMed]
26. Amer, T.; Giovanello, K.S.; Grady, C.L.; Hasher, L. Age differences in memory for meaningful and arbitrary associations: A memory retrieval account. *Psychol. Aging* **2018**, *33*, 74–81. [CrossRef]
27. Turner, R.C.; Seminerio, M.J.; Naser, Z.J.; Ford, J.N.; Martin, S.J.; Matsumoto, R.R.; Rosen, C.L.; Huber, J.D. Effects of aging on behavioral assessment performance: Implications for clinically relevant models of neurological disease. *J. Neurosurg.* **2012**, *117*, 629–637. [CrossRef]
28. Mitchell, S.J.; Scheibye-Knudsen, M.; Longo, D.L.; De Cabo, R. Animal Models of Aging Research: Implications for Human Aging and Age-Related Diseases. *Annu. Rev. Anim. Biosci.* **2015**, *3*, 283–303. [CrossRef]
29. Puzzo, D.; Gulisano, W.; Palmeri, A.; Arancio, O. Rodent models for Alzheimer's disease drug discovery. *Expert Opin. Drug Discov.* **2015**, *10*, 703–711. [CrossRef]
30. Pietropaolo, S.; Feldon, J.; Yee, B.K. Age-dependent phenotypic characteristics of a triple transgenic mouse model of Alzheimer disease. *Behav. Neurosci.* **2008**, *122*, 733–747. [CrossRef] [PubMed]
31. Mastrangelo, M.; Bowers, W.J. Detailed immunohistochemical characterization of temporal and spatial progression of Alzheimer's disease-related pathologies in male triple-transgenic mice. *BMC Neurosci.* **2008**, *9*, 81. [CrossRef] [PubMed]
32. Fahlström, A.; Zeberg, H.; Ulfhake, B. Changes in behaviors of male C57BL/6J mice across adult life span and effects of dietary restriction. *Age* **2012**, *34*, 1435–1452. [CrossRef] [PubMed]
33. Giménez-Llort, L.; Ramírez-Boix, P.; De La Fuente, M. Mortality of septic old and adult male mice correlates with individual differences in premorbid behavioral phenotype and acute-phase sickness behavior. *Exp. Gerontol.* **2019**, *127*, 110717. [CrossRef]
34. Torres-Lista, V.; Giménez-Llort, L. Persistence of behaviours in the Forced Swim Test in 3xTg-AD mice at advanced stages of disease. *Behav. Process.* **2014**, *106*, 118–121. [CrossRef]
35. Giménez-Llort, L.; Arranz, L.; Maté, I.; De La Fuente, M. Gender-Specific Neuroimmunoendocrine Aging in a Triple-Transgenic 3×Tg-AD Mouse Model for Alzheimer's Disease and Its Relation with Longevity. *Neuroimmunomodulation* **2008**, *15*, 331–343. [CrossRef] [PubMed]
36. Muntsant, A.; Jiménez-Altayó, F.; Puertas-Umbert, L.; Jiménez-Xarrie, E.; Vila, E.; Giménez-Llort, L. Sex-Dependent End-of-Life Mental and Vascular Scenarios for Compensatory Mechanisms in Mice with Normal and AD-Neurodegenerative Aging. *Biomedicines* **2021**, *9*, 111. [CrossRef]
37. Van Dijk, P.T.; Dippel, D.W.; Habbema, J.D.F. Survival of Patients with Dementia. *J. Am. Geriatr. Soc.* **1991**, *39*, 603–610. [CrossRef]
38. Zeng, A.; Song, X.; Dong, J.; Mitnitski, A.; Liu, J.; Guo, Z.; Rockwood, K. Mortality in Relation to Frailty in Patients Admitted to a Specialized Geriatric Intensive Care Unit. *J. Gerontol. Ser. A Boil. Sci. Med. Sci.* **2015**, *70*, 1586–1594. [CrossRef] [PubMed]
39. A Brown, M.; Sampson, E.L.; Jones, L.; Barron, A.M. Prognostic indicators of 6-month mortality in elderly people with advanced dementia: A systematic review. *Palliat. Med.* **2012**, *27*, 389–400. [CrossRef] [PubMed]
40. Pike, C.J. Sex and the development of Alzheimer's disease. *J. Neurosci. Res.* **2017**, *95*, 671–680. [CrossRef]
41. Rezzani, R.; Franco, C.; Rodella, L.F. Sex differences of brain and their implications for personalized therapy. *Pharmacol. Res.* **2019**, *141*, 429–442. [CrossRef]
42. Sturchler-Pierrat, C.; Staufenbiel, M. Pathogenic Mechanisms of Alzheimer's Disease Analyzed in the APP23 Transgenic Mouse Model. *Ann. N. Y. Acad. Sci.* **2006**, *920*, 134–139. [CrossRef]
43. Hirata-Fukae, C.; Li, H.-F.; Hoe, H.-S.; Gray, A.J.; Minami, S.S.; Hamada, K.; Niikura, T.; Hua, F.; Tsukagoshi-Nagai, H.; Horikoshi-Sakuraba, Y.; et al. Females exhibit more extensive amyloid, but not tau, pathology in an Alzheimer transgenic model. *Brain Res.* **2008**, *1216*, 92–103. [CrossRef]
44. Rae, E.A.; Brown, R.E. The problem of genotype and sex differences in life expectancy in transgenic AD mice. *Neurosci. Biobehav. Rev.* **2015**, *57*, 238–251. [CrossRef]
45. Kane, A.E.; Shin, S.; Wong, A.A.; Fertan, E.; Faustova, N.S.; Howlett, S.E.; Brown, R.E. Sex Differences in Healthspan Predict Lifespan in the 3xTg-AD Mouse Model of Alzheimer's Disease. *Front. Aging Neurosci.* **2018**, *10*, 172. [CrossRef]
46. Giménez-Llort, L.; Maté, I.; Manassra, R.; Vida, C.; De La Fuente, M. Peripheral immune system and neuroimmune communication impairment in a mouse model of Alzheimer's disease. *Ann. N. Y. Acad. Sci.* **2012**, *1262*, 74–84. [CrossRef] [PubMed]
47. Montacute, R.; Foley, K.; Forman, R.; Else, K.J.; Cruickshank, S.M.; Allan, S.M. Enhanced susceptibility of triple transgenic Alzheimer's disease (3xTg-AD) mice to acute infection. *J. Neuroinflamm.* **2017**, *14*, 1–13. [CrossRef] [PubMed]
48. García-Mesa, Y.; Giménez-Llort, L.; López, L.C.; Venegas, C.; Cristòfol, R.; Escames, G.; Acuña-Castroviejo, D.; Sanfeliu, C. Melatonin plus physical exercise are highly neuroprotective in the 3xTg-AD mouse. *Neurobiol. Aging* **2012**, *33*, 1124.e13–1124.e29. [CrossRef]

49. Sturchler-Pierrat, C.; Abramowski, D.; Duke, M.; Wiederhold, K.-H.; Mistl, C.; Rothacher, S.; Ledermann, B.; Bürki, K.; Frey, P.; Paganetti, P.A.; et al. Two amyloid precursor protein transgenic mouse models with Alzheimer disease-like pathology. *Proc. Natl. Acad. Sci. USA* **1997**, *94*, 13287–13292. [CrossRef]
50. Kilkenny, C.; Browne, W.J.; Cuthill, I.C.; Emerson, M.; Altman, D.G. Improving Bioscience Research Reporting: The ARRIVE Guidelines for Reporting Animal Research. *PLoS Biol.* **2010**, *8*, e1000412. [CrossRef] [PubMed]
51. Baeta-Corral, R.; Giménez-Llort, L. Bizarre behaviors and risk assessment in 3xTg-AD mice at early stages of the disease. *Behav. Brain Res.* **2014**, *258*, 97–105. [CrossRef]
52. Torres-Lista, V.; Parrado-Fernández, C.; Alvarez-Montón, I.; Frontiñán-Rubio, J.; Durán-Prado, M.; Peinado, J.R.; Johansson, B.; Alcaín, F.J.; Giménez-Llort, L. Neophobia, NQO1 and SIRT1 as premorbid and prodromal indicators of AD in 3xTg-AD mice. *Behav. Brain Res.* **2014**, *271*, 140–146. [CrossRef]
53. Chen, Y.; Liang, Z.; Blanchard, J.; Dai, C.-L.; Sun, S.; Lee, M.H.; Grundke-Iqbal, I.; Iqbal, K.; Liu, F.; Gong, C.-X. A Non-transgenic Mouse Model (icv-STZ Mouse) of Alzheimer's Disease: Similarities to and Differences from the Transgenic Model (3xTg-AD Mouse). *Mol. Neurobiol.* **2013**, *47*, 711–725. [CrossRef] [PubMed]
54. Bernier, G.; Nardini, E.; Hogan, R.; Flamier, A. Alzheimer's disease: A tale of two diseases? *Neural Regen. Res.* **2021**, *16*, 1958–1964. [CrossRef] [PubMed]
55. Lalonde, R.; Lewis, T.; Strazielle, C.; Kim, H.; Fukuchi, K. Transgenic mice expressing the βAPP695SWE mutation: Effects on exploratory activity, anxiety, and motor coordination. *Brain Res.* **2003**, *977*, 38–45. [CrossRef]
56. Sinforiani, E.; Citterio, A.; Zucchella, C.; Bono, G.; Corbetta, S.; Merlo, P.; Mauri, M. Impact of Gender Differences on the Outcome of Alzheimer's Disease. *Dement. Geriatr. Cogn. Disord.* **2010**, *30*, 147–154. [CrossRef] [PubMed]
57. Mielke, M.; Vemuri, P.; Rocca, W. Clinical epidemiology of Alzheimer's disease: Assessing sex and gender differences. *Clin. Epidemiol.* **2014**, *6*, 37–48. [CrossRef]
58. Mazure, C.M.; Swendsen, J. Sex differences in Alzheimer's disease and other dementias. *Lancet Neurol.* **2016**, *15*, 451–452. [CrossRef]
59. Pugh, P.L.; Richardson, J.C.; Bate, S.T.; Upton, N.; Sunter, D. Non-cognitive behaviours in an APP/PS1 transgenic model of Alzheimer's disease. *Behav. Brain Res.* **2007**, *178*, 18–28. [CrossRef]
60. Giménez-Llort, L.; Blázquez, G.; Cañete, T.; Rosa, R.; Vivó, M.; Oddo, S.; Navarro, X.; LaFerla, F.M.; Johansson, B.; Tobena, A.; et al. Modeling neuropsychiatric symptoms of Alzheimer's disease dementia in 3xTg-AD mice. In *Alzheimer's Disease: New Advances*; Iqbal, K., Winblad, B., Avila, J., Eds.; Medimond SRL: Pianoro, Italy, 2006; pp. 513–516.
61. Lát, J. The analysis of habituation. *Acta Neurobiol. Exp.* **1973**, *33*, 771–789.
62. King, D.L.; Arendash, G.W. Behavioral characterization of the Tg2576 transgenic model of Alzheimer's disease through 19 months. *Physiol. Behav.* **2002**, *75*, 627–642. [CrossRef]
63. Dumont, M.; Strazielle, C.; Staufenbiel, M.; Lalonde, R. Spatial learning and exploration of environmental stimuli in 24-month-old female APP23 transgenic mice with the Swedish mutation. *Brain Res.* **2004**, *1024*, 113–121. [CrossRef] [PubMed]
64. Giménez-Llort, L.; Ferre, S.; Martínez, E. Effects of the systemic administration of kainic acid and NMDA on exploratory activity in rats. *Pharmacol. Biochem. Behav.* **1995**, *51*, 205–210. [CrossRef]
65. Callisaya, M.L.; Beare, R.; Phan, T.G.; Chen, J.; Srikanth, V.K. Global and Regional Associations of Smaller Cerebral Gray and White Matter Volumes with Gait in Older People. *PLoS ONE* **2014**, *9*, e84909. [CrossRef] [PubMed]
66. Studenski, S.; Perera, S.; Patel, K.; Rosano, C.; Faulkner, K.; Inzitari, M.; Brach, J.; Chandler, J.; Cawthon, P.; Connor, E.B.; et al. Gait speed and survival in older adults. *JAMA* **2011**, *305*, 50–58. [CrossRef] [PubMed]
67. Middleton, A.; Fulk, G.D.; Beets, M.W.; Herter, T.M.; Fritz, S.L. Self-Selected Walking Speed Is Predictive of Daily Ambulatory Activity in Older Adults. *J. Aging Phys. Act.* **2016**, *24*, 214–222. [CrossRef] [PubMed]
68. Artaud, F.; Singh-Manoux, A.; Dugravot, A.; Tzourio, C.; Elbaz, A. Decline in Fast Gait Speed as a Predictor of Disability in Older Adults. *J. Am. Geriatr. Soc.* **2015**, *63*, 1129–1136. [CrossRef] [PubMed]
69. Sabia, S.; Dumurgier, J.; Tavernier, B.; Head, J.; Tzourio, C.; Elbaz, A. Change in Fast Walking Speed Preceding Death: Results from a Prospective Longitudinal Cohort Study. *J. Gerontol. Ser. A Boil. Sci. Med. Sci.* **2013**, *69*, 354–362. [CrossRef]
70. Callisaya, M.L.; Launay, C.P.; Srikanth, V.K.; Verghese, J.; Allali, G.; Beauchet, O. Cognitive status, fast walking speed and walking speed reserve—the Gait and Alzheimer Interactions Tracking (GAIT) study. *GeroScience* **2017**, *39*, 231–239. [CrossRef]
71. Allali, G.; Annweiler, C.; Blumen, H.M.; Callisaya, M.L.; De Cock, A.-M.; Kressig, R.W.; Srikanth, V.; Steinmetz, J.-P.; Verghese, J.; Beauchet, O. Gait phenotype from mild cognitive impairment to moderate dementia: Results from the GOOD initiative. *Eur. J. Neurol.* **2016**, *23*, 527–541. [CrossRef] [PubMed]
72. Nehlig, A.; Daval, J.-L.; DeBry, G. Caffeine and the central nervous system: Mechanisms of action, biochemical, metabolic and psychostimulant effects. *Brain Res. Rev.* **1992**, *17*, 139–170. [CrossRef]
73. Giménez-Llort, L.; Masino, S.A.; Diao, L.; Fernández-Teruel, A.; Tobeña, A.; Halldner, L.; Fredholm, B.B. Mice lacking the adenosine A1 receptor have normal spatial learning and plasticity in the CA1 region of the hippocampus, but they habituate more slowly. *Synapse* **2005**, *57*, 8–16. [CrossRef] [PubMed]
74. King, D.L.; Arendash, G.W. Maintained synaptophysin immunoreactivity in Tg2576 transgenic mice during aging: Correlations with cognitive impairment. *Brain Res.* **2002**, *926*, 58–68. [CrossRef]

75. España, J.; Giménez-Llort, L.; Valero, J.; Miñano, A.; Rábano, A.; Rodriguez-Alvarez, J.; LaFerla, F.M.; Saura, C.A. Intraneuronal β-Amyloid Accumulation in the Amygdala Enhances Fear and Anxiety in Alzheimer's Disease Transgenic Mice. *Biol. Psychiatry* **2010**, *67*, 513–521. [CrossRef]
76. Thompson, R. The comparative effects of anterior and posterior cortical lesions on maze retention. *J. Comp. Physiol. Psychol.* **1959**, *52*, 506–508. [CrossRef]
77. Zhang, W.-N.; Pothuizen, H.; Feldon, J.; Rawlins, J. Dissociation of function within the hippocampus: Effects of dorsal, ventral and complete excitotoxic hippocampal lesions on spatial navigation. *Neuroscience* **2004**, *127*, 289–300. [CrossRef] [PubMed]
78. Deacon, R.M.J.; Rawlins, J.N.P. T-maze alternation in the rodent. *Nat. Protoc.* **2006**, *1*, 7–12. [CrossRef] [PubMed]
79. Giménez-Llort, L.; Schiffmann, S.N.; Shmidt, T.; Canela, L.; Camón, L.; Wassholm, M.; Canals, M.; Terasmaa, A.; Fernández-Teruel, A.; Tobeña, A.; et al. Working memory deficits in transgenic rats overexpressing human adenosine A2A receptors in the brain. *Neurobiol. Learn. Mem.* **2007**, *87*, 42–56. [CrossRef]
80. Guayerbas, N.; Puerto, M.; Ferrández, M.D.; De La Fuente, M. A diet supplemented with thiolic anti-oxidants improves leucocyte function in two strains of prematurely ageing mice. *Clin. Exp. Pharmacol. Physiol.* **2002**, *29*, 1009–1014. [CrossRef]
81. Giménez-Llort, L.; García, Y.; Buccieri, K.; Revilla, S.; Suñol, C.; Cristofol, R.; Sanfeliu, C. Gender-Specific Neuroimmunoendocrine Response to Treadmill Exercise in 3xTg-AD Mice. *Int. J. Alzheimer's Dis.* **2010**, *2010*, 1–17. [CrossRef]
82. García-Mesa, Y.; López-Ramos, J.C.; Giménez-Llort, L.; Revilla, S.; Guerra, R.; Gruart, A.; LaFerla, F.M.; Cristòfol, R.; Delgado-García, J.M.; Sanfeliu, C. Physical Exercise Protects Against Alzheimer's Disease in 3xTg-AD Mice. *J. Alzheimer's Dis.* **2011**, *24*, 421–454. [CrossRef] [PubMed]
83. Ariza, L.; Giménez-Llort, L.; Cubizolle, A.; Pagès, G.; García-Lareu, B.; Serratrice, N.; Cots, D.; Thwaite, R.; Chillón, M.; Kremer, E.J.; et al. Central Nervous System Delivery of Helper-Dependent Canine Adenovirus Corrects Neuropathology and Behavior in Mucopolysaccharidosis Type VII Mice. *Hum. Gene Ther.* **2014**, *25*, 199–211. [CrossRef] [PubMed]
84. Sanderson, D.J.; Bannerman, D.M. The role of habituation in hippocampus-dependent spatial working memory tasks: Evidence from GluA1 AMPA receptor subunit knockout mice. *Hippocampus* **2012**, *22*, 981–994. [CrossRef]
85. Tempier, A.; He, J.; Zhu, S.; Zhang, R.; Kong, L.; Tan, Q.; Luo, H.; Kong, J.; Li, X.-M. Quetiapine Modulates Conditioned Anxiety and Alternation Behavior in Alzheimer's Transgenic Mice. *Curr. Alzheimer Res.* **2013**, *10*, 199–206. [CrossRef] [PubMed]
86. Rinaldi, A.; Mandillo, S.; Oliverio, A.; Mele, A. D1 and D2 Receptor Antagonist Injections in the Prefrontal Cortex Selectively Impair Spatial Learning in Mice. *Neuropsychopharmacology* **2006**, *32*, 309–319. [CrossRef] [PubMed]
87. Delotterie, D.; Ruiz, G.; Brocard, J.; Schweitzer, A.; Roucard, C.; Roche, Y.; Suaud-Chagny, M.-F.; Bressand, K.; Andrieux, A. Chronic administration of atypical antipsychotics improves behavioral and synaptic defects of STOP null mice. *Psychopharmacology* **2010**, *208*, 131–141. [CrossRef]
88. Morris, R.G.M. Developments of a water-maze procedure for studying spatial learning in the rat. *J. Neurosci. Methods* **1984**, *11*, 47–60. [CrossRef]
89. Giménez-Llort, L.; Rivera-Hernández, G.; Marín-Argany, M.; Sánchez-Quesada, J.L.; Villegas, S. Early intervention in the 3xTg-AD mice with an amyloid β-antibody fragment ameliorates first hallmarks of Alzheimer disease. *mAbs* **2013**, *5*, 665–864. [CrossRef]
90. Baeta-Corral, R.; Giménez-Llort, L. Persistent hyperactivity and distinctive strategy features in the Morris water maze in 3xTg-AD mice at advanced stages of disease. *Behav. Neurosci.* **2015**, *129*, 129–137. [CrossRef] [PubMed]
91. Lalonde, R.; Dumont, M.; Staufenbiel, M.; Strazielle, C. Neurobehavioral characterization of APP23 transgenic mice with the SHIRPA primary screen. *Behav. Brain Res.* **2005**, *157*, 91–98. [CrossRef]

biomedicines

MDPI

Review

Psychiatric Neural Networks and Precision Therapeutics by Machine Learning

Hidetoshi Komatsu [1,2,*], Emi Watanabe [3] and Mamoru Fukuchi [4]

1 Medical Affairs, Kyowa Pharmaceutical Industry Co., Ltd., Osaka 530-0005, Japan
2 Department of Biological Science, Graduate School of Science, Nagoya University, Nagoya City 464-8602, Japan
3 Interactive Group, Accenture Japan Ltd., Tokyo 108-0073, Japan; emi-w@ruri.waseda.jp
4 Laboratory of Molecular Neuroscience, Faculty of Pharmacy, Takasaki University of Health and Welfare, Gunma 370-0033, Japan; fukuchi@takasaki-u.ac.jp
* Correspondence: hidetkomatsu@fuji.waseda.jp; Tel.: +81-6-6121-6244; Fax: +81-6-6121-2858

Abstract: Learning and environmental adaptation increase the likelihood of survival and improve the quality of life. However, it is often difficult to judge optimal behaviors in real life due to highly complex social dynamics and environment. Consequentially, many different brain regions and neuronal circuits are involved in decision-making. Many neurobiological studies on decision-making show that behaviors are chosen through coordination among multiple neural network systems, each implementing a distinct set of computational algorithms. Although these processes are commonly abnormal in neurological and psychiatric disorders, the underlying causes remain incompletely elucidated. Machine learning approaches with multidimensional data sets have the potential to not only pathologically redefine mental illnesses but also better improve therapeutic outcomes than DSM/ICD diagnoses. Furthermore, measurable endophenotypes could allow for early disease detection, prognosis, and optimal treatment regime for individuals. In this review, decision-making in real life and psychiatric disorders and the applications of machine learning in brain imaging studies on psychiatric disorders are summarized, and considerations for the future clinical translation are outlined. This review also aims to introduce clinicians, scientists, and engineers to the opportunities and challenges in bringing artificial intelligence into psychiatric practice.

Keywords: psychiatric disorder; machine learning; neural network; antipsychotics; schizophrenia; bipolar disorder; depression; precision medicine; endophenotype; decision making

Citation: Komatsu, H.; Watanabe, E.; Fukuchi, M. Psychiatric Neural Networks and Precision Therapeutics by Machine Learning. *Biomedicines* **2021**, 9, 403. https://doi.org/10.3390/biomedicines9040403

Academic Editor: Masaru Tanaka

Received: 1 February 2021
Accepted: 6 April 2021
Published: 8 April 2021

Publisher's Note: MDPI stays neutral with regard to jurisdictional claims in published maps and institutional affiliations.

1. Introduction

Living organisms have self-sustaining properties that are absent in purely physical systems. They acquire energy from food for sustenance, growth, and reproduction. Another self-sustaining ability of animals is the adaptive behavior. Behavioral strategies that improve their ability to acquire energy and produce successful offspring to help each species proliferating evolutionarily through the process of natural selection [1]. Three essential principles for biological behaviors have been proposed as materiality (an embodied brain embedded in the world), agency (action-perception closed loops and purpose), and historicity (individuality and historical contingencies) [2]. The three principles are arguably unique to life and imperative for neuroscience. We believe that these considerations will shed light on our typical approaches to address not only the conundrum of animal behaviors but also the nature of mental disorders.

The complexity of environment and social dynamics often make it difficult to identify optimal behaviors in the real world. Decision-making in this process involves many different brain areas and circuits that are exacerbated in numerous neurological and psychiatric disorders [3]. Traditional approaches have dominated the studies on optimal behaviors. Among these, a prescriptive approach addresses the question of what is the best choice for a given challenge. For instance, economists and game theorists describe how self-interested rationales should behave individually or in a group [4,5]. However, the real behaviors of animals and humans seldom follow the predictions of such prescriptive theories. Indeed, prospect theory can predict the decision-making of animals as well as humans more accurately than the prescriptive theories [6–8]. Likewise, humans often behave altruistically and thus deviate from the predictions of the game theory [9,10]. Recently, these traditional approaches have merged with neuroscientific theories, in which learning plays a crucial role in choosing optimal behaviors and decisions. Particularly, reinforcement learning theory presents a worthwhile framework to model how an individual's behaviors are tuned by experience [11,12]. Neuroscientists have begun to uncover numerous core mechanisms in the brain responsible for various computational processes of learning and decision-making. Their findings are now frequently featured in the literatures in many disciplines, such as ethics [13], law [14], politics [15], marketing [16], and economic and financial decisions [17,18].

A distinct set of computational algorithms evoked through coordination among myriad brain systems are abnormal in many types of neurological and psychiatric disorders, leading to aberrant and maladaptive behaviors [19–24]. Notwithstanding, psychiatric status is still diagnosed and treated according to the experiential schemes based on symptomatic phenotypes. The definitions of many mental disorders described in the DSM and ICD manuals do not always match well with neuroscientific, psychopathological, and genetic evidences [25,26]. Thus, there is a greater desire to redefine mental illness as a discrete disease. To satisfy this aspect, the Research Domain Criteria (RDoC) initiative has been launched to reconceptualize mental disorders as a dimensional approach that incorporates many different levels of data from molecular factors to social determinants and linked more precisely to interventions for a given individual [27–29]. This approach is more likely to be compatible with the facts that psychiatric patients comprise of clusters of psychopathological symptoms and that many symptoms are shared among different mental disorders. Machine learning approaches are well suited to achieve this goal.

Machine learning approaches for psychiatry feature statistical learning functions from multidimensional data sets to unveil general principles underlying a series of observations without definite guidance. Machine learning algorithms can be generally classified into three categories, namely supervised, unsupervised, and reinforcement learning methods [30,31]. Supervised learning models, such as support vector machines (SVM) and neural-network algorithms, are designed to predict a discrete outcome (e.g., healthy group vs. psychiatric group), or continuous outcome (e.g., psychiatric severity degrees) from the qualitative data on behaviors (e. g., questionnaire), genetics (e. g., single nucleotide polymorphisms, gene expressions), or brain function (e. g., neural activity). Unsupervised learning describes models to discover unknown statistical configurations across subjects without reference to a specific outcome. Reinforcement learning investigates how actions in one's environment (such as treatment) change behaviors [31]. Among these algorithms, supervised learning, especially SVM, is most widely used in psychiatry to classify individuals into groups within a statistical framework. This approach has already shown promising results in neuroimaging-based psychosis prediction and treatment-response estimation [32–34]. With increasing digitized phenotypic data, improved computing power, and less expensive data storage, machine learning, as well as deep learning that is the artificial neural network algorithms to learn complex representations of high-dimensional data patterns such as images and language, would offer findings with important implications for the development of therapeutic interventions, leading to precision psychiatry and stratified clinical trial designs.

A main purpose of this review is to exemplify the new insights provided by recent applications of machine learning in neuroimaging and clinical studies on major psychiatric disorders. To this end, decision-making in real life and mental illness is briefly described. Next, our current knowledge of neuronal circuits or functional connectivity in major psychiatric disorders is summarized. This review also argues that machine learning is predisposed to address many challenges in the era of precision psychiatry.

2. Decision-Making in Real Life and Psychiatric Disorders

The understanding of decision-making processes helps us develop machine learning tools for precision psychiatry. Flawed decision-making has been commonly observed in major psychiatric disorders, often causing poor real-life outcomes. In many cases, flawed decision-making in mental illness results from abnormalities in fundamental neuropsychological processes, including impaired attention, reward processing, associative learning, and working memory. For instance, defects in reward and avoidance learning are reported in patients with depression. Aberrant hedonic capacity and cognitive impairment occur in bipolar disorder and schizophrenia. Flawed decision-making can contribute to abnormal behaviors such as nonadherence to medications or outpatient appointments, failing to exercise, or poor diet. Downstream consequences of poor decisions can lead to worsening of symptoms, reduced life satisfaction, impaired everyday functioning, relapse and rehospitalization, poor physical health, and even more tragic outcomes such as accidental death, homicide, or suicide [35].

Decision-making is a constant process in real life and takes place from when we wake up until we go to bed. Its processes are largely divided into three steps: (1) identification and depiction of all alternatives, (2) assessment of the consequences of each alternative, and (3) a comparison of the accuracy and efficiency of each of these consequences [35]. Different disciplines attempt to systematize the understanding of decision-making. For instance, consumer decision-making has long been of interest to economists. Consumers are viewed as rational decision-makers who are only concerned with self-interest. One of the most prevalent consumer decision models is the Engel-Blackwell-Miniard Model (Figure 1) [36], in which every conceptual step of decision-making is instrumental for developing machine learning algorithms to implement customized advertising tactics [37]. The model has the following decision processes: need recognition followed by a search of information, the evaluation of alternatives, purchase, and finally, post purchase reflection. These decisions can be influenced by two main factors, namely memories of previous experiences and external variables in the form of either environmental influences or individual differences. In other words, this model shows that various computational steps of decision-making can be affected by the environment, individual factors, and memory. Similarly, the environment and individual factors, including polygenic architecture and epigenetic risk elements, underlie the manifestation of psychiatric disorders [38]. The pathophysiology of psychiatric disorders is complex and not well understood. Thus, it will be interesting to illustrate mental illness with common denominators across diagnostic boundaries. One common element in severe mental illness is pervasive poor decision-making. Since innumerable combinations of computational algorithms in the brain are evoked in a flexible manner for optimal decision-making, it would be challenging to elucidate the nature of decision-making impairments in different psychiatric disorders. Therefore, econometric models are becoming valuable tools for computational psychiatry [26,39–42].

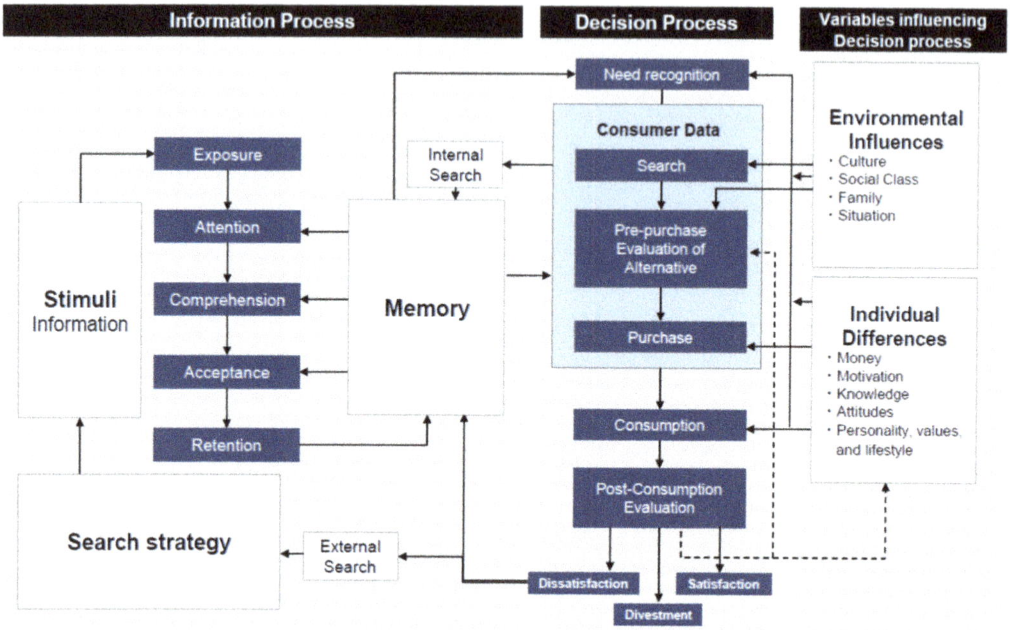

Figure 1. Schematic illustration of the Consumer Decision Model. The Consumer Decision Model (also known as the Engel-Blackwell-Miniard Model) that was originally developed by Engel, Kollat, and Blackwell is modified [36]. This model comprises conceptual steps of decision making in the real world and thus could be extended to be applied for developing precision medicine in psychiatry.

2.1. Schizophrenia

Schizophrenia is a severe psychiatric disorder that affects approximately 1% of the population worldwide. It is characterized by positive symptoms (e.g., delusion, hallucination, and thought disorder), negative symptoms (e.g., apathy, poor social functioning, and emotional blunting), cognitive deficits and other psychopathological symptoms (e.g., psychomotor retardation, lack of insight, poor attention, and impulse control) [43]. These symptoms are likely linked not only to excessive dopaminergic transmissions in the mesolimbic pathway but also to the dopamine release decline in the prefrontal cortex. Although dysfunctions of N-methyl-D-aspartic acid (NMDA) receptor systems and weaker prefrontal GABAergic actions are also implicated, the precise manner in which plural neurotransmitter systems interact with one another in schizophrenia remains elusive [44].

Various types of cognitive functions are impaired in schizophrenia [45]. Altered prefrontal functions might also be responsible for abnormalities in decision-making and reinforcement learning observed in patients with schizophrenia [46]. For instance, during economic decision-making challenges, schizophrenic patients incline to put less weight on potential losses compared to the healthy subjects [47], and also show impairments in feedback-based learning [48,49]. Consistent with these results, activity involved in reward prediction error in striatum and the frontal cortex is attenuated in patients with schizophrenia [50,51]. A pervasive clinical burden in schizophrenia is the high prevalence of comorbidity with substance abuse disorders. Approximately half of patients with schizophrenia exhibit a lifetime history of substance abuse disorders [52], and almost all of them are smokers [53,54]. These unusual high rates of substance-use comorbidity may be attributed to disrupted reward processing [55]. These global cognitive impairments are translated in the devastating functional toll of this disorder.

2.2. Bipolar Disorder

Bipolar disorder and schizophrenia share high levels of polygenic and pleiotropic molecular architecture [38]. In accord with this, these two disorders share similar types of impairments in cognitive domains including processing speed, attention, working memory, and executive function, although bipolar disorder usually exhibits less severe deficits [56]. These cognitive deficits bring about a substantial clinical burden in up to 60% of patients with bipolar disorder and can be observed not only in depressed, manic, and mixed episodes but also in the euthymic state. These pervasive impairment in bipolar disorder indicates that it may be a trait marker linked with genetic vulnerability [57]. In addition to cognitive dysfunctions, emotion processing is severely altered in patients with bipolar disorder. Upregulated processing of positive emotion regardless of the context is central to the manic bipolar episode [58]. Theory of mind and emotion processing are significantly disrupted in the euthymic bipolar state [59]. Thus, bipolar patients display defects in their ability to understand other emotions and intentions, with a resultant impact on everyday functioning. Moreover, euthymic bipolar patients show moderate to severe impairments in a broad range of executive functions including mental manipulation, verbal learning, abstraction, sustained attention, and response inhibition [60–64]. In addition to these deficits, there seems to be specific decision-making biases in bipolar patients including impulsivity and deficits in risk assessment and reward processing. The weights of these aberrant decision-making are evident in depressed bipolar patients [35].

2.3. Depression and Anxiety Disorders

Depression and anxiety disorder are characterized by disturbances in mood and emotion and feature poor concentration and negative mood states, such as sadness and anger, with high levels of their comorbidities [65–67]. However, they have some important differences. Anxiety is needed to improve individual's readiness for impending danger, whereas depression might prohibit previously unsuccessful actions and enhance more reflective cognitive processes. Both depression and anxiety disorder often cause systematic biases in decision-making [67,68]. Patients with anxiety disorders are hypersensitive to threatening cues without apparent memory bias. In contrast, depressed patients show a bias to memorize negative events and ruminate excessively [69].

The symptoms of these two mood disorders have been extensively investigated, and some responsible brain regions have been identified. For instance, symptoms of depression is associated with abnormalities in frontostriatal monoamines involved in reinforcement learning [70]. Meanwhile, the brain regions responsible for anxiety disorders include the amygdala, insula, and anterior cingulate cortex [71,72]. Interestingly, the default network is overactive in patients with depression. The levels of excessive rumination and negative self-referential memory in depressive states are likely to be correlated with the default network function [73]. Indeed, deep brain stimulation in the subgenual cingulate cortex of patients with major depressive disorder produces therapeutic effects [74].

Although the neurochemical mechanism of mood disorders remains unclear, much attention has been paid to the role of changed serotonin metabolism [75]. For instance, it has been hypothesized that future reward is discounted markedly in patients with depression due to a low level of serotonin [76]. Serotonin has been proposed to be primarily involved in the inhibition of thoughts and behaviors associated with aversive outcomes, including the heuristic process of unpromising decision-making [77–79].

2.4. Autism Spectrum Disorder

Autism spectrum disorder (ASD) is a neurodevelopmental disorder, featuring early-onset impairments in social cognition, poor communication abilities, restricted repetitive and stereotyped behaviors, and narrow interests that hurt the individual's ability to function properly in school, work, and other fields of life [80]. Particularly, patients with ASD show impairments in their ability to make inferences about the intentions and beliefs of others, namely, theory of mind [81,82]. Such impaired abilities might underlie differences in socially interactive decision-making tasks between autistic patients and healthy subjects. Autism is known as a "spectrum" disorder because there is a wide range of variations in the type and severity of symptoms [83]. Under the DSM-5 criteria, patients with ASD must display symptoms from early childhood, even if those symptoms are not recognized later. They also may not be fully recognized until social demands surpass their capacity to receive the diagnosis. The earliest symptoms include the lack of attention to faces [84], imitative behaviors [85], and motor deficits [86].

In ASD, a variety of brain architectures are altered, ranging from the brain stem to the cerebellum and cerebral cortex [87–90]. In particular, the connectivity deficit in the parieto-frontal circuit involved in the mirror mechanism has been proposed to underlie some cognitive aspects of ASD [91,92]. Several brain regions affected in ASD have also been shown to be involved in decision-making. Neurobiological studies have revealed that ASD has functional abnormalities in the amygdala, prefrontal cortex, superior temporal sulcus, and fusiform gyrus whose brain regions are thought to constitute the "social brain" [93,94]. Especially, the amygdala, ventral striatum, and prefrontal cortex are implicated in decision-making according to functional neuroimaging and lesion analyses [95–97].

3. Psychiatric Neural Networks

Brain imaging can give important insights into the underlying neural mechanisms of psychiatric disorders. For instance, the resting state functional magnetic resonance imaging (rs-fMRI) analyses in humans have identified a large number of potentially important abnormal functional connections that may underlie psychiatric manifestations [98–101]. Most of MRI-based neuroimaging biomarker studies have applied the machine learning algorithm of SVM to achieve high accuracy with many features and shown that different diagnoses are related to unique patterns of functional connections [102–105].

Functional connectivity (FC) shows how brain regions are temporally coordinated and is becoming more and more used to investigate neuronal network architecture. Resting state FC has been linked with a diverse range of individual traits [106–110]. For instance, whole-brain FC models have revealed that patterns of functional connections across brain regions can predict cognitive abilities not only in healthy individuals but also in individuals with mental illness [111–115]. Intriguingly, a prediction model of working memory on letter three-back task performance using whole-brain FC shows the order of working memory impairment for major psychiatric disorders (i.e., schizophrenia > major depressive disorder > obsessive-compulsive disorder > ASD) [115]. This suggests that specific cognitive processes may be represented by the corresponding FC patterns among distributed neuronal networks. Whole-brain FC-based models also have been shown to predict psychiatric disease, including schizophrenia, ASD, and major depressive disorder, as well as individual clinical severities [105,116,117], suggesting that FC alteration is quantitatively associated with psychiatric abnormality.

MRI-based delineation of psychiatric disorders has been explored as a complement to the current symptom-based diagnoses. While a number of studies have identified numerous disease-specific functional and structural aberrations, none of them are practically used as a credible biomarker mostly because of the lack of its generalizability. Namely, the reliability of the developed classifiers has not been demonstrated with regard to the variety of population demographics and data attributes [118–124]. These elements include different ethnicities, sex, ages, medication profiles, scanner specifications, imaging parameters, and instructions to participants, all of which are known to affect the MRI results [108,125–129]. Thus, little attention has been paid to the neuroimaging-based biomarkers in neuropsychiatry until recently [130,131].

To identify a generalizable classifier, we must surmount the following two major difficulties: over-fitting and nuisance variables (NVs). First, certain situations in data and model properties bring about over-fitting problems where the model fitting to the training data can be so precise that the associated errors become artificially smaller compared with the inherent data variance [130]. Second, any machine learning algorithms used for classification is doomed to employ NVs specific to a given sample data and to falsely choose neuroimaging features that are associated with the NVs. NVs include site-specific conditions in image acquisition and properties in the sample population such as demographic attributes, treatment status, and illness severity. To abrogate the over-fitting and the effects of NVs, advanced approaches with a unique combination of machine learning algorithms across multiple imaging sites have recently identified generalizable FC classifiers correlated with specific psychiatric disorders as described below.

3.1. Functional Connectivity as ASD Classifier

The rs-fMRI studies have revealed a reliable neuroimaging-based classifier for ASD that shows the spatial distribution of the 16 FCs identified from the data at multiple sites in Japan by the machine-learning algorithm (Figure 2 and Table 1) [105]. They also have demonstrated that both a sophisticated machine learning algorithm and a large training data set are prerequisite for identifying a reliable and generalizable classifier. Concerning the hemispheric distribution of the 16 FC related-brain regions, there are significantly more regions in the right hemisphere than in the left. Concerning the functional network attributes of the 32 brain regions constituting these 16 FCs, the 13 brain regions participate in the cingulo-opercular network [105,108,132]. This ASD classifier achieves a diagnosis prediction accuracy of 85% for each individual with balanced sensitivity and specificity of 80% and 89%, respectively [105]. Intriguingly, the ASD classifier is intermediately generalizable to schizophrenia, whereas it hardly exhibits any generalizability to attention-deficit hyperactivity disorder (ADHD) and major depressive disorder (MDD). This suggests that ASD shares more intrinsic neural networks with schizophrenia than with ADHD or MDD [105]. In concordance with this, genome-level studies have found that ASD shares a high degree of polygenic risk with schizophrenia, but not with ADHD or MDD [133,134]. Accumulating evidence by clinical and behavioral studies also has shown a close relationship between ASD and schizophrenia [135,136].

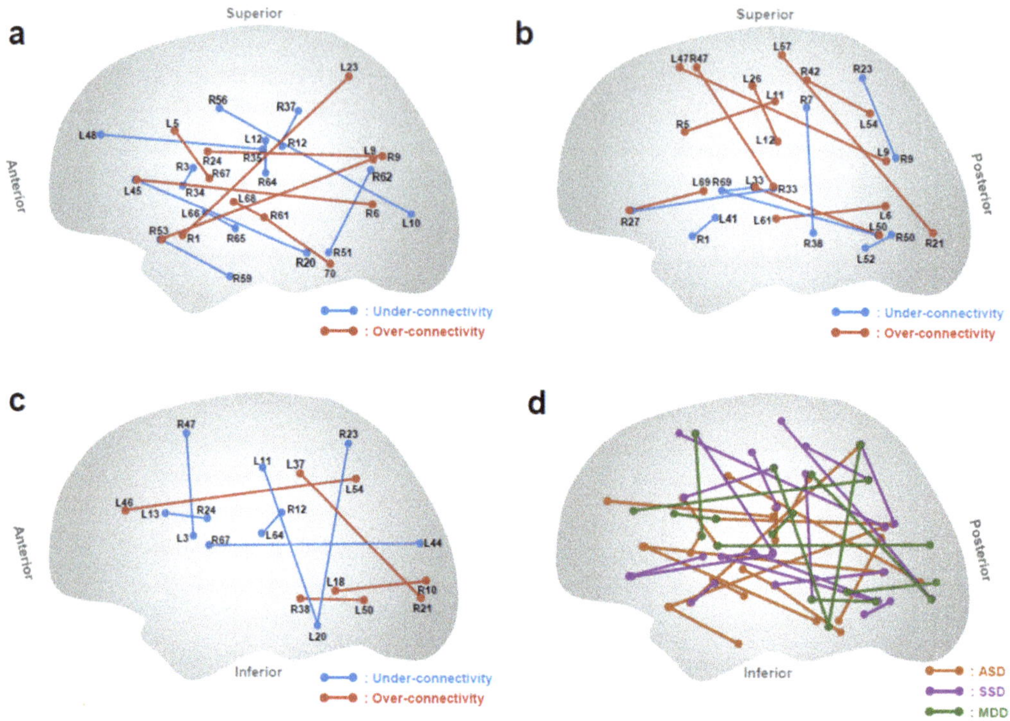

Figure 2. The specific FCs identified for ASD/SSD/MDD classifiers. The 70 terminal regions connected by the FCs are numbered as described in Table 1. The state of FC exhibiting the smaller (more negative) and greater (more positive) correlations than the healthy control is termed under- and over-connectivity, respectively. Specific FCs identified for (**a**) ASD [105], (**b**) SSD [116], and (**c**) MDD classifiers [117], are illustrated. These three classifiers are summarized in (**d**), where they did not overlap.

Table 1. The identified terminal regions in ASD/SSD/MDD classifiers. The terminal regions identified for ASD/SSD/MDD classifiers are numbered. See Figure 2.

No	Anatomical Name	No	Anatomical Name
1	anterior lateral fissure	36	posterior sub-central ramus of the lateral fissure
2	anterior ramus of the lateral fissure	37	calloso-marginal posterior fissure
3	diagonal ramus of the lateral fissure	38	collateral fissure
4	anterior sub-central ramus of the lateral fissure	39	intraparietal sulcus
5	calloso-marginal anterior fissure	40	secondary intermediate ramus of the intraparietal sulcus

Table 1. *Cont.*

No	Anatomical Name	No	Anatomical Name
6	calcarine fissure	41	insula
7	superior postcentral intraparietal superior sulcus	42	paracentral lobule central sulcus
8	primary intermediate ramus of the intraparietal sulcus	43	central sylvian sulcus
9	parieto-occipital fissure	44	cuneal sulcus
10	lobe occipital	45	anterior interior frontal sulcus
11	central sulcus	46	intermediate frontal sulcus
12	subcallosal sulcus	47	median frontal sulcus
13	inferior frontal sulcus	48	polar frontal sulcus
14	internal frontal sulcus	49	sulcus of the supra-marginal gyrus
15	marginal frontal sulcus	50	posterior intra-lingual sulcus
16	orbital frontal sulcus	51	internal occipito-temporal lateral sulcus
17	superior frontal sulcus	52	posterior occipito-temporal lateral sulcus
18	anterior intralingual sulcus	53	olfactory sulcus
19	anterior occipito-temporal lateral sulcus	54	internal parietal sulcus
20	median occipito-temporal lateral sulcus	55	transverse precentral sulcus
21	occipito-polar sulcus	56	intermediate precentral sulcus
22	orbital sulcus	57	median precentral sulcus
23	superior parietal sulcus	58	superior postcentral sulcus
24	interior precentral sulcus	59	rhinal sulcus
25	marginal precentral sulcus	60	posterior inferior temporal sulcus
26	superior precentral sulcus	61	superior temporal sulcus
27	inferior rostral sulcus	62	superior terminal ascending branch of the superior temporal sulcus
28	anterior inferior temporal sulcus	63	sub-parietal sulcus
29	polar temporal sulcus	64	Thalamus
30	anterior terminal ascending branch of the superior temporal sulcus	65	Amygdala
31	paracentral sulcus	66	Accumbens
32	ventricle	67	Caudate
33	posterior lateral fissure	68	Pallidum
34	ascending ramus of the lateral fissure	69	Putamen
35	retro central transverse ramus of the lateral fissure	70	Vermis

3.2. Functional Connectivity as Schizophrenia Spectrum Disorder Classifier

The rs-fMRI studies also have identified a reliable classifier for schizophrenia spectrum disorder (SSD) using L1-norm regularized sparse canonical correlation analyses and sparse logistic regression (SLR) [137,138]. The machine-learning algorithms automatically selected SSD-specific FCs from about 10,000 FCs of whole-brain rs-fMRI [116]. The SSD classifier shows the distinctive 16 FCs that are distributed as interhemispheric (44%), left intra-hemispheric (25%), and right intra-hemispheric connections (31%) (Figure 2 and Table 1) [116]. The classifier differentiates SSD from healthy controls with an accuracy of 76% [116]. The 16 FCs as SSD classifier are different from the 16 FCs as ASD classifier mentioned above (Figure 2d). The weighted linear summation (WLS) of the selected FCs predicts the categorical diagnostic label for each individual. The values of WLS provide a degree of classification certainty, which can be construed as neural classification certainty for the disorders. Then, each biological dimension can be determined based on the WLS [116]. On the basis of the SSD and ASD biological dimensions, the WLS distributions of individuals with SSD and ASD display overlapping but asymmetrical patterns in the two biological dimensions. This suggests that the neuronal network of SSD is characterized by a larger diversity and that it partially shares spatial distributions with the smaller network of ASD. In accord with this, the recent genetic findings demonstrate that ASD shares a significant degree of polygenic architecture with SSD [133], and that common genetic variants explain nearly 50% of total liability to ASD and approximately 30% of total liability to SSD [139,140].

3.3. Functional Connectivity as MDD Classifier

According to the meta-analysis published results of MRI-based biomarkers in depressive disorders [141], approximately 30% of them harnessed rs-fMRI as modality, of which only one-third employed FCs among region of interests (ROIs). As most of those studies have applied the SVM algorithm to achieve high diagnostic accuracy, it remains unknown that which are the most critical FCs in depression across the whole brain. Approximately half of depressed patients are inadequately treated by available interventions, as there are no reliable guidelines to match patients to optimal treatments. This mainly derives from the heterogeneity of depression [142]. Thus, it would be important to pay attention to a specific subtype of depression in order to identify target FCs.

Melancholic major depressive disorder is a subtype of MDD that is considered to be the most drug-responsive [143–146]. The sparse machine learning algorithm identified melancholic MDD-specific 10 FCs from rs-fMRI data of 130 individuals including melancholic MDD patients and healthy controls (Figure 2 and Table 1) [117]. Importantly, this biomarker does not generalize to non-melancholic and treatment-resistant MDD, ASD, and schizophrenia. Out of 10 FCs, the top two FCs as the melancholic MDD-specific classifier includes the FCs (SN-ECN connectivity) with left inferior frontal gyrus (IFG) in executive control network (ECN) and right dorsomedial prefrontal cortex (DMPFC)/frontal eye field (FEF)/supplementary motor area (SMA) in salience network (SN), and the FCs (DMN-ECN connectivity) with left dorsolateral prefrontal cortex (DLPFC)/inferior frontal gyrus (IFG) in executive control network (ECN) and posterior cingulate cortex (PCC)/Precuneus in default mode network (DMN). These brain regions are tightly linked with cognitive flexibility, such as reversal learning tasks, in which patients with depression often have functional impairments [147,148]. In SN-ECN connectivity, activation in IFG and DMPFC leads to empathic accuracy with compassion meditation training [149], and adolescents with depression show reduced connectivity between DMPFC and IFG during cognitive reappraisal of emotional images [150]. Priming transcranial magnetic stimulation (TMS) studies demonstrate that the DMPFC play an essential role in forming social-relevant impression, such as processing verbal emotional stimuli and face-adjective pair [151,152]. In DMN-ECN connectivity, bilateral DLPFC/IFG relate to conflict processing and attention control [153], and PCC/Precuneus are linked with anhedonic anxious arousal and depression [154]. In addition to the accumulated evidence that links the connections of

DLPFC to depression [110,155–161], there is another evidence that supports therapeutic relevance. For instance, DLPFC is a well-known target for repetitive TMS (rTMS) therapy for treatment-resistant depression [162–164]. Besides, neurofeedback therapy targeting DMN-ECN connectivity has been reported to be effective [165–167], suggesting that DLPFC plays a causal role in manifestation of depression.

4. Machine Learning Approach to Predict Therapeutic Outcomes in Psychiatric Disorders

Psychiatric research and treatment are based on a diagnostic system exclusively dependent on human experiential terms rather than on objective biological markers. Psychiatrists use a prolonged trial-and-error process to identify the optimal medications for each patient [168,169]. Although the standard diagnostic classifications have been constructed from expert opinions and defined in DSM and ICD, they are not sufficient for judging an appropriate treatment for each patient. Modern drug treatment choices are only effective in roughly half of the patients [25,141]. This is because of the heterogeneity of psychiatric disorders and the unknown precise mechanism of action of antipsychotic drugs. The psychiatrist's choice from the best-possible treatment options does not rely on what has caused or maintained the mental illness of a given patient. While current clinical research goal is mainly to discover novel treatment options that benefit some majority of a certain patient group, an attractive alternative research goal is to improve the choice from existing treatment options by predicting their effectiveness of individual patients. In fact, a specific drug or psychotherapy treatment has been successful in a particular clinical group and unsuccessful in another patient group labeled even with the identical diagnosis [170]. This approach might help reduce the time spent in trial-and error treatment and accompanying personal and economic burden.

Machine learning methods can offer a set of tools that are especially suited to achieve clinical predictions at the individual level. Predictive models are conceptually positioned between genetic vulnerability as an individual's architecture and clinical symptoms as an individual's behavioral manifestations. The exploitation of various endophenotypes has the translational potential to refine individual clinical management by early diagnosis, disease stratification, optimal choices of drug treatments and dosages, and prognosis for psychiatric care (Figure 3) [99]. Machine learning models have a long-standing focus on prediction as a metric of statistical quality and are able to predict an outcome from single observation, such as behavioral, neural, or genetic measurements of individuals [141,171]. In contrast, traditional statistical methods, such as Student's t test, are often used in medical research to explain variance of group effects.

An observed impact evaluated to be statistically significant by a p value does not always produce a high prediction accuracy in new and independent data. A classical null-hypothesis method takes a one-step procedure. Namely, a given dataset is routinely used to yield a p value or an effect size in a single process. This result itself cannot be used to judge other data in later steps. In a two-step procedure of machine learning models, a learning algorithm is fitted on a larger amount of available data (training data) and the resulting "trained" learning model is evaluated by application to new data (test data). In a first step, structured knowledge in openly available or hospital-provided data sets can be extracted. In a second step, the resulting trained algorithms can be applied with little effort in a large number of individuals in diverse mental health contexts.

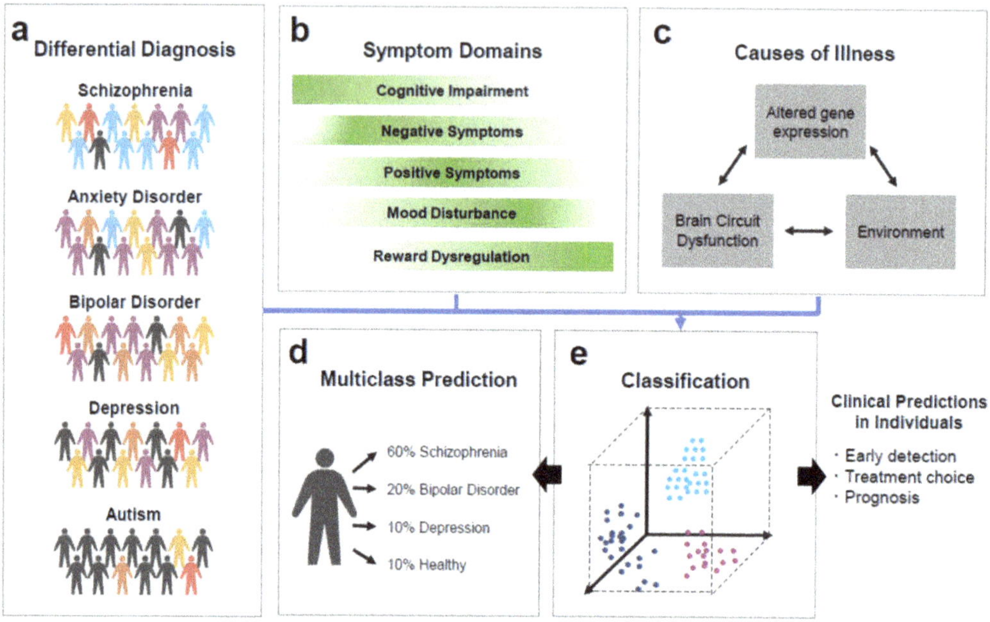

Figure 3. Challenges for precision medicine in psychiatry by artificial intelligence. (**a**) Traditional psychiatric research investigates a given patient group by comparison against the healthy group, possibly creating artificial dichotomies. (**b**) Each psychiatric disorder has various types of the symptoms with their varying degrees. (**c**) The interplay between altered gene expression and neural circuit, and environment such as stress, may elicit psychiatric manifestations. Instead of relying on diagnostic category, a given patient can be classified based on biological and pathological properties (i.e. endophenotypes). (**d**) Artificial intelligence such as machine learning can be extended to compare observations from numerous groups in the same statistical estimation. (**e**) Machine learning algorithms, such as SVM, can automatically extract unknown patterns of variations in individuals simultaneously from heterogenous data labeled with traditional diagnosis. Predictive models could improve patient care by early detection, treatment choice, and prognosis.

4.1. Prediction of Therapeutic Outcomes in Schizophrenia

Despite the established pharmacological treatments for schizophrenia, up to 50% of the patients develop poor disease outcomes [172,173]. Stratifying treatment through the early recognition of outcome indicators might alleviate unfavorable disease progression in these patients [174,175]. Group-level studies have discovered many potential outcome predictors, such as disease course variables, treatment adherence and response, comorbidity, and cognitive impairments [176]. It remains unclear which of these characteristics should be combined for prediction, whether these group-level findings can be used to generate significant predictions for individual patients, or how accurate these predictions might be at another sites. Furthermore, the outcome can be not merely defined by symptomatic remission, but has to include various concepts that focus on restored functioning to widely cover treatment effects [177].

Large multisite treatment databases containing prospective phenotypic data of psychiatric disorders, such as the European First Episode Schizophrenia Trial (EUFEST), enable us to develop powerful machine learning methods to reliably predict treatment outcomes. By using data from EUFEST, the pooled non-linear SVMs predicted patients' 4-week and 52-week outcomes with cross-validated balanced accuracies (BAC) of 75.0% and 73.8%, respectively [34]. This non-linear SVMs surpassed linear SVMs, univariate and multivariate logistic regression, and decision tree ensembles. Intriguingly, the most useful predictors of poor 4-week and 52-week treatment outcome were unemployment, daytime activities, psychological distress, educational difficulties, low educational status of the patient and patient's mother. In patients with good 52-week prognosis, haloperidol was linked with shorter adherence compared with ziprasidone, amisulpride, and olanzapine due to insufficient response and side effects. Olanzapine and amisulpride were associated with higher global assessment of functioning (GAF) scores than quetiapine [34].

Recent machine learning methods have revealed that functional striatal abnormalities (FSA) are significantly correlated with a spectrum of severity across psychiatric disorders, where dysfunction is most severe in schizophrenia, milder in bipolar disorder, and indistinguishable from individuals in obsessive-compulsive disorder (OCD), depression, and ADHD [178]. FSA scores provide a personalized index of striatal dysfunction and distinguish individuals with schizophrenia from healthy controls with an accuracy exceeding 80% (sensitivity, 79.3%; specificity, 81.5%). FSA scores are also significantly linked with antipsychotic treatment response. Interestingly, clozapine, the only drug approved for treatment-resistant schizophrenia, is not associated with FSA scores. This may suggest that FSA can characterize treatment response across different types of antipsychotics, preferentially the types with lower Meltzer's ratio (5-HT2A/D2 affinity ratio) [178].

4.2. Prediction of Therapeutic Outcomes in Depression

Antidepressant medication is the first option for the treatment of MDD. However, remission rates are approximately 30% to 55% after first or second medication trials and then drop with subsequent medication trials [168]. Thus, the patients experience trial and error periods with different treatments before finding the optimal one. One solution is to identify the biological predictors of response to an antidepressant. This may expedite the treatment and lead to faster relief of the symptoms.

Electroencephalography (EEG) and fMRI have been used for predicting treatment response in MDD patients [179–181]. Since EEG is relatively more available and cost-effective than fMRI, it is a good option for developing such treatment biomarkers. The accumulated findings suggest that EEG-derived features before treatment may predict clinical response to antidepressants [182,183]. Several EEG studies have shown that characteristics of resting-state neural oscillations, especially in alpha and theta bands, may predict the drug response [184–188]. For instance, posterior alpha activity is associated with response to amitriptyline and fluoxetine [189,190]; theta activity with imipramine, venlafaxine, and several selective serotonin reuptake inhibitors (SSRI) [188,191,192]; interhemispheric delta asymmetry with fluoxetine [193]; delta activity with paroxetine and imipramine [188,194]; delta activity in rostral anterior cingulate cortex with nortriptyline, venlafaxine, and fluoxetine [195,196]; nonlinear features of EEG signals with clomipramine, escitalopram, citalopram, bupropion, and mirtazapine [197–199].

Although resting-state EEG can be useful for predicting drug response, the aforementioned studies fail to address several questions that are important for translating this finding into a clinical tool. First, they use small and homogeneous sample sets. Second, most of them report low prediction accuracy. Third, their prediction accuracies are biased upward by the lack of an independent testing set. One of the most powerful methods for addressing these questions is applying machine learning techniques. Zhdanov et al. used a SVM classifier to predict EEG-derived escitalopram treatment outcome using data from a large, Canada-wide, multicenter study, the first Canadian Biomarker Integration Network in Depression (CAN-BIND-1) study [200]. This classifier identified responders with an estimated balanced accuracy of 79.2% (sensitivity, 67.3%; specificity, 91.0%) when using EEG data recorded before the treatment, whereas additional EEG data after first 2 weeks of treatment increased the accuracy to 82.4% (sensitivity, 79.2%; specificity, 85.5%). In rTMS, Hasanzadeh et al. used k-nearest neighbors (KNN) classifier to predict its EEG-derived treatment response in MDD [201]. Using beta bands, this classifier discriminated between responders and non-responders to rTMS treatment with the accuracy of 91.3% (sensitivity, 91.3%; specificity, 91.3%) when resting-state EEG data from 46 MDD patients were used.

5. Conclusions

The infusion of economic and machine learning framework into neuroscience has rapidly advanced our understanding of neural mechanisms for various cognitive processes including decision-making. Because flawed decision-making is the most prominent symptoms in numerous psychiatric disorders, it is essential for neuroscientists and psychiatrists to combine their expertise to develop more effective treatment. They also need to redefine mental illness to meet biological and pathological evidence as seen in the RDoC initiative, while DSM/ICD manuals often reflect public values, such as the definition of sexual identity disorders and the advent of internet gaming disorder [202,203], and have been frequently revised so far. Since substantial progress in major mental illness research has been made in understanding the molecular mechanisms through basic and translational approaches, including cell and animal models, those types of big data may also be helpful for reinforcing weakness of RDoC [204]. Following the growing data richness and changing research questions, machine learning or deep learning algorithms could enable clinical translation of empirically trusted prediction for individual patients in a fast, cost-effective, and practical manner. Such artificial intelligence algorithms may be particularly tuned to precision psychiatry because they can directly translate large-scale multidimensional data into clinical relevance. From a long-term and larger perspective, it is particularly challenging to verbalize mechanistic hypotheses for mental disorders at the abstraction level, ranging from molecular mechanisms to urbanization trends in society. Individual consumer decision patterns would be useful for this purpose. Ultimately, we may more effectively impact psychiatric disorders that arise from the interplay between genetic vulnerability and life experience, both of which are unique to each individual.

Author Contributions: H.K. conceived the idea and wrote the manuscript. E.W. and M.F. depicted the figures and table. All authors have read and agreed to the published version of the manuscript.

Funding: This research received no external funding.

Institutional Review Board Statement: Not applicable.

Informed Consent Statement: Not applicable.

Data Availability Statement: Data sharing not applicable. No new data were created or analyzed in this study.

Acknowledgments: We would like to thank Abul K. Azad and Wei-hsuan Yu for reviewing this manuscript.

Conflicts of Interest: The authors declare no conflict of interest.

References

1. Pontzer, H.; Brown, M.H.; Raichlen, D.A.; Dunsworth, H.; Hare, B.; Walker, K.; Luke, A.; Dugas, L.R.; Durazo-Arvizu, R.; Schoeller, D.; et al. Metabolic acceleration and the evolution of human brain size and life history. *Nat. Cell Biol.* **2016**, *533*, 390–392. [CrossRef] [PubMed]
2. Gomez-Marin, A.; Ghazanfar, A.A. The Life of Behavior. *Neuron* **2019**, *104*, 25–36. [CrossRef] [PubMed]
3. Ferguson, B.R.; Gao, W.-J. PV Interneurons: Critical Regulators of E/I Balance for Prefrontal Cortex-Dependent Behavior and Psychiatric Disorders. *Front. Neural Circuits* **2018**, *12*, 37. [CrossRef] [PubMed]
4. Chowdhury, S.M. The attack and defense mechanisms: Perspectives from behavioral economics and game theory. *Behav. Brain Sci.* **2019**, *42*, e121. [CrossRef]
5. Robalino, N.; Robson, A. The economic approach to 'theory of mind'. *Philos. Trans. R. Soc. Lond. B Biol. Sci.* **2012**, *367*, 2224–2233. [CrossRef]
6. Brosnan, S.F.; Jones, O.D.; Lambeth, S.P.; Mareno, M.C.; Richardson, A.S.; Schapiro, S.J. Endowment Effects in Chimpanzees. *Curr. Biol.* **2007**, *17*, 1704–1707. [CrossRef]
7. Lakshminaryanan, V.; Chen, M.K.; Santos, L.R. Endowment effect in capuchin monkeys. *Philos. Trans. R. Soc. B Biol. Sci.* **2008**, *363*, 3837–3844. [CrossRef]
8. Santos, L.R.; Hughes, K.D. Economic cognition in humans and animals: The search for core mechanisms. *Curr. Opin. Neurobiol.* **2009**, *19*, 63–66. [CrossRef]
9. Camerer, C.F. Behavioural studies of strategic thinking in games. *Trends Cogn. Sci.* **2003**, *7*, 225–231. [CrossRef]
10. Camerer, C.F. Psychology and economics. Strategizing in the brain. *Science* **2003**, *300*, 1673–1675. [CrossRef]

11. Mackintosh, N.J. Varieties of perceptual learning. *Learn. Behav.* **2009**, *37*, 119–125. [CrossRef]
12. Laurent, P.A. The emergence of saliency and novelty responses from Reinforcement Learning principles. *Neural Netw.* **2008**, *21*, 1493–1499. [CrossRef]
13. Liao, S.M. Neuroscience and Ethics. *Exp. Psychol.* **2017**, *64*, 82–92. [CrossRef]
14. Jones, O.D.; Marois, R.; Farah, M.J.; Greely, H.T. Law and Neuroscience. *J. Neurosci.* **2013**, *33*, 17624–17630. [CrossRef]
15. Arciniegas, D.B.; Anderson, C.A. Toward a Neuroscience of Politics. *J. Neuropsychiatry Clin. Neurosci.* **2017**, *29*, 84–85. [CrossRef]
16. Appleton, K.M.; Bray, J.; Price, S.; Liebchen, G.; Jiang, N.; Mavridis, I.; Saulais, L.; Giboreau, A.; Perez-Cueto, F.J.A.; Coolen, R.; et al. A Mobile Phone App for the Provision of Personalized Food-Based Information in an Eating-Out Situation: Development and Initial Evaluation. *JMIR Form. Res.* **2019**, *3*, e12966. [CrossRef]
17. Frydman, C.; Camerer, C.F. The Psychology and Neuroscience of Financial Decision Making. *Trends Cogn. Sci.* **2016**, *20*, 661–675. [CrossRef]
18. Padoa-Schioppa, C.; Conen, K.E. Orbitofrontal Cortex: A Neural Circuit for Economic Decisions. *Neuron* **2017**, *96*, 736–754. [CrossRef]
19. Rosenberg, A.; Patterson, J.S.; Angelaki, D.E. A computational perspective on autism. *Proc. Natl. Acad. Sci. USA* **2015**, *112*, 9158–9165. [CrossRef]
20. Dayan, P.; Niv, Y.; Seymour, B.; Daw, N.D. The misbehavior of value and the discipline of the will. *Neural Netw.* **2006**, *19*, 1153–1160. [CrossRef]
21. Rangel, A.; Camerer, C.F.; Montague, P.R. A framework for studying the neurobiology of value-based decision making. *Nat. Rev. Neurosci.* **2008**, *9*, 545–556. [CrossRef] [PubMed]
22. Lee, D.; Seo, H.; Jung, M.W. Neural Basis of Reinforcement Learning and Decision Making. *Annu. Rev. Neurosci.* **2012**, *35*, 287–308. [CrossRef] [PubMed]
23. Van Der Meer, M.; Kurth-Nelson, Z.; Redish, A.D. Information Processing in Decision-Making Systems. *Neuroscience* **2012**, *18*, 342–359. [CrossRef] [PubMed]
24. Delgado, M.R.; Dickerson, K.C. Reward-Related Learning via Multiple Memory Systems. *Biol. Psychiatry* **2012**, *72*, 134–141. [CrossRef]
25. Hyman, S.E. Can neuroscience be integrated into the DSM-V? *Nat. Rev. Neurosci.* **2007**, *8*, 725–732. [CrossRef]
26. Sharp, C.; Monterosso, J.; Montague, P.R. Neuroeconomics: A Bridge for Translational Research. *Biol. Psychiatry* **2012**, *72*, 87–92. [CrossRef]
27. Kelly, J.R.; Clarke, G.; Cryan, J.F.; Dinan, T.G. Dimensional thinking in psychiatry in the era of the Research Domain Criteria (RDoC). *Ir. J. Psychol. Med.* **2017**, *35*, 89–94. [CrossRef]
28. Cuthbert, B.N. The RDoC framework: Facilitating transition from ICD/DSM to dimensional approaches that integrate neuroscience and psychopathology. *World Psychiatry* **2014**, *13*, 28–35. [CrossRef]
29. Insel, T.; Cuthbert, B.; Garvey, M.; Heinssen, R.; Pine, D.S.; Quinn, K.; Sanislow, C.; Wang, P. Research Domain Criteria (RDoC): Toward a New Classification Framework for Research on Mental Disorders. *Am. J. Psychiatry* **2010**, *167*, 748–751. [CrossRef]
30. Tai, A.M.; Albuquerque, A.; Carmona, N.E.; Subramanieapillai, M.; Cha, D.S.; Sheko, M.; Lee, Y.; Mansur, R.; McIntyre, R.S. Machine learning and big data: Implications for disease modeling and therapeutic discovery in psychiatry. *Artif. Intell. Med.* **2019**, *99*, 101704. [CrossRef]
31. Galatzer-Levy, I.R.; Ruggles, K.V.; Chen, Z. Data Science in the Research Domain Criteria Era: Relevance of Machine Learning to the Study of Stress Pathology, Recovery, and Resilience. *Chronic Stress* **2018**, 2. [CrossRef]
32. Koutsouleris, N.; Riecher-Rössler, A.; Meisenzahl, E.M.; Smieskova, R.; Studerus, E.; Kambeitz-Ilankovic, L.; Von Saldern, S.; Cabral, C.; Reiser, M.; Falkai, P.; et al. Detecting the Psychosis Prodrome Across High-Risk Populations Using Neuroanatomical Biomarkers. *Schizophr. Bull.* **2014**, *41*, 471–482. [CrossRef]
33. Chekroud, A.M.; Zotti, R.J.; Shehzad, Z.; Gueorguieva, R.; Johnson, M.K.; Trivedi, M.H.; Cannon, T.D.; Krystal, J.H.; Corlett, P.R. Cross-trial prediction of treatment outcome in depression: A machine learning approach. *Lancet Psychiatry* **2016**, *3*, 243–250. [CrossRef]
34. Koutsouleris, N.; Kahn, R.S.; Chekroud, A.M.; Leucht, S.; Falkai, P.; Wobrock, T.; Derks, E.M.; Fleischhacker, W.W.; Hasan, A. Multisite prediction of 4-week and 52-week treatment outcomes in patients with first-episode psychosis: A machine learning approach. *Lancet Psychiatry* **2016**, *3*, 935–946. [CrossRef]
35. Cáceda, R.; Nemeroff, C.B.; Harvey, P.D. Toward an Understanding of Decision Making in Severe Mental Illness. *J. Neuropsychiatry Clin. Neurosci.* **2014**, *26*, 196–213. [CrossRef]
36. Blackwell, R.D.; Miniard, P.W.; Engel, J.F. *Consumer Behavior*, 9th ed.; Harcourt College Publishers: Ft. Worth, TX, USA, 2001; p. 570.
37. Ammerman, W. *The Invisible Brand: Marketing in the Age of Automation, Big Data, and Machine Learning*; McGraw-Hill Education: New York, NY, USA, 2019; p. xiv.
38. Gandal, M.J.; Haney, J.R.; Parikshak, N.N.; Leppa, V.; Ramaswami, G.; Hartl, C.; Schork, A.J.; Appadurai, V.; Buil, A.; Werge, T.M.; et al. Shared molecular neuropathology across major psychiatric disorders parallels polygenic overlap. *Science* **2018**, *359*, 693–697. [CrossRef] [PubMed]
39. Kishida, K.T.; King-Casas, B.; Montague, P.R. Neuroeconomic Approaches to Mental Disorders. *Neuron* **2010**, *67*, 543–554. [CrossRef]

40. Hasler, G. Can the neuroeconomics revolution revolutionize psychiatry? *Neurosci. Biobehav. Rev.* **2012**, *36*, 64–78. [CrossRef]
41. Montague, P.R.; Dolan, R.J.; Friston, K.J.; Dayan, P. Computational psychiatry. *Trends Cogn. Sci.* **2012**, *16*, 72–80. [CrossRef]
42. Morningstar, J. The Mind Within the Brain: How We Make Decisions and How Those Decisions Go Wrong. *Libr. J.* **2013**, *138*, 94.
43. Andreasen, N.C.; Carpenter, W.T. Diagnosis and Classification of Schizophrenia. *Schizophr. Bull.* **1993**, *19*, 199–214. [CrossRef] [PubMed]
44. Lewis, D.A. Cortical circuit dysfunction and cognitive deficits in schizophrenia—implications for preemptive interventions. *Eur. J. Neurosci.* **2012**, *35*, 1871–1878. [CrossRef] [PubMed]
45. Barch, D.M.; Ceaser, A. Cognition in schizophrenia: Core psychological and neural mechanisms. *Trends Cogn. Sci.* **2012**, *16*, 27–34. [CrossRef] [PubMed]
46. Weinberger, D.R.; Berman, K.F.; Zec, R.F. Physiologic dysfunction of dorsolateral prefrontal cortex in schizophrenia. I. Regional cerebral blood flow evidence. *Arch. Gen. Psychiatry* **1986**, *43*, 114–124. [CrossRef]
47. Heerey, E.A.; Bell-Warren, K.R.; Gold, J.M. Decision-Making Impairments in the Context of Intact Reward Sensitivity in Schizophrenia. *Biol. Psychiatry* **2008**, *64*, 62–69. [CrossRef]
48. Waltz, J.A.; Frank, M.J.; Robinson, B.M.; Gold, J.M. Selective Reinforcement Learning Deficits in Schizophrenia Support Predictions from Computational Models of Striatal-Cortical Dysfunction. *Biol. Psychiatry* **2007**, *62*, 756–764. [CrossRef]
49. Strauss, G.P.; Frank, M.J.; Waltz, J.A.; Kasanova, Z.; Herbener, E.S.; Gold, J.M. Deficits in Positive Reinforcement Learning and Uncertainty-Driven Exploration Are Associated with Distinct Aspects of Negative Symptoms in Schizophrenia. *Biol. Psychiatry* **2011**, *69*, 424–431. [CrossRef]
50. Corlett, P.R.; Murray, G.K.; Honey, G.D.; Aitken, M.R.F.; Shanks, D.R.; Robbins, T.; Bullmore, E.; Dickinson, A.; Fletcher, P.C. Disrupted prediction-error signal in psychosis: Evidence for an associative account of delusions. *Brain* **2007**, *130*, 2387–2400. [CrossRef]
51. Gradin, V.B.; Kumar, P.; Waiter, G.; Ahearn, T.; Stickle, C.; Milders, M.; Reid, I.; Hall, J.; Steele, J.D. Expected value and prediction error abnormalities in depression and schizophrenia. *Brain* **2011**, *134*, 1751–1764. [CrossRef]
52. Volkow, N.D. Substance Use Disorders in Schizophrenia—Clinical Implications of Comorbidity. *Schizophr. Bull.* **2009**, *35*, 469–472. [CrossRef]
53. Goff, D.C.; Henderson, D.C.; Amico, E. Cigarette smoking in schizophrenia: Relationship to psychopathology and med-ication side effects. *Am. J. Psychiatry* **1992**, *149*, 1189–1194. [PubMed]
54. De Leon, J.; Dadvand, M.; Canuso, C.; White, A.O.; Stanilla, J.K.; Simpson, G.M. Schizophrenia and smoking: An epi-demiological survey in a state hospital. *Am. J. Psychiatry* **1995**, *152*, 453–455. [PubMed]
55. Krystal, J.H.; D'Souza, D.C.; Gallinat, J.; Driesen, N.; Abi-Dargham, A.; Petrakis, I.; Heinz, A.; Pearlson, G. The vulner-ability to alcohol and substance abuse in individuals diagnosed with schizophrenia. *Neurotox. Res.* **2006**, *10*, 235–252. [CrossRef] [PubMed]
56. Harvey, P.D.; Wingo, A.P.; Burdick, K.E.; Baldessarini, R.J. Cognition and disability in bipolar disorder: Lessons from schizophrenia research. *Bipolar Disord.* **2010**, *12*, 364–375. [CrossRef]
57. Martino, D.J.; Strejilevich, S.A.; Scápola, M.; Igoa, A.; Marengo, E.; Ais, E.D.; Perinot, L. Heterogeneity in cognitive functioning among patients with bipolar disorder. *J. Affect. Disord.* **2008**, *109*, 149–156. [CrossRef]
58. Gruber, J. A Review and Synthesis of Positive Emotion and Reward Disturbance in Bipolar Disorder. *Clin. Psychol. Psychother.* **2011**, *18*, 356–365. [CrossRef]
59. Samame, C.; Martino, D.J.; Strejilevich, S.A. Social cognition in euthymic bipolar disorder: Systematic review and me-ta-analytic approach. *Acta Psychiatr. Scand.* **2012**, *125*, 266–280. [CrossRef]
60. Robinson, L.J.; Thompson, J.M.; Gallagher, P.; Goswami, U.; Young, A.H.; Ferrier, I.N.; Moore, P.B. A meta-analysis of cognitive deficits in euthymic patients with bipolar disorder. *J. Affect. Disord.* **2006**, *93*, 105–115. [CrossRef]
61. Thompson, J.M.; Gallagher, P.; Hughes, J.H.; Watson, S.; Gray, J.M.; Ferrier, I.N.; Young, A.H. Neurocognitive im-pairment in euthymic patients with bipolar affective disorder. *Br. J. Psychiatry* **2005**, *186*, 32–40. [CrossRef]
62. Torres, I.J.; Boudreau, V.G.; Yatham, L.N. Neuropsychological functioning in euthymic bipolar disorder: A meta-analysis. *Acta Psychiatr. Scand.* **2007**, *116*, 17–26. [CrossRef]
63. Rau, G.; Blair, K.S.; Berghorst, L.; Knopf, L.; Skup, M.; Luckenbaugh, D.A.; Pine, D.S.; Blair, R.J.; Leibenluft, E. Processing of Differentially Valued Rewards and Punishments in Youths with Bipolar Disorder or Severe Mood Dysregulation. *J. Child. Adolesc. Psychopharmacol.* **2008**, *18*, 185–196. [CrossRef]
64. Ernst, M.; Dickstein, D.P.; Munson, S.; Eshel, N.; Pradella, A.; Jazbec, S.; Pine, D.S.; Leibenluft, E. Reward-related pro-cesses in pediatric bipolar disorder: A pilot study. *J. Affect. Disord.* **2004**, *82* (Suppl. 1), S89–S101. [CrossRef]
65. Kovacs, M.; Devlin, B. Internalizing disorders in childhood. *J. Child Psychol. Psychiatry* **1998**, *39*, 47–63. [CrossRef]
66. Krueger, R.F. Internalization and Externalization and the Structure of Common Mental Disorders. *Psycextra Dataset* **2004**, *56*, 921–926. [CrossRef]
67. Mineka, S.; Watson, D.; Clark, L.A. Comorbidity of anxiety and unipolar mood disorders. *Annu. Rev. Psychol.* **1998**, *49*, 377–412. [CrossRef]
68. Paulus, M.P.; Yu, A.J. Emotion and decision-making: Affect-driven belief systems in anxiety and depression. *Trends Cogn. Sci.* **2012**, *16*, 476–483. [CrossRef] [PubMed]
69. Nolen-Hoeksema, S. The role of rumination in depressive disorders and mixed anxiety/depressive symptoms. *J. Abnorm. Psychol.* **2000**, *109*, 504–511. [CrossRef]

70. Eshel, N.; Roiser, J.P. Reward and Punishment Processing in Depression. *Biol. Psychiatry* **2010**, *68*, 118–124. [CrossRef]
71. Craske, M.G.; Rauch, S.L.; Ursano, R.; Prenoveau, J.; Pine, D.S.; Zinbarg, R.E. What is an anxiety disorder? *Depress. Anxiety* **2009**, *26*, 1066–1085. [CrossRef]
72. Hartley, C.A.; Phelps, E.A. Anxiety and Decision-Making. *Biol. Psychiatry* **2012**, *72*, 113–118. [CrossRef]
73. Sheline, Y.I.; Barch, D.M.; Price, J.L.; Rundle, M.M.; Vaishnavi, S.N.; Snyder, A.Z.; Mintun, M.A.; Wang, S.; Coalson, R.S.; Raichle, M.E. The default mode network and self-referential processes in depression. *Proc. Natl. Acad. Sci. USA* **2009**, *106*, 1942–1947. [CrossRef]
74. Mayberg, H.S.; Lozano, A.M.; Voon, V.; McNeely, H.E.; Seminowicz, D.; Hamani, C.; Schwalb, J.M.; Kennedy, S.H. Deep brain stimulation for treatment-resistant depression. *Neuron* **2005**, *45*, 651–660. [CrossRef] [PubMed]
75. Dayan, P.; Huys, Q.J.M. Serotonin in Affective Control. *Annu. Rev. Neurosci.* **2009**, *32*, 95–126. [CrossRef] [PubMed]
76. Doya, K. Metalearning and neuromodulation. *Neural Netw.* **2002**, *15*, 495–506. [CrossRef]
77. Daw, N.D.; Kakade, S.; Dayan, P. Opponent interactions between serotonin and dopamine. *Neural Netw.* **2002**, *15*, 603–616. [CrossRef]
78. Dayan, P.; Huys, Q.J. Serotonin, inhibition, and negative mood. *PLoS Comput. Biol.* **2008**, *4*, e4. [CrossRef]
79. Huys, Q.J.M.; Eshel, N.; O'Nions, E.; Sheridan, L.; Dayan, P.; Roiser, J.P. Bonsai Trees in Your Head: How the Pavlovian System Sculpts Goal-Directed Choices by Pruning Decision Trees. *PLoS Comput. Biol.* **2012**, *8*, e1002410. [CrossRef]
80. Geschwind, D.H.; Levitt, P. Autism spectrum disorders: Developmental disconnection syndromes. *Curr. Opin. Neurobiol.* **2007**, *17*, 103–111. [CrossRef]
81. Baron-Cohen, S.; Leslie, A.M.; Frith, U. Does the autistic child have a "theory of mind"? *Cognition* **1985**, *21*, 37–46. [CrossRef]
82. Frith, U. Mind Blindness and the Brain in Autism. *Neuron* **2001**, *32*, 969–979. [CrossRef]
83. Wiggins, L.D.; Rice, C.E.; Barger, B.; Soke, G.N.; Lee, L.-C.; Moody, E.; Edmondson-Pretzel, R.; Levy, S.E. DSM-5 criteria for autism spectrum disorder maximizes diagnostic sensitivity and specificity in preschool children. *Soc. Psychiatry Psychiatr. Epidemiol.* **2019**, *54*, 693–701. [CrossRef] [PubMed]
84. Hadjikhani, N.; Joseph, R.M.; Snyder, J.; Tager-Flusberg, H. Abnormal activation of the social brain during face perception in autism. *Hum. Brain Mapp.* **2006**, *28*, 441–449. [CrossRef] [PubMed]
85. Nebel, M.B.; Joel, S.E.; Muschelli, J.; Barber, A.D.; Caffo, B.S.; Pekar, J.J.; Mostofsky, S.H. Disruption of functional organization within the primary motor cortex in children with autism. *Hum. Brain Mapp.* **2012**, *35*, 567–580. [CrossRef] [PubMed]
86. Staples, K.L.; Reid, G. Fundamental Movement Skills and Autism Spectrum Disorders. *J. Autism Dev. Disord.* **2010**, *40*, 209–217. [CrossRef]
87. Breveglieri, R.; Galletti, C.; Gamberini, M.; Passarelli, L.; Fattori, P. Somatosensory Cells in Area PEc of Macaque Posterior Parietal Cortex. *J. Neurosci.* **2006**, *26*, 3679–3684. [CrossRef]
88. Courchesne, E. Brainstem, cerebellar and limbic neuroanatomical abnormalities in autism. *Curr. Opin. Neurobiol.* **1997**, *7*, 269–278. [CrossRef]
89. Frith, U. *Autism: Explaining the Enigma*, 2nd ed.; Blackwell Pub.: New York, NY, USA, 2003.
90. Müller, R.-A.; Kleinhans, N.; Kemmotsu, N.; Pierce, K.; Courchesne, E. Abnormal Variability and Distribution of Functional Maps in Autism: An fMRI Study of Visuomotor Learning. *Am. J. Psychiatry* **2003**, *160*, 1847–1862. [CrossRef]
91. Hadjikhani, N.; Joseph, R.M.; Snyder, J.; Tager-Flusberg, H. Anatomical Differences in the Mirror Neuron System and Social Cognition Network in Autism. *Cereb. Cortex* **2005**, *16*, 1276–1282. [CrossRef]
92. Williams, J.; Whiten, A.; Suddendorf, T.; Perrett, D. Imitation, mirror neurons and autism. *Neurosci. Biobehav. Rev.* **2001**, *25*, 287–295. [CrossRef]
93. Baron-Cohen, S.; Ring, H.; Bullmore, E.; Wheelwright, S.; Ashwin, C.; Williams, S. The amygdala theory of autism. *Neurosci. Biobehav. Rev.* **2000**, *24*, 355–364. [CrossRef]
94. Brothers, L. Brain mechanisms of social cognition. *J. Psychopharmacol.* **1996**, *10*, 2–8. [CrossRef]
95. Ernst, M.; Bolla, K.; Mouratidis, M.; Contoreggi, C.; Matochik, J.A.; Kurian, V.; Cadet, J.-L.; Kimes, A.S.; London, E.D. Decision-making in a Risk-taking Task A PET Study. *Neuropsychopharmacol.* **2002**, *26*, 682–691. [CrossRef]
96. Bar-On, R.; Tranel, D.; Denburg, N.L.; Bechara, A. Exploring the neurological substrate of emotional and social intelli-gence. *Brain* **2003**, *126*, 1790–1800. [CrossRef]
97. Bechara, A. The role of emotion in decision-making: Evidence from neurological patients with orbitofrontal damage. *Brain Cogn.* **2004**, *55*, 30–40. [CrossRef]
98. Cao, H.; Plichta, M.M.; Schafer, A.; Haddad, L.; Grimm, O.; Schneider, M.; Esslinger, C.; Kirsch, P.; Meyer-Lindenberg, A.; Tost, H. Test-retest reliability of fMRI-based graph theoretical properties during working memory, emotion processing, and resting state. *NeuroImage* **2014**, *84*, 888–900. [CrossRef]
99. Drysdale, A.T.; Grosenick, L.; Downar, J.; Dunlop, K.; Mansouri, F.; Meng, Y.; Fetcho, R.N.; Zebley, B.; Oathes, D.J.; Etkin, A.; et al. Resting-state connectivity biomarkers define neurophysio-logical subtypes of depression. *Nat. Med.* **2017**, *23*, 28–38. [CrossRef]
100. Sundermann, B.; Feder, S.; Wersching, H.; Teuber, A.; Schwindt, W.; Kugel, H.; Heindel, W.; Arolt, V.; Berger, K.; Pfleiderer, B. Diagnostic classification of unipolar depression based on resting-state functional connectivity MRI: Effects of generali-zation to a diverse sample. *J. Neural. Transm.* **2017**, *124*, 589–605. [CrossRef]
101. Kupfer, D.J.; Frank, E.; Phillips, M.L. Major depressive disorder: New clinical, neurobiological, and treatment perspectives. *Lancet* **2012**, *379*, 1045–1055. [CrossRef]

102. Baker, J.T.; Holmes, A.J.; Masters, G.A.; Yeo, B.T.T.; Krienen, F.; Buckner, R.L.; Öngür, D. Disruption of Cortical Association Networks in Schizophrenia and Psychotic Bipolar Disorder. *JAMA Psychiatry* **2014**, *71*, 109–118. [CrossRef]
103. Harrison, B.J.; Soriano-Mas, C.; Pujol, J.; Ortiz, H.; Lopez-Sola, M.; Hernandez-Ribas, R.; Deus, J.; Alonso, P.; Yucel, M.; Pantelis, C.; et al. Altered corticostriatal functional connectivity in obsessive-compulsive disorder. *Arch. Gen. Psychiatry* **2009**, *66*, 1189–1200. [CrossRef]
104. Kaiser, R.H.; Andrews-Hanna, J.R.; Wager, T.D.; Pizzagalli, D.A. Large-Scale Network Dysfunction in Major Depressive Disorder: A Meta-analysis of Resting-State Functional Connectivity. *JAMA Psychiatry* **2015**, *72*, 603–611. [CrossRef]
105. Yahata, N.; Morimoto, J.; Hashimoto, R.; Lisi, G.; Shibata, K.; Kawakubo, Y.; Kuwabara, H.; Kuroda, M.; Yamada, T.; Megumi, F.; et al. A small number of abnormal brain connections predicts adult autism spectrum disorder. *Nat. Commun.* **2016**, *7*, 11254. [CrossRef]
106. Shaposhnyk, V.; Villa, A.E. Reciprocal projections in hierarchically organized evolvable neural circuits affect EEG-like signals. *Brain Res.* **2012**, *1434*, 266–276. [CrossRef]
107. Baldassarre, A.; Lewis, C.M.; Committeri, G.; Snyder, A.Z.; Romani, G.L.; Corbetta, M. Individual variability in functional connectivity predicts performance of a perceptual task. *Proc. Natl. Acad. Sci. USA* **2012**, *109*, 3516–3521. [CrossRef]
108. Dosenbach, N.U.F.; Nardos, B.; Cohen, A.L.; Fair, D.A.; Power, J.D.; Church, J.A.; Nelson, S.M.; Wig, G.S.; Vogel, A.C.; Lessov-Schlaggar, C.N.; et al. Prediction of Individual Brain Maturity Using fMRI. *Science* **2010**, *329*, 1358–1361. [CrossRef]
109. Lewis, C.M.; Baldassarre, A.; Committeri, G.; Romani, G.L.; Corbetta, M. Learning sculpts the spontaneous activity of the resting human brain. *Proc. Natl. Acad. Sci. USA* **2009**, *106*, 17558–17563. [CrossRef]
110. Seeley, W.W.; Menon, V.; Schatzberg, A.F.; Keller, J.; Glover, G.H.; Kenna, H.; Reiss, A.L.; Greicius, M.D. Dissociable Intrinsic Connectivity Networks for Salience Processing and Executive Control. *J. Neurosci.* **2007**, *27*, 2349–2356. [CrossRef]
111. Finn, E.S.; Shen, X.; Scheinost, D.; Rosenberg, M.D.; Huang, J.; Chun, M.M.; Papademetris, X.; Constable, R.T. Functional connectome fingerprinting: Identifying individuals using patterns of brain connectivity. *Nat. Neurosci.* **2015**, *18*, 1664–1671. [CrossRef]
112. Rosenberg, M.D.; Finn, E.S.; Scheinost, D.; Papademetris, X.; Shen, X.; Constable, R.T.; Chun, M.M. A neuromarker of sustained attention from whole-brain functional connectivity. *Nat. Neurosci.* **2016**, *19*, 165–171. [CrossRef]
113. Smith, S.M.; Nichols, T.E.; Vidaurre, D.; Winkler, A.M.; Behrens, T.E.J.; Glasser, M.F.; Ugurbil, K.; Barch, D.M.; Van Essen, D.C.; Miller, K.L. A positive-negative mode of population covariation links brain connectivity, demographics and behavior. *Nat. Neurosci.* **2015**, *18*, 1565–1567. [CrossRef]
114. Yamashita, M.; Kawato, M.; Imamizu, H. Predicting learning plateau of working memory from whole-brain intrinsic network connectivity patterns. *Sci. Rep.* **2015**, *5*, 7622. [CrossRef] [PubMed]
115. Yamashita, M.; Yoshihara, Y.; Hashimoto, R.; Yahata, N.; Ichikawa, N.; Sakai, Y.; Yamada, T.; Matsukawa, N.; Okada, G.; Tanaka, S.C.; et al. A prediction model of working memory across health and psychiatric disease using whole-brain functional connectivity. *eLife* **2018**, *7*, e38844. [CrossRef] [PubMed]
116. Yoshihara, Y.; Lisi, G.; Yahata, N.; Fujino, J.; Matsumoto, Y.; Miyata, J.; Sugihara, G.-I.; Urayama, S.-I.; Kubota, M.; Yamashita, M.; et al. Overlapping but Asymmetrical Relationships Between Schizophrenia and Autism Revealed by Brain Connectivity. *Schizophr. Bull.* **2020**, *46*, 1210–1218. [CrossRef] [PubMed]
117. Ichikawa, N.; Lisi, G.; Yahata, N.; Okada, G.; Takamura, M.; Hashimoto, R.I.; Yamada, T.; Yamada, M.; Suhara, T.; Moriguchi, S.; et al. Primary functional brain connections associated with melancholic major depressive disorder and modulation by antidepressants. *Sci. Rep.* **2020**, *10*, 3542. [CrossRef]
118. Ecker, C.; Marquand, A.; Mourao-Miranda, J.; Johnston, P.; Daly, E.M.; Brammer, M.J.; Maltezos, S.; Murphy, C.M.; Robertson, D.; Williams, S.C.; et al. Describing the brain in autism in five dimensions–magnetic resonance im-aging-assisted diagnosis of autism spectrum disorder using a multiparameter classification approach. *J. Neurosci.* **2010**, *30*, 10612–10623. [CrossRef]
119. Ecker, C.; Rocha-Rego, V.; Johnston, P.; Mourao-Miranda, J.; Marquand, A.; Daly, E.M.; Brammer, M.J.; Murphy, C.; Murphy, D.G. Investigating the predictive value of whole-brain structural MR scans in autism: A pattern classification approach. *NeuroImage* **2010**, *49*, 44–56. [CrossRef]
120. Uddin, L.Q.; Menon, V.; Young, C.B.; Ryali, S.; Chen, T.; Khouzam, A.; Minshew, N.J.; Hardan, A.Y. Multivariate Searchlight Classification of Structural Magnetic Resonance Imaging in Children and Adolescents with Autism. *Biol. Psychiatry* **2011**, *70*, 833–841. [CrossRef]
121. Anderson, J.S.; Nielsen, J.A.; Froehlich, A.L.; DuBray, M.B.; Druzgal, T.J.; Cariello, A.N.; Cooperrider, J.R.; Zielinski, B.A.; Ravichandran, C.; Fletcher, P.T.; et al. Functional connectivity magnetic resonance imaging classification of autism. *Brain* **2011**, *134*, 3742–3754. [CrossRef]
122. Ingalhalikar, M.; Parker, D.; Bloy, L.; Roberts, T.P.; Verma, R. Diffusion based abnormality markers of pathology: Toward learned diagnostic prediction of ASD. *NeuroImage* **2011**, *57*, 918–927. [CrossRef]
123. Wang, H.; Chen, C.; Fushing, H. Extracting Multiscale Pattern Information of fMRI Based Functional Brain Connectivity with Application on Classification of Autism Spectrum Disorders. *PLoS ONE* **2012**, *7*, e45502. [CrossRef]
124. Edeshpande, G.; Libero, L.E.; Sreenivasan, K.R.; Deshpande, H.D.; Kana, R.K. Identification of neural connectivity signatures of autism using machine learning. *Front. Hum. Neurosci.* **2013**, *7*, 670. [CrossRef]
125. Tomasi, D.; Volkow, N.D. Gender differences in brain functional connectivity density. *Hum. Brain Mapp.* **2011**, *33*, 849–860. [CrossRef]

126. Klaassens, B.L.; Van Gorsel, H.C.; Khalili-Mahani, N.; Van Der Grond, J.; Wyman, B.T.; Whitcher, B.; Rombouts, S.A.; Van Gerven, J.M. Single-dose serotonergic stimulation shows widespread effects on functional brain connectivity. *NeuroImage* **2015**, *122*, 440–450. [CrossRef]
127. Friedman, L.; Glover, G.H.; Fbirn, C. Reducing interscanner variability of activation in a multicenter fMRI study: Con-trolling for signal-to-fluctuation-noise-ratio (SFNR) differences. *NeuroImage* **2006**, *33*, 471–481. [CrossRef]
128. Thulborn, K.R.; Chang, S.Y.; Shen, G.X.; Voyvodic, J.T. High-resolution echo-planar fMRI of human visual cortex at 3.0 tesla. *Nmr Biomed.* **1997**, *10*, 183–190. [CrossRef]
129. Van Dijk, K.R.A.; Hedden, T.; Venkataraman, A.; Evans, K.C.; Lazar, S.W.; Buckner, R.L. Intrinsic Functional Connectivity as a Tool for Human Connectomics: Theory, Properties, and Optimization. *J. Neurophysiol.* **2010**, *103*, 297–321. [CrossRef]
130. Whelan, R.; Garavan, H. When Optimism Hurts: Inflated Predictions in Psychiatric Neuroimaging. *Biol. Psychiatry* **2014**, *75*, 746–748. [CrossRef]
131. The IMAGEN Consortium; Whelan, R.J.; Watts, R.; Orr, C.A.; Althoff, R.R.; Artiges, E.; Banaschewski, T.; Barker, G.J.; Bokde, A.L.W.; Büchel, C.; et al. Neuropsychosocial profiles of current and future adolescent alcohol misusers. *Nat. Cell Biol.* **2014**, *512*, 185–189. [CrossRef]
132. Tu, P.-C.; Hsieh, J.-C.; Li, C.-T.; Bai, Y.-M.; Su, T.-P. Cortico-striatal disconnection within the cingulo-opercular network in schizophrenia revealed by intrinsic functional connectivity analysis: A resting fMRI study. *NeuroImage* **2012**, *59*, 238–247. [CrossRef]
133. Cross-Disorder Group of the Psychiatric Genomics Consortium. Identification of risk loci with shared effects on five major psychiatric disorders: A genome-wide analysis. *Lancet* **2013**, *381*, 1371–1379.
134. Geschwind, D.H.; Flint, J. Genetics and genomics of psychiatric disease. *Science* **2015**, *349*, 1489–1494. [CrossRef] [PubMed]
135. King, B.H.; Lord, C. Is schizophrenia on the autism spectrum? *Brain Res.* **2011**, *1380*, 34–41. [CrossRef] [PubMed]
136. Pinkham, A.E.; Hopfinger, J.B.; Pelphrey, K.A.; Piven, J.; Penn, D.L. Neural bases for impaired social cognition in schizophrenia and autism spectrum disorders. *Schizophr. Res.* **2008**, *99*, 164–175. [CrossRef]
137. Witten, D.M.; Tibshirani, R.; Hastie, T. A penalized matrix decomposition, with applications to sparse principal compo-nents and canonical correlation analysis. *Biostatistics* **2009**, *10*, 515–534. [CrossRef] [PubMed]
138. Yamashita, O.; Sato, M.-A.; Yoshioka, T.; Tong, F.; Kamitani, Y. Sparse estimation automatically selects voxels relevant for the decoding of fMRI activity patterns. *NeuroImage* **2008**, *42*, 1414–1429. [CrossRef] [PubMed]
139. Gaugler, T.; Klei, L.; Sanders, S.J.; Bodea, C.A.; Goldberg, A.P.; Lee, A.B.; Mahajan, M.C.; Manaa, D.; Pawitan, Y.; Reichert, J.G.; et al. Most genetic risk for autism resides with common variation. *Nat. Genet.* **2014**, *46*, 881–885. [CrossRef] [PubMed]
140. Sullivan, P.F.; Magnusson, C.; Reichenberg, A.; Boman, M.; Dalman, C.; Davidson, M.; Fruchter, E.; Hultman, C.M.; Lundberg, M.; Långström, N.; et al. Family History of Schizophrenia and Bipolar Disorder as Risk Factors for Autism. *Arch. Gen. Psychiatry* **2012**, *69*, 1099–1103. [CrossRef]
141. Arbabshirani, M.R.; Plis, S.; Sui, J.; Calhoun, V.D. Single subject prediction of brain disorders in neuroimaging: Promises and pitfalls. *NeuroImage* **2017**, *145*, 137–165. [CrossRef]
142. Akil, H.; Gordon, J.; Hen, R.; Javitch, J.; Mayberg, H.; McEwen, B.; Meaney, M.J.; Nestler, E.J. Treatment resistant de-pression: A multi-scale, systems biology approach. *Neurosci. Biobehav. Rev.* **2018**, *84*, 272–288. [CrossRef]
143. Kendler, K.S. The Diagnostic Validity of Melancholic Major Depression in a Population-Based Sample of Female Twins. *Arch. Gen. Psychiatry* **1997**, *54*, 299–304. [CrossRef]
144. Sun, N.; Li, Y.; Cai, Y.; Chen, J.; Shen, Y.; Sun, J.; Zhang, Z.; Zhang, J.; Wang, L.; Guo, L.; et al. A comparison of melancholic and nonmelan-cholic recurrent major depression in Han Chinese women. *Depress. Anxiety* **2012**, *29*, 4–9. [CrossRef]
145. Consortium, C. Sparse whole-genome sequencing identifies two loci for major depressive disorder. *Nature* **2015**, *523*, 588–591. [CrossRef]
146. Hyett, M.P.; Breakspear, M.J.; Friston, K.J.; Guo, C.C.; Parker, G.B. Disrupted Effective Connectivity of Cortical Systems Supporting Attention and Interoception in Melancholia. *JAMA Psychiatry* **2015**, *72*, 350–358. [CrossRef]
147. Greening, S.G.; Finger, E.C.; Mitchell, D.G. Parsing decision making processes in prefrontal cortex: Response inhibition, overcoming learned avoidance, and reversal learning. *NeuroImage* **2011**, *54*, 1432–1441. [CrossRef]
148. Dombrovski, A.Y.; Szanto, K.; Clark, L.; Aizenstein, H.J.; Chase, H.W.; Reynolds, C.F., 3rd; Siegle, G.J. Corticostria-tothalamic reward prediction error signals and executive control in late-life depression. *Psychol. Med.* **2015**, *45*, 1413–1424. [CrossRef]
149. Mascaro, J.S.; Rilling, J.K.; Negi, L.T.; Raison, C.L. Compassion meditation enhances empathic accuracy and related neural activity. *Soc. Cogn. Affect. Neurosci.* **2013**, *8*, 48–55. [CrossRef]
150. LeWinn, K.Z.; Strigo, I.A.; Connolly, C.G.; Ho, T.C.; Tymofiyeva, O.; Sacchet, M.D.; Weng, H.Y.; Blom, E.H.; Simmons, A.N.; Yang, T.T. An exploratory examination of reappraisal success in depressed adolescents: Preliminary evidence of functional differences in cognitive control brain regions. *J. Affect. Disord.* **2018**, *240*, 155–164. [CrossRef]
151. Ferrari, C.; Lega, C.; Vernice, M.; Tamietto, M.; Mende-Siedlecki, P.; Vecchi, T.; Todorov, A.; Cattaneo, Z. The Dorsomedial Prefrontal Cortex Plays a Causal Role in Integrating Social Impressions from Faces and Verbal Descriptions. *Cereb. Cortex* **2014**, *26*, 156–165. [CrossRef]
152. Mattavelli, G.; Cattaneo, Z.; Papagno, C. Transcranial magnetic stimulation of medial prefrontal cortex modulates face expressions processing in a priming task. *Neuropsychology* **2011**, *49*, 992–998. [CrossRef]

153. Jonides, J.; Nee, D. Brain mechanisms of proactive interference in working memory. *Neuroscience* **2006**, *139*, 181–193. [CrossRef]
154. Engels, A.S.; Heller, W.; Spielberg, J.M.; Warren, S.L.; Sutton, B.P.; Banich, M.T.; Miller, G.A. Co-occurring anxiety influences patterns of brain activity in depression. *Cogn. Affect. Behav. Neurosci.* **2010**, *10*, 141–156. [CrossRef] [PubMed]
155. Ardila, A.; Bernal, B.; Rosselli, M. How Localized are Language Brain Areas? A Review of Brodmann Areas Involvement in Oral Language. *Arch. Clin. Neuropsychol.* **2016**, *31*, 112–122. [CrossRef] [PubMed]
156. Pascual-Leone, A.; Rubio, B.; Pallardó, F.; Catalá, M.D. Rapid-rate transcranial magnetic stimulation of left dorsolateral prefrontal cortex in drug-resistant depression. *Lancet* **1996**, *348*, 233–237. [CrossRef]
157. Brzezicka, A.; Kamiński, J.; Kamińska, O.K.; Wołyńczyk-Gmaj, D.; Sedek, G. Frontal EEG alpha band asymmetry as a predictor of reasoning deficiency in depressed people. *Cogn. Emot.* **2016**, *31*, 868–878. [CrossRef]
158. Mennella, R.; Patron, E.; Palomba, D. Frontal alpha asymmetry neurofeedback for the reduction of negative affect and anxiety. *Behav. Res.* **2017**, *92*, 32–40. [CrossRef] [PubMed]
159. Zotev, V.; Yuan, H.; Misaki, M.; Phillips, R.; Young, K.D.; Feldner, M.T.; Bodurka, J. Correlation between amygdala BOLD activity and frontal EEG asymmetry during real-time fMRI neurofeedback training in patients with depression. *NeuroImage Clin.* **2016**, *11*, 224–238. [CrossRef] [PubMed]
160. Okada, G.; Okamoto, Y.; Morinobu, S.; Yamawaki, S.; Yokota, N. Attenuated Left Prefrontal Activation during a Verbal Fluency Task in Patients with Depression. *Neuropsychobiology* **2003**, *47*, 21–26. [CrossRef] [PubMed]
161. Takamura, M.; Okamoto, Y.; Okada, G.; Toki, S.; Yamamoto, T.; Yamamoto, O.; Jitsuiki, H.; Yokota, N.; Tamura, T.; Kurata, A.; et al. Disrupted Brain Activation and Deactivation Pattern during Semantic Verbal Fluency Task in Patients with Major Depression. *Neuropsychobiology* **2016**, *74*, 69–77. [CrossRef] [PubMed]
162. Chen, A.C.; Oathes, D.J.; Chang, C.; Bradley, T.; Zhou, Z.-W.; Williams, L.M.; Glover, G.H.; Deisseroth, K.; Etkin, A. Causal interactions between fronto-parietal central executive and default-mode networks in humans. *Proc. Natl. Acad. Sci. USA* **2013**, *110*, 19944–19949. [CrossRef]
163. Cho, S.S.; Strafella, A.P. rTMS of the Left Dorsolateral Prefrontal Cortex Modulates Dopamine Release in the Ipsilateral Anterior Cingulate Cortex and Orbitofrontal Cortex. *PLoS ONE* **2009**, *4*, e6725. [CrossRef]
164. Fox, M.D.; Buckner, R.L.; White, M.P.; Greicius, M.D.; Pascual-Leone, A. Efficacy of Transcranial Magnetic Stimulation Targets for Depression Is Related to Intrinsic Functional Connectivity with the Subgenual Cingulate. *Biol. Psychiatry* **2012**, *72*, 595–603. [CrossRef]
165. Bassett, D.S.; Khambhati, A.N. A network engineering perspective on probing and perturbing cognition with neu-rofeedback. *Ann. N. Y. Acad. Sci.* **2017**, *1396*, 126–143. [CrossRef]
166. Orndorff-Plunkett, F.; Singh, F.; Aragón, O.R.; Pineda, J.A. Assessing the Effectiveness of Neurofeedback Training in the Context of Clinical and Social Neuroscience. *Brain Sci.* **2017**, *7*, 95. [CrossRef]
167. Yamada, T.; Hashimoto, R.I.; Yahata, N.; Ichikawa, N.; Yoshihara, Y.; Okamoto, Y.; Kato, N.; Takahashi, H.; Kawato, M. Resting-State Functional Connectivity-Based Biomarkers and Functional MRI-Based Neurofeedback for Psychiatric Dis-orders: A Challenge for Developing Theranostic Biomarkers. *Int. J. Neuropsychopharmacol.* **2017**, *20*, 769–781. [CrossRef]
168. Rush, A.J.; Trivedi, M.H.; Wisniewski, S.R.; Nierenberg, A.A.; Stewart, J.W.; Warden, D.; Niederehe, G.; Thase, M.E.; Lavori, P.W.; Lebowitz, B.D.; et al. Acute and longer-term outcomes in depressed outpatients requiring one or several treatment steps: A STAR*D report. *Am. J. Psychiatry* **2006**, *163*, 1905–1917. [CrossRef]
169. Arroll, B.; Macgillivray, S.; Ogston, S.; Reid, I.; Sullivan, F.; Williams, B.; Crombie, I. Efficacy and tolerability of tricyclic antidepressants and SSRIs compared with placebo for treatment of depression in primary care: A meta-analysis. *Ann. Fam. Med.* **2005**, *3*, 449–456. [CrossRef]
170. Gabrieli, J.D.; Ghosh, S.S.; Whitfield-Gabrieli, S. Prediction as a Humanitarian and Pragmatic Contribution from Human Cognitive Neuroscience. *Neuron* **2015**, *85*, 11–26. [CrossRef]
171. Stephan, K.; Schlagenhauf, F.; Huys, Q.; Raman, S.; Aponte, E.; Brodersen, K.; Rigoux, L.; Moran, R.; Daunizeau, J.; Dolan, R.; et al. Computational neuroimaging strategies for single patient predictions. *NeuroImage* **2017**, *145*, 180–199. [CrossRef]
172. Freyhan, F.A. Course and outcome of schizophrenia. *Am. J. Psychiatry* **1955**, *112*, 161–169. [CrossRef]
173. Häfner, H.; Der Heiden, W.A. The course of schizophrenia in the light of modern follow-up studies: The ABC and WHO studies. *Eur. Arch. Psychiatry Clin. Neurosci.* **1999**, *249*, S14–S26. [CrossRef]
174. Kane, J.M.; Correll, C.U. Past and Present Progress in the Pharmacologic Treatment of Schizophrenia. *J. Clin. Psychiatry* **2010**, *71*, 1115–1124. [CrossRef] [PubMed]
175. Mourao-Miranda, J.; Reinders, A.A.T.S.; Rocha-Rego, V.; Lappin, J.; Rondina, J.; Morgan, C.; Morgan, K.D.; Fearon, P.; Jones, P.B.; Doody, G.A.; et al. Individualized prediction of illness course at the first psychotic episode: A support vector machine MRI study. *Psychol. Med.* **2011**, *42*, 1037–1047. [CrossRef] [PubMed]
176. Tsang, H.W.H.; Leung, A.Y.; Chung, R.C.K.; Bell, M.; Cheung, W.-M. Review on vocational predictors: A systematic review of predictors of vocational outcomes among individuals with schizophrenia: An update since 1998. *Aust. N. Z. J. Psychiatry* **2010**, *44*, 495–504.
177. Jääskeläinen, E.; Juola, P.; Hirvonen, N.; McGrath, J.J.; Saha, S.; Isohanni, M.; Veijola, J.; Miettunen, J. A Systematic Review and Meta-Analysis of Recovery in Schizophrenia. *Schizophr. Bull.* **2013**, *39*, 1296–1306. [CrossRef]
178. Li, A.; Zalesky, A.; Yue, W.; Howes, O.; Yan, H.; Liu, Y.; Fan, L.; Whitaker, K.J.; Xu, K.; Rao, G.; et al. A neu-roimaging biomarker for striatal dysfunction in schizophrenia. *Nat. Med.* **2020**, *26*, 558–565. [CrossRef]

179. Patel, M.J.; Andreescu, C.; Price, J.C.; Edelman, K.L.; Reynolds, C.F., 3rd; Aizenstein, H.J. Machine learning approaches for integrating clinical and imaging features in late-life depression classification and response prediction. *Int. J. Geriatr. Psychiatry* **2015**, *30*, 1056–1067. [CrossRef]
180. Redlich, R.; Opel, N.; Grotegerd, D.; Dohm, K.; Zaremba, D.; Bürger, C.; Münker, S.; Mühlmann, L.; Wahl, P.; Heindel, W.; et al. Prediction of Individual Response to Electroconvulsive Therapy via Machine Learning on Structural Magnetic Resonance Imaging Data. *JAMA Psychiatry* **2016**, *73*, 557–564. [CrossRef]
181. Wade, B.S.C.; Joshi, S.H.; Njau, S.; Leaver, A.M.; Vasavada, M.; Woods, R.P.; A Gutman, B.; Thompson, P.M.; Espinoza, R.; Narr, K.L. Effect of Electroconvulsive Therapy on Striatal Morphometry in Major Depressive Disorder. *Neuropsychopharmacology* **2016**, *41*, 2481–2491. [CrossRef]
182. Iosifescu, D.V. Electroencephalography-Derived Biomarkers of Antidepressant Response. *Harv. Rev. Psychiatry* **2011**, *19*, 144–154. [CrossRef]
183. Baskaran, A.; Milev, R.; McIntyre, R.S. The neurobiology of the EEG biomarker as a predictor of treatment response in depression. *Neuropharmacology* **2012**, *63*, 507–513. [CrossRef]
184. Leuchter, A.F.; Cook, I.A.; Uijtdehaage, S.H.; Dunkin, J.; Lufkin, R.B.; Anderson-Hanley, C.; Abrams, M.; Rosenberg-Thompson, S.; O'Hara, R.; Simon, S.L.; et al. Brain structure and function and the outcomes of treatment for depression. *J. Clin. Psychiatry* **1997**, *58*, 22–31.
185. Rabinoff, M.; Kitchen, C.; Cook, I.; Leuchter, A. Evaluation of Quantitative EEG by Classification and Regression Trees to Characterize Responders to Antidepressant and Placebo Treatment. *Open Med. Inform. J.* **2011**, *5*, 1–8. [CrossRef]
186. Bareš, M.; Brunovsky, M.; Kopecek, M.; Novak, T.; Stopkova, P.; Kožený, J.; Šóš, P.; Krajca, V.; Höschl, C. Early reduction in prefrontal theta QEEG cordance value predicts response to venlafaxine treatment in patients with resistant depressive disorder. *Eur. Psychiatry* **2008**, *23*, 350–355. [CrossRef]
187. Cook, I.A.; Leuchter, A.F.; Morgan, M.L.; Stubbeman, W.; Siegman, B.; Abrams, M. Changes in prefrontal activity characterize clinical response in SSRI nonresponders: A pilot study. *J. Psychiatr. Res.* **2005**, *39*, 461–466. [CrossRef]
188. Knott, V.J.; I Telner, J.; Lapierre, Y.D.; Browne, M.; Horn, E.R. Quantitative EEG in the prediction of antidepressant response to imipramine. *J. Affect. Disord.* **1996**, *39*, 175–184. [CrossRef]
189. Bruder, G.E.; Sedoruk, J.P.; Stewart, J.W.; McGrath, P.J.; Quitkin, F.M.; Tenke, C.E. Electroencephalographic Alpha Measures Predict Therapeutic Response to a Selective Serotonin Reuptake Inhibitor Antidepressant: Pre- and Post-Treatment Findings. *Biol. Psychiatry* **2008**, *63*, 1171–1177. [CrossRef]
190. Ulrich, G.; Renfordt, E.; Zeller, G.; Frick, K. Interrelation between Changes in the EEG and Psychopathology under Pharmacotherapy for Endogenous Depression. *Pharmacopsychiatry* **1984**, *17*, 178–183. [CrossRef] [PubMed]
191. Iosifescu, D.V.; Greenwald, S.; Devlin, P.; Mischoulon, D.; Denninger, J.W.; Alpert, J.E.; Fava, M. Frontal EEG predictors of treatment outcome in major depressive disorder. *Eur. Neuropsychopharmacol.* **2009**, *19*, 772–777. [CrossRef]
192. Iosifescu, D.V.; Nierenberg, A.A.; Mischoulon, D.; Perlis, R.H.; Papakostas, G.I.; Ryan, J.L.; Alpert, J.E.; Fava, M. An open study of triiodothyronine augmentation of selective serotonin reuptake inhibitors in treatment-resistant major de-pressive disorder. *J. Clin. Psychiatry* **2005**, *66*, 1038–1042. [CrossRef]
193. Bruder, G.E.; Stewart, J.W.; Tenke, C.E.; McGrath, P.J.; Leite, P.; Bhattacharya, N.; Quitkin, F.M. Electroencephalo-graphic and perceptual asymmetry differences between responders and nonresponders to an SSRI antidepressant. *Biol. Psychiatry* **2001**, *49*, 416–425. [CrossRef]
194. Knott, V.; Mahoney, C.; Kennedy, S.; Evans, K. Pre-treatment EEG and it's relationship to depression severity and par-oxetine treatment outcome. *Pharmacopsychiatry* **2000**, *33*, 201–205. [CrossRef] [PubMed]
195. Korb, A.S.; Hunter, A.M.; Cook, I.A.; Leuchter, A.F. Rostral anterior cingulate cortex theta current density and response to antidepressants and placebo in major depression. *Clin. Neurophysiol.* **2009**, *120*, 1313–1319. [CrossRef] [PubMed]
196. Pizzagalli, D.; Pascual-Marqui, R.D.; Nitschke, J.B.; Oakes, T.R.; Larson, C.L.; Abercrombie, H.C.; Schaefer, S.M.; Koger, J.V.; Benca, R.M.; Davidson, R.J. Anterior cingulate activity as a predictor of degree of treatment response in major de-pression: Evidence from brain electrical tomography analysis. *Am. J. Psychiatry* **2001**, *158*, 405–415. [CrossRef]
197. Méndez, M.A.; Zuluaga, P.; Hornero, R.; Gómez, C.; Escudero, J.; Rodríguez-Palancas, A.; Ortiz, T.; Fernández, A. Complexity analysis of spontaneous brain activity: Effects of depression and antidepressant treatment. *J. Psychopharmacol.* **2011**, *26*, 636–643. [CrossRef]
198. Jaworska, N.; Wang, H.; Smith, D.M.; Blier, P.; Knott, V.; Protzner, A.B. Pre-treatment EEG signal variability is associated with treatment success in depression. *NeuroImage Clin.* **2018**, *17*, 368–377. [CrossRef]
199. Thomasson, N.; Pezard, L. Dynamical systems and depression: A framework for theoretical perspectives. *Acta Biotheor.* **1999**, *47*, 209–218. [CrossRef]
200. Zhdanov, A.; Atluri, S.; Wong, W.; Vaghei, Y.; Daskalakis, Z.J.; Blumberger, D.M.; Frey, B.N.; Giacobbe, P.; Lam, R.W.; Milev, R.; et al. Use of Machine Learning for Predicting Escitalopram Treatment Outcome From Electroencephalography Recordings in Adult Patients With Depression. *JAMA Netw. Open* **2020**, *3*, e1918377. [CrossRef]

201. Hasanzadeh, F.; Mohebbi, M.; Rostami, R. Prediction of rTMS treatment response in major depressive disorder using machine learning techniques and nonlinear features of EEG signal. *J. Affect. Disord.* **2019**, *256*, 132–142. [CrossRef]
202. Garg, G.; Elshimy, G.; Marwaha, R. *Gender Dysphoria (Sexual Identity Disorders)*; StatPearls: Treasure Island, FL, USA, 2020.
203. Petry, N.M.; Rehbein, F.; Ko, C.-H.; O'Brien, C.P. Internet Gaming Disorder in the DSM-5. *Curr. Psychiatry Rep.* **2015**, *17*, 1–9. [CrossRef]
204. Ross, C.A.; Margolis, R.L. Research Domain Criteria: Strengths, Weaknesses, and Potential Alternatives for Future Psy-chiatric Research. *Mol. Neuropsychiatry* **2019**, *5*, 218–236. [CrossRef]

biomedicines

MDPI

Review

Crosstalk between Existential Phenomenological Psychotherapy and Neurological Sciences in Mood and Anxiety Disorders

Lehel Balogh [1,*], Masaru Tanaka [2,3], Nóra Török [2,3], László Vécsei [2,3] and Shigeru Taguchi [4]

1. Center for Applied Ethics and Philosophy, Hokkaido University, North 10, West 7, Kita-ku, Sapporo 060-0810, Japan
2. MTA-SZTE, Neuroscience Research Group, Semmelweis u. 6, H-6725 Szeged, Hungary; tanaka.masaru.1@med.u-szeged.hu (M.T.); toroknora85@gmail.com (N.T.); vecsei.laszlo@med.u-szeged.hu (L.V.)
3. Department of Neurology, Interdisciplinary Excellence Centre, Faculty of Medicine, University of Szeged, Semmelweis u. 6, H-6725 Szeged, Hungary
4. Faculty of Humanities and Human Sciences & Center for Human Nature, Artificial Intelligence, and Neuroscience (CHAIN), Hokkaido University, Kita 12, Nishi 7, Kita-ku, Sapporo 060-0812, Japan; tag@let.hokudai.ac.jp

* Correspondence: lehel7@gmail.com; Tel.: +81-80-8906-4263

Citation: Balogh, L.; Tanaka, M.; Török, N.; Vécsei, L.; Taguchi, S. Crosstalk between Existential Phenomenological Psychotherapy and Neurological Sciences in Mood and Anxiety Disorders. *Biomedicines* **2021**, *9*, 340. https://doi.org/10.3390/biomedicines9040340

Academic Editors: Verinder Sharma and Rochelle M. Hines

Received: 24 December 2020
Accepted: 25 March 2021
Published: 27 March 2021

Abstract: Psychotherapy is a comprehensive biological treatment modifying complex underlying cognitive, emotional, behavioral, and regulatory responses in the brain, leading patients with mental illness to a new interpretation of the sense of self and others. Psychotherapy is an art of science integrated with psychology and/or philosophy. Neurological sciences study the neurological basis of cognition, memory, and behavior as well as the impact of neurological damage and disease on these functions, and their treatment. Both psychotherapy and neurological sciences deal with the brain; nevertheless, they continue to stay polarized. Existential phenomenological psychotherapy (EPP) has been in the forefront of meaning-centered counseling for almost a century. The phenomenological approach in psychotherapy originated in the works of Martin Heidegger, Ludwig Binswanger, Medard Boss, and Viktor Frankl, and it has been committed to accounting for the existential possibilities and limitations of one's life. EPP provides philosophically rich interpretations and empowers counseling techniques to assist mentally suffering individuals by finding meaning and purpose to life. The approach has proven to be effective in treating mood and anxiety disorders. This narrative review article demonstrates the development of EPP, the therapeutic methodology, evidence-based accounts of its curative techniques, current understanding of mood and anxiety disorders in neurological sciences, and a possible converging path to translate and integrate meaning-centered psychotherapy and neuroscience, concluding that the EPP may potentially play a synergistic role with the currently prevailing medication-based approaches for the treatment of mood and anxiety disorders.

Keywords: depression; anxiety disorders; existential psychotherapy; logotherapy; meaning-centered psychotherapy; functional magnetic resonance imaging; biomarker; kynurenines; Martin Heidegger; Viktor Frankl

1. Introduction

Mood and anxiety disorders are one of the most common diagnoses categorized in Diagnostic and Statistical Manual of Mental Disorders, 5th Edition (DSM-5) and the 11th revision of the International Statistical Classification of Diseases and Related Health Problems (ICD-11). Mental disorders account for almost 65 percent of psychiatric conditions worldwide and nearly 30 percent of the population is affected by mental illness during their lifetime [1]. A selective serotonin reuptake inhibitor (SSRI) fluoxetine is the most effective pharmacotherapy for the acute treatment of moderate-to-severe depressive disorder in children and adolescents [2]. However, only 40–60% of individuals relieved their symptoms with antidepressants within six to eight weeks [3]. Furthermore, intervention for treatment-resistant depression (TRD) and prevention of suicide attempt are a major challenge. Mood and anxiety disorders elevate morbidity and mortality, present a high rate of comorbidity with medical conditions, and impose a great social burden. The comorbidity complicates symptoms, limits choice of pharmacological treatments, lowers treatment adherence, increases the use of healthcare service, and thus increases costs [4]. Treatment options for psychological symptoms are even more limited for post-myocardial infarction patients and patients in terminal care due to advanced cancer [5,6].

A meta-analysis reported once that pharmacotherapy with SSRIs was significantly more effective than psychotherapy in patients with major depressive disorder [7]. However, a network analysis revealed that combined pharmacotherapy and psychotherapy was superior to monotherapy, while no significant difference was found between pharmacotherapy and psychotherapy in the treatment of depression [8]. An increasing number of therapists pay more attention to psychotherapy as an effective adjunct in interventions for psychiatric disorders. Psychotherapy has presented successful clinical outcomes, which are consistent with less than five percent variance among skillful psychotherapists. Psychotherapy has also given deeper insights into human behavior, but it still stands in need of empirical assessments and methodologies [8]. It would undoubtedly be useful to investigate in what way and how psychotherapy modifies the complex brain responses underlying mental illness, which may lead to the development of new therapeutic interventions. Existential phenomenological psychotherapy (EPP) has been at the forefront of meaning-centered psychotherapy (MCP). Meanwhile, the progress in neuroimaging research such as functional magnetic resonance imaging (fMRI) techniques has provided more and more knowledge of brain functions, which leads to deeper understanding of psychopathologies and the development of therapeutic interventions for mental disorders [9]. Neuroscience in vitro and in animal models have allowed us to test hypotheses, reveal pathogenesis, and develop new drugs for psychiatric disorders [10]. Therefore, translating and integrating methods and knowledge of psychotherapy and neurological sciences can certainly lead to deeper understanding of disease mechanisms, testing new hypotheses, and searching for novel treatments of mental illness [11]. This review article presents the development and methods of EPP, clinical evidence of its efficacy, current understanding of mood and anxiety disorders in neurosciences, and the need for convergence of this expertise to translate and integrate MCP and neurological sciences (Figure 1).

2. Existential Phenomenological Psychotherapy

Phenomenology as a philosophical approach of grasping and explaining reality appeared on the European intellectual scene some 130 years ago. Although G.W.F. Hegel already talked and wrote extensively about the "phenomenology of spirit" in the early 19th century, it was not until Edmund Husserl's adaptation of the term in the early 1900s that it came to gain its philosophically characteristic, nuanced meaning. Husserl, a mathematician and philosopher, was strongly influenced in the construction of his methodology by philosopher and psychologist Franz Brentano and by historian and hermeneutic philosopher Wilhelm Dilthey. From Brentano he took over arguments regarding the structure of consciousness as well as the general task of critiquing psychologism in the domain of philosophical logic, whereas from Dilthey he appropriated the "attempt to develop a more descriptive approach to the human sciences" [12]. Having carefully designed his innovative philosophical methodology, which he believed "could discover the structures common to all mental acts", he had high hopes that the systematic utilization of this methodology could turn philosophy into a "rigorous science" on par with the natural sciences. Thus, was born phenomenology, a novel philosophical approach whose concise programmatic ideal was aptly conveyed in the following famous slogan: "back to the things themselves".

What does Husserl mean by "back to the things themselves"? This motto involves a call, an appeal to turn away and leave behind concepts and theories, and instead to experientially encounter all phenomena of the pure consciousness just as they present themselves, without the conceptual burden with which language and tradition weighs them down. An eminent historian of the phenomenological movement, Herbert Spiegelberg, noted that transcendental phenomenology attempted to reveal "the structures of pure consciousness, [which were] made accessible by a special suspension of belief in the reality of our natural and scientific world, the so-called phenomenological reduction, in which the constitution of the phenomena according to intending acts and intended contents was studied in detail" [13]. This phenomenological reduction is essential to understanding how Husserl's phenomenology was intended to operate. As Husserl explained, the main objective of phenomenology's undertaking was to intuitively discern eidetic essences that lay beyond the singular expressions of individual phenomena [14]. While descriptive phenomenology's primary goal was to "intuit, analyze, and describe the data of direct experience in a fresh and systematic manner", essential or eidetic phenomenology's responsibility was to explore "essential structures on the basis of imaginative variation of the data" [13].

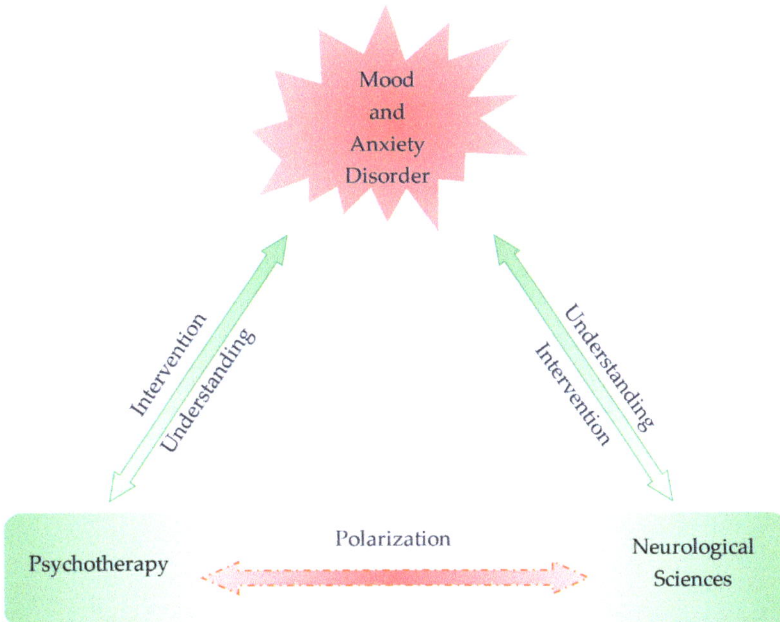

Figure 1. Polarization of two fields of expertise: psychotherapy and neurological sciences. Both psychotherapy and neurological sciences explore the pathomechanism and interventional opportunity of psychiatric disorders. Translational studies are scarce, and each area of expertise stays polarized.

The phenomenological approach had progressively become influential in psychological and psychiatric circles from the second third of the last century; especially after it successfully wed itself with the newly emerging philosophical and ethical concerns of existentialism. Martin Heidegger, who was originally an assistant of Husserl, and whose philosophical reputation by the 1930s came to match his distinguished former teacher's considerable intellectual stature, was the one who, albeit unwittingly and increasingly unwillingly, facilitated this fruitful philosophical nuptial. In his famous 1927 work 'Being and Time', Heidegger critically transformed Husserl's insights and carried them over to the spheres of ontology [13]. Ontology as a specialized philosophical field deals with the existence—or being—of all beings, and tries to find answers to such questions as what "being" means, what separates being from non-being, what levels of existence and various classes of entities there are, etc. Heidegger's quest for the forgotten meaning of "being", and particularly the "existential analytic" of Being and Time that expounded on the self's—or as Heidegger had called it, Dasein's—existential possibilities and limitations, initiated a prominent philosophical and literary movement that came to be called "existentialism". Among the proponents of existentialism influential figures customarily counted are Jean-Paul Sartre, Albert Camus, Simone de Beauvoir, Karl Jaspers, Maurice Merleau-Ponty, and so forth. Nevertheless, the rapidly growing existentialist movement of the 1940s and 1950s also began to claim an outstanding philosophical ancestry that ranged from the works of Arthur Schopenhauer to Soren Kierkegaard and from Fyodor Dostoevsky to Friedrich Nietzsche. What was common in this exceptionally diverse bunch of thinkers was the circumstance that they were all deeply intrigued by the "subjective" experiences and the inwardness of the self, at the same time looking distrustfully upon the claims for scientific hegemony of the positivist, reductionist, and objectifying approaches of the natural sciences (Figure 2a).

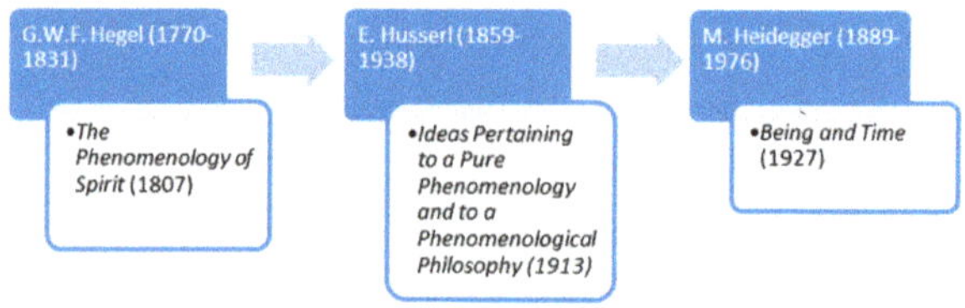

(a) The milestones of philosophical phenomenology.

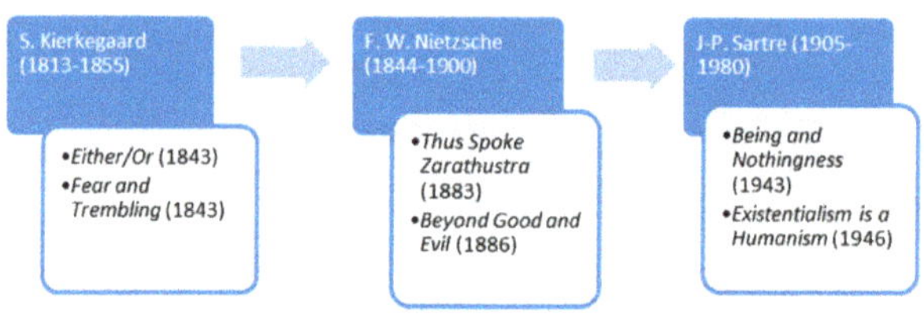

(b) The milestones of philosophical existentialism.

Figure 2. The milestones of philosophical phenomenology and philosophical existentialism. (**a**) The milestones of philosophical phenomenology. (**b**) The milestones of philosophical existentialism.

Discovering the meaning of human existence was the first and foremost task which the existentialist thinkers set for themselves. As Wrathall and Dreyfus eloquently put it: "For existentialist thinkers, the focus is on uncovering what is unique to that individual, rather than treating her as a manifestation of a general type (...) With their focus on the individual and a denial of any meaningful sense of what constitutes an essential or absolute goal for human existence, existentialists emphasize human freedom and responsibility, and hold that the only goal consistent with that freedom and responsibility is to live authentically" [12]. When phenomenology began to merge with existentialism, first in Heidegger's, then in a prestigious line of other up-and-coming philosophers' work, the rigorousness of phenomenology and the existential concerns of existentialism generated a unique blend of philosophizing. As Spiegelberg rightly points out, this new combined approach was in palpable contrast with the methodologically less scrupulous early existentialist writings of for instance Kierkegaard or Nietzsche. The new phenomenological-existential approach firmly maintained "that existence *can* be approached phenomenologically and studied as one phenomenon among others in its essential structures" [12]. Wrathall and Dreyfus add to this that since phenomenology and existentialism share many of their concerns, their joint focus tends to be on these concerns, rather than on numerous other issues that they would disagree on. "Like the phenomenology of Heidegger, Merleau-Ponty, and Sartre, existentialism as a movement starts its analysis with the existing individual—the individual engaged in a particular world with a characteristic form of life. Thus, an emphasis on the body and on the affective rather than rational side of human being are characteristic of existentialism" (Figure 2b) [12].

This is the tradition upon which existential psychiatry and psychotherapy has established its theory and practice. Existential psychotherapy is a unique approach in that it scrutinizes psychic phenomena from an existentialist point of view. This entails that existential therapists understand man not as a substantive subject that is torn from objective, "external" reality, but as a Being-in-the-World (Heidegger's term) or existence. Existential psychiatry began forming shortly after the first reception of Heidegger's Being and Time—that is, in the early 1930s—, but it became influential only from the 1950s and 1960s. In the beginning, such psychiatrists as Ludwig Binswanger and Medard Boss had attempted to elaborate the putting into practice of what Heidegger had to say about Dasein's fundamental ontological structures [15]. Under the name of 'Daseinsanalysis', both Binswanger and Boss had worked out a theory as to how one might utilize phenomenology's insights in understanding and curing the mentally ill. Around the same time Austrian-born Viktor Frankl also established a distinct existential school of psychiatry and psychotherapy for which he coined the name Logotherapy (Figure 3a).

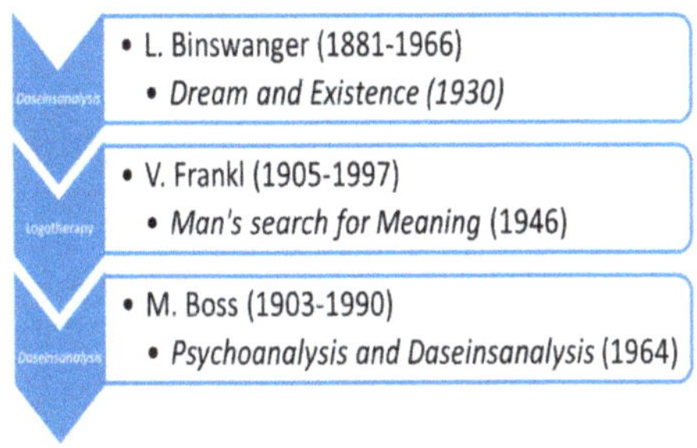

(a) Main figures of early existential psychotherapy (Daseinsanalysis and Logotherapy)

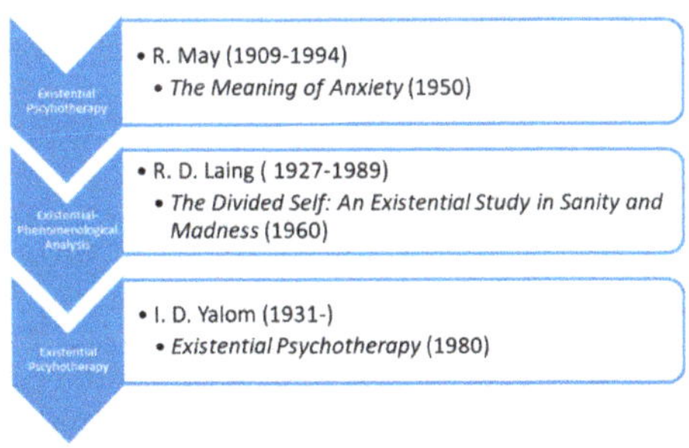
• R. May (1909-1994)
• The Meaning of Anxiety (1950)
• R. D. Laing (1927-1989)
• The Divided Self: An Existential Study in Sanity and Madness (1960)
• I. D. Yalom (1931-)
• Existential Psychotherapy (1980)

(b) Main figures of later existential psychotherapy (British and American).

Figure 3. Main figures of early existential psychotherapy and later existential psychotherapy. (**a**) Main figures of early existential psychotherapy (Daseinsanalysis and Logotherapy). (**b**) Main figures of later existential psychotherapy (British and American).

It is important to keep in mind that existential-phenomenological psychiatry and psychotherapy were born out of the elemental dissatisfaction with the ways psychiatrists tried to cure conventionally conceived "diseases" of conventionally conceived human "subjects": for existentialists it seemed that neither of these were adequate modes of either grasping human reality or of trying to advance the well-being of the individual [16]. By the end of the 1950s, the existential approach to psychiatry and psychotherapy arrived and started to grow in the US. Along with the so-called humanistic movement in psychology, it has gained considerable influence after a relatively brief period of time. Rollo May and Irvin D. Yalom are the most well-known and acknowledged representatives of the American school of existential therapy. Meanwhile in Great Britain, it was Ronald David Laing who first offered analyses of psychopathological and psychotherapeutic phenomena from an existential-phenomenological stance. Somewhat later, several members of the British School of Existential Analysis came to reform the principles of existential therapy. Their objective was to strip the therapeutic setting from the urge to diagnose the "disease" of the client, along with the removal of the habitual pathologization of various "abnormal" psychological phenomena and the moral evaluation of medical data. Instead, they suggested that therapy should focus on the phenomenological description of the "lived world" of the patient. Ernesto Spinelli, leading representative of the British School of Existential Analysis, asserted that existential psychotherapy's "primary task is *not* one of seeking to direct change in the worldview of the client. Rather, existential psychotherapy's principal concerns lie with its attempts to descriptively clarify that worldview so that its explicit and implicit, sedimented dispositional stances can be re-examined inter-relationally" [17] (Figure 3b).

2.1. *Existential Psychotherapy's Approach for the Treatment of Mood and Anxiety Disorders*

The aim of existential analysis is to guide a person towards experiencing their life authentically and freely. This is done through practical methods that help an individual to live with 'inner consent', or the ability to affirm what he or she is doing [18].

As Viktor Frankl, the founder of the Vienna School of Existential Analysis maintained, existential analysis is the search for meaning: the meaning of a given individual's unique existence with its goals and values, amidst its limitations and situatedness [19]. However, this approach to the human psyche comprises other essential facets as well that point beyond a mere psychological analysis of contingent factors. Frankl claimed that "existential analysis is (...) not only the explication of ontic existence, but also the ontological explication of what existence is. In this sense, existential analysis is the attempt at a psychotherapeutic anthropology, an anthropology that precedes all psychotherapy, not only logotherapy." The establishment of such an anthropology is the ultimate goal of existential psychology and psychiatry as a theory of the human psyche and its dysfunctions. It is exceedingly important to clarify such an anthropology, because, as Frankl goes on to explain: "every psychotherapy plays itself out against an a priori horizon. There is always an anthropological conception at its foundation, no matter how little aware of this the psychotherapy may be" [19].

Frankl, an Austrian-born Holocaust survivor, believed that the root cause of the majority of our psychological problems was a general feeling of meaninglessness: an "existential vacuum" which leads one to despair and believe that life no longer has any meaning [19]. Therefore, the goal of his therapeutic approach is to assist rediscovering meaning in one's life (logotherapy: meaning therapy). One might wonder why meaning appears crucial for psychiatry and psychopathology. The answer lies in the fact that mental health and the perceived meaningfulness of personal existence seem to be both coemerging and codependent. Numerous studies have demonstrated that the absence of a comprehensive framework of meaning which includes goals, values, and priorities in an individual's life is strongly correlated with the formation of depressive disorders [20]. On the other hand, the presence of meaning has been shown to be an active and potent protective factor against the emergence of suicidal tendencies which are among the most dangerous potential consequences of depression [21,22].

Besides depression, other psychological illnesses such as anxiety disorders can also be directly linked with a lack of a sense of overall meaning in life. "Although skeptical scholars criticize meaning in life as a tenuous construct, research shows that many individuals perceive there to be a larger direction and orientation in their daily lives, and when they lack this experience, they seem more prone to developing depression, anxiety, and other psychological problems" [23].

Regarding some of the concrete techniques that EPP routinely employs to treat mental disorders, the following two are of special interest: paradoxical intention and dereflection [19] (Table 1). Frankl argued that both with anxiety disorders and with obsessive-compulsive disorders, the technique of paradoxical intention can be effectively utilized. As he wrote, "we define paradoxical intention in the following way: the patient will be directed to wish (in the case of anxiety neuroses) or to resolve to do (in the case of compulsive neuroses) precisely that which the patient fears so much" [19]. In other words, paradoxical intention is a technique whereby the individual resolves themselves to opt for an attitude that is diametrically opposed to that which they would originally want to adopt as a "natural" reaction to their perceived psychological difficulty. For example, if one is pathologically anxious and is terrified of having a panic attack when speaking in front of an audience (glossophobia), then Frankl would suggest that instead of trying to avoid the anxiety-inducing thoughts, on the contrary, they should engage these troubling thoughts head-on and even exaggerate them. As Vos elucidates, "paradoxical intentions are based on the assumption that individuals can choose the stance they take towards their psychological difficulties and that their symptoms are exacerbated by avoiding problems or feeling saddened or anxious. Frankl invited clients to deliberately practice or exaggerate a neurotic habit or thought, so that they stopped fighting and instead identified and undermined their problems. This technique has proven to be particularly effective in anxiety disorders [23] (Table 1).

Table 1. Techniques of existential psychotherapy.

Name of the Technique	How Does It Work?	Application
Paradoxical intention	Resolves to opt for an attitude that is diametrically opposed to that which they would originally want to adopt as a "natural" reaction to perceived psychological difficulty	Anxiety disorders Depression [18].
Dereflection	Redirect the attention from the self, towards other people or other phenomena in the world	Anxiety disorders Depression [18].

The other technique of EPP is called dereflection. It follows the opposite route of paradoxical intention: instead of directly engaging the issues with which the individual is principally preoccupied, the attention gets redirected, away from the self, towards other people or other phenomena in the world. As a rule, this technique is used when the client becomes overly self-absorbed with their own goals and problems. The excessive absorption with one's own problems is what Frankl called hyperreflection. In the following passage he refers to the example of sexual impotence which is caused by psychological dysfunction. "In logotherapy we counter hyperreflection with a dereflection. To treat the specific hyperintention that is so pathological in cases of impotence we have developed a special technique, which dates back to 1947. We recommend that the patient be encouraged 'not to engage in sex, but rather to acquiesce to fragmentary acts of tenderness, like a mutual sexual foreplay" [19]. Consequently, by the drawing away of the attention from the perceived problem—sexual impotence—and thus from the self towards the other person—by giving tenderness and caring, as well as by other gentle forms of mutual pleasuring—the psychological block can be gradually lifted, and the sexual functioning can become normal once again (Table 1).

2.2. Clinical Evidence of Meaning-Centered Psychotherapy

The EPP is practiced as a MCP in general. MCP has proved its efficacy against depressive and anxiety symptoms in patients with a wide range of diseases from psychiatric disorders, cardiovascular disease to terminal cancer. Systematic search was conducted in PubMed/Medline with keywords "meaning-centered" and "psychotherapy" on 16 December 2020. Fifty-three articles were retrieved, and twelve articles were eventually deemed appropriate for synthesis (Supplement Figure S1).

An exploratory pilot study reported that advanced cancer patients receiving home palliative care showed a significant decrease in levels of despair, anxiety, depression, and emotional distress by receiving individual MCP (IMCP), compared to those who received only counseling [24]. Randomized control trials showed the efficacy of IMCP and meaning-centered group psychotherapy (MCGP) for psychological and existential distress in patients with advanced cancer. The IMCP and MCGP were superior to enhanced usual care and supportive psychotherapy [25–28]. In MCGP the improvements of quality of life, depression, hopelessness, and desire for hastened death in advanced cancer patients were mediated by an enhanced sense of meaning and peace in life [29]. A longitudinal mixed-effects model also showed significant increases in alleviating burden, anxiety, and depression and finding meaning, benefit, and spiritual well-being among cancer caregivers in response to web-based MCP [30]. A one-year follow-up study showed that cancer survivors who completed MCGP presented more personal growth than those who received supportive group psychotherapy. A two-year follow-up study reported that MCGP cancer survivors showed better positive relations than usual care receivers, suggesting that MCGP carries higher efficacy in the long term [31]. The effectiveness and cost-effectiveness measurements of MCGP for cancer survivors have been designed to compare meaning making, quality of life, anxiety and depression, hopelessness, optimism, adjustment to cancer, and costs with supportive group psychotherapy and usual care [32].

The results may reinforce the evidence of the efficacy and determine the cost-benefit ratio of MCGP. Furthermore, an open trial study reported the preliminary results that meaning-centered grief therapy for parents who lost a child to cancer presented improvements in prolonged grief, sense of meaning, depression, hopelessness, continuing bonds with their child, posttraumatic growth, positive affect, and quality of life. The treatment gains were maintained or improved after three months [33]. The meaning-centered intervention was shown to provide perceived benefits to palliative care nurses who faced recurrent burden, but improvement of spiritual and emotional quality of life remains unclear [34].

A meta-analysis which included 60 trials and 3713 samples reported that MCP had large effect sizes on quality of life and psychological stress in the immediate time frame and follow-up compared to controls. Quality of life is larger in effect size in the immediate time frame than meaning in life, hope and optimism, self-efficacy, and social well-being. Moreover, meta-regression analysis revealed that meaning in life is a predictor of psychological stress [35].

In summary, both IMCP and MCGP are more effective than supportive psychotherapy, counselling, or supportive care. MCGP nurtures personal growth and positive relations. MCGP is effective in the long term and more cost-effective. However, most MCP studies mentioned above dealt with terminal cancer patients presenting mood symptoms. MCP analysis targeting a population of neurologic or psychiatric diseases, MCP for individuals without comorbidity, and comparison with patients under pharmacotherapy will further reveal the efficacy, the applicability, and the limits of MCP for the treatment of a wide range of diseases.

3. Neurological Sciences' Approach to Mood and Anxiety Disorders

3.1. Neuroimaging

Recent advances in neuroimaging technology have facilitated the investigation of brain structure and function. Among magnetic resonance imaging, computed tomography, and positron emission tomography, functional MRI (fMRI) provides information on the properties of functional connectivity (FC). Resting-state fMRI investigates behavioral characteristics such as psychological states, sustained attention, personality, temperament traits, creative ability, and cognitive ability including working memory and motor performance [36–39]. Furthermore, the patterns of resting-state fMRI are correlated with specific symptoms and respond to treatment [40,41]. Analytical methods of resting-state network connectivity include seed-based analysis, the amplitude of low-frequency fluctuation (ALFF) and fractional

ALFF techniques, regional homogeneity (ReHo), independent component analysis (ICA), and graph theory.

3.1.1. Functional Magnetic Resonance Imaging

The Default Mode Network

The default mode network (DMN) is a network of interacting brain regions which shows synchronized activation and deactivation during tasks [42]. DMN includes the medial prefrontal cortices (mPFC), the posterior cingulate cortex (PCC), precuneus, inferior parietal lobule, lateral temporal cortex, and hippocampal formation [43,44]. DMN activity is associated with internal processes including self-referential thinking, autobiographical memory, or thinking about the future [45–47]. The DMN is divided into an anterior subdivision centered in the mPFC and a posterior subdivision centered in the PCC. The anterior DMN is more related to self-referential processing, and emotion regulation through its strong connections with limbic areas. The posterior DMN is associated with consciousness and memory processing through its connection with hippocampal formation [48,49] (Figure 4).

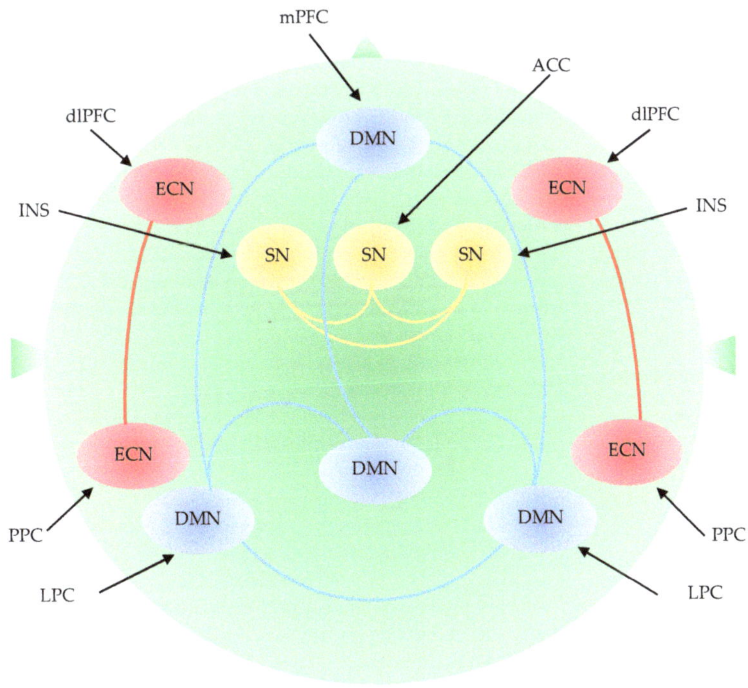

Figure 4. Large-scale brain network including the default mode network, the executive control network, and the salience network. DMN: default mode network; ECN: executive control network; SN: salience network; ACC: anterior cingulate cortex; dlPFC: dorsolateral prefrontal cortex; INS: insular cortex; LPC: lateral parietal cortex; mPFC: medial prefrontal cortex; PPC: posterior parietal cortex.

A relative increase in DMN connectivity and significant ReHo reduction were observed in the posterior DMN of patients with late-life depression (LLD) [50–53]. ICA studies revealed an increased connectivity within the anterior DMN of patients with depression compared to healthy controls [54]. The dissociation between the anterior and posterior DMN subdivisions was observed in patients with major depressive disorder [55]. Antidepressant treatment restored FC abnormality in the posterior DMN but did not correct the FC abnormality in the anterior DMN. Network homogeneity was increased in the anterior DMN but decreased in the posterior DMN [56]. Seed-based analysis using mPFC showed the dissociation between the anterior and posterior DMN and increased connectivity between the anterior DMN and the salience network (SN) in depression [57,58]. Decreased PCC connectivity and increased connectivity in the anterior DMN were observed in depressive patients without medication and 12-weeks treatment of paroxetine partially restored the decreased connectivity [59]. In general, FC between PCC and left medial frontal gyrus decreased in patients with depression and 12-weeks of antidepressant treatment increased FC between PCC to the bilateral medial frontal gyrus [60]. Psychedelics are known to disrupt the activity of the DMN. Serotonergic psychedelic psilocybin-assisted therapy significantly reduced the depression scores of patients with severe depression [61].

The Executive Control Network

The executive control network (ECN) plays an important role in the integration of sensory and memory information, the regulation of cognition and behavior, and the process of working memory [62]. The ECN consists of the dorsolateral prefrontal cortex (dlPFC), medial frontal cortex, lateral parietal cortex, cerebellum, and supplementary motor area [63]. Changes in the ECN were reported in ageing and in patients with LLD, mild cognitive impairment, Alzheimer's disease, and Parkinson's disease [64–68] (Figure 4).

Disruptions of the ECN were reported in non-demented elders with LLD [69–71]. Seed-based analyses using the dlPFC showed decreased FC in the frontoparietal areas in patients with LLD and current depression [72]. Seed-based analyses of the cerebellum presented decreased FC in ECN nodes in dlPFC and the parietal cortex and DMN nodes [73,74]. ICA analyses reported decreased FC in the dlPFC and superior frontal areas, which is consistent with other resting-state fMRI studies with ReHo and ALFF [52,75–77]. Decreased FC in the frontal-parietal cortex was also reported in LLD remitters 3 months after remission [78]. Alteration of the ECN was associated with susceptibility to distraction, and difficulty in sustaining attention, multi-tasking, organizational skills, and concrete thinking [79]. The FC between the dlPFC and other bilateral regions was negatively associated with executive function in patients with LLD [80]. Furthermore, the levels of functional disability were positively correlated with executive dysfunction in LLD [81,82]. Low and slow response to antidepressants and relapse were correlated with deficits in word-list generation and response inhibition which are governed by the executive function network [83,84]. In addition, dissociation between the posterior DMN and ECN was also reported in patients with LLD and current depression [85,86].

The Salience Network

The SN detects and filters salient stimuli and recruits relevant functional networks [87]. The SN is responsible for detecting and incorporating sensory and emotional stimuli, allocating attention, and switching inward and outward cognition. The SN is located in the ventral anterior insula and includes nodes in the amygdala, hypothalamus, ventral striatum, and thalamus [88]. The ventral components play a role in emotional control, while the dorsal components play a role in cognitive control [89]. Cognitive tasks activate the dorsal components including the dorsal anterior cingulate cortex and the right anterior insula. During cognitive tasks, the SN engages ECN and disengages DMN, but vice versa in rest [89–91]. Dissociation between the ECN and SN is correlated with cognitive task performance [92] (Figure 4).

Decreased FC from the amygdala to the hippocampus was observed in patients with depression and individuals at high risk of depression [93,94]. A disrupted pattern of SN connectivity was reported in depression, especially in the insula and amygdala [95]. Elevated connectivity was found between the insula and DMN in patients with LLD [96]. Seed-based analysis using the amygdala as a seed region was positively associated with increased amygdala FC with DMN nodes and long-term negative emotions [97]. Increased FC between the SN and DMN is considered to predispose individuals to depression but decreased FC between the amygdala and precuneus was reported in patients with depression [70,98,99]. Decreased negative FC between the ECN and the SN was associated with cognitive impairment and severity of depression in patients with LLD. Disrupted standard SN pattern was associated with a worse treatment response [100].

3.1.2. Task-Related Functional Magnetic Resonance Imaging

Mood disorders, anxiety disorders, and posttraumatic stress disorder (PTSD) share neurobiologically common characteristics in task-related fMRI. A meta-analysis was conducted using articles studying stereotactic coordinates of whole-brain-based activation in task-related fMRI as between adult patients and controls [101]. Patients with mood disorders, anxiety disorders, or PTSD shared abnormalities in convergence of task-related brain activity in regions associated with inhibitory control and salience processing [101]. Patients who suffered from mood and anxiety disorders presented abnormally lower activity in the inferior prefrontal and parietal cortex, the insula, and the putamen [101]. These regions are responsible for cognitive and motional control, and inhibition of and switching to new mental activities. The patients also showed higher activity in the anterior cingulate cortex, the left amygdala, and the thalamus which process emotional thoughts and feelings [101].

3.2. Other Relevant Biomarkers and Therapeutic Targets

Besides the large-scale brain network, natural products, endogenous metabolites, neuropeptides, receptor agonists, their synthetic analogues, plasma proteins, and lipids are under extensive study in search of biomarkers and novel drugs for mental disorders [102–109]. In addition, the disruption of neural circuitry-neurogenesis coupling was observed in depression [109]. Several neurotransmitters including serotonin, dopamine, adrenaline, histamine, gamma-aminobutyric acid, and peptides play an important role in the pathogenesis of mood and anxiety disorders. Selective serotonin reuptake inhibitors (SSRIs), selective norepinephrine reuptake inhibitors (SNRIs), and monoamine oxidase inhibitors (MAOIs) are major classes of antidepressants currently prescribed for the treatment of depression and anxiety. SSRIs, SNRIs, and MAORs all act on components of neurotransmission. Serotonergic psychedelics are a subclass of hallucinogens that act on the serotonin 5-HT_{2A} receptors. The naturally occurring psychedelic prodrug psylocibin was reported to alleviate depression and anxiety in patients with life-threating diseases [106]. Glutamatergic neural transmission is drawing increasing attention because normal human brain functions are maintained in balance of 80% of excitatory neuronal and 20% of inhibitory neuronal activities [110]. Excitatory neurotransmission is governed by glutamatergic neurons with the N-methyl-D-aspartate (NMDA) receptor [111]. NMDA receptor antagonists are under extensive study for the treatment of TRD [112]. The subanesthetic dose of NMDA receptor antagonist ketamine rapidly improves depressive symptoms and leads to the resolution of suicidal ideation in patients with serious depression [113]. However, the NMDA receptor appears not to be a single pharmacological target of ketamine in the alleviation of depression [114].

Kynurenines (KYNs) are intermediate metabolites of the tryptophan (TRP)-KYN metabolic pathway, which exhibit a wide range of bioactivity such as neurotoxic, neuroprotective, oxidative, antioxidative, and/or immunological actions [115]. The KYN metabolites include a NMDA receptor agonist as well as a NMDA antagonist [116]. Furthermore, the KYN pathway supplies neuroactive metabolites which trigger biological functions not only in synaptic spaces, but also in the non-synaptic microenvironment around the neurons [117]. Moreover, increasing attention has been paid to the KYN pathway since over 95 percent of TRP is metabolized through the KYN pathway, leaving about one percent to the synthesis of serotonin that plays an important role in mood disorders. Kynurenic acid (KYNA) is found to be a diagnostic as well as predicative biomarker for depression, while KYN and KYNA are potential predictive biomarkers for escitalopram treatment in depression [118]. KYNs are agonists or antagonists at the NMDA receptor of the glutamatergic nervous system. Thus, the glutamatergic nervous system has been proposed to be a target for mood disorders [110]. A meta-analysis concluded that an increased risk of depression was correlated with inflammation in chronic illness through the TRP-KYN metabolic pathway [119]. A systematic review reported KYN metabolism abnormalities in TRD and suicidal behavior, proposing the KYN enzymes as novel targets in TRD and suicidality [120].

Gastrointestinal microbiota were observed to participate in development of visceral pain, anxiety, depression, cognitive disturbance, and social behavior and microbiota composition was proposed to be a potential biomarker and target [121,122]. Serum plasma profiles may serve as a potential predictive biomarker for the choice of antidepressants [123]. Foods, or fortified food products beneficial to physiological body functions, were proposed for the treatment of metabolic dysfunction in ageing neurodegenerative diseases [124]. In addition to biomolecules, any measurable indicators are important for risk, diagnosis, prognostic, and predictive biomarkers and interventional targets. Depression was found to be a risk factor for Alzheimer's disease and dementia. Dyslipidemia treatment reduced the risk of development of dementia in diabetics [125]. The presence of depressive symptoms following acute stroke or transient ischemic attack increased mortality and disability within the following 12-month period, suggesting that depression is a prognostic biomarker in cerebral ischemia [126]. Therefore, the treatment of depression is a crucial measure to avoid the development of comorbid conditions and psychotherapy is certainly able to contribute to the prevention of disease progression and complications for a better quality of life. In addition, depression is a measurable psychobehavioral component of dementia, which can be ameliorated by animal-assisted and pet-robot interventions in patients with dementia [127] (Figure 5).

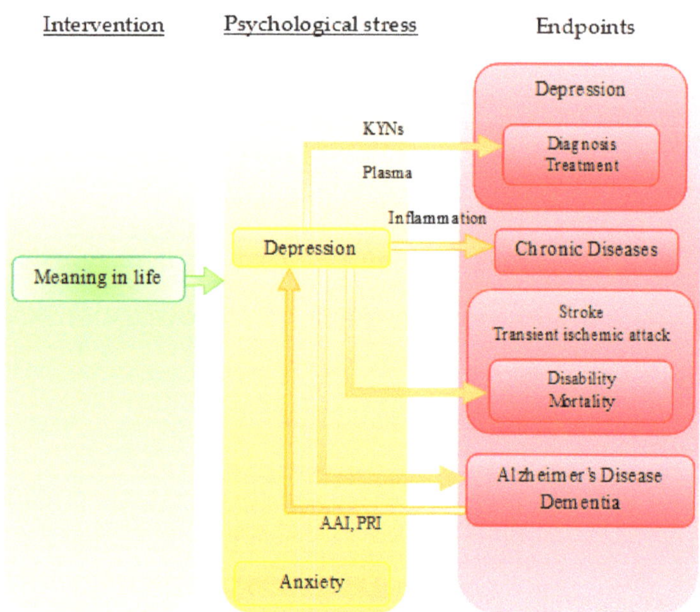

Figure 5. Meaning-centered psychotherapy, its effective targets, and endpoints. Meaning in life is a predictor of psychological stress. Psychological stress causes depression, anxiety, and cognitive impairment. Depression is a measurable indicator which predicts diagnosis and/or treatment of depression with kynurenines (KYNs), chronic diseases with inflammation, disability and mortality of stroke and transient ischemic attack, and Alzheimer's disease and dementia. Depression of Alzheimer's diseases and dementia can be ameliorated by AAI (animal-assisted intervention) and pet-robot intervention (PRI).

4. Future Perspective: Bridging the Expertise

Clinical evidence including randomized-controlled clinical trials and meta-analysis presented solid evidence that EPP, which is generally practiced as MCP, provides substantial relief to individuals under psychological stress such as depression and anxiety. MCP improves quality of life and ameliorates psychological stress, while meaning in life predicts the degree of psychological stress in patients with advanced cancer.

Neurological sciences have shed more light on the understanding of the pathomechanisms of depression and anxiety and explores possible interventional targets. Imaging studies and various network analyses have provided enormous data on and presented possible mechanisms of mood and anxiety disorders, but changes in the networks in individuals under psychotherapy have been rarely reported. Neither have been measurable biomarkers in individuals under psychotherapy. Recent research revealed that depression itself is a risk, diagnostic, prognostic, and/or predictive biomarker for various diseases such Alzheimer's disease, dementia, strokes, major depressive disorders, and chronic diseases (Figure 5). Thus, depression may be a desirable interventional target to reduce the risk, morbidity, disability, and mortality of illness. It has been observed that neurologic diseases are commonly associated with psychiatric comorbidities, exposing neurologic patients to a sense of hopelessness and consequently a higher risk of suicidal ideation and suicidal behavior. Thus, neurologic diseases may be the ideal territory for bridging existential psychotherapy and neurological sciences from the side of clinical medicine [21,22]. Meanwhile, characterizing the behavior traits of animal models of neurologic and psychiatric diseases and developing animal models of happiness and wellbeing to assess hedonic and eudaimonic components, if there are any, may pave an approach toward the converging point from the side of laboratory medicine. On the other hand, the introduction of DSM-5 and ICD-11 has accelerated a trend toward discounting the psychological and social factors of psychiatric disorders. The roles of transdisciplinary psychiatry are expected to be explored and refined to fill the gap between psychiatry and neuroscience [128].

Further translational and integrative research on both psychotherapy and neuroscience is expected in order to provide symptomatic relief from psychological stress, to prevent the development of comorbidity, and to avoid exacerbation of diseases, especially for individuals contraindicated to pharmacotherapy, making available more options for treatment and realizing a possible individualized combination therapy based on psychotherapy and pharmacotherapy.

Supplementary Materials: The following are available online at https://www.mdpi.com/article/10.3390/biomedicines9040340/s1, Figure S1: Preferred reporting items for systematic reviews and meta-analysis (PRISMA) flow diagram for systematic review.

Author Contributions: Data collection: L.B. and M.T., writing—original draft preparation L.B. and M.T.; writing—review and editing, L.B., M.T., N.T., L.V., and S.T.; visualization L.B., and M.T.; supervision, L.V. and S.T.; funding acquisition, L.V. All authors have read and agreed to the published version of the manuscript.

Funding: The current work was supported by GINOP 2.3.2-15-2016-00034, GINOP 2.3.2-15-2016-00048 (Stay Alive), TUDFO/47138-1/2019-ITM, TKP2020 Thematic Excellence Programme 2020, University of Szeged Open Access Fund (4909).

Institutional Review Board Statement: Not applicable.

Informed Consent Statement: Not applicable.

Data Availability Statement: The data that support the findings of this study are available from the corresponding author, L.B., upon reasonable request.

Conflicts of Interest: The authors declare no conflict of interest.

Abbreviations

AAI	animal-assisted intervention
ALFF	amplitude of low-frequency fluctuation
dlPFC	dorsolateral prefrontal cortex
DMN	default mode network
ECN	executive control network
EPP	existential phenomenological psychotherapy
FC	functional connectivity
fMRI	functional magnetic resonance imaging
ICA	independent component analysis
IMCP	individual meaning-centered psychotherapy
KYN	kynurenines
KYNA	kynurenic acid
LLD	late-life depression
MAOI	monoamine oxidase inhibitors
MCGP	meaning-centered group psychotherapy
MCP	meaning-centered psychotherapy
NMDA	N-methyl-D-aspartate
mPFC	medial prefrontal cortices
PCC	posterior cingulate cortex
PRI	pet-robot intervention
PTSD	posttraumatic stress disorder
ReHo	regional homogeneity
SNRI	selective norepinephrine reuptake inhibitor
SSRI	selective serotonin reuptake inhibitor
SN	salience network
TRD	treatment-resistant depression
TRP	tryptophan

References

1. Mental Health—Our World in Data. Available online: https://ourworldindata.org/mental-health#:~{}:text=Globally%20an%20estimated%20284%20million,experience%20anxiety%20disorders%20than%20men (accessed on 14 December 2020).
2. Zhou, X.; Teng, T.; Zhang, Y.; Del Giovane, C.; Furukawa, T.A.; Weisz, J.R.; Li, X.; Cuijpers, P.; Coghill, D.; Xiang, Y.; et al. Comparative efficacy and acceptability of antidepressants, psychotherapies, and their combination for acute treatment of children and adolescents with depressive disorder: A systematic review and network meta-analysis. *Lancet Psychiatry* **2020**, *7*, 581–601. [CrossRef]
3. InformedHealth.org. Cologne, Germany: Institute for Quality and Efficiency in Health Care (IQWiG). Depression: How Effective Are Antidepressants? 2020. Available online: https://www.ncbi.nlm.nih.gov/books/NBK361016/ (accessed on 14 December 2020).
4. Depression and Other Common Mental Disorders Global Health Estimates. Available online: https://apps.who.int/iris/bitstream/handle/10665/254610/WHO-MSD-MER-2017.2-eng.pdf (accessed on 14 December 2020).
5. Smolderen, K.G.; Buchanan, D.M.; Gosch, K.; Whooley, M.; Chan, P.S.; Vaccarino, V.; Parashar, S.; Shah, A.J.; Ho, P.M.; Spertus, J.A. Depression Treatment and 1-Year Mortality After Acute Myocardial Infarction: Insights from the TRIUMPH Registry (Translational Research Investigating Underlying Disparities in Acute Myocardial Infarction Patients' Health Status). *Circulation* **2017**, *135*, 1681–1689. [CrossRef] [PubMed]
6. Ahmed, E. Antidepressants in Patients with Advanced Cancer: When They're Warranted and How to Choose Therapy. *Oncol. Williston Park* **2019**, *33*, 62–68.
7. Cuijpers, P.; van Straten, A.; van Oppen, P.; Andersson, G. Are psychological and pharmacologic interventions equally effective in the treatment of adult depressive disorders? A meta-analysis of comparative studies. *J. Clin. Psychiatry* **2008**, *69*, 1675–1685. [CrossRef] [PubMed]
8. Cuijpers, P.; Noma, H.; Karyotaki, E.; Vinkers, C.H.; Cipriani, A.; Furukawa, T.A. A network meta-analysis of the effects of psychotherapies, pharmacotherapies and their combination in the treatment of adult depression. *World Psychiatry* **2020**, *19*, 92–107. [CrossRef] [PubMed]
9. Castanheira, L.; Silva, C.; Cheniaux, E.; Telles-Correia, D. Neuroimaging Correlates of Depression-Implications to Clinical Practice. *Front. Psychiatry* **2019**, *10*, 703. [CrossRef] [PubMed]
10. Pound, P. Are Animal Models Needed to Discover, Develop and Test Pharmaceutical Drugs for Humans in the 21st Century? *Animals* **2020**, *10*, 2455. [CrossRef] [PubMed]
11. Javanbakht, A.; Alberini, C.M. Editorial: Neurobiological Models of Psychotherapy. *Front. Behav. Neurosci.* **2019**, *13*, 144. [CrossRef] [PubMed]

12. Wrathall, M.A.; Dreyfus, H.L.; Dreyfus, H.L. A Brief Introduction to Phenomenology and Existentialism. In *A Companion to Phenomenology and Existentialism*; Dreyfus, H.L., Wrathall, M.A., Eds.; Malden Blackwell Publishing: Oxford, UK, 2006; pp. 1–6.
13. Spiegelberg, H. *Phenomenology in Psychology and Psychiatry: A Historical Introduction*; Northwestern University Press: Evanston, IL, USA, 1972.
14. Moran, D. *Introduction to Phenomenology*; Routledge: London, UK; New York, NY, USA, 2000.
15. Wiggins, O.P.; Schwartz, M.A. Psychiatry. In *Encyclopedia of Phenomenology*; Embree, L., Ed.; Springer Science + Business Media: Dordrecht, The Netherlands, 1997; pp. 562–568.
16. Wertz, F.J. Phenomenological Currents in Twentieth-Century Psychology. In *A Companion to Phenomenology and Existentialism*; Dreyfus, H.L., Wrathall, M.A., Eds.; Malden Blackwell Publishing: Oxford, UK, 2006; pp. 394–411.
17. Spinelli, E. *Practising Existential Psychotherapy: The Relational World*; SAGE Publications: Los Angeles, CA, USA; London, UK; New Delhi, India; Singapore, 2007.
18. Längle, A. The Viennese School of Existential Analysis: The Search for Meaning and Affirmation of Life. In *Existential Therapy: Legacy, Vibrancy and Dialogue*; Barnett, L., Madison, G., Eds.; Routledge: London, UK; New York, NY, USA, 2012; pp. 159–170.
19. Frankl, E.V. *On the Theory and Therapy of Mental Disorders: An Introduction to Logotherapy and Existential Analysis*; Dubois, J.M., Ed.; Brunner Routledge: New York, NY, USA, 2004.
20. Ameli, M. Reason, Meaning, and Resilience in the Treatment of Depression: Logotherapy as a Bridge Between Cognitive-Behavior Therapy and Positive Psychology. In *Clinical Perspectives on Meaning: Positive and Existential Psychotherapy*; Russo-Netzer, P., Schulenberg, S.E., Batthyany, A., Eds.; Springer: Cham, Switzerland, 2016; pp. 223–244.
21. Costanza, A.; Baertschi, M.; Weber, K.; Canuto, A. Maladies neurologiques et suicide: De la neurobiologie au manque d'espoir [Neurological diseases and suicide: From neurobiology to hopelessness]. *Rev. Med. Suisse* **2015**, *11*, 402–405.
22. Costanza, A.; Amerio, A.; Aguglia, A.; Escelsior, A.; Serafini, G.; Berardelli, I.; Pompili, M.; Amore, M. When Sick Brain and Hopelessness Meet: Some Aspects of Suicidality in the Neurological Patient. *CNS Neurol Disord Drug Targets* **2020**, *19*, 257–263. [CrossRef]
23. Vos, J. Working with Meaning in Life in Mental Health Care: A Systematic Literature Review of the Practices and Effectiveness of Meaning-Centred Therapies. In *Clinical Perspectives on Meaning: Positive and Existential Psychotherapy*; Russo-Netzer, P., Schulenberg, S.E., Batthyany, A., Eds.; Springer: Cham, Switzerland, 2016; pp. 59–87.
24. Fraguell-Hernando, C.; Limonero, J.T.; Gil, F. Psychological intervention in patients with advanced cancer at home through Individual Meaning-Centered Psychotherapy-Palliative Care: A pilot study. *Support Care Cancer* **2020**, *28*, 4803–4811. [CrossRef]
25. Breitbart, W.; Poppito, S.; Rosenfeld, B.; Vickers, A.J.; Li, Y.; Abbey, J.; Olden, M.; Pessin, H.; Lichtenthal, W.; Sjoberg, D.; et al. Pilot randomized controlled trial of individual meaning-centered psychotherapy for patients with advanced cancer. *J. Clin. Oncol.* **2012**, *30*, 1304–1309. [CrossRef]
26. Breitbart, W.; Rosenfeld, B.; Gibson, C.; Pessin, H.; Poppito, S.; Nelson, C.; Tomarken, A.; Timm, A.K.; Berg, A.; Jacobson, C.; et al. Meaning-centered group psychotherapy for patients with advanced cancer: A pilot randomized controlled trial. *Psychooncology* **2010**, *19*, 21–28. [CrossRef]
27. Breitbart, W.; Pessin, H.; Rosenfeld, B.; Applebaum, A.J.; Lichtenthal, W.G.; Li, Y.; Saracino, R.M.; Marziliano, A.M.; Masterson, M.; Tobias, K.; et al. Individual meaning-centered psychotherapy for the treatment of psychological and existential distress: A randomized controlled trial in patients with advanced cancer. *Cancer* **2018**, *124*, 3231–3239. [CrossRef]
28. Breitbart, W.; Rosenfeld, B.; Pessin, H.; Applebaum, A.; Kulikowski, J.; Lichtenthal, W.G. Meaning-centered group psychotherapy: An effective intervention for improving psychological well-being in patients with advanced cancer. *J. Clin. Oncol.* **2015**, *33*, 749–754. [CrossRef]
29. Rosenfeld, B.; Cham, H.; Pessin, H.; Breitbart, W. Why is Meaning-Centered Group Psychotherapy (MCGP) effective? Enhanced sense of meaning as the mechanism of change for advanced cancer patients. *Psychooncology* **2018**, *27*, 654–660. [CrossRef]
30. Applebaum, A.J.; Buda, K.L.; Schofield, E.; Farberov, M.; Teitelbaum, N.D.; Evans, K.; Cowens-Alvarado, R.; Cannady, R.S. Exploring the cancer caregiver's journey through web-based Meaning-Centered Psychotherapy. *Psychooncology* **2018**, *27*, 847–856. [CrossRef] [PubMed]
31. Holtmaat, K.; van der Spek, N.; Lissenberg-Witte, B.; Breitbart, W.; Cuijpers, P.; Verdonck-de Leeuw, I. Long-term efficacy of meaning-centered group psychotherapy for cancer survivors: 2-Year follow-up results of a randomized controlled trial. *Psychooncology* **2020**, *29*, 711–718. [CrossRef] [PubMed]
32. Van der Spek, N.; Vos, J.; van Uden-Kraan, C.F.; Breitbart, W.; Cuijpers, P.; Knipscheer-Kuipers, K.; Willemsen, V.; Tollenaar, R.A.; van Asperen, C.J.; Verdonck-de Leeuw, I.M. Effectiveness and cost-effectiveness of meaning-centered group psychotherapy in cancer survivors: Protocol of a randomized controlled trial. *BMC Psychiatry* **2014**, *14*, 22. [CrossRef]
33. Lichtenthal, W.G.; Catarozoli, C.; Masterson, M.; Slivjak, E.; Schofield, E.; Roberts, K.E.; Neimeyer, R.A.; Wiener, L.; Prigerson, H.G.; Kissane, D.W.; et al. An open trial of meaning-centered grief therapy: Rationale and preliminary evaluation. *Palliat. Support Care* **2019**, *17*, 2–12. [CrossRef] [PubMed]
34. Fillion, L.; Duval, S.; Dumont, S.; Gagnon, P.; Tremblay, I.; Bairati, I.; Breitbart, W.S. Impact of a meaning-centered intervention on job satisfaction and on quality of life among palliative care nurses. *Psychooncology* **2009**, *18*, 1300–13310. [CrossRef]
35. Vos, J.; Vitali, D. The effects of psychological meaning-centered therapies on quality of life and psychological stress: A metaanalysis. *Palliat Support Care* **2018**, *16*, 608–632. [CrossRef] [PubMed]

36. Rosenberg, M.D.; Finn, E.S.; Scheinost, D.; Papademetris, X.; Shen, X.; Constable, R.T.; Chun, M.M. A neuromarker of sustained attention from whole-brain functional connectivity. *Nat. Neurosci.* **2016**, *19*, 165–171. [CrossRef]
37. Hsu, W.-T.; Rosenberg, M.D.; Scheinost, D.; Constable, R.T.; Chun, M.M. Resting-state functional connectivity predicts neuroticism and extraversion in novel individuals. *Soc. Cogn. Affect. Neurosci.* **2018**, *13*, 224–232. [CrossRef]
38. Jiang, R.; Calhoun, V.D.; Zuo, N.; Lin, D.; Li, J.; Fan, L.; Qi, S.; Sun, H.; Fu, Z.; Song, M.; et al. Connectome-based individualized prediction of temperament trait scores. *Neuroimage* **2018**, *183*, 366–374. [CrossRef] [PubMed]
39. Beaty, R.E.; Kenett, Y.N.; Christensen, A.P.; Rosenberg, M.D.; Benedek, M.; Chen, Q.; Fink, A.; Qiu, J.; Kwapil, T.R.; Kane, M.J.; et al. Robust prediction of individual creative ability from brain functional connectivity. *Proc. Natl. Acad. Sci. USA* **2018**, *115*, 1087–1092. [CrossRef] [PubMed]
40. Kühn, S.; Vanderhasselt, M.-A.; De Raedt, R.; Gallinat, J. Why ruminators won't stop: The structural and resting state correlates of rumination and its relation to depression. *J. Affect. Disord.* **2012**, *141*, 352–360. [CrossRef]
41. Brakowski, J.; Spinelli, S.; Dörig, N.; Bosch, O.G.; Manoliu, A.; Holtforth, M.G.; Seifritz, E. Resting state brain network function in major depression—Depression symptomatology, antidepressant treatment effects, future research. *J. Psychiatr. Res.* **2017**, *92*, 147–159. [CrossRef]
42. Raichle, M.E.; MacLeod, A.M.; Snyder, A.Z.; Powers, W.J.; Gusnard, D.A.; Shulman, G.L. A default mode of brain function. *Proc. Natl. Acad. Sci. USA* **2001**, *98*, 676–682. [CrossRef]
43. Buckner, R.L.; Andrews-Hanna, J.R.; Schacter, D.L. The Brain's Default Network. *Ann. N. Y. Acad. Sci.* **2008**, *1124*, 1–38. [CrossRef]
44. Mohan, A.; Roberto, A.J.; Mohan, A.; Lorenzo, A.; Jones, K.; Carney, M.J.; Liogier-Weyback, L.; Hwang, S.; Lapidus, K.A.B. The Significance of the Default Mode Network (DMN) in Neurological and Neuropsychiatric Disorders: A Review. *Yale J. Biol. Med.* **2016**, *89*, 49–57.
45. Kyeong, S.; Kim, J.; Kim, J.; Kim, E.J.; Kim, H.E.; Kim, J.-J. Differences in the modulation of functional connectivity by self-talk tasks between people with low and high life satisfaction. *Neuroimage* **2020**, *217*, 116929. [CrossRef]
46. Spreng, R.N.; Mar, R.A.; Kim, A.S.N. The common neural basis of autobiographical memory, prospection, navigation, theory of mind, and the default mode: A quantitative meta-analysis. *J. Cogn. Neurosci.* **2009**, *21*, 489–510. [CrossRef] [PubMed]
47. Raichle, M.E. The Brain's Default Mode Network. *Annu. Rev. Neurosci.* **2015**, *38*, 433–447. [CrossRef] [PubMed]
48. Andrews-Hanna, J.R.; Smallwood, J.; Spreng, R.N. The default network and self-generated thought: Component processes, dynamic control, and clinical relevance. *Ann. N. Y. Acad. Sci.* **2014**, *1316*, 29–52. [CrossRef] [PubMed]
49. Leech, R.; Sharp, D.J. The role of the posterior cingulate cortex in cognition and disease. *Brain* **2014**, *137*, 12–32. [CrossRef]
50. Posner, J.; Hellerstein, D.J.; Gat, I.; Mechling, A.; Klahr, K.; Wang, Z.; McGrath, P.J.; Stewart, J.W.; Peterson, B.S. Antidepressants Normalize the Default Mode Network in Patients with Dysthymia. *JAMA Psychiatry* **2013**, *70*, 373–382. [CrossRef]
51. Zhou, J.; Greicius, M.D.; Gennatas, E.D.; Growdon, M.E.; Jang, J.Y.; Rabinovici, G.D.; Kramer, J.H.; Weiner, M.; Miller, B.L.; Seeley, W.W. Divergent network connectivity changes in behavioural variant frontotemporal dementia and Alzheimer's disease. *Brain* **2010**, *133*, 1352–1367. [CrossRef]
52. Yuan, Y.; Zhang, Z.; Bai, F.; Yu, H.; Shi, Y.; Qian, Y.; Liu, W.; You, J.; Zhang, X.; Liu, Z. Abnormal neural activity in the patients with remitted geriatric depression: A resting-state functional magnetic resonance imaging study. *J. Affect. Disord.* **2008**, *111*, 145–152. [CrossRef]
53. Chen, J.; Liu, F.; Xun, G.; Chen, H.; Hu, M.; Guo, X.; Xiao, C.; Wooderson, S.C.; Guo, W.; Zhao, J. Early and late onset, first-episode, treatment-naive depression: Same clinical symptoms, different regional neural activities. *J. Affect. Disord.* **2012**, *143*, 56–63. [CrossRef] [PubMed]
54. Mulders, P.C.; van Eijndhoven, P.F.; Schene, A.H.; Beckmann, C.F.; Tendolkar, I. Resting-state functional connectivity in major depressive disorder: A review. *Neurosci. Biobehav. Rev.* **2015**, *56*, 330–344. [CrossRef]
55. Li, B.; Liu, L.; Friston, K.J.; Shen, H.; Wang, L.; Zeng, L.-L.; Hu, D. A Treatment-Resistant Default Mode Subnetwork in Major Depression. *Biol. Psychiatry* **2013**, *74*, 48–54. [CrossRef]
56. Guo, W.; Liu, F.; Zhang, J.; Zhang, Z.; Yu, L.; Liu, J.; Chen, H.; Xiao, C. Abnormal default-mode network homogeneity in first-episode, drug-naive major depressive disorder. *PLoS ONE* **2014**, *9*, e91102. [CrossRef]
57. Sheline, Y.I.; Price, J.L.; Yan, Z.; Mintun, M.A. Resting-state functional MRI in depression unmasks increased connectivity between networks via the dorsal nexus. *Proc. Natl. Acad. Sci. USA* **2010**, *107*, 11020–11025. [CrossRef]
58. Van Tol, M.J.; Li, M.; Metzger, C.D.; Hailla, N.; Horn, D.I.; Li, W.; Heinze, H.J.; Bogerts, B.; Steiner, J.; He, H.; et al. Local cortical thinning links to resting-statedisconnectivity in major depressive disorder. *Psychol. Med.* **2014**, *44*, 2053–2065. [CrossRef]
59. Wu, M.; Andreescu, C.; Butters, M.A.; Tamburo, R.; Reynolds, C.F.; Aizenstein, H. Default-mode network connectivity and white matter burden in late-life depression. *Psychiatry Res. Neuroimaging* **2011**, *194*, 39–46. [CrossRef]
60. Andreescu, C.; Tudorascu, D.L.; Butters, M.A.; Tamburo, E.; Patel, M.; Price, J.; Karp, J.F.; Reynolds, C.F.; Aizenstein, H. Resting state functional connectivity and treatment response in late-life depression. *Psychiatry Res. Neuroimaging* **2013**, *214*, 313–321. [CrossRef]
61. Davis, A.K.; Barrett, F.S.; May, D.G.; Cosimano, M.P.; Sepeda, N.D.; Johnson, M.W.; Finan, P.H.; Griffiths, R.G. Effects of Psilocybin-Assisted Therapy on Major Depressive Disorder: A Randomized Clinical Trial. *JAMA Psychiatry* **2020**. [CrossRef]
62. Duffau, H. Functional Mapping before and after Low-Grade Glioma Surgery: A New Way to Decipher Various Spatiotemporal Patterns of Individual Neuroplastic Potential in Brain Tumor Patients. *Cancers* **2020**, *12*, 2611. [CrossRef]

63. Shen, K.K.; Welton, T.; Lyon, M.; McCorkindale, A.N.; Sutherland, G.T.; Burnham, S.; Fripp, J.; Martins, R.; Grieve, S.M. Structural core of the executive control network: A high angular resolution diffusion MRI study. *Hum. Brain Mapp.* **2020**, *41*, 1226–1236. [CrossRef]
64. Zhu, Z.; Johnson, N.F.; Kim, C.; Gold, B.T. Reduced frontal cortex efficiency is associated with lower white matter integrity in aging. *Cereb. Cortex* **2015**, *25*, 138–146. [CrossRef]
65. Rosenberg-Katz, K.; Herman, T.; Jacob, Y.; Mirelman, A.; Giladi, N.; Hendler, T.; Hausdorff, J.M. Fall risk is associated with amplified functional connectivity of the central executive network in patients with Parkinson's disease. *J. Neurol.* **2015**, *262*, 2448–2456. [CrossRef]
66. Cai, S.; Peng, Y.; Chong, T.; Zhang, Y.; von Deneen, K.M.; Huang, L. Differentiated Effective Connectivity Patterns of the Executive Control Network in Progressive MCI: A Potential Biomarker for Predicting AD. *Curr. Alzheimer Res.* **2017**, *14*, 937–950. [CrossRef]
67. Zhao, Q.; Lu, H.; Metmer, H.; Li, W.X.Y.; Lu, J. Evaluating functional connectivity of executive control network and frontoparietal network in Alzheimer's disease. *Brain Res.* **2018**, *1678*, 262–272. [CrossRef]
68. Cieri, F.; Esposito, R.; Cera, N.; Pieramico, V.; Tartaro, A.; Di Giannantonio, M. Late-life depression: Modifications of brain resting state activity. *J. Geriatr. Psychiatry Neurol.* **2017**, *30*, 140–150. [CrossRef]
69. Respino, M.; Hoptman, M.J.; Victoria, L.W.; Alexopoulos, G.S.; Solomonov, N.; Stein, A.T.; Coluccio, M.; Morimoto, S.S.; Blau, C.J.; Abreu, L.; et al. Cognitive Control Network Homogeneity and Executive Functions in Late-Life Depression. *Biol. Psychiatry Cogn. Neurosci. Neuroimaging* **2020**, *5*, 213–221. [CrossRef]
70. Manning, K.; Wang, L.; Steffens, D. Recent advances in the use of imaging in psychiatry: Functional magnetic resonance imaging of large-scale brain networks in late-life depression. *F1000Research* **2019**, *8*, 1–9. [CrossRef]
71. Lockwood, K.A.; Alexopoulos, G.S.; van Gorp, W.G. Executive dysfunction in geriatric depression. *Am. J. Psychiatry* **2002**, *159*, 1119–1126. [CrossRef]
72. Alexopoulos, G.S.; Hoptman, M.J.; Kanellopoulos, D.; Murphy, C.F.; Lim, K.O.; Gunning, F.M. Functional connectivity in the cognitive control network and the default mode network in late-life depression. *J. Affect. Disord.* **2012**, *139*, 56–65. [CrossRef]
73. Alalade, E.; Denny, K.; Potter, G.; Steffens, D.; Wang, L. Altered Cerebellar-Cerebral Functional Connectivity in Geriatric Depression. *PLoS ONE* **2011**, *6*, e20035. [CrossRef]
74. Yin, Y.; Hou, Z.; Wang, X.; Sui, Y.; Yuan, Y. Association between altered resting-state cortico-cerebellar functional connectivity networks and mood/cognition dysfunction in late-onset depression. *J. Neural Transm.* **2015**, *122*, 887–889. [CrossRef]
75. Li, W.; Wang, Y.; Ward, B.D.; Antuono, P.G.; Li, S.-J.; Goveas, J.S. Intrinsic inter-network brain dysfunction correlates with symptom dimensions in late-life depression. *J. Psychiatr. Res.* **2017**, *87*, 71–80. [CrossRef]
76. Yue, Y.; Jia, X.; Hou, Z.; Zang, Y.; Yuan, Y. Frequency-dependent amplitude alterations of resting-state spontaneous fluctuations in late-onset depression. *Biomed. Res. Int.* **2015**, *2015*, 1–9. [CrossRef] [PubMed]
77. Yue, Y.; Yuan, Y.; Hou, Z.; Jiang, W.; Bai, F.; Zhang, Z. Abnormal Functional Connectivity of Amygdala in Late- Onset Depression Was Associated with Cognitive Deficits. *PLoS ONE* **2013**, *8*, e75058. [CrossRef] [PubMed]
78. Wang, Z.; Yuan, Y.; Bai, F.; Shu, H.; You, J.; Li, L.; Zhang, Z. Altered functional connectivity networks of hippocampal subregions in remitted late-onset depression: A longitudinal resting-state study. *Neurosci. Bull.* **2015**, *31*, 13–21. [CrossRef] [PubMed]
79. Manning, K.J.; Alexopoulos, G.S.; Mcgovern, A.R.; Morimoto, S.S.; Yuen, G.; Kanellopoulos, T.; Gunning, F.M. Executive functioning in late-life depression. *Psychiatr. Ann.* **2014**, *44*, 143–146. [CrossRef]
80. Gandelman, J.A.; Albert, K.; Boyd, B.D.; Park, J.W.; Riddle, M.; Woodward, N.D.; Kang, H.; Landman, B.A.; Taylor, W.D. Intrinsic Functional Network Connectivity Is Associated With Clinical Symptoms and Cognition in Late-Life Depression. *Biol. Psychiatry Cogn. Neurosci. Neuroimaging* **2019**, *4*, 160–170. [CrossRef]
81. Alexopoulos, G.S.; Kiosses, D.N.; Klimstra, S.; Kalayam, B.; Bruce, M.L. Clinical Presentation of the "Depression–Executive Dysfunction Syndrome" of Late Life. *Am. J. Geriatr. Psychiatry* **2002**, *10*, 98–106. [PubMed]
82. Alexopoulos, G.S.; Kiosses, D.N.; Heo, M.; Murphy, C.F.; Shanmugham, B.; Gunning-Dixon, F. Executive Dysfunction and the Course of Geriatric Depression. *Biol. Psychiatry* **2005**, *58*, 204–210. [CrossRef]
83. Manning, K.J.; Alexopoulos, G.S.; Banerjee, S.; Morimoto, S.S.; Seirup, J.K.; Klimstra, S.A.; Yuen, G.; Kanellopoulos, T.; Gunning-Dixon, F. Executive functioning complaints and escitalopram treatment response in late-life depression. *Am. J. Geriatr. Psychiatry* **2015**, *23*, 440–445. [CrossRef]
84. Morimoto, S.S.; Kanellopoulos, D.; Manning, K.J.; Alexopoulos, G.S. Diagnosis and treatment of depression and cognitive impairment in late life. *Ann. N. Y. Acad. Sci.* **2015**, *1345*, 36–46. [CrossRef]
85. Yin, Y.; He, X.; Xu, M.; Hou, Z.; Song, X.; Sui, Y.; Liu, Z.; Jiang, W.; Yue, Y.; Zhang, Y.; et al. Structural and functional connectivity of default mode network underlying the cognitive impairment in late-onset depression. *Sci. Rep.* **2016**, *6*, 1–10. [CrossRef]
86. Kim, J.; Kim, Y.-K. Crosstalk between Depression and Dementia with Resting-State fMRI Studies and Its Relationship with Cognitive Functioning. *Biomedicines* **2021**, *9*, 82. [CrossRef] [PubMed]
87. Menon, V.; Uddin, L.Q. Saliency, switching, attention and control: A network model of insula function. *Brain Struct. Funct.* **2010**, *214*, 655–667. [CrossRef] [PubMed]
88. Seeley, X.W.W. The Salience Network: A Neural System for Perceiving and Responding to Homeostatic Demands. *J. Neurosci.* **2019**, *39*, 9878–9882. [CrossRef] [PubMed]
89. Touroutoglou, A.; Hollenbeck, M.; Dickerson, B.C.; Feldman Barrett, L. Dissociable large-scale networks anchored in the right anterior insula subserve affective experience and attention. *Neuroimage* **2012**, *60*, 1947–1958. [CrossRef]

90. Seeley, W.W.; Menon, V.; Schatzberg, A.F.; Keller, J.; Glover, G.H.; Kenna, H.; Reiss, A.L.; Greicius, M.D. 973 Dissociable Intrinsic Connectivity Networks for Salience Processing and Executive Control. *J. Neurosci.* **2007**, *27*, 2349–2356. [CrossRef]
91. Chand, G.B.; Wu, J.; Hajjar, I.; Qiu, D. Interactions of the Salience Network and Its Subsystems with the Default-Mode and the Central-Executive. *Brain Connect.* **2017**, *7*, 401–412. [CrossRef]
92. Elton, A.; Gao, W. Divergent task-dependent functional connectivity of executive control and salience networks. *Cortex* **2014**, *51*, 56–66. [CrossRef]
93. Cullen, K.R.; Westlund, M.K.; Klimes-Dougan, B.; Mueller, B.A.; Houri, A.; Eberly, L.E.; Lim, K.O. Abnormal Amygdala Resting-State Functional Connectivity in Adolescent Depression. *JAMA Psychiatry* **2014**, *71*, 1138–1147. [CrossRef]
94. Luking, K.R.; Repovs, G.; Belden, A.C.; Gaffrey, M.S.; Botteron, K.N.; Luby, J.L.; Barch, D.M. Functional Connectivity of the Amygdala in Early-Childhood-Onset Depression. *J. Am. Acad. Child Adolesc. Psychiatry* **2011**, *50*, 1027–1041. [CrossRef]
95. Dai, L.; Zhou, H.; Xu, X.; Zuo, Z. Brain structural and functional changes in patients with major depressive disorder: A literature review. *PeerJ* **2019**, *7*, e8170. [CrossRef]
96. Connolly, C.G.; Wu, J.; Ho, T.C.; Hoeft, F.; Wolkowitz, O.; Eisendrath, S.; Frank, G.; Hendren, R.; Max, J.E.; Paulus, M.P.; et al. Resting-state functional connectivity of subgenual anterior cingulate cortex in depressed adolescents. *Biol. Psychiatry* **2013**, *74*, 898–907. [CrossRef]
97. Davey, C.G.; Whittle, S.; Harrison, B.J.; Simmons, J.G.; Byrne, M.L.; Schwartz, O.S.; Allen, N.B. Functional brain-imaging correlates of negative affectivity and the onset of first-episode depression. *Psychol. Med.* **2015**, *45*, 1001–1009. [CrossRef]
98. Yuen, G.S.; Gunning-Dixon, F.M.; Hoptman, M.J.; AbdelMalak, B.; McGovern, A.R.; Seirup, J.K.; Alexopoulos, G.S. The salience network in the apathy of late-life depression. *Int. J. Geriatr. Psychiatry* **2014**, *29*, 1116–1124. [CrossRef]
99. Zhang, H.; Li, L.; Wu, M.; Chen, Z.; Hu, X.; Chen, Y.; Zhu, H.; Jia, Z.; Gong, Q. Brain gray matter alterations in first episodes of depression: A meta-analysis of whole-brain studies. *Neurosci. Biobehav. Rev.* **2016**, *60*, 43–50. [CrossRef]
100. Steffens, D.C.; Wang, L.; Pearlson, G.D. Functional connectivity predictors of acute depression treatment outcome. *Int. Psychogeriatr.* **2019**, *31*, 1831–1835. [CrossRef]
101. Janiri, D.; Moser, D.A.; Doucet, G.E.; Luber, M.J.; Rasgon, A.; Lee, W.H.; Murrough, J.W.; Sani, G.; Eickhoff, S.B.; Frangou, S. Shared Neural Phenotypes for Mood and Anxiety Disorders: A Meta-analysis of 226 Task-Related Functional Imaging Studies. *JAMA Psychiatry* **2020**, *77*, 172–179. [CrossRef]
102. Tanaka, M.; Telegdy, G. Neurotransmissions of antidepressant-like effects of neuromedin U-23 in mice. *Behav. Brain Res.* **2014**, *259*, 196–199. [CrossRef]
103. Tanaka, M.; Kádár, K.; Tóth, G.; Telegdy, G. Antidepressant-like effects of urocortin 3 fragments. *Brain Res. Bull.* **2011**, *84*, 414–418. [CrossRef]
104. Telegdy, G.; Tanaka, M.; Schally, A.V. Effects of the LHRH antagonist Cetrorelix on the brain function in mice. *Neuropeptides* **2009**, *43*, 229–234. [CrossRef]
105. Tanaka, M.; Schally, A.V.; Telegdy, G. Neurotransmission of the antidepressant-like effects of the growth hormone-releasing hormone antagonist MZ-4-71. *Behav. Brain Res.* **2012**, *228*, 388–391. [CrossRef] [PubMed]
106. Vargas, A.S.; Luís, Â.; Barroso, M.; Gallardo, E.; Pereira, L. Psilocybin as a New Approach to Treat Depression and Anxiety in the Context of Life-Threatening Diseases—A Systematic Review and Meta-Analysis of Clinical Trials. *Biomedicines* **2020**, *8*, 331. [CrossRef] [PubMed]
107. Ibos, K.E.; Bodnár, É.; Bagosi, Z.; Bozsó, Z.; Tóth, G.; Szabó, G.; Csabafi, K. Kisspeptin-8 Induces Anxiety-Like Behavior and Hypolocomotion by Activating the HPA Axis and Increasing GABA Release in the Nucleus Accumbens in Rats. *Biomedicines* **2021**, *9*, 112. [CrossRef] [PubMed]
108. Caruso, G.; Godos, J.; Castellano, S.; Micek, A.; Murabito, P.; Galvano, F.; Ferri, R.; Grosso, G.; Caraci, F. The Therapeutic Potential of Carnosine/Anserine Supplementation against Cognitive Decline: A Systematic Review with Meta-Analysis. *Biomedicines* **2021**, *9*, 253. [CrossRef]
109. Kim, I.B.; Park, S.-C. Neural Circuitry–Neurogenesis Coupling Model of Depression. *Int. J. Mol. Sci.* **2021**, *22*, 2468. [CrossRef]
110. Małgorzata, P.; Paweł, K.; Iwona, M.L.; Brzostek, T.; Andrzej, P. Glutamatergic dysregulation in mood disorders: Opportunities for the discovery of novel drug targets. *Expert Opin. Ther. Targets* **2020**, *3*, 1–23.
111. Tanaka, M.; Bohár, Z.; Vécsei, L. Are Kynurenines Accomplices or Principal Villains in Dementia? Maintenance of Kynurenine Metabolism. *Molecules* **2020**, *25*, 564. [CrossRef]
112. Pochwat, B.; Nowak, G.; Szewczyk, B. An update on NMDA antagonists in depression. *Expert Rev. Neurother.* **2019**, *19*, 1055–1067. [CrossRef]
113. Shin, C.; Kim, Y.K. Ketamine in Major Depressive Disorder: Mechanisms and Future Perspectives. *Psychiatry Investig.* **2020**, *17*, 181–192. [CrossRef]
114. Zanos, P.; Gould, T.D. Mechanisms of ketamine action as an antidepressant. *Mol. Psychiatry* **2018**, *23*, 801–811. [CrossRef]
115. Encyclopedia. The Tryptophan-Kynurenine Metabolic Pathway. Available online: https://encyclopedia.pub/8633 (accessed on 24 March 2021).
116. Tanaka, M.; Toldi, J.; Vécsei, L. Exploring the Etiological Links behind Neurodegenerative Diseases: Inflammatory Cytokines and Bioactive Kynurenines. *Int. J. Mol. Sci.* **2020**, *21*, 2431. [CrossRef]
117. Török, N.; Tanaka, M.; Vécsei, L. Searching for Peripheral Biomarkers in Neurodegenerative Diseases: The Tryptophan-Kynurenine Metabolic Pathway. *Int. J. Mol. Sci.* **2020**, *21*, 9338. [CrossRef]

118. Erabi, H.; Okada, G.; Shibasaki, C.; Setoyama, D.; Kang, D.; Takamura, M.; Yoshino, A.; Fuchikami, M.; Kurata, A.; Kato, T.A.; et al. Kynurenic acid is a potential overlapped biomarker between diagnosis and treatment response for depression from metabolome analysis. *Sci. Rep.* **2020**, *10*, 16822. [CrossRef]
119. Hunt, C.; Macedo e Cordeiro, T.; Suchting, R.; de Dios, C.; Cuellar Leal, V.A.; Soares, J.C.; Dantzer, R.; Teixeira, A.L.; Selvaraj, S. Effect of immune activation on the kynurenine pathway and depression symptoms—A systematic review and meta-analysis. *Neurosci. Biobehav. Rev.* **2020**, *118*, 514. [CrossRef] [PubMed]
120. Serafini, G.; Adavastro, G.; Canepa, G.; Capobianco, L.; Conigliaro, C.; Pittaluga, F.; Murri, M.B.; Valchera, A.; De Berardis, D.; Pompili, M.; et al. Abnormalities in Kynurenine Pathway Metabolism in Treatment-Resistant Depression and Suicidality: A Systematic Review. *CNS Neurol. Disord. Drug Targets* **2017**, *16*, 440–453. [CrossRef] [PubMed]
121. Kennedy, P.J.; Cryan, J.F.; Dinan, T.G.; Clarke, G. Kynurenine pathway metabolism and the microbiota-gut-brain axis. *Neuropharmacology* **2017**, *112*, 399–412. [CrossRef]
122. Kim, E.Y.; Ahn, H.-S.; Lee, M.Y.; Yu, J.; Yeom, J.; Jeong, H.; Min, H.; Lee, H.J.; Kim, K.; Ahn, Y.M. An Exploratory Pilot Study with Plasma Protein Signatures Associated with Response of Patients with Depression to Antidepressant Treatment for 10 Weeks. *Biomedicines* **2020**, *8*, 455. [CrossRef] [PubMed]
123. López-Gambero, A.J.; Sanjuan, C.; Serrano-Castro, P.J.; Suárez, J.; Rodríguez de Fonseca, F. The Biomedical Uses of Inositols: A Nutraceutical Approach to Metabolic Dysfunction in Aging and Neurodegenerative Diseases. *Biomedicines* **2020**, *8*, 295. [CrossRef]
124. Cantón-Habas, V.; Rich-Ruiz, M.; Romero-Saldaña, M.; Carrera-González, M.P. Depression as a Risk Factor for Dementia and Alzheimer's Disease. *Biomedicines* **2020**, *8*, 45. [CrossRef]
125. Kowalska, K.; Krzywoszański, Ł.; Droś, J.; Pasińska, P.; Wilk, A.; Klimkowicz-Mrowiec, A. Early Depression Independently of Other Neuropsychiatric Conditions, Influences Disability and Mortality after Stroke (Research Study—Part of PROPOLIS Study). *Biomedicines* **2020**, *8*, 509. [CrossRef] [PubMed]
126. Carrillo-Mora, P.; Pérez-De la Cruz, V.; Estrada-Cortés, B.; Toussaint-González, P.; Martínez-Cortéz, J.A.; Rodríguez-Barragán, M.; Quinzaños-Fresnedo, J.; Rangel-Caballero, F.; Gamboa-Coria, G.; Sánchez-Vázquez, I.; et al. Serum Kynurenines Correlate with Depressive Symptoms and Disability in Poststroke Patients: A Cross-sectional Study. *Neurorehabilit. Neural Repair* **2020**, 154596832095367.
127. Park, S.; Bak, A.; Kim, S.; Nam, Y.; Kim, H.; Yoo, D.-H.; Moon, M. Animal-Assisted and Pet-Robot Interventions for Ameliorating Behavioral and Psychological Symptoms of Dementia: A Systematic Review and Meta-Analysis. *Biomedicines* **2020**, *8*, 150. [CrossRef] [PubMed]
128. Di Nicola, V.; Stoyanov, D.S. *Psychiatry in Crisis At the Crossroads of Social Sciences, the Humanities, and Neuroscience*; Springer Nature Switzerland AG: Cham, Switzerland, 2021. [CrossRef]

biomedicines

MDPI

Article

The Therapeutic Potential of Carnosine/Anserine Supplementation against Cognitive Decline: A Systematic Review with Meta-Analysis

Giuseppe Caruso [1], Justyna Godos [2], Sabrina Castellano [3], Agnieszka Micek [4], Paolo Murabito [5], Fabio Galvano [2], Raffaele Ferri [6], Giuseppe Grosso [2,*] and Filippo Caraci [1,6]

[1] Department of Drug and Health Sciences, University of Catania, 95125 Catania, Italy; forgiuseppecaruso@gmail.com (G.C.); f.caraci@unict.it (F.C.)
[2] Department of Biomedical and Biotechnological Sciences, University of Catania, 95123 Catania, Italy; justyna.godos@gmail.com (J.G.); fgalvano@unict.it (F.G.)
[3] Department of Educational Sciences, University of Catania, 95124 Catania, Italy; sabrina.castellano@unict.it
[4] Department of Nursing Management and Epidemiology Nursing, Faculty of Health Sciences, Jagiellonian University Medical College, 31-501 Krakow, Poland; agnieszka.micek@uj.edu.pl
[5] Department of General Surgery and Medical-Surgical Specialties, Section of Anesthesia and Intensive Care, University of Catania, 95123 Catania, Italy; paolo.murabito@unict.it
[6] Oasi Research Institute—IRCCS, 94018 Troina, Italy; rferri@oasi.en.it
* Correspondence: giuseppe.grosso@unict.it; Tel.: +39-0954-781-187

Abstract: Carnosine is a natural occurring endogenous dipeptide that was proposed as an anti-aging agent more than 20 years ago. Carnosine can be found at low millimolar concentrations at brain level and different preclinical studies have demonstrated its antioxidant, anti-inflammatory, and anti-aggregation activity with neuroprotective effects in animal models of Alzheimer's disease (AD). A selective deficit of carnosine has also been linked to cognitive decline in AD. Different clinical studies have been conducted to evaluate the impact of carnosine supplementation against cognitive decline in elderly and AD subjects. We conducted a systematic review with meta-analysis, in accordance with the PRISMA guidelines coupled to the PICOS approach, to investigate the therapeutic potential of carnosine against cognitive decline and depressive symptoms in elderly subjects. We found five studies matching the selection criteria. Carnosine/anserine was administered for 12 weeks at a dose of 1 g/day and improved global cognitive function, whereas no effects were detected on depressive symptoms. These data suggest a preliminary evidence of clinical efficacy of carnosine against cognitive decline both in elderly subjects and mild cognitive impairment (MCI) patients, although larger and long-term clinical studies are needed in MCI patients (with or without depression) to confirm the therapeutic potential of carnosine.

Keywords: carnosine; cognitive function; depressive symptoms; age-related cognitive decline; Alzheimer's disease; neuroinflammation; oxidative stress

Citation: Caruso, G.; Godos, J.; Castellano, S.; Micek, A.; Murabito, P.; Galvano, F.; Ferri, R.; Grosso, G.; Caraci, F. The Therapeutic Potential of Carnosine/Anserine Supplementation against Cognitive Decline: A Systematic Review with Meta-Analysis. *Biomedicines* **2021**, *9*, 253. https://doi.org/10.3390/biomedicines9030253

Academic Editor: Masaru Tanaka

Received: 29 December 2020
Accepted: 27 February 2021
Published: 4 March 2021

1. Introduction

Carnosine is a natural occurring endogenous dipeptide discovered by Gulewitsch and Amiradžibi during the analysis of a meat extract more than 100 years ago [1]. The synthesis of this molecule starting from its constituting amino acids, β-alanine and L-histidine, through an enzyme-catalyzed reaction requiring Mg^{++} and adenosine triphosphate (ATP) was first described in 1950s [2,3]. Carnosine has been found in the tissues and organs of vertebrates [4] as well as in the tissues of some invertebrate species [5,6]. With regard to mammalian, this widely distributed molecule is present in different organs, such as spleen and kidney [7], and can be found at low millimolar (mM) concentrations at brain level [8], while it reaches high mM concentrations (up to 20 mM) in cardiac and skeletal muscles [9]. In a study by Fonteh et al., a selective deficit of carnosine has been related to cognitive decline in probable Alzheimer's disease (pAD) subjects [10]. In this study, where the free amino acid and dipeptide changes in the body fluids from pAD subjects were analyzed, carnosine levels were significantly lower in pAD (328.4 ± 91.31 nmol/dl) than in plasma of healthy subjects (654.23 ± 100.61nmol/dl); this deficit of carnosine correlated with reduced global cognitive function measured by Mini-Mental State Examination (MMSE) and Alzheimer's Disease Assessment Scale cognitive subscale (ADAS-cog).

The decrease of carnosine levels in AD is also favored by the age-related increase in the serum-circulating (CNDP1 or CN1) activity in specific brain regions [11]. In fact the concentrations of carnosine in human tissues and biological fluids are regulated by the activity of two dipeptidases: CNDP1 [12] and the cytosolic (CNDP2 or CN2) carnosinase [13], both of them members of the M20 metalloprotease family [14]. As it has been shown for the first time by Perry and colleagues, patients with carnosinase deficiency, a condition also known as carnosinemia, present an excess of carnosine in the urine (carnosinuria) and develop a progressive neurologic disorder characterized by severe mental defects and intellectual disability [15–17].

Different mechanisms have been identified that can explain the hypothesized protective activity of carnosine against cognitive decline [18]. In fact, it can act as neurotransmitter [19], immune system enhancer [20], nitric oxide metabolism modulator [21,22], heavy metal chelator [23,24], cell energy metabolism enhancer [25,26], anti-glycation, and anti-aging agent [27,28]. Carnosine has also been shown to modulate glutamatergic system by upregulating the glutamate transporter 1 and reducing glutamate concentrations in the central nervous system (CNS) [29].

It is becoming increasingly evident that neuroinflammation [30–32] and oxidative stress [33,34], along with the abnormal accumulation of proteins at brain level [35,36], significantly contribute to the cognitive decline associated to different pathologies of CNS. According to this scenario, the well-known antioxidant, anti-inflammatory, and anti-aggregation activities of carnosine have been recently reconsidered [37], to better understand the therapeutic potential of this peptide in the treatment of cognitive disorders. In a preclinical study by Herculano et al., the treatment with carnosine (5 mg/day for six weeks) was able to rescue cognitive deficits and revert oxidative stress and microglial activation induced by an high fat diet in the hippocampus of a transgenic mouse model of AD [38]. The rescue of cognitive deficit by carnosine was also demonstrated in streptozotocin-induced diabetic rats [39], as well as in subcortical ischemic vascular dementia [40] and transgenic 3 × Tg-AD mice, showing both amyloid beta (Aβ)- and tau-dependent pathology [41]. Preclinical studies in mice have demonstrated that this dipeptide is essentially non-toxic [42]; additionally, it is well tolerated in humans [43,44] without known drug interactions and dangerous side effects.

Moving from mice to humans, different clinical trials have been conducted to explore the therapeutic effects of carnosine in cognitive disorders. In a randomized double-blind placebo controlled 12-week dose escalation study, involving 25 Gulf War illness subjects, carnosine (1500 mg/day) gave beneficial cognitive effects [45]. In a study carried out by Masuoka et al., the potential protective effects of anserine/carnosine (3:1) supplementation against cognitive decline in APOE4 (+) mild cognitive impairment (MCI) subjects were shown, possibly by preventing a transition from MCI to AD [46]. Improvements on cognitive functioning have also been observed in two different studies, using a pill-based nutraceutical (NT-020) containing carnosine in older adults [47] or a formulation (formula F) including carnosine administered along with donepezil to moderate probable AD subjects [48].

Carnosine was proposed as an anti-aging agent more than 20 years ago [28]. During the following years, several human studies have been carried out to test its possible positive effects in the elderly. It has been shown that dietary supplementation of carnosine (250–350 mg/daily) in combination with its methylated analogue anserine (β-alanyl-1-N-methyl-L-histidine) (650–750 mg/daily) for about 13 weeks is able to improve cognitive function [49,50] and physical activity [50], to preserve verbal episodic memory and brain perfusion [49,51], and to modulate network connectivity changes associated with cognitive function [49] in elderly people.

Despite numerous preclinical and clinical studies that have been carried out, the effects of carnosine supplementation in preventing and/or counteracting cognitive decline in humans have not yet been completely understood. Recent reviews provide a comprehensive overview of the role of carnosine in neurological, neurodegenerative, and psychiatric disorders [52], although no specific meta-analyses have been conducted to analyze the clinical efficacy of carnosine in different double-blind randomized placebo-controlled trials.

With the present study, we aimed to address this specific gap in the knowledge of the therapeutic potential of carnosine against cognitive decline by conducting a systematic review with meta-analysis, in accordance with the PRISMA guidelines coupled to the PICOS approach, to investigate the effects of this peptide with a multimodal pharmacodynamic profile on cognitive function and depressive symptoms in elderly subjects.

2. Methods

The design, analysis, and reporting of this study followed Preferred Reporting Items for Systematic Reviews and Meta-Analysis (PRISMA) (Supplementary Table S1) [53]. Moreover, eligibility criteria for the search and meta-analyses were specified using the PICOS approach: Determination of the population (P), intervention (I), comparison (C), outcomes (O), study design (S) (Table 1).

Table 1. PICOS criteria.

PICOS	Description
P (Population)	Men and/or women, adults.
I (Intervention)	Carnosine supplementation (carnosine alone or combined with other treatment).
C (Comparison)	Carnosine supplementation group (carnosine alone or combined with other treatment) versus placebo/control group.
O (Outcomes)	Changes in cognitive function, depressive symptoms, and overall mental health. Long term changes rather than acute effect.
S (Study design)	Systematic review with meta-analysis.

2.1. Study Selection

A systematic search on PubMed (http://www.ncbi.nlm.nih.gov/pubmed/ (accessed on 4 March 2021)), EMBASE (http://www.embase.com/ (accessed on 4 March 2021)), and Web of Science (www.webofknowledge.com (accessed on 4 March 2021)) databases of studies published up to April 2020 was performed using the following search strategy: (carnosine OR l-carnosine OR n-acetyl-carnosine OR n-acetyl-l-carnosine OR histidine OR beta-alanyl-l-histidine OR b-alanyl-l-histidine OR L-Histidine OR l-alpha-alanyl-l-histidine OR beta-alanine OR β-alanine OR beta alanyl 3 methylhistidine OR 3-aminopropionic-acid OR anserine) AND (cognitive OR cognition OR mental OR mood OR memory OR learning OR attention OR depression OR depressive OR schizophrenia OR Alzheimer OR Alzheimer's OR autism OR sleep) AND (randomized clinical trial OR controlled clinical trial OR randomized OR placebo OR clinical trial OR trial OR randomly OR intervention OR enrolled). The search was restricted to the studies conducted in humans. Studies were eligible if they met the following inclusion criteria: (i) were intervention studies with control group; (ii) were conducted on adults; (iii) evaluated the effect of carnosine supplementation on cognitive function and/or depression; (iv) evaluated long term effects of carnosine rather than acute effects. Studies which evaluated the effect of carnosine on cognitive performance were excluded. Finally, the studies that provided sufficient statistical data were further considered for the meta-analysis. Reference lists of eligible studies were scanned for any additional study not previously identified. If more than one study reported results on the same individuals, only the study including the larger sample size, the longest follow-up, or the most comprehensive statistical data was included in the meta-analysis. The systematic search and study selection was performed by two independent authors (J.G. and G.C.).

2.2. Data Extraction

Data were extracted using a standardized extraction form. The following information was collected: (i) First author name and publication year; (ii) study design and country; (iii) sample size and intervention duration; (iv) sex and mean age of participants; (v) type of intervention and its main characteristics; (vi) outcome scores, including means and standard deviations or standard errors or 95% confidence intervals (Cis) for each score at baseline and after follow-up for each group (intervention and control) or *p*-value for significance of this change (from paired t-test or Wilcoxon test).

2.3. Study Quality and Risk of Bias Assessment

The quality of each eligible study was assessed according to the NIH Quality Assessment of Controlled Intervention Studies (Supplementary Table S2). This tool allows the rater to assign a three-level quality score ("good", "fair", or "poor"), based on the consideration of 14 items. The tool for controlled intervention studies evaluates the following: adequate randomization, treatment allocation and blinding, similarity of groups at the baseline, dropout rates, adherence to the treatment, avoidance of other interventions, outcome measures assessment, sample size and power calculation, pre-specified outcomes, and intention-to-treat analysis. Risk of bias across included studies was assessed using Cochrane risk-of-bias tool for randomized trials (RoB-2) [54].

2.4. Statistical Analysis

All studies identified during systematic search had the independent-group pre-test–post-test design (i.e., the outcome was measured before and after intervention, and different groups received the experimental intervention or served as control group) [55]. We used standardized mean difference (SMD) due to necessity of harmonizing different scores measuring the same outcome with different tools. We used the so-called raw score metric to focus on group differences (i.e., the effect size for SMD in each intervention group was defined as the pre-test–post-test change divided by the pre-test standard deviation, due to likeness being more consistent across studies as not being influenced by the experimental manipulations) [56]. Transforming effect sizes into raw score metric required an estimate of the population correlation between pre- and post-test, which was [55]. Fixed-effects models were used to perform all meta-analyses irrespectively of heterogeneity due to small number of trials. In order to compare tools with differences in the direction of the scale, the mean values from one set of studies was multiplied by -1. Finally, in order to test whether variation between studies in effect size was associated with differences in methodology of the studies or in characteristics of participants, meta-regression analyses were performed taking into account age, sex, sample size, length of trial, and baseline scores value. A two-sided *p*-value 0.05 was set as the level of significance for comparisons of SMD. Data were analyzed using R software version 3.6.1 (Development Core Team, Vienna, Austria).

3. Results

3.1. Study Identification and Selection Process

The systematic search yielded 516 studies, out of which 403 and 77 were excluded based on the title and abstract evaluation, respectively. Thirty-six articles were assessed based on the full-text version, and 31 studies did not meet the pre-specified inclusion criteria. In particular, the studies were excluded as they (i) reported on the acute effects of carnosine supplementation, (ii) reported results on children, (iii) reported on other outcomes, such as quality of life of cognitive performance, (iv) did not explore the outcomes of interest, and (v) were conducted on partially same patients (thus, only the latest report was included). Finally, five studies [46,48,50,57,58] were included in the systematic review, out of which three provided sufficient statistical data and were included in the quantitative analysis (Figure 1).

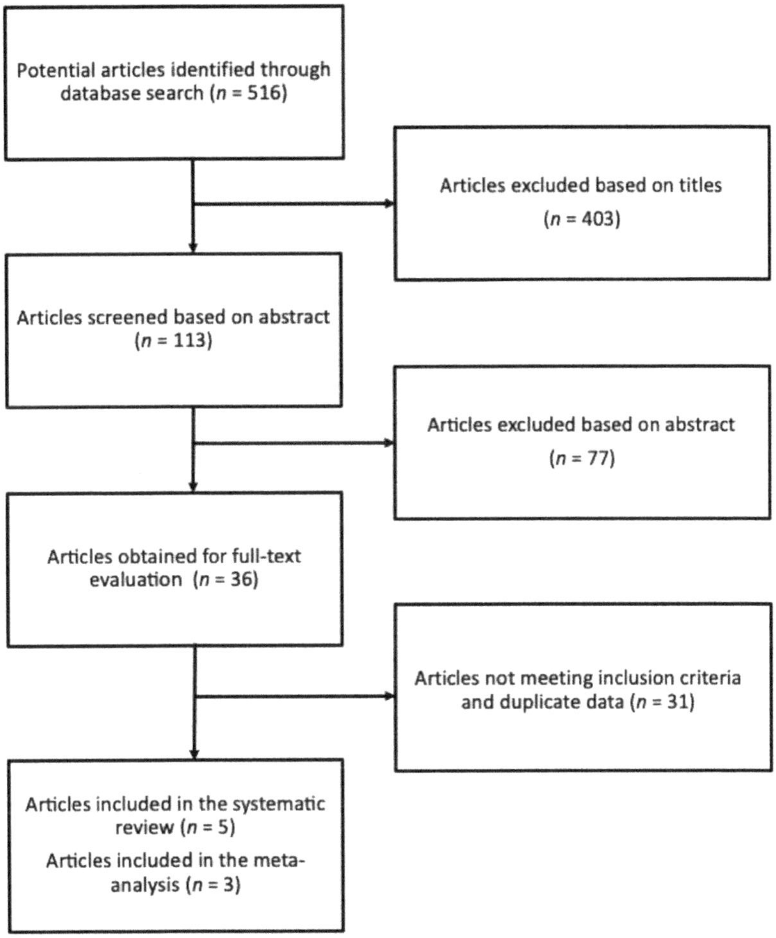

Figure 1. Study selection process.

The main characteristics of the studies included in the systematic review and meta-analysis are presented in Table 2.

Table 2. Main characteristics of the studies included in the systematic review and meta-analysis.

Author and Publication Year	Study Design, Country	Sample Size, Trial Duration	Sex, Age (mean ± SD)	Population Characteristics	Intervention (and Doses)	Measured Outcomes of Interest	NIH Quality Assessment
Szcześniak et al. 2014	Double-blind randomized placebo-controlled trial, Poland	51, 13 weeks	MF, 81.0 ± 7.0 y intervention group, 80.5 ± 7.5 y control group	Nursing home residents, MMSE score >15	1 g of anserine/carnosine (2:1 ratio); once a day	Cognitive function (MMSE, STMS), depressive symptoms (GDS), dementia (CDR)	Good
Cornelli 2010	Double-blind randomized controlled trial, USA	48, 6 months	MF, 75.0 ± 4.2 y intervention group, 74.0 ± 4.9 y control group	Patients with diagnosis of probable AD, MMSE score >21	Formula F (100 mg carnosine and antioxidant compounds: vitamins B, vitamin C and E, coenzyme Q10, beta-carotene, selenium, l-cysteine, Ginko biloba); once per day	Cognitive function (MMSE)	Good
Katakura et al. 2017	Double-blind randomized placebo-controlled trial, Japan	60, 3 months	MF, 60.4 ± 2.1 y intervention group, 65.3 ± 1.6 y control group	Healthy elderly volunteers	1 g of anserine/carnosine (3:1 ratio); twice a day	Cognitive function (MMSE, MCS), Alzheimer's disease (ADAS), memory (WMS-LM1, WMS-LM2), depressive symptoms (BDI)	Good
Masuoka et al. 2019	Double-blind randomized placebo-controlled trial, Japan	50, 12 weeks	MF, 72.9 ± 8.8 y intervention group, 73.6 ± 6.1 y control group	Outpatients with MCI, MMSE >23	750 mg anserine and 250 mg carnosine; once a day	Cognitive function (MMSE), Alzheimer's disease (ADAS), dementia (CDR), memory (WMS), depressive symptoms (GDS),	Good
Shirotsuki et al. 2017	Randomized placebo-controlled trial, Japan	72, 6 weeks	MF, 37.88 ± 9.15 y intervention group, 38.35 ± 8.83 y control group	Healthy full-time office workers	Supplement drink with 200 mg carnosine and computerized cognitive behavior therapy; once a day	Mood (POMS)	Fair

Abbreviations: AD (Alzheimer's disease); ADAS (Alzheimer's Disease Assessment Scale); AVLT (Auditory Verbal Learning Test); BDI (Beck Depression Inventory); CCBT (computerized cognitive behavior therapy); CDR (Clinical Dementia Rating); CES-D (Centers for Epidemiologic Studies Depression Scale); F (female); GDS (Geriatric Depression Scale); M (male); MCI (mild cognitive impairment); MCS (Mental health Component Summary); MMSE (Mini Mental State Examination); POMS (Profile of Mood Scale); RCT (randomized controlled trial); STMS (Short Test of Mental Status); WMS-LM (Wechsler Memory Scale Logical Memory); y (years).

One study was conducted in USA [48], three in Asia [46,57,58], and one in Europe [50]. The outcome measures explored in the studies included Mini Mental State Examination (MMSE) [46,48,50,57], Alzheimer's Disease Assessment Scale (ADAS) [46,57], Clinical Dementia Rating (CDR) [46,50], Geriatric Depression Scale (GDS) [46,50], Beck Depression Inventory (BDI) [57], Wechsler Memory Scale Logical Memory (WMS-LM) [46,49], Profile of Mood Scale (POMS) [58], Mental health Component Summary (MCS) [57], and Short Test of Mental Status (STMS) [50]. Sample size and trial length ranged from 48 to 72 individuals and six to 13 weeks, respectively.

3.2. Study Quality Assessment

Based on the NIH Quality Assessment of Controlled Intervention Studies, four of the studies reached a "good" quality score, while one scored as "fair" quality. The main limitation was that the studies did not use intention-to-treat analysis and in several cases the sample size was not sufficiently large to be able to detect a difference in the main outcome between groups with at least 80% power.

3.3. Risk of Bias

According to the Cochrane RoB-2, most of the studies had low risk of selection and attrition bias (Figure 2, Supplementary Figure S1).

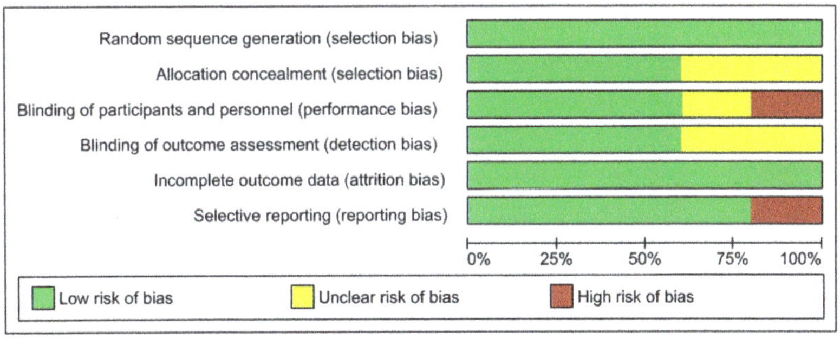

Figure 2. Summary of the risk of bias assessment according to the Cochrane risk-of-bias tool for randomized trials (RoB-2).

However, one study demonstrated high risk of performance bias due to the lack of blinding [58], and one study high reporting bias as some of the data were not reported in the manuscript [48].

3.4. Carnosine Supplementation and Cognitive and Memory Function

Four individual studies explored whether carnosine supplementation did affect cognitive function [46,48,50,57]. The study of Cornelli [48] involved 52 patients (mean age about 75 years old) affected with moderate probable Alzheimer's disease already being treated with donepezil (5 mg/day for at least two months); the authors reported that the MMSE remained stable in the group treated with standard therapy and placebo, while significant improvements were found in the intervention group with donepezil plus a formula containing 100 g of carnosine (among other antioxidants). In the study of Szcześniak et al. [50], 56 healthy subjects (age 65+ years old) were administered chicken meat extract containing 40% of anserine and carnosine components or a placebo for a 13 weeks of supplementation; the mean values of the Short Test of Mental Status (STMS) scores showed a significant increase in the intervention group, specifically in the sub scores of construction/copying, abstraction, and recall. The study of Katakura et al. [57] involved 60 healthy elderly volunteers administered 1 g carnosine/anserine or a placebo for three months; preservation of verbal memory, assessed by the WMS-LM, was observed in the intervention group (especially among older participants), while no significant changes were observed in other cognitive function measures. A significant correlation was also found between the preservation of verbal memory and suppression of C-C Motif Chemokine Ligand 24 (CCL24; an inflammatory chemokine) expression in the group that was in their 70s. The last published trial from Masouka et al. [46] on 54 subjects with MCI, randomized to an active group receiving a dose of 1 g per day of carnosine/anserine or a placebo for 12 weeks, showed improvement in the global Clinical Dementia Rating in the active group, as compared for placebo, but no significant results in the other psychometric tests, including the MMSE and the ADAS. The authors did not detect improvements in verbal episodic memory, but, interestingly, when they separated APOE4 positive (APOE4 (+)) or negative (APOE4 (−)) subjects, a clinically-relevant change was observed in the APOE4 (+) subjects both in MMSE and in gloCDR scores.

Out of the four studies, three provided sufficient data to be eligible for quantitative comparison of cognitive outcomes. The meta-analysis included two studies testing cognitive function through the MMSE [46,50] and one through the ADAS tool [57]. Although the results from individual studies did not show significant differences between intervention and control groups, results from the meta-analysis (presented in Figure 3) revealed that supplementation with carnosine led to a SMD of -0.25 (95% CI = −0.46, −0.04) in favor of the intervention compared to the control group, indicating an improvement in cognitive function.

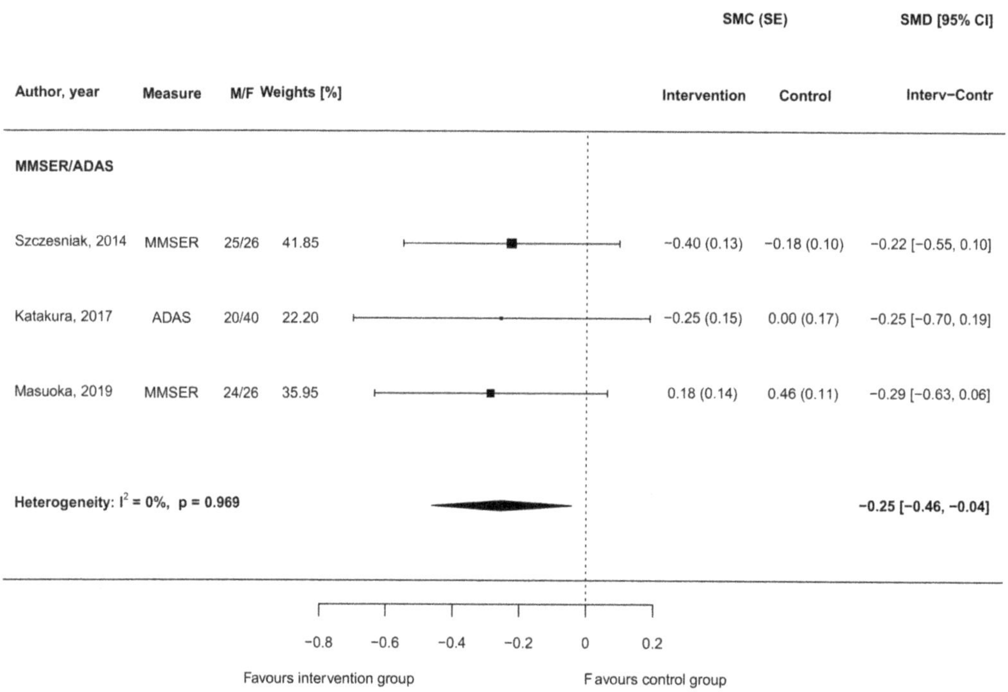

Figure 3. Standardized mean differences in cognitive outputs between intervention groups supplemented with carnosine and control groups in randomized controlled trials. Abbreviations: ADAS (Alzheimer's Disease Assessment Scale), CI (confidence interval), F (female), M (male), MMSER (Mini Mental State Examination), SE (standard error), SMC (standardized mean change), SMD (standardized mean difference).

No evidence of heterogeneity between studies (I2 = 0%, $p = 0.969$) nor asymmetry on funnel plots (Supplementary Figure S2) were found.

Meta-regression analyses were conducted to test whether study-related characteristics may have affected the results; however, none of the other variables investigated as moderators substantially influenced the overall effect size (Supplementary Table S3).

Results from the two studies reporting comparable quantitative data on verbal memory, assessed through the Wechsler memory scale–revised logical memory immediate recall (WMS-LM1) and delayed recall (WMS-LM2) tests, are shown in Figure 4.

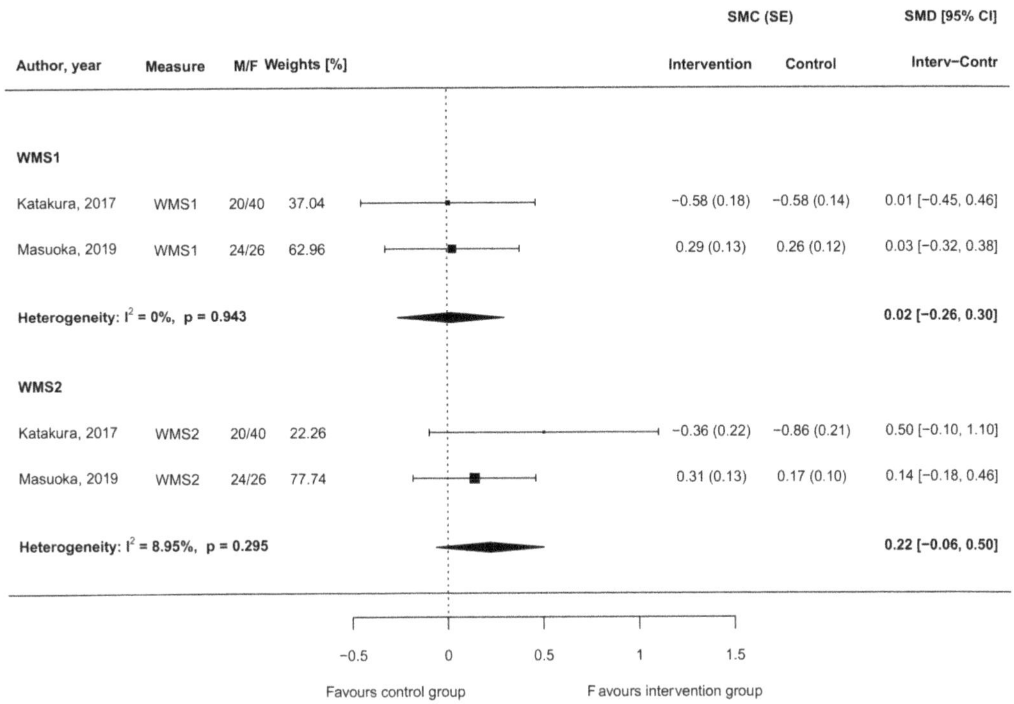

Figure 4. Standardized mean differences in verbal memory outputs between intervention groups supplemented with carnosine and control groups in randomized controlled trials. Abbreviations: CI (confidence interval), F (female), M (male), SE (standard error), SMC (standardized mean change), SMD (standardized mean difference), WMS (Wechsler Memory Scale).

While nearly no differences could be observed for the WMS-LM1, an improvement, yet not significant, in the WMS-LM2 was found in the intervention compared to the control group (SMD = 0.22, 95 CI: −0.06, 0.50), with no evidence of heterogeneity between studies (I2 = 8.95%, p = 0.295; Figure 4).

All studies but one lasted less than 12 weeks, thus no meta-regression was conducted on length of trial. None of the other variables investigated as moderators substantially influenced the overall effect size (Supplementary Table S3).

3.5. Carnosine Supplementation and Depressive Symptoms

The effect of carnosine supplementation toward depressive symptoms was investigated in three studies [46,50,57]. One of these studies reported no improvement of depressive symptoms among all subjects measured with the GDS, also authors did not observe any altering of the distribution of ratings of depressive symptoms in the carnosine supplemented individuals [50]. Additionally, Masuoka et al. reported null results when considering depressive symptoms as an outcome [46]. However, in another study, a weak trend towards improvement in the BDI test for assessing the level of depression following three-month supplementation was observed [57]. When pooling together results from all investigations, no significant results were found (SMD = −0.01, 95% CI: −0.20, 0.18; Figure 5).

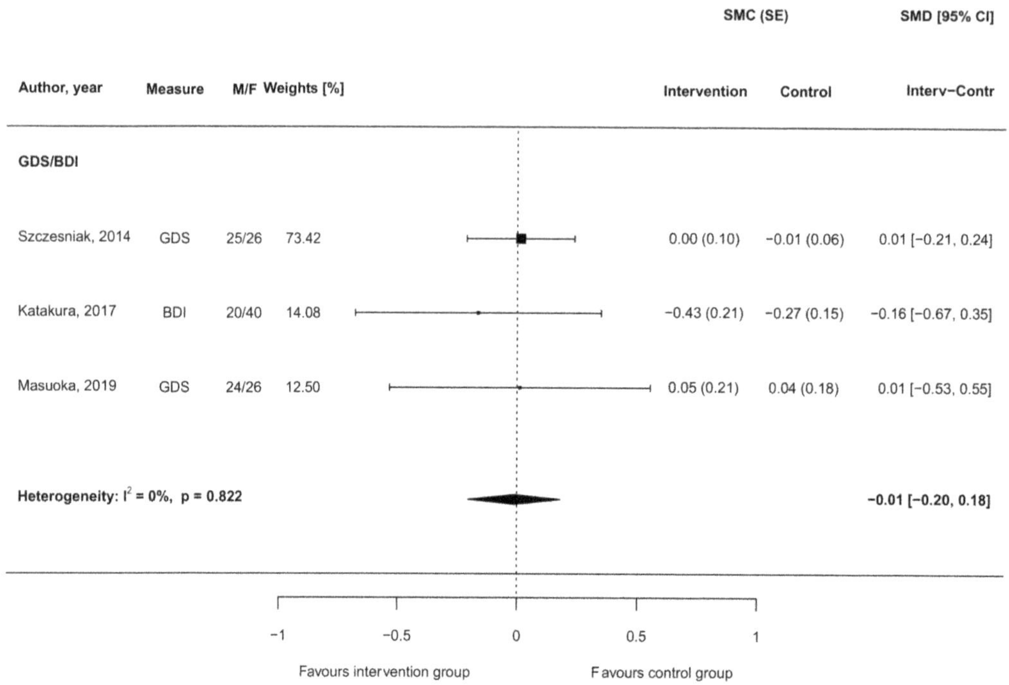

Figure 5. Standardized mean differences in depressive symptoms outputs between intervention groups supplemented with carnosine and control groups in randomized controlled trials. Abbreviations: BDI (Beck Depression Inventory), CI (confidence interval), F (female), GDS (Geriatric Depression Scale), M (male), SE (standard error), SMC (standardized mean change), SMD (standardized mean difference).

No findings are to be reported concerning meta-regression analysis on the role of potential moderators on results (Supplementary Table S3).

3.6. Carnosine Supplementation and Mood

Solely one eligible study explored the effect of carnosine supplementation on mood (measured using POMS questionnaire). The study enrolled 72 healthy full-time office workers and randomized them into either treatment group, which received a daily supplement drink with 200 g of carnosine together with computer cognitive behavior treatment (CCBT), or placebo group. After a six-week follow-up period, the study demonstrated that the carnosine and CCBT group showed significant improvements in fatigue [58].

4. Discussion

Carnosine is a natural occurring dipeptide and an over-the-counter food supplement that has been shown to exert multimodal and neuroprotective activity, including the detoxification of free radicals [59], the down-regulation of pro-inflammatory markers [60], as well as the modulation of immune cells (e.g., macrophages and microglia [25,26,61,62]), including the synthesis and the release of neurotrophins such as transforming growth factor beta-1 (TGF-β1) [62].

Interestingly, carnosine is able to counteract different factors, such as neuroinflammation, oxidative stress, and the deficit of neurotrophic factors which are strictly connected with aging-related cognitive decline and the risk to develop dementia [37] (Figure 6).

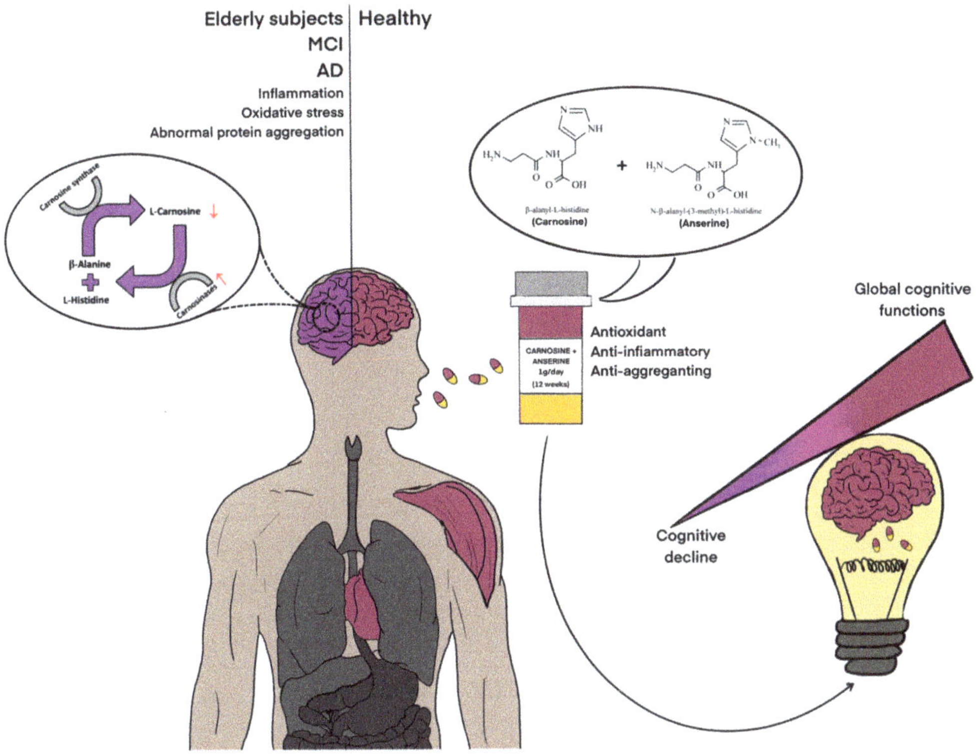

Figure 6. Improvement of global cognitive functions following carnosine/anserine supplementation. Carnosine can be found at mM concentrations at brain level as well as in cardiac and skeletal muscles (indicated in fuchsia). A selective deficit of carnosine and an age-related increase in the serum-circulating carnosinase have been linked to cognitive decline in elderly, MCI and AD subjects (indicated in purple). Red ↑ indicates an increase of carnosinase activity; red ↓ indicates a decrease of carnosine bioavailability. Abbreviations: AD (Alzheimer's disease); MCI (mild cognitive impairment).

There is evidence that dietary factors may modulate oxidative stress, which in turn play a role on cognitive decline with aging in healthy adults [63]. A review written by Gorelick, including observational epidemiological studies and clinical trials, strongly suggests that inflammation also significantly contribute to cognitive impairment and dementia [64]. Last on the background, it has been demonstrated that immune system dysfunction and the impairment of neurotrophins signaling, such as brain-derived neurotrophic factor (BDNF) and TGF-β1, could promote cognitive decline [65] and neurogenesis [66], while the activation of immune cells (e.g., group 2 innate lymphoid cells) alleviates aging-associated cognitive decline [67].

Starting from the strong preclinical evidence, the therapeutic potential of carnosine to enhance cognition in elderly people as well as in patients suffering of brain-related disorders has been recently considered [52], but the question on the clinical impact of carnosine on cognitive decline still remains open.

We conducted the present systematic review with meta-analysis, in accordance with the PRISMA guidelines coupled to the PICOS approach, to examine the clinical efficacy of carnosine on cognitive function and depressive symptoms in elderly subjects. We first examined the effects of carnosine on cognitive function. When considering all the available studies evaluating the impact of carnosine supplementation on cognitive function, we found that only three trials provided sufficient data to be eligible for quantitative comparison of cognitive decline (Figure 1).

The studies included in our meta-analysis involved partially elderly patients with age-related cognitive decline and MCI patients, a population at high risk of developing AD [46,50,57]. All studies reported, to a various extent, improvements in certain measurements of cognitive status. Another two studies [49,51] conducted on a subgroup sample of Masuoka et al., not included in our meta-analysis, showed similar results as for the main study. It is noteworthy to underline that when restricting the analysis to psychometric tools for the evaluation of global cognitive function (i.e., MMSE and ADAS, specifically), individual studies failed to report significant changes, while an overall effect could have been observed when pooling the results. This observation might have different explanations. First, it may be possible that carnosine might affect specific cognitive functions, perhaps observable in the clinical context with more specific tools rather than a general assessment of cognitive status. However, we were not able to detect clinically-relevant effects of carnosine on verbal memory as assessed by WMS-LM in 2 different clinical trials (Katakura et al. [57], Masuoka et al. [46]). Verbal memory deficits are associated with age-related cognitive decline and, most importantly, with MCI [68]. If we consider the increased effects detected by Masuoka et al. in the APOE4 (+) MCI subjects [69], larger long term (i.e., six months) double-blind, randomized, placebo-controlled trials in amnestic MCI patients are needed to confirm this preliminary evidence of clinical efficacy of carnosine. Second, as individual studies reported improvements in cognitive function of individuals in the intervention groups compared to placebo, but failed showing significant results, it may be possible that larger sample sizes are needed to achieve statistical significance in individual intervention trials.

Most of the studies selected in the present meta-analysis elderly patients received a formula containing 500 mg of carnosine/anserine or 1 g carnosine/anserine. Anserine is a natural derivative of carnosine, usually adopted because it is not cleaved by human carnosinase, which is abundant in human serum and is known to reduce carnosine bioavailability [70]. Anserine and carnosine have equivalent reported physiological functions [7], but the high preclinical evidence on the procognitive effects of carnosine suggest that further clinical studies with carnosine alone (1 g/die) vs. placebo are needed to better understand the therapeutic potential of carnosine against cognitive decline.

Carnosine could prevent and/or counteract the cognitive decline observed in MCI and AD patients through its anti-aggregation activity [71,72]. Insoluble protein aggregates have been found in MCI and AD brain [73], and carnosine might exert its precognitive effects by preventing the transition from Aβ monomers to Aβ oligomers [37]. Furthermore, it cannot be excluded that carnosine can exert its therapeutic potential against cognitive decline, by rescuing BDNF and TGF-β1 signaling [62,74], two neurotrophins whose impairment has been linked to age-related cognitive decline and MCI [65,75,76]. In addition to the well-known antioxidant, anti-inflammatory, and anti-aggregation activities, it has also been shown that carnosine is able to reduce advanced glycation end products (AGEs) and tumor necrosis factor-α (TNF-α) levels in patients with type 2 diabetes mellitus (T2DM) [77]. T2DM is known to be a risk factor for MCI and AD [78], and different neurobiological links have been identified between T2DM and AD such as insulin resistance, low-grade inflammation, increased oxidative stress, and accumulation of AGEs [79,80]. When considering the preliminary evidence of clinical efficacy of carnosine in T2DM patients on insulin resistance, AGEs, and TNF-α, future clinical studies should be conducted in T2DM patients with MCI to better understand the therapeutic potential of carnosine against cognitive decline.

In the present systematic review and meta-analysis, we also examined the effects of carnosine on depressive symptoms, starting from a large body of evidence which shows a strong link between depression and cognitive deficits both in elderly depressed patients and MCI patients [81]. In the present study we failed to find any effect of carnosine supplementation on depressive symptoms, as assessed by different and validated psychometric tools in the elderly, such as the Geriatric Depression Scale (GDS). These results can be explained by considering the high heterogeneity of psychometric tools adopted in the selected studies, as well as the exclusion from these trials of patients with major depressive disorder (MDD). Cognitive dysfunction represents a distinct biological and clinical dimension in MDD that strongly affects psychosocial functioning in MDD patients [82]. A recent study conducted by Araminia et al. [83] found the first evidence of clinical efficacy of L-Carnosine (400 mg twice daily) against affective symptoms as add-on therapy in MDD patients, but the authors did not analyze the impact of the peptide on cognitive symptoms. Further double-blind, randomized, placebo-controlled trials are needed in elderly MDD patients or depressed MCI patients to evaluate the clinical efficacy of carnosine both on cognitive and affective symptoms in MDD.

5. Conclusions

A selective deficit of carnosine has been linked to cognitive decline in AD, also promoted by the age-related increase in CN1 activity in the brain. Along this line, different preclinical studies have demonstrated the neuroprotective and procognitive effects of carnosine in experimental models of AD. It is; therefore, expected that carnosine supplementation can improve cognitive function in elderly subjects with age-related cognitive decline as well as in MCI patients with a high risk to develop AD. We conducted the present systematic review with meta-analysis to investigate the therapeutic potential of carnosine against cognitive decline and depressive symptoms in elderly subjects. We found that carnosine/anserine administered for 12 weeks, at a dose of 500 mg^{-1} g/day, improved global cognitive function and verbal memory in the four selected double-blind, randomized, placebo-controlled trials, whereas no effects were detected on depressive symptoms. These data suggest preliminary evidence of the clinical efficacy of carnosine against cognitive decline, both in elderly subjects and MCI patients, although larger and long-term clinical studies are needed in MCI patients (with or without depression) to confirm the therapeutic potential of carnosine.

Supplementary Materials: The following are available online at https://www.mdpi.com/2227-9059/9/3/253/s1, Supplementary Figure S1: Risk of bias assessment of the included studies according to the Cochrane risk-of-bias tool for randomized trials (RoB-2), Supplementary Figure S2: Funnel plots of studies for cognitive (A), verbal memory (B,C), and depressive symptoms (D) outputs, Supplementary Table S1: Preferred Reporting Items for Systematic Reviews and Meta-Analysis (PRISMA) checklist, Supplementary Table S2: NIH Quality Assessment of Controlled Intervention Studies, Supplementary Table S3: Meta-regression analysis for investigated outcomes.

Author Contributions: Conceptualization G.C., G.G., F.C.; methodology J.G., S.C., A.M., G.G.; formal analysis, A.M.; writing—original draft preparation, G.C., J.G., A.M., G.G., F.C.; writing—review and editing, G.C., J.G., S.C., A.M., P.M., F.G., R.F., G.G., F.C.; supervision, F.G., R.F., G.G., F.C. All authors listed have made a substantial, direct, and intellectual contribution to the work and approved it in its final format. All authors have read and agreed to the published version of the manuscript.

Funding: This research received no external funding.

Acknowledgments: The study is a part of the staring grant project ADICOS (Association between Dietary Factors and Cognitive Status; Giuseppe Grosso).

Conflicts of Interest: The authors declare no conflict of interest.

References

1. Gulewitsch, W.; Amiradžibi, S. Ueber das carnosin, eine neue organische base des fleischextractes. *Ber. Dtsch. Chem. Ges.* **1900**, *33*, 1902–1903. [CrossRef]
2. Kalyankar, G.D.; Meister, A. Enzymatic synthesis of carnosine and related β-alanyl and γ-aminobutyryl peptides. *J. Biol. Chem.* **1959**, *234*, 3210–3218. [CrossRef]
3. Winnick, R.; Winnick, T. Carnosine-anserine synthetase of muscle i. Preparation and properties of a soluble enyzme from chick muscle. *Biochim. Biophys. Acta* **1959**, *31*, 47–55. [CrossRef]
4. Menon, K.; Mousa, A.; de Courten, B. Effects of supplementation with carnosine and other histidine-containing dipeptides on chronic disease risk factors and outcomes: Protocol for a systematic review of randomised controlled trials. *BMJ Open* **2018**, *8*, e020623. [CrossRef]

5. Parker, C.J., Jr.; Ring, E. A comparative study of the effect of carnosine on myofibrillar-atpase activity of vertebrate and invertebrate muscles. *Comp. Biochem. Physiol.* **1970**, *37*, 413–419. [CrossRef]
6. Drozak, J.; Veiga-da-Cunha, M.; Vertommen, D.; Stroobant, V.; Van Schaftingen, E. Molecular identification of carnosine synthase as atp-grasp domain-containing protein 1 (atpgd1). *J. Biol. Chem.* **2010**, *285*, 9346–9356. [CrossRef]
7. Boldyrev, A.A.; Aldini, G.; Derave, W. Physiology and pathophysiology of carnosine. *Physiol. Rev.* **2013**, *93*, 1803–1845. [CrossRef]
8. Hipkiss, A.R.; Preston, J.E.; Himsworth, D.T.; Worthington, V.C.; Keown, M.; Michaelis, J.; Lawrence, J.; Mateen, A.; Allende, L.; Eagles, P.A.; et al. Pluripotent protective effects of carnosine, a naturally occurring dipeptide. *Ann. N. Y. Acad. Sci.* **1998**, *854*, 37–53. [CrossRef]
9. Mannion, A.F.; Jakeman, P.M.; Dunnett, M.; Harris, R.C.; Willan, P.L. Carnosine and anserine concentrations in the quadriceps femoris muscle of healthy humans. *Eur. J. Appl. Physiol. Occup. Physiol.* **1992**, *64*, 47–50. [CrossRef]
10. Fonteh, A.N.; Harrington, R.J.; Tsai, A.; Liao, P.; Harrington, M.G. Free amino acid and dipeptide changes in the body fluids from alzheimer's disease subjects. *Amino Acids* **2007**, *32*, 213–224. [CrossRef] [PubMed]
11. Bellia, F.; Calabrese, V.; Guarino, F.; Cavallaro, M.; Cornelius, C.; De Pinto, V.; Rizzarelli, E. Carnosinase levels in aging brain: Redox state induction and cellular stress response. *Antioxid. Redox Signal.* **2009**, *11*, 2759–2775. [CrossRef] [PubMed]
12. Lenney, J.F.; George, R.P.; Weiss, A.M.; Kucera, C.M.; Chan, P.W.; Rinzler, G.S. Human serum carnosinase: Characterization, distinction from cellular carnosinase, and activation by cadmium. *Clin. Chim. Acta* **1982**, *123*, 221–231. [CrossRef]
13. Lenney, J.F.; Peppers, S.C.; Kucera-Orallo, C.M.; George, R.P. Characterization of human tissue carnosinase. *Biochem. J.* **1985**, *228*, 653–660. [CrossRef]
14. Teufel, M.; Saudek, V.; Ledig, J.P.; Bernhardt, A.; Boularand, S.; Carreau, A.; Cairns, N.J.; Carter, C.; Cowley, D.J.; Duverger, D.; et al. Sequence identification and characterization of human carnosinase and a closely related non-specific dipeptidase. *J. Biol. Chem.* **2003**, *278*, 6521–6531. [CrossRef] [PubMed]
15. Perry, T.L.; Hansen, S.; Tischler, B.; Bunting, R.; Berry, K. Carnosinemia. A new metabolic disorder associated with neurologic disease and mental defect. *N. Engl. J. Med.* **1967**, *277*, 1219–1227. [CrossRef] [PubMed]
16. Bessman, S.P.; Baldwin, R. Imidazole aminoaciduria in cerebromacular degeneration. *Science* **1962**, *135*, 789–791. [CrossRef]
17. Levenson, J.; Lindahl-Kiessling, K.; Rayner, S. Carnosine excretion in juvenile amaurotic idiocy. *Lancet* **1964**, *284*, 756–757. [CrossRef]
18. Banerjee, S.; Poddar, M.K. Carnosine research in relation to aging brain and neurodegeneration: A blessing for geriatrics and their neuronal disorders. *Arch. Gerontol. Geriatr.* **2020**, *91*, 104239. [CrossRef]
19. Tiedje, K.; Stevens, K.; Barnes, S.; Weaver, D. B-alanine as a small molecule neurotransmitter. *Neurochem. Int.* **2010**, *57*, 177–188. [CrossRef]
20. Mal'tseva, V.V.; Sergienko, V.V.; Stvolinskii, S.L. The effect of carnosine on hematopoietic stem cell activity in irradiated animals. *Biokhimiia* **1992**, *57*, 1378–1382. [PubMed]
21. Fresta, C.G.; Chakraborty, A.; Wijesinghe, M.B.; Amorini, A.M.; Lazzarino, G.; Lazzarino, G.; Tavazzi, B.; Lunte, S.M.; Caraci, F.; Dhar, P.; et al. Non-toxic engineered carbon nanodiamond concentrations induce oxidative/nitrosative stress, imbalance of energy metabolism, and mitochondrial dysfunction in microglial and alveolar basal epithelial cells. *Cell Death Dis.* **2018**, *9*, 245. [CrossRef]
22. Caruso, G.; Fresta, C.G.; Martinez-Becerra, F.; Antonio, L.; Johnson, R.T.; de Campos, R.P.S.; Siegel, J.M.; Wijesinghe, M.B.; Lazzarino, G.; Lunte, S.M. Carnosine modulates nitric oxide in stimulated murine raw 264.7 macrophages. *Mol. Cell Biochem.* **2017**, *431*, 197–210. [CrossRef]
23. Hasanein, P.; Felegari, Z. Chelating effects of carnosine in ameliorating nickel-induced nephrotoxicity in rats. *Can. J. Physiol. Pharm.* **2017**, *95*, 1426–1432. [CrossRef] [PubMed]
24. Brown, C.E.; Antholine, W.E. Chelation chemistry of carnosine. Evidence that mixed complexes may occur in vivo. *J. Phys. Chem.* **1979**, *83*, 3314–3319. [CrossRef]
25. Fresta, C.G.; Fidilio, A.; Lazzarino, G.; Musso, N.; Grasso, M.; Merlo, S.; Amorini, A.M.; Bucolo, C.; Tavazzi, B.; Lazzarino, G.; et al. Modulation of pro-oxidant and pro-inflammatory activities of m1 macrophages by the natural dipeptide carnosine. *Int. J. Mol. Sci.* **2020**, *21*, 776. [CrossRef] [PubMed]
26. Caruso, G.; Fresta, C.G.; Fidilio, A.; O'Donnell, F.; Musso, N.; Lazzarino, G.; Grasso, M.; Amorini, A.M.; Tascedda, F.; Bucolo, C.; et al. Carnosine decreases pma-induced oxidative stress and inflammation in murine macrophages. *Antioxidants* **2019**, *8*, 281. [CrossRef] [PubMed]
27. Pepper, E.D.; Farrell, M.J.; Nord, G.; Finkel, S.E. Antiglycation effects of carnosine and other compounds on the long-term survival of escherichia coli. *Appl. Environ. Microbiol.* **2010**, *76*, 7925–7930. [CrossRef] [PubMed]
28. Boldyrev, A.A.; Gallant, S.C.; Sukhich, G.T. Carnosine, the protective, anti-aging peptide. *Biosci. Rep.* **1999**, *19*, 581–587. [CrossRef]
29. Ouyang, L.; Tian, Y.; Bao, Y.; Xu, H.; Cheng, J.; Wang, B.; Shen, Y.; Chen, Z.; Lyu, J. Carnosine decreased neuronal cell death through targeting glutamate system and astrocyte mitochondrial bioenergetics in cultured neuron/astrocyte exposed to ogd/recovery. *Brain Res. Bull.* **2016**, *124*, 76–84. [CrossRef]
30. Marsland, A.L.; Gianaros, P.J.; Kuan, D.C.; Sheu, L.K.; Krajina, K.; Manuck, S.B. Brain morphology links systemic inflammation to cognitive function in midlife adults. *Brain Behav. Immun.* **2015**, *48*, 195–204. [CrossRef]

31. Caruso, G.; Fresta, C.G.; Grasso, M.; Santangelo, R.; Lazzarino, G.; Lunte, S.M.; Caraci, F. Inflammation as the common biological link between depression and cardiovascular diseases: Can carnosine exert a protective role? *Curr. Med. Chem.* **2019**, *27*, 1782–1880. [CrossRef]
32. Bettcher, B.M.; Kramer, J.H. Longitudinal inflammation, cognitive decline, and alzheimer's disease: A mini-review. *Clin. Pharmacol. Ther.* **2014**, *96*, 464–469. [CrossRef] [PubMed]
33. Morrison, C.D.; Pistell, P.J.; Ingram, D.K.; Johnson, W.D.; Liu, Y.; Fernandez-Kim, S.O.; White, C.L.; Purpera, M.N.; Uranga, R.M.; Bruce-Keller, A.J.; et al. High fat diet increases hippocampal oxidative stress and cognitive impairment in aged mice: Implications for decreased nrf2 signaling. *J. Neurochem.* **2010**, *114*, 1581–1589. [CrossRef]
34. Droge, W.; Schipper, H.M. Oxidative stress and aberrant signaling in aging and cognitive decline. *Aging Cell* **2007**, *6*, 361–370. [CrossRef]
35. Irvine, G.B.; El-Agnaf, O.M.; Shankar, G.M.; Walsh, D.M. Protein aggregation in the brain: The molecular basis for alzheimer's and parkinson's diseases. *Mol. Med.* **2008**, *14*, 451–464. [CrossRef] [PubMed]
36. Espa, E.; Clemensson, E.K.H.; Luk, K.C.; Heuer, A.; Björklund, T.; Cenci, M.A. Seeding of protein aggregation causes cognitive impairment in rat model of cortical synucleinopathy. *Mov. Disord.* **2019**, *34*, 1699–1710. [CrossRef]
37. Caruso, G.; Caraci, F.; Jolivet, R.B. Pivotal role of carnosine in the modulation of brain cells activity: Multimodal mechanism of action and therapeutic potential in neurodegenerative disorders. *Prog. Neurobiol.* **2019**, *175*, 35–53. [CrossRef] [PubMed]
38. Herculano, B.; Tamura, M.; Ohba, A.; Shimatani, M.; Kutsuna, N.; Hisatsune, T. Beta-alanyl-l-histidine rescues cognitive deficits caused by feeding a high fat diet in a transgenic mouse model of alzheimer's disease. *J. Alzheimers Dis.* **2013**, *33*, 983–997. [CrossRef] [PubMed]
39. Ahshin-Majd, S.; Zamani, S.; Kiamari, T.; Kiasalari, Z.; Baluchnejadmojarad, T.; Roghani, M. Carnosine ameliorates cognitive deficits in streptozotocin-induced diabetic rats: Possible involved mechanisms. *Peptides* **2016**, *86*, 102–111. [CrossRef]
40. Ma, J.; Xiong, J.Y.; Hou, W.W.; Yan, H.J.; Sun, Y.; Huang, S.W.; Jin, L.; Wang, Y.; Hu, W.W.; Chen, Z. Protective effect of carnosine on subcortical ischemic vascular dementia in mice. *CNS Neurosci. Ther.* **2012**, *18*, 745–753. [CrossRef]
41. Corona, C.; Frazzini, V.; Silvestri, E.; Lattanzio, R.; La Sorda, R.; Piantelli, M.; Canzoniero, L.M.; Ciavardelli, D.; Rizzarelli, E.; Sensi, S.L. Effects of dietary supplementation of carnosine on mitochondrial dysfunction, amyloid pathology, and cognitive deficits in 3xtg-ad mice. *PLoS ONE* **2011**, *6*, e17971.
42. Boldyrev, A.A. *Carnosine and Oxidative Stress in Cells and Tissues*; Nova Publishers: Hauppauge, NY, USA, 2007.
43. Gardner, M.L.; Illingworth, K.M.; Kelleher, J.; Wood, D. Intestinal absorption of the intact peptide carnosine in man, and comparison with intestinal permeability to lactulose. *J. Physiol.* **1991**, *439*, 411–422. [CrossRef]
44. Goto, K.; Maemura, H.; Takamatsu, K.; Ishii, N. Hormonal responses to resistance exercise after ingestion of carnosine and anserine. *J. Strength Cond. Res.* **2011**, *25*, 398–405. [CrossRef]
45. Baraniuk, J.N.; El-Amin, S.; Corey, R.; Rayhan, R.; Timbol, C. Carnosine treatment for gulf war illness: A randomized controlled trial. *Glob. J. Health Sci.* **2013**, *5*, 69–81. [CrossRef]
46. Masuoka, N.; Yoshimine, C.; Hori, M.; Tanaka, M.; Asada, T.; Abe, K.; Hisatsune, T. Effects of anserine/carnosine supplementation on mild cognitive impairment with apoe4. *Nutrients* **2019**, *11*, 1626. [CrossRef]
47. Small, B.J.; Rawson, K.S.; Martin, C.; Eisel, S.L.; Sanberg, C.D.; McEvoy, C.L.; Sanberg, P.R.; Shytle, R.D.; Tan, J.; Bickford, P.C. Nutraceutical intervention improves older adults' cognitive functioning. *Rejuvenation Res.* **2014**, *17*, 27–32. [CrossRef]
48. Cornelli, U. Treatment of alzheimer's disease with a cholinesterase inhibitor combined with antioxidants. *Neurodegener. Dis.* **2010**, *7*, 193–202. [CrossRef] [PubMed]
49. Rokicki, J.; Li, L.; Imabayashi, E.; Kaneko, J.; Hisatsune, T.; Matsuda, H. Daily carnosine and anserine supplementation alters verbal episodic memory and resting state network connectivity in healthy elderly adults. *Front. Aging Neurosci.* **2015**, *7*, 219. [CrossRef] [PubMed]
50. Szcześniak, D.; Budzeń, S.; Kopeć, W.; Rymaszewska, J. Anserine and carnosine supplementation in the elderly: Effects on cognitive functioning and physical capacity. *Arch. Gerontol. Geriatr.* **2014**, *59*, 485–490. [CrossRef]
51. Hisatsune, T.; Kaneko, J.; Kurashige, H.; Cao, Y.; Satsu, H.; Totsuka, M.; Katakura, Y.; Imabayashi, E.; Matsuda, H. Effect of anserine/carnosine supplementation on verbal episodic memory in elderly people. *J. Alzheimers Dis.* **2016**, *50*, 149–159. [CrossRef] [PubMed]
52. Schön, M.; Mousa, A.; Berk, M.; Chia, W.L.; Ukropec, J.; Majid, A.; Ukropcová, B.; de Courten, B. The potential of carnosine in brain-related disorders: A comprehensive review of current evidence. *Nutrients* **2019**, *11*, 1196. [CrossRef] [PubMed]
53. Moher, D.; Liberati, A.; Tetzlaff, J.; Altman, D.G. Preferred reporting items for systematic reviews and meta-analyses: The prisma statement. *BMJ* **2009**, *339*, b2535. [CrossRef]
54. Sterne, J.A.C.; Savović, J.; Page, M.J.; Elbers, R.G.; Blencowe, N.S.; Boutron, I.; Cates, C.J.; Cheng, H.Y.; Corbett, M.S.; Eldridge, S.M.; et al. Rob 2: A revised tool for assessing risk of bias in randomised trials. *BMJ* **2019**, *366*, l4898. [CrossRef] [PubMed]
55. Morris, S.B.; DeShon, R.P. Combining effect size estimates in meta-analysis with repeated measures and independent-groups designs. *Psychol. Methods* **2002**, *7*, 105–125. [CrossRef] [PubMed]
56. Becker, B.J. Synthesizing standardized mean-change measures. *Br. J. Math. Stat. Psychol.* **1988**, *41*, 257–278. [CrossRef]
57. Katakura, Y.; Totsuka, M.; Imabayashi, E.; Matsuda, H.; Hisatsune, T. Anserine/carnosine supplementation suppresses the expression of the inflammatory chemokine ccl24 in peripheral blood mononuclear cells from elderly people. *Nutrients* **2017**, *9*, 1199. [CrossRef] [PubMed]

58. Shirotsuki, K.; Nonaka, Y.; Abe, K.; Adachi, S.I.; Adachi, S.; Kuboki, T.; Nakao, M. The effect for japanese workers of a self-help computerized cognitive behaviour therapy program with a supplement soft drink. *Biopsychosoc. Med.* **2017**, *11*, 23. [CrossRef]
59. Prokopieva, V.D.; Yarygina, E.G.; Bokhan, N.A.; Ivanova, S.A. Use of carnosine for oxidative stress reduction in different pathologies. *Oxid. Med. Cell Longev.* **2016**, *2016*, 2939087. [CrossRef]
60. Kubota, M.; Kobayashi, N.; Sugizaki, T.; Shimoda, M.; Kawahara, M.; Tanaka, K.-i. Carnosine suppresses neuronal cell death and inflammation induced by 6-hydroxydopamine in an in vitro model of parkinson's disease. *PLoS ONE* **2020**, *15*, e0240448. [CrossRef]
61. Fresta, C.G.; Hogard, M.L.; Caruso, G.; Melo Costa, E.E.; Lazzarino, G.; Lunte, S.M. Monitoring carnosine uptake by raw 264.7 macrophage cells using microchip electrophoresis with fluorescence detection. *Anal. Methods* **2017**, *9*, 402–408. [CrossRef]
62. Caruso, G.; Fresta, C.G.; Musso, N.; Giambirtone, M.; Grasso, M.; Spampinato, S.F.; Merlo, S.; Drago, F.; Lazzarino, G.; Sortino, M.A.; et al. Carnosine prevents aβ-induced oxidative stress and inflammation in microglial cells: A key role of tgf-β1. *Cells* **2019**, *8*, 64. [CrossRef] [PubMed]
63. Godos, J.; Currenti, W.; Angelino, D.; Mena, P.; Castellano, S.; Caraci, F.; Galvano, F.; Del Rio, D.; Ferri, R.; Grosso, G. Diet and mental health: Review of the recent updates on molecular mechanisms. *Antioxidants* **2020**, *9*, 346. [CrossRef] [PubMed]
64. Gorelick, P.B. Role of inflammation in cognitive impairment: Results of observational epidemiological studies and clinical trials. *Ann. N. Y. Acad. Sci.* **2010**, *1207*, 155–162. [CrossRef]
65. Caraci, F.; Spampinato, S.F.; Morgese, M.G.; Tascedda, F.; Salluzzo, M.G.; Giambirtone, M.C.; Caruso, G.; Munafò, A.; Torrisi, S.A.; Leggio, G.M.; et al. Neurobiological links between depression and ad: The role of tgf-β1 signaling as a new pharmacological target. *Pharm. Res.* **2018**, *130*, 374–384. [CrossRef] [PubMed]
66. Marin, I.; Kipnis, J. Learning and memory ... And the immune system. *Learn Mem.* **2013**, *20*, 601–606. [CrossRef]
67. Fung, I.T.H.; Sankar, P.; Zhang, Y.; Robison, L.S.; Zhao, X.; D'Souza, S.S.; Salinero, A.E.; Wang, Y.; Qian, J.; Kuentzel, M.L.; et al. Activation of group 2 innate lymphoid cells alleviates aging-associated cognitive decline. *J. Exp. Med.* **2020**, *217*, 217. [CrossRef]
68. Constantinidou, F.; Zaganas, I.; Papastefanakis, E.; Kasselimis, D.; Nidos, A.; Simos, P.G. Age-related decline in verbal learning is moderated by demographic factors, working memory capacity, and presence of amnestic mild cognitive impairment. *J. Int. Neuropsychol. Soc.* **2014**, *20*, 822–835. [CrossRef] [PubMed]
69. Ali, J.I.; Smart, C.M.; Gawryluk, J.R. Subjective cognitive decline and apoe ϵ4: A systematic review. *J. Alzheimers Dis.* **2018**, *65*, 303–320. [CrossRef] [PubMed]
70. Kubomura, D.; Matahira, Y.; Masui, A.; Matsuda, H. Intestinal absorption and blood clearance of l-histidine-related compounds after ingestion of anserine in humans and comparison to anserine-containing diets. *J. Agric. Food Chem.* **2009**, *57*, 1781–1785. [CrossRef] [PubMed]
71. Attanasio, F.; Convertino, M.; Magno, A.; Caflisch, A.; Corazza, A.; Haridas, H.; Esposito, G.; Cataldo, S.; Pignataro, B.; Milardi, D.; et al. Carnosine inhibits aβ(42) aggregation by perturbing the h-bond network in and around the central hydrophobic cluster. *Chembiochem* **2013**, *14*, 583–592. [CrossRef]
72. Aloisi, A.; Barca, A.; Romano, A.; Guerrieri, S.; Storelli, C.; Rinaldi, R.; Verri, T. Anti-aggregating effect of the naturally occurring dipeptide carnosine on aβ1-42 fibril formation. *PLoS ONE* **2013**, *8*, e68159. [CrossRef] [PubMed]
73. Kepchia, D.; Huang, L.; Dargusch, R.; Rissman, R.A.; Shokhirev, M.N.; Fischer, W.; Schubert, D. Diverse proteins aggregate in mild cognitive impairment and alzheimer's disease brain. *Alzheimers Res. Ther.* **2020**, *12*, 75. [CrossRef] [PubMed]
74. Kadooka, K.; Fujii, K.; Matsumoto, T.; Sato, M.; Morimatsu, F.; Tashiro, K.; Kuhara, S.; Katakura, Y. Mechanisms and consequences of carnosine-induced activation of intestinal epithelial cells. *J. Funct. Foods* **2015**, *13*, 32–37. [CrossRef]
75. Bosco, P.; Ferri, R.; Salluzzo, M.G.; Castellano, S.; Signorelli, M.; Nicoletti, F.; Nuovo, S.D.; Drago, F.; Caraci, F. Role of the transforming-growth-factor-β1 gene in late-onset alzheimer's disease: Implications for the treatment. *Curr. Genom.* **2013**, *14*, 147–156. [CrossRef] [PubMed]
76. Siuda, J.; Patalong-Ogiewa, M.; Żmuda, W.; Targosz-Gajniak, M.; Niewiadomska, E.; Matuszek, I.; Jędrzejowska-Szypułka, H.; Lewin-Kowalik, J.; Rudzińska-Bar, M. Cognitive impairment and bdnf serum levels. *Neurol. Neurochir. Polska* **2017**, *51*, 24–32. [CrossRef]
77. Houjeghani, S.; Kheirouri, S.; Faraji, E.; Jafarabadi, M.A. L-carnosine supplementation attenuated fasting glucose, triglycerides, advanced glycation end products, and tumor necrosis factor-alpha levels in patients with type 2 diabetes: A double-blind placebo-controlled randomized clinical trial. *Nutr. Res.* **2018**, *49*, 96–106. [CrossRef]
78. Cheng, G.; Huang, C.; Deng, H.; Wang, H. Diabetes as a risk factor for dementia and mild cognitive impairment: A meta-analysis of longitudinal studies. *Intern. Med. J.* **2012**, *42*, 484–491. [CrossRef] [PubMed]
79. Shinohara, M.; Sato, N. Bidirectional interactions between diabetes and alzheimer's disease. *Neurochem. Int.* **2017**, *108*, 296–302. [CrossRef] [PubMed]
80. Caruso, G.; Distefano, D.A.; Parlascino, P.; Fresta, C.G.; Lazzarino, G.; Lunte, S.M.; Nicoletti, V.G. Receptor-mediated toxicity of human amylin fragment aggregated by short- and long-term incubations with copper ions. *Mol. Cell Biochem.* **2017**, *425*, 85–93. [CrossRef] [PubMed]
81. Mourao, R.J.; Mansur, G.; Malloy-Diniz, L.F.; Castro Costa, E.; Diniz, B.S. Depressive symptoms increase the risk of progression to dementia in subjects with mild cognitive impairment: Systematic review and meta-analysis. *Int. J. Geriatr. Psychiatry* **2016**, *31*, 905–911. [CrossRef]

82. Baune, B.T.; Sluth, L.B.; Olsen, C.K. The effects of vortioxetine on cognitive performance in working patients with major depressive disorder: A short-term, randomized, double-blind, exploratory study. *J. Affect. Disord.* **2018**, *229*, 421–428. [CrossRef] [PubMed]
83. Araminia, B.; Shalbafan, M.; Mortezaei, A.; Shirazi, E.; Ghaffari, S.; Sahebolzamani, E.; Mortazavi, S.H.; Shariati, B.; Ardebili, M.E.; Aqamolaei, A.; et al. L-carnosine combination therapy for major depressive disorder: A randomized, double-blind, placebo-controlled trial. *J. Affect. Disord.* **2020**, *267*, 131–136. [CrossRef] [PubMed]

biomedicines

Article

Effects of Psychostimulants and Antipsychotics on Serum Lipids in an Animal Model for Schizophrenia

Banny Silva Barbosa Correia [1], João Victor Nani [2,3], Raniery Waladares Ricardo [1], Danijela Stanisic [1], Tássia Brena Barroso Carneiro Costa [1], Mirian A. F. Hayashi [2,3,*] and Ljubica Tasic [1,*]

1 Instituto de Química, Universidade Estadual de Campinas (UNICAMP), Campinas 13083-970, Brazil; banny.barbosa@gmail.com (B.S.B.C.); raniery014@gmail.com (R.W.R.); danijela@unicamp.br (D.S.); tassiabrena@gmail.com (T.B.B.C.C.)
2 Departamento de Farmacologia, Escola Paulista de Medicina (EPM), Universidade Federal de São Paulo (UNIFESP), São Paulo 04044-020, Brazil; joaoonanii@gmail.com
3 National Institute for Translational Medicine (INCT-TM, CNPq), Faculdade de Medicina de Ribeirão Preto da Universidade de São Paulo (FMRP-USP), São Paulo 14049-900, Brazil
* Correspondence: mhayashi@unifesp.br (M.A.F.H.); ljubica@unicamp.br (L.T.); Tel.: +55-11-5576-4447 (M.A.F.H.); +55-19-3521-1106 (L.T.); Fax: +55-11-5576-4499 (M.A.F.H.); +55-19-3521-3023 (L.T.)

Abstract: Schizophrenia (SCZ) treatment is essentially limited to the use of typical or atypical antipsychotic drugs, which suppress the main symptoms of this mental disorder. Metabolic syndrome is often reported in patients with SCZ under long-term drug treatment, but little is known about the alteration of lipid metabolism induced by antipsychotic use. In this study, we evaluated the blood serum lipids of a validated animal model for SCZ (Spontaneously Hypertensive Rat, SHR), and a normal control rat strain (Normotensive Wistar Rat, NWR), after long-term treatment (30 days) with typical haloperidol (HAL) or atypical clozapine (CLZ) antipsychotics. Moreover, psychostimulants, amphetamine (AMPH) or lisdexamfetamine (LSDX), were administered to NWR animals aiming to mimic the human first episode of psychosis, and the effects on serum lipids were also evaluated. Discrepancies in lipids between SHR and NWR animals, which included increased total lipids and decreased phospholipids in SHR compared with NWR, were similar to the differences previously reported for SCZ patients relative to healthy controls. Administration of psychostimulants in NWR decreased omega-3, which was also decreased in the first episode of psychosis of SCZ. Moreover, choline glycerophospholipids allowed us to distinguish the effects of CLZ in SHR. Thus, changes in the lipid metabolism in SHR seem to be reversed by the long-term treatment with the atypical antipsychotic CLZ, which was under the same condition described to reverse the SCZ-like endophenotypes of this validated animal model for SCZ. These data open new insights for understanding the potential influence of the treatment with typical or atypical antipsychotics on circulating lipids. This may represent an outcome effect from metabolic pathways that regulate lipids synthesis and breakdown, which may be reflecting a cell lipids dysfunction in SCZ.

Keywords: lipidomics; schizophrenia; animal models; antipsychotics

Citation: Correia, B.S.B.; Nani, J.V.; Waladares Ricardo, R.; Stanisic, D.; Costa, T.B.B.C.; Hayashi, M.A.F.; Tasic, L. Effects of Psychostimulants and Antipsychotics on Serum Lipids in an Animal Model for Schizophrenia. *Biomedicines* **2021**, *9*, 235. https://doi.org/10.3390/biomedicines9030235

Academic Editor: Masaru Tanaka

Received: 4 December 2020
Accepted: 2 February 2021
Published: 26 February 2021

1. Introduction

Schizophrenia (SCZ) is a severe, complex and chronic mental disorder (MD), with a serious impact on patients and their families and caretakers. This highly disabling MD imposes an unemployment rate of about 80%, in addition to an important reduction in the life expectancy of patients, which is estimated to be shortened up by about 20 years compared to the general population without psychiatric dysfunctions [1]. In general, SCZ patients are characterized by positive symptoms such as delusions, hallucinations, psychosis, or negative symptoms, which include impaired motivation, reduction in spontaneous speech and social withdrawal, emotional processing/cognitive deficits, and may possibly include impaired neurocognitive deficits, confused speech or behavior alterations [2,3].

The most accepted theory to explain the neurobiology of SCZ is based on abnormalities in neurotransmission, as for instance, the alterations in dopaminergic, serotoninergic, glutamatergic, among other signaling pathways [1,4]. The main drugs used to treat SCZ symptoms are antipsychotic drugs, which are usually employed to normalize the dysfunctions in neurotransmission. Although antipsychotic drugs can control the main symptoms of SCZ, the disease progression is not stopped by long-term treatments with antipsychotics [5]. Another pathway implicated in SCZ pathophysiology is the kynurenine pathway (KP), which involves the tryptophan metabolism [6]. The KP metabolites modulate neurotransmitters related to cognition [7]. Individuals with MDs presented lower levels of kynurenines, which may be involved in cognitive impairment [8], while conversely, SCZ patients showed increased kynurenine levels [6,8]. Therefore, tryptophan–kynurenine metabolism in psychiatric disease is well established, and disturbance of the tryptophan–kynurenine metabolic pathway might be a promising target to unravel the therapeutic effects of psychoactive drugs. Additionally, the KP is also related to lipid metabolism [6,7].

Several studies have pointed to some abnormalities in cell membranes and brain lipids that compromise the structural integrity and functional properties of neurons in patients with MD [9,10]. Moreover, insufficient uptake, excessive breakdown and/or changes in membrane phospholipids composition are all associated with SCZ and dysfunctional synapses [9–11]. The analytical evaluation of the effects of drugs currently employed in clinics is of utmost importance for the progress in the knowledge in the field. For this purpose, optimized animal models have the power to contribute for understanding the pharmacological effects of each class of antipsychotics on animal metabolism and, consequently, to the discovery of new pathways underlying complex diseases such as MDs [12].

The Spontaneously Hypertensive Rat (SHR) strain was recognized as a reliable animal model for studying SCZ due to the depicted SCZ-like behaviors, which were reversed by the treatment with typical and atypical antipsychotics [13,14]. It is worth mentioning that these animal behavior alterations following the treatment with antipsychotics were not associated with the high blood pressure of adult SHR [15], although they were associated with differences in biochemical biomarkers in blood serum and brain from SHR compared with normotensive Wistar rats (NWR) [14,16]. Moreover, these altered levels of biochemical biomarkers in SHR relative to NWR were also observed in SCZ compared with healthy control subjects [17–19], reinforcing the validity of this animal model for studying pathophysiological pathways associated with this psychiatric disorder.

The power of analytical approaches for lipid metabolism in neuropsychiatric disorders is increasingly recognized [20–23], and a better understanding of blood lipids could potentially add important knowledge. Nuclear magnetic resonance (NMR) spectroscopy is a powerful analytical tool that provides relevant information for comparison of different samples, and allows the identification of lipids [24]. In the present study, we tested the alterations in the lipid content by comparing the effects of typical haloperidol (HAL) and atypical clozapine (CLZ) antipsychotic drugs after 30 days of treatment of a validated animal model for studying SCZ (namely SHR), which were compared with a control normal strain (namely NWR). In addition, to mimic the increases of dopamine release, expected to occur in episodes of psychosis, NWR animals were challenged by acute administration of psychostimulants–amphetamine (AMPH) or lisdexamfetamine (LSDX) [16]—for blood lipid contents evaluation. Herein, the lipidomics by NMR analyses aimed to identify potential changes in lipids that could provide insights into the metabolic consequences of the pharmacological interventions with pro-psychotic psychostimulants or antipsychotics employing animal models. These results may contribute to the understanding of the metabolic effects of the treatments of SCZ patients with typical or atypical antipsychotics under clinical conditions.

2. Materials and Methods

2.1. Animals

Spontaneously Hypertensive Rat (SHR) and normotensive Wistar rat (NWR) strains were treated under previously described conditions [13–16]. Male 4–5 months-old animals, from our own local colony, were housed in groups of 3–4 animals per cage (41 × 34 × 16.5 cm^3), under controlled temperature (22–23 °C) and 12/12 h light/dark cycle conditions, with lights on at 07:00 AM, and with free access to water and a normocaloric Nuvilab CR-1 irradiated diet (Quimtia®, Curitiba, Brazil). The animals were maintained following the guidelines of the Committee on Care and Use of Laboratory Animal Resources, National Research Council, USA. This study was approved by the Ethical Committee of the Universidade Federal de São Paulo (UNIFESP/EPM), identification CEUA N° 7290170315, approved on 15 March 2015.

2.2. Reagents and Drugs

The solvents (chloroform, methanol, and acetone) used for lipids extraction were from LabSynth Products Laboratories (Diadema, SP, Brazil), and deuterated chloroform ($CDCl_3$, with 99.8% of D) was from Cambridge Isotope Laboratories, Inc. (Tewksbury, MA, USA). Other reagents were of analytical grade from Sigma-Aldrich (St. Louis, MI, USA). Antipsychotics haloperidol (HAL, Sigma-Aldrich, St. Louis, MO, USA) and clozapine (CLZ, Pinazan, Laboratório Cristália, São Paulo, Brazil), as well as the psychostimulants amphetamine (AMPH, Sigma-Aldrich) and lisdexamfetamine dimesylate (LSDX, Vynvase™, Shire LLC, São Paulo, Brazil), were dissolved in saline solution, and they were injected by intraperitoneal (ip) route in a volume of 1 mL/kg of animal body weight. The volume of the vehicle administered for the negative controls was also 1 mL/kg of animal body weight.

2.3. Drug-Naïve Animals

The blood samples of drug-naïve NWR and SHR male animals (5 months-old) were collected in dry blood tubes, soon after the animal euthanasia by decapitation, strictly following the standards described in the Guidelines for Ethical Conduct in the Care and Use of Animals.

2.4. Treatment with Psychostimulants

Male NWR (5 months-old) were grouped in each cage with 4–5 animals, and a single dose of the propsychotic psychostimulants (0.5 or 5.0 mg/kg), namely AMPH or LSDX, was administered by ip route, aiming to mimic the SCZ-like psychotic episodes [13]. Before (baseline) and 2 h after this single ip injection of either psychostimulants, the blood of the animals was collected in heparin tubes by tail punction.

2.5. Treatment with Antipsychotics

Male NWR and SHR (4 months-old) animals were kept in cages for a month to acclimate before starting the daily treatment for 30 days. This treatment was performed exactly as previously described to evaluate and reverse the characteristic SCZ-like behavioral and biochemical changes [13,14,16]. Then, animals were grouped into: Group I—control animals receiving vehicle (saline 0.9%, 0.1 mL/kg, ip); Group II: animals treated with HAL (0.5 mg/kg, ip); and Group III: animals treated daily with CLZ (2.5 mg/kg, ip). At the end of the treatments, one day after the last administration of antipsychotics (experimental groups) or saline vehicle (negative control group), the blood was collected in dry blood tubes, soon after the euthanasia of animals by decapitation.

Sixty-one animal serum samples underwent lipids extraction and subsequent proton NMR (^{1}H-NMR) analysis. The serum samples from animals were:

(a) non-treated animal strains, NWR (control group, N = 4), and SHR (SCZ group, N = 4), with a total animal serum sample equal to 8;

(b) NWR animals challenged with psychostimulants (AMPH or LSDX) and controls receiving saline, in which:

(1) NWR receiving saline 0.9% (N = 5); (2) NWR receiving single administration of 0.5 mg/kg (N = 5) or 5.0 mg/kg (N = 5) of AMPH; (3) NWR receiving single administration of 0.5 mg/kg (N = 5) or 5.0 mg/kg (N = 5) of LSDX, with a total animal serum samples equal to 25;

(c) treatment with antipsychotics for 30 days: (1) NWR receiving saline 0.9% (N = 4); (2) SHR receiving saline 0.9% (N = 4); (3) NWR treated with CLZ (N = 5); (4) NWR treated with HAL (N = 5); (5) SHR treated with CLZ (N = 5); (6) SHR treated with HAL (N = 5), with a total animal serum samples equal to 28.

2.6. Extraction of Lipids from Serum Samples and NMR Analysis

Animal serum (0.5 mL) was mixed for 1 min, using a vortex, with 2.4 mL of the solvent mixture composed of methanol: chloroform: sodium chloride solution (0.15 mol/L) in a ratio of 1:2:2 (*v*/*v*/*v*). Then, the mixture was centrifuged for 20 min at 2200× *g* at 10 °C, and the chloroform phase that contained serum lipids was carefully separated from the hydro-alcoholic phase. Chloroform was evaporated and obtained samples were weighted and stored at −20 °C until the analysis by NMR [24].

Lipids (10 mg) were dissolved in 600 µL of 99.8% deuterated chloroform ($CDCl_3$, Cambridge Isotope Laboratories, Inc.) and were transferred into the NMR tubes (5 mm) and kept at 4 °C, to avoid the chloroform evaporation and/or lipid oxidation. ^{1}H-NMR analyses were conducted in a Bruker Avance III NMR 600 MHz spectrometer equipped with the Triple Resonance Broad Band NMR probe (Bruker Corp., Billerica, MA, USA). ^{1}H-NMR spectra were recorded at 25 °C with the acquisition time of 2.66 s, spectral window width of 26.564 Hz, relaxation time decay (relaxation delay) of 2 s, and 128 number of scans.

For quantitative analysis, some representative samples were chosen and prepared by adding 100 µL of the standard solution of 1,2,4,5-tetrachloro-3-nitrobenzene (5 mg/mL, 99.86% purity; Sigma-Aldrich) into a solution of 10 mg of lipids previously dissolved in 500 µL of deuterated chloroform ($CDCl_3$) with tetramethylsilane (TMS) [25]. ^{1}H-NMR spectra were recorded using 90° pulse sequence at 25 °C, acquisition time of 8.19 s, spectral window width of 9.9955 Hz, 64 k, relaxation delay of 40 s (5 times T_1), and 56 scans. ^{1}H-NMR data were assigned in accordance with the previously reported NMR data for lipids [26].

2.7. Data Processing

^{1}H-NMR (600 MHz) spectra for statistical and quantitative analyses were first processed using the TopSpin software (Bruker Corp.). Free induction decays were multiplied by a 0.3 Hz exponential multiplication function prior to Fourier transformation; the tetramethylsilane (TMS) signal was calibrated at δ 0.00, and only a zero-order phase correction was allowed.

For statistical analysis of spectra, the binning of 0.04 ppm was applied to spectral data using MestreNova software, and spectra were transformed into a data matrix. The MetaboAnalyst 3.0 platform (http://www.metaboanalyst.ca/faces/home.xhtml accessed on 1 December 2020) was used for principal component analysis (PCA) and partial least squares discriminant analysis (PLS-DA). No data filtering, no sample normalization, and Pareto scaling (mean-centered and divided by the square root of the standard deviation of each variable) were used in data preprocessing. Leave-one-out cross-validation (LOOCV) was applied in PLS-DA. The accuracy, variable importance in projection (VIP) and clustering results shown as heatmaps (distance measure using euclidean, clustering algorithm using ward.D, view options only group aver-ages of top 15 PLS-DA VIP) were also assessed.

For quantitative purposes, specific ^{1}H-NMR signals were manually integrated, and the concentrations of omega-3 (L–linolenic acid) and omega-6 (Ln–linoleic acid) type fatty acids were calculated following the method previously reported by others [26,27]. The concentrations of fatty acids were expressed in molar percentages according to Equations (1) and (2).

$$Ln\% = 100 \times A_{\text{omega }3}/3 \times A_G \quad (1)$$

$$L\% = 100 \times 2 \times A_{omega\,6}/3 \times A_G \qquad (2)$$

in which $A_{omega\text{-}3}$ and $A_{omega\text{-}6}$ are the areas of the bis-allylic proton peaks for omega-3 and omega-6 fatty acids, respectively, and A_G is the area of the proton peaks of glyceryl groups; L refers to omega-3, linolenic acid, and Ln refers to omega-6, linoleic acid.

For statistical analysis of the ratio of omega-3/omega-6, data analyses were performed using the GraphPad Prism version 7.0 for Windows (GraphPad Software Corp., La Jolla, CA, USA). Standard parametric (Student's t-test and one-way Analysis of variance, ANOVA) tests were applied accordingly to variables type and distribution, with post-hoc test Dunnett's for multiple comparisons. All distribution was checked using a Shapiro–Wilk test. All results are expressed as the value of mean ± standard deviation (SD). The significance threshold was considered at $p \leq 0.05$.

3. Results

3.1. Identification of Lipids

^{1}H-NMR data of serum lipids (Table 1) were assigned according to the peak numbers (1–25), as indicated in Figure S1 (Supplementary Information). Chemical shifts, peak multiplicity, and coupling constants for the 1–25 compounds were checked against databases and lipids NMR libraries. Lipids from the animal serum samples showed peaks of cholesterol, saturated fatty acids, unsaturated fatty acids, i.e., omega-3 and omega-6 fatty acids, phosphocholines, cardiolipins, and sphingomyelines. Additionally, glycerol esters, glycerolipids (triacylglycerols), glycerophospholipids, and saccharolipids were identified in lipid samples of drug-naïve and treated animals, receiving acute administration of psychostimulants or treated for 30 days with typical or atypical antipsychotics. It is worth mentioning that the lipids identified in the present study are in agreement with the previously described downregulation of phosphatidylcholine [10,28,29], and upregulation of triacylglycerols [30,31] in SCZ patients compared with healthy control volunteers. In addition, low levels of polyunsaturated fatty acids phospholipid content, specifically in phosphatidylcholine and phosphatidylethanolamine, were reported in first-episode psychosis of SCZ [32,33].

Table 1. Rat serum ^{1}H-NMR spectral assignments. The NMR peaks were numbered as illustrated in Figure S1 (Supplementary Information). Legend: ^{a} omega-6, ^{b} omega-3, and ^{c} glycerol (see Equations (1) and (2) in Methods Section).

Peak	Chemical Shift (ppm)	Assignment
1	0.58–0.70	Terminal methyl group in cholesterol -CH_3
2	0.75–1.00	-CH_3 protons of saturated, oleic and linoleic acyls (omega-6)
3	0.93–1.02	-CH_3 protons of linolenyl chain (omega-3)
4	1.20–1.50	Methylene protons of aliphatic chains -$(CH_2)_n$
5	1.50–1.75	β–methylene protons of the carbonyl –OC(O)-CH_2-CH_2-
6	1.95–2.10	Methylene protons in the α-position of double bonds –CH_2-CH=CH-
7	2.20–2.50	Methylene protons in the carbonyl α-position –OC(O)-CH_2-
8	2.70–2.84	CH_2-*bis*-allyllic protons of polyunsaturated fatty acid (PUFA) chains
9	2.80–2.90 ^{a}	Divinyl methylene protons =HC-CH_2-CH= of omega-6 including linoleyl chain
10	2.79 ^{b}	Divinyl methylene protons =HC-CH_2-CH= of omega-3 including linolenyl chain
11	3.10–3.20	Methylene protons α to the heteroatom –CH_2-OH
12	3.20–3.40	Methyl protons of charged nitrogen –$^+N(CH_3)_3$
13	3.40–3.60	Heteroatom proton –**OH**
14	3.44–3.59	CH of cholesterol relative to the C-3 proton
15	3.50–3.85	Methylene protons α to a charged nitrogen CH_2-$N^+(CH_3)_3$
16	3.65–3.75	Hexoses protons on α-carbon to the heteroatom
17	3.88	Methine proton at C-4 of galactose
18	4.00–4.30	Protons on α-carbon to the heteroatom
19	4.10–4.40	Protons on α-carbon to the heteroatom (OH) and β to the amine -O-CH_2-CH_2-$N^+(CH_3)_3$
20	3.90–4.40	Methylene protons α to the heteroatom in phosphorus CH_2-O-P
21	4.10–4.30 ^{c}	Sn-1 and Sn-3 protons of glycerol -CH_2-OC(O)R
22	5.00	Anomeric carbon protons of galactose
23	5.20–5.40	Amine protons –**HN**$(CH_3)_2$
24	5.25–5.50	Sn-2 protons of glycerol > **CH**-O-C(O)R
25	5.27–5.38	Protons of double bonds with conformation Z-**CH**=HC-

3.2. Comparison of Lipids among Drug-Naïve NWR and SHR Animals, and NWR Receiving Psychostimulants

Blood serum lipidomes of drug-naïve NWR animals were significantly different compared to drug-naïve SHR or NWR under psychostimulants effects, as presented in Figure 1. In fact, the lipids isolated from drug-naïve NWR and SHR animals were different from each other, and formed distinct groups (Figure 1A, Supplementary Information Table S1). The drug-naïve NWR lipids showed to be richer in unsaturated fatty acids (UFA), cholesterol (chol), phospholipids (PL)-saccharolipids, and choline glycerophospholipids (ChoGpl) (Figure 1C). On the other hand, the serum lipids in SHR showed different patterns with high quantities of PUFA and fatty acids in general (Figure 1C). In addition, the drug-naïve SHR strain presented lower amounts of PL compared with drug-naïve NWR, but with increased amounts of PUFA (Supplementary Information Figure S2). Further investigation may clarify if omega-3 PUFA works in compensation of phospholipids loss, as previously described by others [26,27]. The main observation is that the amounts of phospholipids are stable in the SCZ animal model (SHR), but differences in the chemical structures of these phospholipids, as the ratio between omega-3 and omega-6, could be crucial for the disease and treatments, as we will further discuss.

The lipids from drug-naïve NWR animals suffered alterations under the effects of psychoactive drugs, and they were exposed to psychostimulants (AMPH or LSDX) at different doses (0.5 or 5.0 mg/kg), forming the sub-groups NWR-AMPH*, NWR-AMPH**, NWR-LSDX*, and NWR-LSDX** (Figure 1B,D). Cross-validation of the obtained model is presented in Supplementary Information (Table S2). Curiously, serum lipids from the AMPH and LSDX were more similar when the dose dependence was analyzed, and lower doses of psychostimulants determined different effects on NWR lipids compared to higher doses (Figure 1D). However, similarly to the findings for the differences between drug-naïve NWR vs. SHR strains, the ^{1}H-NMR signals representing the phospholipids (PL) were less intense in NWR animals receiving AMPH or LSDX compared with control drug-naïve NWR. Additionally, NWR under psychostimulant effects presented higher levels of PUFA. The evaluation of omega-3 and omega-6 concentrations allowed calculating the omega-6 to omega-3 ratio (Table 2). Excessive amounts of omega-6 polyunsaturated fatty acids (PUFA), and high omega-6/omega-3 ratio are both often associated with eicosanoids production in many diseases [34].

The animals receiving LSDX presented the highest concentrations of omega-6 among all studied groups, although the omega-6/omega-3 ratio was not different from NWR receiving AMPH. Moreover, NWR animals receiving psychostimulants showed a remarkable different blood serum lipidome patterns compared with untreated drug-naïve NWR, with a dose-independent decrease in omega-3, as observed for 10-fold different doses of psychostimulants (0.5 and 5.0 mg/kg).

It is important to point that the decrease of omega-3 and of omega-6 acids were statistically significant ($p = 0.0019$ and $p = 0.0002$, respectively), as well as the omega-6/omega-3 ratio ($p = 0.0042$), compared with drug-naïve SHR or drug-naïve NWR. However, only omega-3 (decrease) and omega-6/omega-3 (increase) ratio were significantly changed ($p < 0.0001$) in NWR after administration of psychostimulants. Thus, we suggest that the omega-3 acid levels could be used as a parameter to evaluate the effects of psychostimulant drugs on lipid changes in animal models.

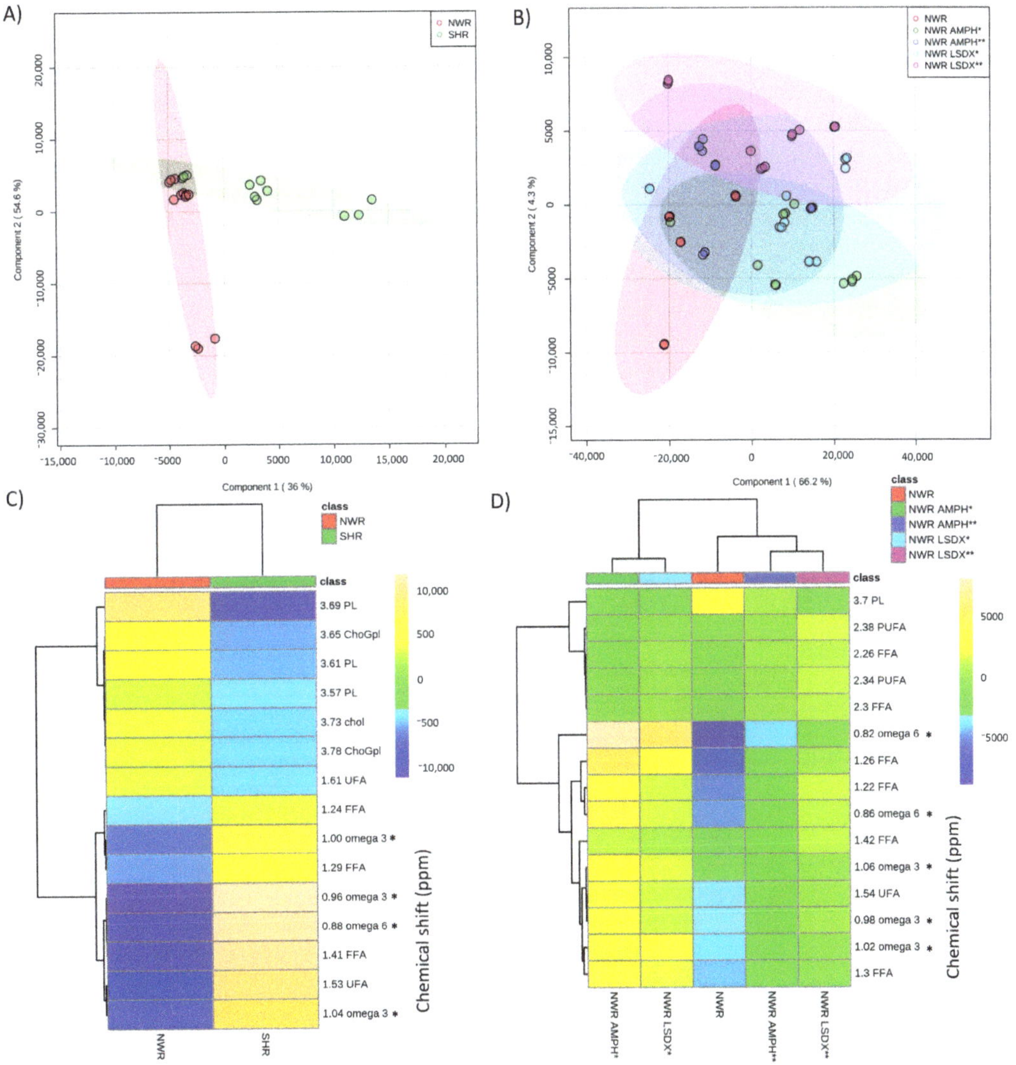

Figure 1. Partial least squares discriminant analysis (PLS-DA) on animal serum lipids ^{1}H-NMR data: (**A**) schizophrenia (SCZ) model (spontaneously hypertensive rat, SHR) vs. control (normotensive Wistar rat, NWR) score plot in PC 1 and PC 2. A total of 23 spectra were used for PLS-DA analysis of SHR against NWR, being four samples of each treatment in triplicate excluding one outlier (SHR group). (**B**) 3D score plot for evaluation in NWR of the effects on lipids of psychostimulants amphetamine (AMPH) or lisdexamfetamine (LSDX) with doses of (*) 0.5 mg/kg and (**) 5.0 mg/kg. A total of 62 spectra were used for PLS-DA analysis of NWR after AMPH or LSDX administration, with five samples for each treatment (four samples for NWR), performed in triplicate, but excluding three outliers in NWR-LSDX* group, three outliers in NWR-AMPH* group, two outliers of NWR-LSDX** group, and two outliers in NWR-AMPH** group. (**C**) Heatmap for SHR vs. NWR shows relative concentrations of the 15 most important variables in projection (VIP). (**D**) Heatmap for NWR vs. AMPH or LSDX shows the relative concentrations of the fifteen variables (VIP) before and after psychostimulants administration. In (**C**,**D**), chemical shifts marked for omega 3 *, omega 6 *, may come from other acyl groups. PL: phospholipids, ChoGpl: choline glycerophospholipids, chol: cholesterol, FFA: free fatty acids, PUFA: polyunsaturated fatty acids, UFA: unsaturated fatty acids.

Table 2. Changes in omega-3 and omega-6 acids determination using the ^{1}H-NMR data from control NWR animals after the administration of psychostimulants (mean values ± SD).

		Omega 3 (%)	Omega 6 (%)	Omega 6/3
Groups	NWR	50.16 ± 9.04	25.74 ± 5.18	0.52 ± 0.05
	SHR	26.37 ± 5.39	7.43 ± 1.06	0.29 ± 0.10
	NWR-AMPH *	5.41 ± 1.56	22.28 ± 7.68	4.12 ± 1.30
	NWR-AMPH **	6.03 ± 2.52	25.86 ± 3.10	4.66 ± 1.25
	NRW-LSDX *	10.10 ± 3.75	43.50 ± 17.40	4.33 ± 0.81
	NRW-LSDX **	10.13 ± 2.55	33.65 ± 6.05	3.49 ± 1.05
***p*-Values**	NWR × SHR	0.0025 (t = 5.24)	0.0002 (t = 6.85)	0.0042 (t = 4.16)
	NWR × NWR-AMPH *	<0.0001 (t = 10.90)	0.5400 (t = 0.83)	0.0003 (t = 6.15)
	NWR × NWR-AMPH **	<0.0001 (t = 10.51)	0.9992 (t = 0.042)	< 0.0001 (t = 7.41)
	NWR × NWR-AMPH * + NWR-AMPH **	<0.0001 (F (2, 14) = 109.0)	0.5403 (F (2, 14) = 0.64)	< 0.0001 (F (2, 14) = 23.26)
	NWR × NWR-LSDX*	<0.0001 (t = 9.14)	0.0467 (t = 2.57)	< 0.0001 (t = 10.42)
	NWR × NWR-LSDX **	<0.0001 (t = 9.52)	0.4440 (t = 2.31)	< 0.0001 (t = 6.28)
	NWR × NWR-LSDX * + NWR-LSDX **	<0.0001 (F (2, 14) = 78.27)	0.0749 (F (2, 14) = 3.24)	< 0.0001 (F (2, 14) = 33.74)
	SHR × NWR-AMPH * + NWR-AMPH **	<0.0001 (F (2, 14) = 54.64)	0.0005 (F (2, 14) = 16.30)	0.0002 (F (2, 14) = 20.37)
	SHR × NWR-LSDX * + NWR-LSDX **	<0.0001 (F (2, 14) = 24.42)	0.0016 (F (2, 14) = 12.18)	< 0.0001 (F (2, 14) = 29.97)

Note: Normal Wistar rat (NWR); Spontaneously Hypertensive rat (SHR); amphetamine (AMPH) and lisdexamfetamine (LSDX) (* 0.5 and ** 5.0 mg/kg); standard deviation (SD). Student's t-test for NWR × SHR; NWR × NWR-AMPH *; NWR × NWR-AMPH **; NWR × NWR-LSDX * and NWR × NWR-LSDX **. One-way ANOVA, post-hoc test Dunnett's for multiple comparisons for NWR × NWR-AMPH * × NWR × AMPH **, NWR × NWR-LSDX * × NWR × LSDX **, SHR × NWR-AMPH * × NWR × AMPH ** and SHR × NWR-LSDX * × NWR × LSDX **. Values are significantly different for $p \leq 0.05$ (N = 5).

3.3. *Influences of Antipsychotics HAL and CLZ on Lipids in SHR and NWR Animals*

The PLS-DA based on the ^{1}H-NMR spectra of lipids extracted from the serum of animals treated with typical HAL or atypical CLZ antipsychotics showed significant differences in lipids composition in antipsychotics-treated SHR compared with control SHR receiving vehicle (Figure 2A,C, and Supplementary Information—Table S3, and Figure S3A,B). The atypical antipsychotic CLZ modified serum lipids to a greater extent relative to the effects determined by the treatment with HAL (Figure 2A), with greater variations in the most chemical shifts (Figure 2C, VIP) compared with the effects determined by the treatment of SHR animals with HAL. Additionally, increases in 4/15, and decreases in 11/15 lipids levels after treatment with CLZ (see dendogram in Figure 2C) were among the most prominent effects. Analysis in the variations in PUFA and omega-3 chemical shifts (Figure S3B) showed important decreases with CLZ treatment. It is also important to point to omega-3, and phospholipids (PL) levels decrease in SHR strain, following the treatment with CLZ (Figure 2C), in addition to the decrease in omega-6 (0.84 ppm), and increase in fatty acids (1.24 ppm). However, an increment in membrane omega-6 fatty acids in SCZ patients after treatment with CLZ was described by others [35].

Moreover, CLZ treatment showed the greatest lipids variations for comparisons between antipsychotic-treated and control NWR animals receiving vehicle (Figure 2B,D, Supplementary Information Table S4). Treatment with HAL slightly increased PUFA and phospholipids (PL) in NWR. In addition to the decreases in PUFAs levels (particularly omega-6), and phospholipids levels observed after the treatment with CLZ, choline glycerophospholipids (ChoGpl) were also identified as an important lipid subclass of phospholipids to distinguish the effects of CLZ in NWR, as ChoGpl were also decreased by CLZ treatment (Figure 2D and Supplementary Information Figure S4D). This last effect was opposite to that observed for SHR strain treated with CLZ, as illustrated in Figure S4C, in which ChoGpl increased in SHR animals after CLZ treatment. In addition, the CLZ effect on omega-3 and omega-6 levels and their ratio in NWR strain were also observed. CLZ determined decreases in omega-3 and omega-6 in both NWR and SHR strains.

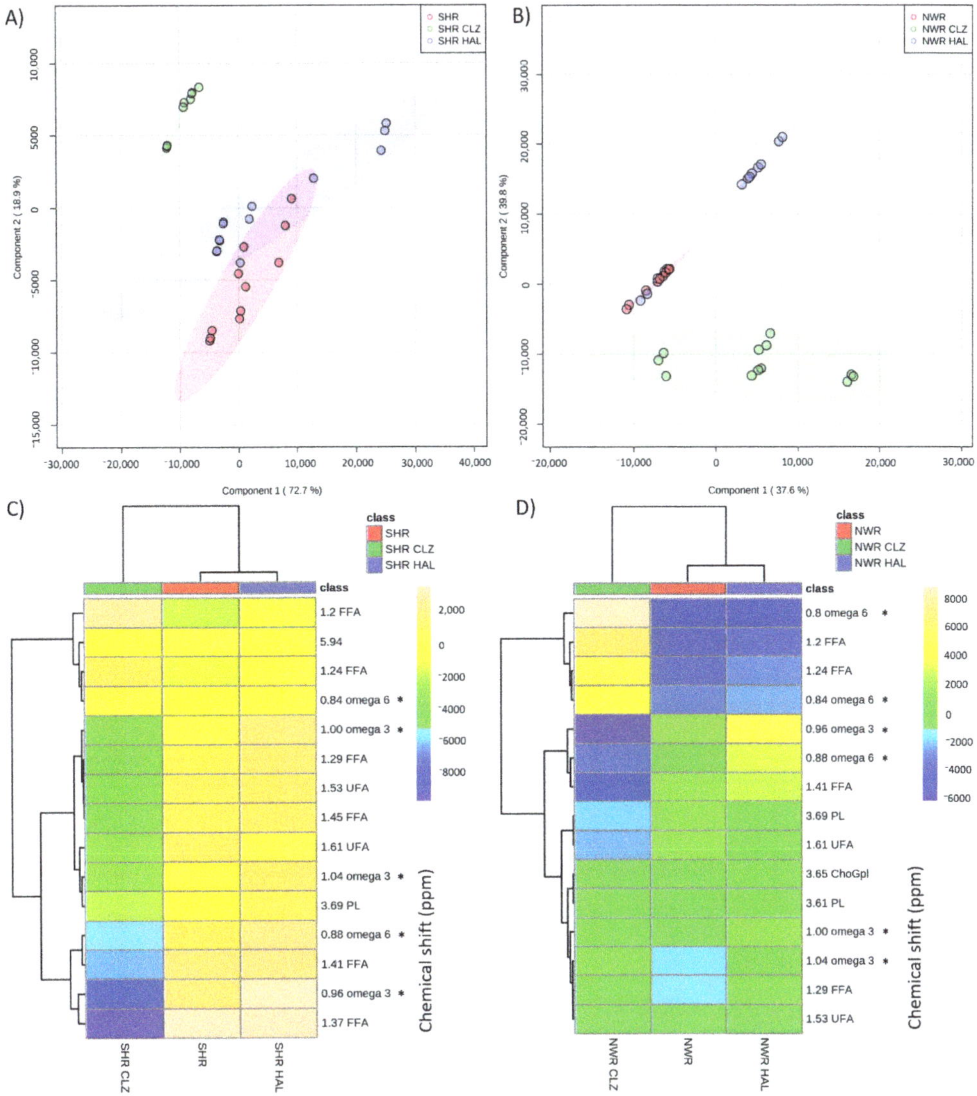

Figure 2. PLS-DA charts obtained for ^{1}H-NMR of lipids isolated from drug-naïve SHR (**A**,**C**) and drug-naïve NWR animals (**B**,**D**) after the treatment with typical haloperidol (HAL) or atypical atypical clozapine (CLZ) antipsychotic drugs. SHR lipid profile changes are shown as PLS-DA scores (**A**) or heatmap (**C**) with the relative concentrations of the 15 best-ranked chemical shifts (VIP scores). NWR lipid profile changes are shown as PLS-DA scores (**B**) or heatmap (**D**) with the relative concentrations of the 15 best-ranked chemical shifts (VIP scores). A total of 34 spectra were used for PLS-DA analysis of SHR after treatment with typical HAL or atypical CLZ antipsychotic drugs, with five samples for each treatment (4 samples for SHR), performed in triplicate, but excluding one outlier of SHR, five outliers of SHR CLZ, and two outliers of SHR-HAL. A total of 34 spectra were used for PLS-DA analysis of NWR treated with typical HAL or atypical CLZ antipsychotic drugs, with five samples for each treatment (four samples for NWR), performed in triplicate, but excluding two outliers of NWR-CLZ, and five outliers of NWR-HAL. In (**C**,**D**), chemical shifts marked for omega 3 *, omega 6 *, may come from other unsaturated acyl groups. PL: phospholipids, ChoGpl: choline glycerophospholipids, chol: cholesterol, FFA: free fatty acids, PUFA: polyunsaturated fatty acids, UFA: unsaturated fatty acids.

The treatment with the atypical antipsychotic CLZ modified the blood serum lipid profiles in SHR animals by causing a different trend compared with what was observed in NWR. Changes in omega-3 and omega-6 determined by the treatment with (typical or atypical) antipsychotic drugs in NWR and SHR (mean values ± SD) are shown in Table 3.

Table 3. Changes in omega-3 and omega-6 determined by ^{1}H-NMR in NWR and SHR after the treatment with (typical or atypical) antipsychotic drugs (mean values ± SD).

		Omega-3 (%)	**Omega-6 (%)**	**Omega 6/3**
Groups	NWR	50.16 ± 9.04	25.74 ± 5.18	0.52 ± 0.05
	SHR	26.37 ± 5.39	7.43 ± 1.06	0.29 ± 0.10
	NWR-HAL	0.75 ± 0.26	2.15 ± 0.54	3.02 ± 0.71
	SHR-HAL	0.92 ± 0.09	2.96 ± 0.77	3.16 ± 0.62
	NWR-CLZ	0.90 ± 0.44	2.69 ± 1.48	2.87 ± 1.42
	SHR-CLZ	1.00 ± 0.57	1.07 ± 0.50	2.60 ± 2.08
***p*-Values**	NWR × SHR	0.0019 (t = 5.24)	0.0002 (t = 7.83)	0.0042 (t = 3.74)
	NWR × NWR-HAL	< 0.0001 (t = 14.05)	<0.0001 (t = 11.48)	0.0037 (t = 6.89)
	NWR × NWR-CLZ	< 0.0001 (t = 14.03)	<0.0001 (t = 10.71)	0.0163 (t = 3.31)
	NWR × NWR-HAL + NWR-CLZ	<0.0001 (F (2, 14) =195.4)	<0.0001 (F (2, 14) = 114.4)	0.0708 (F (2, 14) = 3.41)
	SHR × SHR-HAL	<0.0001 (t = 10.73)	0.0002 (t = 7.27)	0.0110 (t = 8.92)
	SHR × SHR-CLZ	<0.0001 (t = 10.68)	<0.0001 (t = 10.75)	0.0456 (t = 2.66)
	SHR × SHR-HAL + SHR-CLZ	<0.0001 (F (2, 14) = 114.6)	<0.0001 (F (2, 14) = 64.81)	0.0143 (F (2, 14) = 6.69)

Note: Normal Wistar rats (NWR); Spontaneously Hypertensive rats (SHR); haloperidol (HAL); clozapine (CLZ); standard deviation (SD). Student's t-test for NWR × SHR; NWR × NWR-HAL; NWR × NWR-CLZ; SHR × SHR-HAL and SHR × SHR-CLZ, and One-way ANOVA, post-hoc test Dunnett's for multiple comparisons for NWR × NWR-HAL × NWR-CLZ and SHR × SHR-HAL × SHR-CLZ. Values are significantly different for $p \leq 0.05$ (N = 5).

The levels of omega-3 and omega-6 were both significantly different between NWR and SHR lipidomes (p = 0.0019 and p = 0.0002, respectively). The levels of omega-3 decreased with the treatment with antipsychotic drugs (HAL or CLZ) (p < 0.0001), while the omega-6/omega-3 ratios were significantly increased in SHR and NWR after the treatment with HAL or CLZ.

The levels of omega-3, omega-6, and phospholipids may suggest that these important PUFAs were incorporated into ChoGpl, which play important roles in cell membranes. ChoGpl were decreased in NWR treated with CLZ, and were increased in SHR treated with CLZ, and ChoGpl levels in SHR after the treatment with this atypical antipsychotic were closer to those in control NWR receiving vehicle (Supplementary Information Figure S4).

The differences in the effects of typical and atypical antipsychotics were evidenced by the greater lipid changes observed for the treatment with CLZ compared with HAL, as one could expect based on the well-known general pharmacological superiority of CLZ compared to typical antipsychotics, as reported by many [36–38]. In addition, CLZ is approximately 30% more effective in controlling schizophrenic episodes in treatment-resistant patients than other antipsychotic drugs [1]. However, both typical HAL and atypical CLZ antipsychotic drugs equally induced changes in omega-6/omega-3 values in both NWR and SHR strains (Table 3).

4. Discussion

The presence of cholesterol in the serum samples from SCZ-animal model studied here could be associated with the accumulation of cholesterol in the nigrostriatal pathway, which was suggested to contribute to the dopaminergic neurodegeneration in mice brain [39], or to induce cognitive dysfunctions in rats [40]. Additionally, dysfunctions in brain cholesterol homeostasis have been extensively correlated to several other brain disorders, such as autism, Alzheimer's, Parkinson's and Huntington's diseases [35,41–43].

In addition, polyunsaturated fatty acids (PUFAs) are reported to be significantly correlated with the negative SCZ symptoms, and their incorporation into plasma membrane phospholipids can remodel the molecular organization of cholesterol-enriched lipid microdomains [44,45]. Some changes in the composition of membrane phospholipids could be associated with SCZ, since the abnormal composition of esterified fatty acids, such as phospholipids, has been reported in plasma, red blood cells, fibroblasts and in *post-mortem* prefrontal cerebral cortical tissues of SCZ patients. Then, the storage and release of neurotransmitters may also be affected by the changes in the lipid composition of neuronal cell membranes [9–11,28,30,46–49]. Interestingly, omega-3 PUFA deficiency in blood was reported to be a trigger of the effects on the dopamine system, and this blood PUFA deficiency was also associated with SCZ [50]. In addition, omega-3 PUFA deficiency was associated with cognitive impairment, which directly impacts the social functioning in patients with SCZ [51]. Thus, the decreases of phospholipids in SHR animals, and also in NWR animals after receiving psychostimulants (such as AMPH and LSDX) possibly validate the SCZ animal model adopted here. However, the decreased amounts of omega-3 and omega -6 fatty acids in SCZ animal models compared with control NWR strain could point out to possible compensation mechanisms [52].

The differences between animals receiving AMPH or LSDX, including the highest concentrations of omega-6 observed after LSDX administration, could be explained by the fact that psychostimulant effects of AMPH are immediate, while LSDX is a prodrug of AMPH and requires its conversion to the active metabolite AMPH, explaining the differences in their action onset [53]. However, despite the same mechanisms of action of these psychostimulants, they also differ in the determination of blood pressure increases, which is more evident for AMPH compared with LSDX, even when used at same doses [1], but which was not correlated with the changes in biochemical biomarkers or in SCZ-like animal behavior [13–15,54]. Taking this into account, two different doses of psychostimulants were evaluated here, as they could potentially lead to different effects on lipids metabolism, as we, in fact, observed here.

The linoleic (omega-6) and alpha-linolenic (omega-3) fatty acids are two essential PUFAs that must come from diet, and they are also constituents of neuronal membrane phospholipids with a reported contribution to proliferation and differentiation of neural stem cells [55]. Moreover, the importance of omega-3 fatty acids for the structure and function of neuronal membranes is also well-known [56,57]. Therefore, the increased levels of omega-3 in drug-naïve control NWR compared to drug-naïve SHR strain may point out a possible "healthier" cerebral condition in NWR animals. There are some recognized differences in susceptibility to psychostimulant-induced neurotoxicity [58], as for instance, the psychostimulant-induced release of dopamine into the extracellular space, from the newly synthesized pool of transmitter, which plays an essential role in drug-induced neurotoxicity [59]. And this may possibly explain the differences observed for the effects of different doses of AMPH or LSDX evaluated here. Furthermore, lipid metabolism in SCZ might be related not just to the aberration of neural pathways, but also to disturbances in the tryptophan–kynurenine metabolic pathway [6–8], which may warrant future investigation.

Again, since phospholipids are essential constituents of the brain cell membranes, their metabolism might be of great importance in SCZ, as the structural integrity and functional properties of neurons are strongly affected in SCZ patients [9,10]. Moreover, insufficient uptake and biosynthesis or even excessive breakdown of phospholipids from the brain membrane were all hypothesized to be associated with SCZ and dysfunctional synapses [9–11]. Thus, the greater levels of phospholipids in the SCZ animal model treated with antipsychotics HAL or CLZ might be indicative of a possible de novo stimulated synthesis of phospholipids aiming to supply the deficiency of these phospholipids.

Ward and collaborators suggested that the exposure to atypical antipsychotics may not differentiate metabolic phenotypes of patients with SCZ [36], in spite of the several other reports suggesting the neurotoxicity of antipsychotics [37–39,60]. In addition, we also need to consider that these antipsychotics could possibly inhibit the intracellular traffic of lipids [61]. Therefore, in general, we can suggest that typical and atypical antipsychotic drugs had opposite effects on lipid changes, as both HAL and CLZ increased the relative concentrations of omega-6/omega-3 ratio in SHR, although also increasing the levels of ChoGpl.

Considering the well-known importance of omega-3 fatty acids for the structure and function of neuronal membranes [56,57], the decreases in omega-3 and phospholipids in SHR after the treatment with HAL may suggest a possible negative effect of typical antipsychotics in the lipid profile of SCZ patients. However, the increases in omega-6/omega-3 ratios, and the decreases of omega-3 and phospholipids (mainly ChoGpl) levels after the treatment with CLZ, may both suggest a good correlation with the recognized general pharmacological superiority of CLZ compared to typical antipsychotics [36–38]. Moreover, more evident changes in lipid profiles in both rat strains were observed for the treatments with the atypical antipsychotic CLZ compared with typical antipsychotic HAL.

5. Conclusions

Taken together, the results presented here support a concept of altered lipids metabolism in a validated animal model for schizophrenia (SCZ), namely SHR. Acute administration of psychostimulants in control animal strain (NWR) showed similar lipid composition alterations as observed in SHR serum samples, and as also observed in the first episode of psychosis or SCZ patients. In addition, the SCZ-like serum lipids profile was reversed more efficiently by the long-term treatment with the atypical antipsychotic drug clozapine (CLZ), relative to the typical antipsychotic haloperidol (HAL). Considering that CLZ is approximately 30% more effective in controlling schizophrenic episodes in treatment-resistant patients than other antipsychotic drugs, it would be possible to hypothesize that CLZ effects on SCZ symptoms could also benefit from the serum lipids alterations as described herein. Moreover, the treatment with the HAL did not determine significant turnover in serum lipids in the present animal model for SCZ, as the lipids remained almost unaltered even after long-term treatment with this typical antipsychotic drug. Therefore, although metabolic syndrome has been more often correlated with the long-term treatment with atypical antipsychotic drug CLZ, it seems to be a better option to minimize the alteration in serum lipids in SCZ patients.

Supplementary Materials: The following are available online at https://www.mdpi.com/2227-9059/9/3/235/s1.

Author Contributions: Conceptualization, L.T. and M.A.F.H.; methodology, B.S.B.C., J.V.N., R.W.R., D.S.; data treatment, B.S.B.C., J.V.N., D.S., T.B.B.C.C.; writing—original draft preparation, B.S.B.C., J.V.N., D.S., T.B.B.C.C.; writing—review and editing, L.T., M.A.F.H.; supervision, L.T., M.A.F.H. All authors have read and agreed to the published version of the manuscript.

Funding: Mirian A. F. Hayashi is supported by FAPESP (Grants 2017/02413-1, 2019/13112-8), CNPq (477760/2010-4; 557753/2010-4; 508113/2010-5; 311815/2012-0; 475739/2013-2; 309337/2016-0), and National Institute for Translational Medicine (INCT-TM). João V. Nani is a recipient of a fellowship from FAPESP (2019/09207-3). Ljubica Tasic received FAPESP Grants (2014/50867-3, 2018/24069-3), thanks to CNPq, INCTBio, and *grant #2021/01051-4 from FAPESP. This study was financed in part by the Coordenação de Aperfeiçoamento de Pessoal de Nível Superior (CAPES), Brazil–Finance Code 001. We thank the support from FAPESP, grant number 2021/01051-4.

Institutional Review Board Statement: The study was conducted according to the guidelines of the Committee on Care and Use of Laboratory Animal Resources, National Research Council, USA. This study was approved by the Ethical Committee of the Universidade Federal de São Pau-lo (UNIFESP/EPM), identification CEUA No 7290170315, approved on 15 March 2015.

Informed Consent Statement: Not applicable.

Acknowledgments: We thank the executive secretary Rosemary Alves de Oliveira for the great administrative support and Marcela Nering for the extraordinary technical assistance.

Conflicts of Interest: The authors declare no conflict of interest.

Abbreviations

^{1}H NMR	Proton NMR
AMPH	Amphetamine
ANOVA	Analysis of variance
ChoGpl	Choline glycerophospholipids
Chol	Cholesterol
CLZ	Clozapine
FFA	Free fatty acids
HAL	Haloperidol
LOOCV	Leave-one-out cross-validation
LSDX	Lisdexamfetamine
MD	Mental disorder
NMR	Nuclear magnetic resonance
NWR	Normotensive Wistar rat
PCA	Principal component analysis
PL	Phospholipids
PLS-DA	Partial least squares discriminant analysis
PUFA	Polyunsaturated fatty acid
SCZ	Schizophrenia
SD	Standard deviation
SHR	Spontaneously hypertensive rat
UFA	Unsaturated fatty acids
VIP	Variable importance in projection

References

1. Patel, K.R.; Cherian, J.; Gohil, K.; Atkinson, D. Schizophrenia: Overview and treatment options. *Pharm. Ther.* **2014**, *39*, 638–645.
2. Murray, R.M.; Lappin, J.; Di Forti, M. Schizophrenia: From developmental deviance to dopamine dysregulation. *Eur. Neuropsychopharmacol.* **2008**, *18*, S129–S134. [CrossRef] [PubMed]
3. Owen, M.J.; Sawa, A.; Mortensen, P.B. Schizophrenia. *Lancet* **2016**, *388*, 86–97. [CrossRef]
4. Rodríguez, B.; Nani, J.V.; Almeida, P.G.C.; Brietzke, E.; Lee, R.S.; Hayashi, M.A.F. Neuropeptides and oligopeptidases in schizophrenia. *Neurosci. Biobehav. Rev.* **2020**, *108*, 679–693. [CrossRef]
5. Nucifora, F.C.; Woznica, E.; Lee, B.J.; Cascella, N.; Sawa, A. Treatment resistant schizophrenia: Clinical, biological, and therapeutic perspectives. *Neurobiol. Dis.* **2019**, *131*, 104257. [CrossRef] [PubMed]
6. Ulivieri, M.; Wierońska, J.M.; Lionetto, L.; Martinello, K.; Cieslik, P.; Chocyk, A.; Curto, M.; Di Menna, L.; Iacovelli, L.; Traficante, A.; et al. The trace kynurenine, cinnabarinic acid, displays potent antipsychotic-like activity in mice and its levels are reduced in the prefrontal cortex of individuals affected by schizophrenia. *Schizophr. Bull.* **2020**, *46*, 1471–1481. [CrossRef] [PubMed]
7. Koola, M.M. Alpha7 nicotinic-*N*-methyl-D-aspartate hypothesis in the treatment of schizophrenia and beyond. *Hum. Psychopharmacol. Clin. Exp.* **2021**, *36*, 1–16. [CrossRef]
8. Tanaka, M.; Bohár, Z.; Vécsei, L. Are kynurenines accomplices or principal villains in dementia? Maintenance of kynurenine metabolism. *Molecules* **2020**, *25*, 564. [CrossRef]
9. Ghosh, S.; Dyer, R.A.; Beasley, C.L. Evidence for altered cell membrane lipid composition in postmortem prefrontal white matter in bipolar disorder and schizophrenia. *J. Psychiatr. Res.* **2017**, *95*, 135–142. [CrossRef]
10. Wood, P.L.; Unfried, G.; Whitehead, W.; Phillipps, A.; Wood, J.A. Dysfunctional plasmalogen dynamics in the plasma and platelets of patients with schizophrenia. *Schizophr. Res.* **2015**, *161*, 506–510. [CrossRef] [PubMed]
11. Tessier, C.; Sweers, K.; Frajerman, A.; Bergaoui, H.; Ferreri, F.; Delva, C.; Lapidus, N.; Lamaziere, A.; Roiser, J.P.; De Hert, M.; et al. Membrane lipidomics in schizophrenia patients: A correlational study with clinical and cognitive manifestations. *Transl. Psychiatry* **2016**, *6*, e906. [CrossRef] [PubMed]
12. Nani, J.V.; Rodríguez, B.; Cruz, F.; Hayashi, M.A.F. Animal Models in Psychiatric Disorder Studies. In *Animal Models in Medicine and Biology*; Tvrdá, E., Yenisetti, S.C., Eds.; IntechOpen: London, UK, 2019; pp. 1–18.
13. Calzavara, M.B.; Medrano, W.A.; Levin, R.; Kameda, S.R.; Andersen, M.L.; Tufik, S.; Silva, R.H.; Frussa-Filho, R; Abilio, V.C. Neuroleptic drugs revert the contextual fear conditioning deficit presented by spontaneously hypertensive rats: A potential animal model of emotional context processing in schizophrenia? *Schizophr. Bull.* **2009**, *35*, 748–759.
14. Levin, R.; Calzavara, M.B.; Santos, C.M.; Medrano, W.A.; Niigaki, S.T.; Abílio, V.C. Spontaneously hypertensive Rats (SHR) present deficits in prepulse inhibition of startle specifically reverted by clozapine. *Prog. Neuro-Psychopharmacol. Biol. Psychiatry* **2011**, *35*, 1748–1752. [CrossRef]

15. Nani, J.V.; Yonamine, C.M.; Castro Musial, D.; Dal Mas, C.; Mari, J.J.; Hayashi, M.A.F. ACE activity in blood and brain axis in an animal model for schizophrenia: Demonstration of face validity related to ACE and predictive validity in response to antipsychotics. *World J. Biol. Psychiatry* **2019**, *21*, 1–11.
16. Calzavara, M.B.; Levin, R.; Medrano, W.A.; Almeida, V.; Sampaio, A.P.F.; Barone, L.C.; Frussa-Filho, R.; Abílio, V.C. Effects of antipsychotics and amphetamine on social behaviors in spontaneously hypertensive rats. *Behav. Brain Res.* **2011**, *225*, 15–22. [CrossRef] [PubMed]
17. Gadelha, A.; Machado, M.F.M.; Yonamine, C.M.; Sato, J.R.; Juliano, M.A.; Oliveira, V.; Bressan, R.A.; Hayashi, M.A.F. Plasma Ndel1 enzyme activity is reduced in patients with schizophrenia—a potential biomarker? *J. Psychiatr. Res.* **2013**, *47*, 657–663. [CrossRef]
18. Gadelha, A.; Yonamine, C.M.; Ota, V.K.; Oliveira, V.; Sato, J.R.; Belangero, S.I.; Bressan, R.A.; Hayashi, M.A.F. ACE I/D genotype-related increase in ACE plasma activity is a better predictor for schizophrenia diagnosis than the genotype alone. *Schizophr. Res.* **2015**, *164*, 109–114. [CrossRef] [PubMed]
19. Dal Mas, C.; Nani, J.V.; Noto, C.; Yonamine, C.M.; da Cunha, G.R.; Mansur, R.B.; Ota, V.K.; Belangero, S.I.; Cordeiro, Q.; Kapczinski, F.; et al. Ndel1 oligopeptidase activity as a potential biomarker of early stages of schizophrenia. *Schizophr. Res.* **2019**, *208*, 202–208. [CrossRef] [PubMed]
20. Sethi, S.; Hayashi, M.A.F.; Barbosa, B.S.; Pontes, J.G.M.; Tasic, L.; Brietzke, E. Lipidomics, Biomarkers, and Schizophrenia: A Current Perspective. In *Metabolomics: From Fundamentals to Clinical Applications. Advances in Experimental Medicine and Biology*; Sussulini, A., Ed.; Springer International Publishing: Cham, Switzerland, 2017; Volume 965, pp. 265–290.
21. Sethi, S.; Hayashi, M.A.F.; Sussulini, A.; Tasic, L.; Brietzke, E. Analytical approaches for lipidomics and its potential applications in neuropsychiatric disorders. *World J. Biol. Psychiatry* **2017**, *18*, 506–520. [CrossRef]
22. Sethi, S.; Pedrini, M.; Rizzo, L.B.; Zeni-Graiff, M.; Mas, C.D.; Cassinelli, A.C.; Noto, M.N.; Asevedo, E.; Cordeiro, Q.; Pontes, J.G.M.; et al. ^{1}H-NMR, ^{1}H-NMR T_2-edited, and 2D-NMR in bipolar disorder metabolic profiling. *Int. J. Bipolar Disord.* **2017**, *5*, 1–9. [CrossRef]
23. Tasic, L.; Pontes, J.G.M.; Carvalho, M.S.; Cruz, G.; Dal Mas, C.; Sethi, S.; Pedrini, M.; Rizzo, L.B.; ZeniGraiff, M.; Asevedo, E.; et al. Metabolomics and lipidomics analyses by ^{1}H nuclear magnetic resonance of schizophrenia patient serum reveal potential peripheral biomarkers for diagnosis. *Schizophr. Res.* **2017**, *185*, 182–189. [CrossRef] [PubMed]
24. Tukiainen, T.; Tynkkynen, T.; Makinen, V.P.; Jylanki, P.; Kangas, A.; Hokkanen, J.; Vehtari, A.; Gröhn, O.; Hallikainen, M.; Soininen, H.; et al. A multi-metabolite analysis of serum by ^{1}H NMR spectroscopy: Early systemic signs of Alzheimer's disease. *Biochem. Biophys. Res. Commun.* **2008**, *375*, 356–361. [CrossRef]
25. Mor, N.C.; Correia, B.S.B.; Val, A.L.; Tasic, L. A protocol for fish lipid analysis using nuclear magnetic resonance spectroscopy. *J. Braz. Chem. Soc.* **2020**, *31*, 662–672. [CrossRef]
26. Li, J.; Vosegaard, T.; Guo, Z. Applications of nuclear magnetic resonance in lipid analyses: An emerging powerful tool for lipidomics studies. *Prog. Lipid Res.* **2017**, *68*, 37–56. [CrossRef] [PubMed]
27. Vidal, N.P.; Manzanos, M.J.; Goicoechea, E.; Guillén, M.D. Quality of farmed and wild sea bass lipids studied by ^{1}H NMR: Usefulness of this technique for differentiation on a qualitative and a quantitative basis. *Food Chem.* **2012**, *135*, 1583–1591. [CrossRef]
28. Kaddurah-Daouk, R.; McEvoy, J.; Baillie, R.A.; Lee, D.; Yao, J.K.; Doraiswamy, P.M.; Krishnan, K.R.R. Metabolomic mapping of atypical antipsychotic effects in schizophrenia. *Mol. Psychiatry* **2007**, *12*, 934–945. [CrossRef]
29. He, Y.; Yu, Z.; Xie, I.G.L.; Hartmann, A.M.; Prehn, C.; Adamski, J.; Kahn, R.; Li, Y.; Illig, T.; WangSattler, R.; et al. Schizophrenia shows a unique metabolomics signature in plasma. *Transl. Psychiatry* **2012**, *2*, e149. [CrossRef]
30. Orešič, M.; Tang, J.; Seppänen-Laakso, T.; Mattila, I.; Saarni, S.E.; Saarni, S.I.; Lönnqvist, J.; Sysi-Aho, M.; Hyötyläinen, T.; Perälä, J.; et al. Metabolome in schizophrenia and other psychotic disorders: A general population-based study. *Genome Med.* **2011**, *3*, 1–14. [CrossRef]
31. Orešič, M.; Seppänen-Laakso, T.; Sun, D.; Tang, J.; Therman, S.; Viehman, R.; Mustonen, U.; van Erp, T.G.; Hyötyläinen, T.; Thompson, P.; et al. Phospholipids and insulin resistance in psychosis: A lipidomics study of twin pairs discordant for schizophrenia. *Genome Med.* **2012**, *4*, 1–10. [CrossRef]
32. McEvoy, J.; Baillie, R.A.; Zhu, H.; Buckley, P.; Keshavan, M.S.; Nasrallah, H.A.; Dougherty, G.G.; Yao, J.K.; Kaddurah-Daouk, R. Lipidomics reveals early metabolic changes in subjects with schizophrenia: Effects of atypical antipsychotics. *PLoS ONE* **2013**, *8*, e68717. [CrossRef]
33. Yao, J.K.; Stanley, J.A.; Reddy, R.D.; Keshavan, M.S.; Pettegrew, J.W. Correlations between peripheral polyunsaturated fatty acid content and in vivo membrane phospholipid metabolites. *Biol. Psychiatry* **2002**, *52*, 823–830. [CrossRef]
34. Simopoulos, A. The importance of the ratio of omega-6/omega-3 essential fatty acids. *Biomed. Pharmacother* **2002**, *56*, 365–379. [CrossRef]
35. Paul, R.; Choudhury, A.; Kumar, S.; Giri, A.; Sandhir, R.; Borah, A. Cholesterol contributes to dopamine-neuronal loss in MPTP mouse model of Parkinson's disease: Involvement of mitochondrial dysfunctions and oxidative stress. *PLoS ONE* **2017**, *12*, e0171285. [CrossRef]
36. Ward, K.M.; Yeoman, L.; McHugh, C.; Kraal, A.Z.; Flowers, S.A.; Rothberg, A.E.; Karnovsky, A.; Das, A.K.; Ellingrod, V.L.; Stringer, K.A. Atypical antipsychotic exposure may not differentiate metabolic phenotypes of patients with schizophrenia. *Pharmacother. J. Hum. Pharmacol. Drug Ther.* **2018**, *38*, 638–650. [CrossRef]

37. Nandra, K.S.; Agius, M. The differences between typical and atypical antipsychotics: The effects on neurogenesis. *Psychiatr. Danub.* **2012**, *24*, S95–S99. [PubMed]
38. Nasrallah, H.; Chen, A. Multiple neurotoxic effects of haloperidol resulting in neuronal death. *Ann. Clin. Psychiatry* **2017**, *29*, 195–202. [PubMed]
39. Paul, R.; Dutta, A.; Phukan, B.C.; Mazumder, M.K.; Justin-Thenmozhi, A.; Manivasagam, T.; Bhattacharya, P.; Borah, A. Accumulation of cholesterol and homocysteine in the nigrostriatal pathway of brain contributes to the dopaminergic neurodegeneration in mice. *Neuroscience* **2018**, *388*, 347–356. [CrossRef]
40. Zhao, S.; Liao, W.; Xu, N.; Xu, H.; Yu, C.; Liu, X.; Li, C. Polar metabolite of cholesterol induces rat cognitive dysfunctions. *Neuroscience* **2009**, *164*, 398–403. [CrossRef]
41. Leoni, V.; Caccia, C. Study of cholesterol metabolism in Huntington's disease. *Biochem. Biophys. Res. Commun.* **2014**, *446*, 697–701. [CrossRef] [PubMed]
42. Moutinho, M.; Nunes, M.J.; Rodrigues, E. Cholesterol 24-hydroxylase: Brain cholesterol metabolism and beyond. *Biochim. Biophys. Acta Mol. Cell Biol. Lipids* **2016**, *1861*, 1911–1920. [CrossRef] [PubMed]
43. Petrov, A.M.; Kasimov, M.R.; Zefirov, A.L. Cholesterol in the pathogenesis of Alzheimer's, Parkinson's diseases and Autism: Link to synaptic dysfunction. *Acta Nat.* **2017**, *9*, 26–37. [CrossRef]
44. Solberg, D.K.; Bentsen, H.; Refsum, H.; Andreassen, O.A. Lipid profiles in schizophrenia associated with clinical traits: A five year follow-up study. *BMC Psychiatry* **2016**, *16*, 299. [CrossRef]
45. Shaikh, S.R.; Kinnun, J.J.; Leng, X.; Williams, J.A.; Wassall, S.R. How polyunsaturated fatty acids modify molecular organization in membranes: Insight from NMR studies of model systems. *Biochim. Biophys. Acta Biomembr.* **2015**, *1848*, 211–219. [CrossRef]
46. Horrobin, D.F. The membrane phospholipid hypothesis as a biochemical basis for the neurodevelopmental concept of schizophrenia. *Schizophr. Res.* **1998**, *30*, 193–208. [CrossRef]
47. Keshavan, M.S.; Mallinger, A.G.; Pettegrew, J.W.; Dippold, C. Erythrocyte membrane phospholipids in psychotic patients. *Psychiatry Res.* **1993**, *49*, 89–95. [CrossRef]
48. Mahadik, S.P.; Mukherjee, S.; Correnti, E.E.; Kelkar, H.S.; Wakade, C.G.; Costa, R.M.; Scheffer, R. Plasma membrane phospholipid and cholesterol distribution of skin fibroblasts from drug-naive patients at the onset of psychosis. *Schizophr. Res.* **1994**, *13*, 239–247. [CrossRef]
49. Yang, J.; Chen, T.; Sun, L.; Zhao, Z.; Qi, X.; Zhou, K.; Cao, Y.; Wang, X.; Qiu, Y.; Su, M.; et al. Potential metabolite markers of schizophrenia. *Mol. Psychiatry* **2013**, *18*, 67–78. [CrossRef]
50. Schneider, M.; Levant, B.; Reichel, M.; Gulbins, E.; Kornhuber, J.; Müller, C.P. Lipids in psychiatric disorders and preventive medicine. *Neurosci. Biobehav. Rev.* **2017**, *76*, 336–362. [CrossRef]
51. Satogami, K.; Takahashi, S.; Yamada, S.; Ukai, S.; Shinosaki, K. Omega-3 fatty acids related to cognitive impairment in patients with schizophrenia. *Schizophr. Res. Cogn.* **2017**, *9*, 8–12. [CrossRef]
52. Rog, J.; Blazewicz, A.; Juchnowicz, D.; Ludwiczuk, A.; Stelmach, E.; Kozioł, M.; Karakula, M.; Nizinski, P.; Karakula-Juchnowicz, H. The role of GPR120 receptor in essential fatty acids metabolism in schizophrenia. *Biomedicines* **2020**, *8*, 243. [CrossRef] [PubMed]
53. Ward, K.; Citrome, L. Lisdexamfetamine: Chemistry, pharmacodynamics, pharmacokinetics, and clinical efficacy, safety, and tolerability in the treatment of binge eating disorder. *Expert Opin. Drug Metab. Toxicol.* **2018**, *14*, 229–238. [CrossRef] [PubMed]
54. Nani, J.V.; Lee, R.S.; Yonamine, C.; Dal Mas, C.; Sant'Anna, O.; Juliano, M.A.; Gadelha, A.; Mari, J.J.; Hayashi, M.A.F. Evaluation of NDEL1 oligopeptidase activity in blood and brain in an animal model of schizophrenia: Effects of psychostimulants and antipsychotics. *Sci. Rep.* **2020**, *10*, 18513. [CrossRef] [PubMed]
55. Hejr, H.; Ghareghani, M.; Zibara, K.; Ghafari, M.; Sadri, F.; Salehpour, Z.; Hamedi, A.; Negintaji, K.; Azari, H.; Ghanbari, A. The ratio of 1/3 linoleic acid to alpha linolenic acid is optimal for oligodendrogenesis of embryonic neural stem cells. *Neurosci. Lett.* **2017**, *651*, 216–225. [CrossRef]
56. Bourre, J.M.; Dumont, O. Dietary oleic acid not used during brain development and in adult in rat, in contrast with sciatic nerve. *Neurosci. Lett.* **2003**, *336*, 180–184. [CrossRef]
57. Bourre, J.M. Roles of unsaturated fatty acids (especially omega-3 fatty acids) in the brain at various ages and during ageing. *J. Nutr. Health Aging* **2004**, *8*, 163–174. [PubMed]
58. Berman, S.M.; Kuczenski, R.; McCracken, J.T.; London, E.D. Potential adverse effects of amphetamine treatment on brain and behavior: A review. *Mol. Psychiatry* **2009**, *14*, 123–142. [CrossRef]
59. Thomas, D.M.; Francescutti-Verbeem, D.M.; Kuhn, D.M. The newly synthesized pool of dopamine determines the severity of methamphetamine-induced neurotoxicity. *J. Neurochem.* **2008**, *105*, 605–616. [CrossRef] [PubMed]
60. Park, S.W.; Seo, M.K.; McIntyre, R.S.; Mansur, R.B.; Lee, Y.; Lee, J.-H.; Park, S.-C.; Huh, L.; Lee, J.G. Effects of olanzapine and haloperidol on mTORC1 signaling dendritic outgrowth, and synaptic proteins in rat primary hippocampal neurons under toxic conditions. *Neurosci. Lett.* **2018**, *686*, 59–66. [CrossRef]
61. Tessier, C.; Nuss, P.; Staneva, G.; Wolf, C. Modification of membrane heterogeneity by antipsychotic drugs: An X-ray diffraction comparative study. *J. Colloid Interface Sci.* **2008**, *320*, 469–479. [CrossRef]

MDPI
St. Alban-Anlage 66
4052 Basel
Switzerland
Tel. +41 61 683 77 34
Fax +41 61 302 89 18
www.mdpi.com

Biomedicines Editorial Office
E-mail: biomedicines@mdpi.com
www.mdpi.com/journal/biomedicines

www.ingramcontent.com/pod-product-compliance
Lightning Source LLC
Chambersburg PA
CBHW061617220926
51850CB00005B/528
* 9 7 8 3 0 3 6 5 8 2 5 3 5 *